Health in Humanitarian Emergencies

Health in Humanitarian Emergencies

Principles and Practice for Public Health and Healthcare Practitioners

Edited by

David A. Townes
Centers for Disease Control and Prevention, Atlanta, GA

Mike Gerber
Centers for Disease Control and Prevention, Atlanta, GA

Mark Anderson
Centers for Disease Control and Prevention, Atlanta, GA

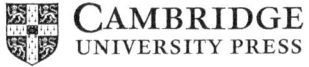

CAMBRIDGE
UNIVERSITY PRESS

University Printing House, Cambridge CB2 8BS, United Kingdom

One Liberty Plaza, 20th Floor, New York, NY 10006, USA

477 Williamstown Road, Port Melbourne, VIC 3207, Australia

314–321, 3rd Floor, Plot 3, Splendor Forum, Jasola District Centre, New Delhi – 110025, India

79 Anson Road, #06–04/06, Singapore 079906

Cambridge University Press is part of the University of Cambridge.

It furthers the University's mission by disseminating knowledge in the pursuit of education, learning, and research at the highest international levels of excellence.

www.cambridge.org
Information on this title: www.cambridge.org/9781107062689
DOI: 10.1017/9781107477261

© Cambridge University Press 2018

This publication is in copyright. Subject to statutory exception and to the provisions of relevant collective licensing agreements, no reproduction of any part may take place without the written permission of Cambridge University Press.

First published 2018

Printed in the United Kingdom by Clays, St Ives plc

A catalogue record for this publication is available from the British Library.

Library of Congress Cataloging-in-Publication Data
Names: Townes, David A., editor.
Title: Health in humanitarian emergencies : principles and practice for public health and healthcare practitioners / edited by David Townes.
Description: Cambridge, United Kingdom ; New York, NY : Cambridge University Press, 2018. | Includes bibliographical references and index.
Identifiers: LCCN 2018012021| ISBN 9781107062689 (hardback) | ISBN 9781107477261 (Cambridge Core)
Subjects: | MESH: Disaster Planning | Public Health | Relief Work | Refugees | Disaster Victims | Needs Assessment
Classification: LCC HV553 | NLM WA 295 | DDC 363.34/8–dc23
LC record available at https://lccn.loc.gov/2018012021

ISBN 978-1-107-06268-9 Hardback

Cambridge University Press has no responsibility for the persistence or accuracy of URLs for external or third-party internet websites referred to in this publication and does not guarantee that any content on such websites is, or will remain, accurate or appropriate.

Every effort has been made in preparing this book to provide accurate and up-to-date information that is in accord with accepted standards and practice at the time of publication. Although case histories are drawn from actual cases, every effort has been made to disguise the identities of the individuals involved. Nevertheless, the authors, editors, and publishers can make no warranties that the information contained herein is totally free from error, not least because clinical standards are constantly changing through research and regulation. The authors, editors, and publishers therefore disclaim all liability for direct or consequential damages resulting from the use of material contained in this book. Readers are strongly advised to pay careful attention to information provided by the manufacturer of any drugs or equipment that they plan to use.

The findings and conclusions in this report are those of the authors and do not necessarily represent the official position of the Centers for Disease Control and Prevention.

The authors' views expressed in this publication do not necessarily reflect the views of the United States Agency for International Development or the United States Government.

Contents

List of Contributors   ix
Foreword   xv
List of Abbreviations   xx

Section 1–Humanitarian Emergencies

1. **Introduction to Humanitarian Emergencies**   1
   Mark Anderson and Michael Gerber

2. **History of Humanitarian Emergencies**   9
   Mark Anderson, Kristin Becknell, and Joanna Taliano

3. **Who's Who in Humanitarian Emergencies**   25
   Cyrus Shahpar and Thomas D. Kirsch

4. **Response to Humanitarian Emergencies**   35
   David A. Townes, Andre Griekspoor, Peter Mala, Ian Norton, and Anthony D. Redmond

5. **Epidemiology**   53
   Christine Dubray and Debarati Guha-Sapir

6. **Ethics**   68
   Barbara Tomczyk and Aun Lor

Section 2–Public Health Principles

7. **Needs Assessments**   79
   Richard Garfield, Johan von Schreeb, Anneli Eriksson, and Patrice Chataigner

8. **Surveys**   91
   Oleg O. Bilukha, Olivier Degomme, and Eva Leidman

9. **Surveillance**   109
   Farah Husain and Peter Mala

10. **Monitoring and Evaluation**   122
    Goldie MacDonald, Lori A. Wingate, and Susan Temporado Cookson

11. **Water, Sanitation, and Hygiene (WASH)**   136
    Nicole Weber, Anu Rajasingham, Molly Patrick, Andrea Martinsen, and Thomas Handzel

12. **Nutrition**   161
    Leisel E. Talley and Erin Boyd

13. **Food Security**   181
    Silke Pietzsch, Leisel E. Talley, and Carlos Navarro-Colorado

14. **Reproductive Health**   198
    Barbara Tomczyk, Diane Morof, and Malcolm Potts

15. **Protection**   214
    Wendy Wheaton, Dabney P. Evans, and Mark Anderson

16. **Vaccine-Preventable Diseases**   227
    Eugene Lam, Henri Van Hombergh, Allen Gidraf Kahindo Maina, Lisandro Torre, and Muireann Brennan

17. **Camp Management**   244
    Paul J. Giannone, Mohamed Hilmi, and Mark Anderson

18. **Shelter and Settlements**   257
    Charles A. Setchell, Eddie J. Argeñal, LeGrand L. Malany, and Paul J. Giannone

19. **Logistics**   270
    Rebecca Turner, Travis Vail Betz, George A. Roark, and Darrell Morris Lester

20. **Disaster Risk Reduction**   284
    Lise D. Martel, Qudsia Huda, Kimberly M. Hanson, and Ali Ardalan

Contents

Section 3–Illness and Injury

21 **Acute Respiratory Infection** 295
Nina Marano and Jamal A. Ahmed

22 **Diarrheal Disease** 310
Ciara O'Reilly, Kathryn Alberti, David Olson, and Eric Mintz

23 **HIV** 336
Kevin R. Clarke and Nathan Ford

24 **Malaria in Humanitarian Emergencies** 348
Holly Williams, Marian Schilperoord, David A. Townes, and S. Patrick Kachur

25 **Acute Malnutrition** 362
Carlos Navarro-Colorado, Eva Leidman, and Maureen L. Gallagher

26 **Measles** 386
Eugene Lam, Allen Gidraf Kahindo Maina, Lisandro Torre, Muireann Brennan, and James L. Goodson

27 **Meningococcal Disease** 400
Sarah Mbaeyi, Amanda Cohn, and Matthew Coldiron

28 **Mental Health** 408
Barbara Lopes Cardozo and Richard Francis Mollica

29 **Tuberculosis** 425
Michelle Gayer and Susan Temporado Cookson

30 **Injuries and Trauma** 441
Benjamin Levy, David Sugerman, Mark Anderson, and Charles Mock

31 **Noncommunicable Diseases** 460
Bayard Roberts, Holly Williams, and Sonia Angell

Index 474

Contributors

Jamal A. Ahmed, MD, MSc, DLSHTM
Public Health Section
Office of the United Nations High Commissioner for Refugees

Kathryn Alberti, MSc
Senior Programme Specialist – Cholera
UNICEF – Health Section

Mark Anderson, MD, MPH
Emergency Response and Recovery Branch
Centers for Disease Control and Prevention
Atlanta, GA

Sonia Angell, MD, MPH, DTM&H
Deputy Commissioner
NYC Department of Health and Mental Hygiene
Long Island City, NY

Ali Ardalan, MD, PhD
Senior HHI Fellow
Visiting Scientist, Harvard T. H. Chan School of Public Health
Boston, MA

Eddie J. Argeñal, MS
Shelter and Settlements Advisor
US Agency for International Development,
Office of US Foreign Disaster Assistance (USAID/OFDA)
Washington, DC

Kristin Becknell, MPH
Emergency Response and Recovery Branch
Centers for Disease Control and Prevention
Atlanta, GA

Travis Vail Betz
Humanitarian Aid Advisor
United States Agency for International Development
Office of US Foreign Disaster Assistance
Washington, DC

Oleg O. Bilukha, MD, PhD
Emergency Response and Recovery Branch
Centers for Disease Control and Prevention
Atlanta, GA

Erin Boyd, MS
Nutrition Advisor
US Agency for International Development
Office of US Foreign Disaster Assistance (USAID/OFDA)
Washington, DC

Muireann Brennan, MD, MPH
Emergency Response and Recovery Branch
Centers for Disease Control and Prevention
Atlanta, GA

Barbara Lopes Cardozo, MD, MPH
Emergency Response and Recovery Branch
Centers for Disease Control and Prevention
Atlanta, GA

Patrice Chataigner, MPH, BA Law, MS, MA
Head of Research and Analysis
Okular Analytics
Geneva, Switzerland

Kevin R. Clarke, MD, CTropMed
Center for Global Health
Centers for Disease Control and Prevention
Atlanta, GA

Amanda Cohn, MD
National Center for Immunization and Respiratory Diseases
Centers for Disease Control and Prevention
Atlanta, GA

List of Contributors

Matthew E. Coldiron, MD, MPH
Epicentre
Paris, France

Susan Temporado Cookson, MD, MPH
Global Tuberculosis Branch
Centers for Disease Control and Prevention
Atlanta, GA

Olivier Degomme, MD, MPH, PhD
Scientific Director
International Centre for Reproductive Health
Faculty of Medicine and Health Sciences
Ghent University
Ghent, Belgium

Christine Dubray, MD, MSc
Centers for Disease Control and Prevention
Atlanta, GA

Anneli Eriksson, RN, MSc, MIH International Health
Project Manager
Centre for Research on Health Care in Disasters
Health Systems and Policy Research group
Department of Public Health Sciences
Karolinska Institutet
Stockholm, Sweden

Dabney P. Evans, PhD, MPH
Center for Humanitarian Emergencies
Rollins School of Public Health, Emory University
Atlanta, GA

Nathan Ford, PhD, MPH, FRCPE
Dept HIV & Global Hepatitis Programme
World Health Organization
Geneva, Switzerland

Maureen L. Gallagher, MSc
Nutrition Specialist
United Nations Emergency Response Team
New York, NY

Richard Garfield, RN, MS, DrPH
Emergency Response and Recovery Branch
Centers for Disease Control and Prevention
Atlanta, GA

Michelle Gayer, MBBS, MPH
Director, Emergency Health
International Rescue Committee
Geneva, Switzerland

Michael Gerber, MPH
Emergency Response and Recovery Branch
Centers for Disease Control and Prevention
Atlanta, GA

Paul J. Giannone, MPH
Centers for Disease Control and Prevention
Atlanta, GA

James L. Goodson, MPH
Global Immunization Division
Centers for Disease Control and Prevention
Atlanta, GA

Andre Griekspoor, MD, MPH
Senior Policy Adviser, Emergency Operations
WHO Health Emergencies Programme
World Health Organization
Geneva, Switzerland

Debarati Guha-Sapir
Professor
Institute of Health and Society
Université Catholique de Louvain

Thomas Handzel, PhD
Emergency Response and Recovery Branch
Centers for Disease Control and Prevention
Atlanta, GA

Kimberly M. Hanson, MPH, AEM
Centers for Disease Control and Prevention
Atlanta, GA

Mohamed Hilmi, BSc(Hons), ME
Shelter and Settlements, and DRR
Humanitarian Policy and Practice
InterAction
Washington, DC

Henri Van Hombergh, MD
The United Nations Children's Fund (UNICEF)
New York, NY

List of Contributors

Qudsia Huda, MBBS, MPH
Team Lead
Health Emergency Preparedness, Planning and Operational Readiness
WHO Health Emergency Program
WHO Headquarters
Geneva, Switzerland

Farah Husain, DMD, MPH
Emergency Response and Recovery Branch
Centers for Disease Control and Prevention
Atlanta, GA

S. Patrick Kachur, MD, MPH
Malaria Branch
Centers for Disease Control and Prevention
Atlanta, GA

Thomas D. Kirsch, MD, MPH
Professor and Director
National Center for Disaster Medicine and Public Health
Uniformed Services University
Bethesda, MD

Eugene Lam, MD, MPH, MSc
Emergency Response and Recovery Branch
Centers for Disease Control and Prevention
Atlanta, GA

Eva Leidman, MSPH
Emergency Response and Recovery Branch
Centers for Disease Control and Prevention
Atlanta, GA

Darrell Morris Lester, MS HR/Economics
Division of Global Health and Protection
Centers for Disease Control and Prevention
Atlanta, GA

Benjamin Levy, MD
Department of Graduate Medical Education
Wellstar Kennestone Regional Medical Center
Marietta, GA

Aun Lor, PhD, MPH
Office of the Director
Centers for Disease Control and Prevention
Atlanta, GA

Goldie MacDonald, PhD
Center for Surveillance, Epidemiology, and Laboratory Services
Centers for Disease Control and Prevention
Atlanta, GA

Allen Gidraf Kahindo Maina, MD, MPH
The United Nations High Commissioner for Refugees (UNHCR)
Geneva, Switzerland

Peter Mala, MD, PHD, MPH
Medical Officer
World Health Organization
Geneva, Switzerland

LeGrand L. Malany, PE, JD
Disaster Response and Mitigation Engineer
US Agency for International Development Office of US Foreign Disaster Assistance
Springfield, Illinois

Nina Marano, DVM, MPH
Division of Global Migration and Quarantine
Centers for Disease Control and Prevention
Atlanta, GA

Lise D. Martel, PhD, MPH, MEd
Division of Global Health Protection
Centers for Disease Control and Prevention
Atlanta, GA

Andrea Martinsen, MPH
Emergency Response and Recovery Branch
Centers for Disease Control and Prevention
Atlanta, GA

Sarah Mbaeyi, MD MPH
National Center for Immunization and Respiratory Diseases
Centers for Disease Control and Prevention
Atlanta, GA

Eric Mintz, MD, MPH
Waterborne Diseases Prevention Branch
Centers for Disease Control and Prevention
Atlanta GA

Charles Mock, MD, PhD
Professor of Surgery
University of Washington Seattle, WA

List of Contributors

Richard Francis Mollica, MD, MAR
Director, Harvard Program in Refugee Trauma
Massachusetts General Hospital
Professor of Psychiatry, Harvard Medical School
Boston, MA

Diane Morof, MD, MSc, FACOG
Division of Reproductive Health
Centers for Disease Control and Prevention
Atlanta, GA

Carlos Navarro-Colorado, MD, PhD, MSc
Emergency Response and Recovery Branch
Centers for Disease Control and Prevention
Atlanta, GA

Ian Norton, MD
Manager, Emergency Medical Teams
Emergency Management and Operations
World Health Organization
Geneva, Switzerland

David Olson, MD
Cholera referent-Operational Center, Paris
Doctors Without Borders/MSF
New York, NY

Ciara O'Reilly, PhD
Waterborne Diseases Prevention Branch
Centers for Disease Control and Prevention
Atlanta, GA

Molly Patrick, MEng
National Center for Emerging and Zoonotic
Infectious Diseases, Centers for Disease Control
and Prevention
Atlanta, GA

Silke Pietzsch, MSc, MPH
Technical Director
Action Against Hunger USA
New York, NY

Malcolm Potts, MB, BChir, PhD, FRCOG
Professor and Former Chair
Bixby Center for Population, Health and
Sustainability
University of California, Berkeley
Berkeley, CA

Anu Rajasingham, MPH
Emergency Response and Recovery Branch
Centers for Disease Control and Prevention
Atlanta, GA

Anthony D. Redmond
Professor of International Emergency Medicine
Head, WHO Collaborating Centre for
Emergency Medical Teams and Emergency
Capacity Building
Deputy Director, Humanitarian and
Conflict Response Institute
University of Manchester, UK

George A. Roark, MHRE, MHCA
Division of Emergency Operations
Centers for Disease Control and Prevention
Atlanta, GA

Bayard Roberts PhD, MSc, MA
Professor of Health Systems and Policy
London School of Hygiene and Tropical Medicine,
United Kingdom.

Marian Schilperoord, MA, RN
Senior Project Manager Global Cash Operations
Division of Programme Support and Management
UNHCR

Johan von Schreeb, MD, PhD
Associate Professor and
Director, Centre for Research on Health Care in
Disasters
Health Systems and Policy Research Group
Department of Public Health Sciences
Karolinska Institutet
Stockholm, Sweden

Charles A. Setchell, MCP
Senior Shelter, Settlements, and Hazard Mitigation
Advisor
US Agency for International Development Office of
US Foreign Disaster Assistance (USAID/OFDA)
Washington, DC

Cyrus Shahpar, MD, MBA, MPH
Emergency Response and Recovery Branch
Centers for Disease Control and Prevention
Atlanta, GA

David Sugerman, MD, MPH, FACEP
Workforce and Institute Development Branch
Centers for Disease Control and Prevention
Atlanta, GA

Joanna Taliano, MA, MLS
Library Science Branch
Centers for Disease Control and Prevention
Atlanta, GA

Leisel E. Talley, MPH
Emergency Response and Recovery Branch
Centers for Disease Control and Prevention
Atlanta, GA

Barbara Tomczyk, DrPH, MPH, MS, RN, FAAN
Center for Global Health
Centers for Disease Control and Prevention
Atlanta, GA

Lisandro Torre, MPH
Emergency Response and Recovery Branch
Centers for Disease Control and Prevention
Atlanta, GA

David A. Townes MD, MPH, DTM&H
Emergency Response and Recovery Branch
Centers for Disease Control and Prevention
Atlanta, GA
Public Health and Medical Technical Advisor
US Agency for International Development,
Office of US Foreign Disaster Assistance (USAID/OFDA), Washington, DC
Professor of Emergency Medicine
Adjunct Professor of Global Health
University of Washington
Seattle, WA

Rebecca Turner, MSc
Country Director Global Health Supply Chain
Procurement and Supply Management
Chemonics International, Inc.
Luanda, Angola

Nicole Weber, MPH
Emergency Response and Recovery
Branch, Centers for Disease
Control and Prevention
Atlanta, GA

Wendy Wheaton, MIA, PhD(c)
Adjunct Faculty, Georgetown University
Director of Education South Sudan
Mission, US Agency for International
Development

Holly Ann Williams, PhD, MN, RN
Division of Violence Prevention
Centers for Disease Control and Prevention
Atlanta, GA

Lori A. Wingate, PhD
The Evaluation Center
Western Michigan University
Kalamazoo, MI

Foreword

Background

In 1976, soon after completing a Diploma of Tropical Medicine and Hygiene in London, I found myself at the remote camp of Ban Nam Yao in the mountains of northern Thailand. I had just been employed by a small American NGO to be director of the health program for fifteen thousand Laotian refugees, including a 60-bed hospital that was under construction when I arrived. Starting with two Australian physicians and two Thai nurses, our team gradually expanded to a peak of six doctors, ten nurses, and a laboratory technician, from six countries, including two Lao nurses from the refugee camp. In addition, a number of refugees were trained as nurse aides, some of whom had been medics in the Lao Army. Of historical interest, this was the first refugee setting where doctors and nurses were mobilized by the new French organization, Médecins sans Frontières (MSF), which had been founded five years earlier.

All of us had clinical backgrounds, and our work focused almost exclusively on the hospital outpatients and inpatients. Once a week, we would conduct a mobile clinic for one of the Thai villages in the area. None of us had training in public health let alone epidemiology, a discipline some of us had never heard of. At that time, there were no reference texts, manuals, or guidelines that focused on health in refugee camps, and even if we had been able to access the published literature we would have found almost no articles relevant to the context we were working in.

Confined to clinical roles, we conducted no surveys of nutritional status or any other key indicators of population health. We only collected statistics on hospital inpatients and outpatients, and routine vaccination was limited to children who accessed the hospital. Following outbreaks of typhoid fever and gastroenteritis, we eventually trained a cadre of volunteers who conducted health education in the camp. We paid little attention to the quantity and quality of food rations and drinking water. After all, we were doctors and nurses.

In 1980, around one million ethnic Somalis fled conflict in Ethiopia into 35 camps throughout Somalia. After having worked for five years in Ban Nam Yao, I was recruited by the Somali Ministry of Health's Refugee Health Unit (RHU) as the senior medical adviser. This time, I found an opportunity to take a public health approach to a refugee population and apply the concepts of Primary Health Care (launched in Alma Ata two years earlier) to a refugee situation for the first time. Also for the first time, I encountered CDC epidemiologists who conducted population surveys and advised the RHU on establishing an appropriate disease surveillance system.

Refugee community health workers were trained in large numbers, and standardized treatment protocols, information systems, and essential drugs were agreed to by the 20 or more international NGOs working in the camps. In 1981, the RHU developed a manual – Guidelines for Health Care in Refugee Camps in the Somali Democratic Republic – the first such manual of its kind. A large scurvy outbreak occurred in Somali camps, with thousands of cases – the largest documented outbreak of scurvy in the twentieth century.[1] The epidemiology training provided by CDC staff formed the basis of the outbreak investigation.

In 1986, I was awarded a Fogarty Fellowship to do epidemiologic research at CDC, focusing on morbidity and mortality in refugee populations. I discovered that my CDC colleagues in Somalia were members of just the third response by the agency to a refugee crisis. For the subsequent ten years I was privileged to be part of the growth in CDC's capacity to respond to humanitarian emergencies and to the development of epidemiologic methods, tools, and indicators that contributed to the body of knowledge that is the basis of this book. This in turn was part of a global transformation of the health response to humanitarian emergencies from an attitude of "Do the best you can...," when I was in Thailand 40 years earlier, to an evidence-based framework supported by comprehensive technical guidelines and minimum standards.

History of CDC Responses to Humanitarian Emergencies

The first example of CDC engagement in a humanitarian crisis was during the Nigeria-Biafra civil war when, at the request of the International Committee of the Red Cross (ICRC), CDC participated in refugee support for two years by providing disease control and nutrition assistance. During this effort, the CDC assisted the diagnosis and treatment of five hundred thousand children who were affected by severe malnutrition. Dr. William H. Foege was CDC's first epidemiologist in the Biafran effort, and he served from September until November, 1967. He would later serve as CDC director. In all, around two dozen CDC staff were mobilized. Tragically, in 1968, Paul Schnitker became the first and only Epidemic Intelligence Service (EIS) officer to die in the line of duty when his plane crashed en route to Nigeria.

At this time, there were no international guidelines or assessment tools available for humanitarian emergencies, such as the Biafran crisis. Nor had CDC developed specific methodologies for working in these settings. CDC staff applied and adapted the principles and practices of the field epidemiology that the agency had developed in large part to address public health issues and outbreaks in the United States.

More than a decade later, in 1979, hundreds of thousands of Cambodian refugees fled into Eastern Thailand, initially in Sakaeo camp where early mortality rates were extremely high. Then CDC director William Foege accompanied First Lady Rosalynn Carter to the camp, and soon after CDC epidemiologists were deployed. Again, it was the ICRC that requested CDC assistance. CDC established routine surveillance for the first time in a refugee setting, identifying outbreaks of malaria, measles, and meningitis.[2]

The crude monthly mortality rate in October 1979 in Sakaeo camp was 31.9 per 1000, compared with a baseline in Cambodia of 2.5 per 1000.[3] Within seven weeks, mortality rates returned to normal. CDC expanded surveillance to other camps, such as the massive Khao-I-Dang, with a population of greater than 100,000 refugees. In 1983, the data gathered and analyzed were published in a CDC Monograph – at the time the most comprehensive descriptive epidemiology of a refugee population.[4]

Starting in 1980, CDC sent a number of epidemiologists to Somalia to conduct mortality and nutrition surveys, establish surveillance, train Somali staff in field epidemiology, and contribute to standard operational guidelines. These epidemiologists were embedded within the RHU, described earlier. The large epidemic of scurvy in the Somali refugee camps led to sustained technical advocacy by CDC to ensure that refugees everywhere received food rations containing the full complement of essential nutrients, including vitamin C.

Reinforcing CDC's Internal Capacity

Starting in 1987, I occupied the sole designated position to support CDC responses to conflict-related emergencies within the Technical Support Division of the International Health Program Office. Further analyses of data from refugee camps in Thailand, Somalia, Sudan, and Ethiopia led to a series of papers on the public health impact of forced displacement.[5] The first EIS officer was assigned in 1990, and his first mission was to conduct a health needs assessment of Liberian refugees in the Forest Region of Guinea.

In subsequent years, CDC provided epidemiologic assistance in the following settings: Somali refugees in eastern Ethiopia (1989)[6]; internally displaced persons in Southern Sudan (1989); Afghan refugees in Pakistan (1991); and Mozambican refugees in Malawi and Zimbabwe (1990–93), where there were repeated cholera outbreaks and a major outbreak of pellagra in Malawi due to the removal of peanuts, the main source of niacin, from the food ration.[7]

In the aftermath of the First Gulf War in 1991, half a million Iraqis, mainly Kurds, fled to the Turkish border. A number of CDC epidemiologists were attached to the US military in Turkey and Northern Iraq where they helped to establish camp mortality and morbidity surveillance, investigated a cholera outbreak, conducted a mortality and nutrition survey, and liaised with the military on appropriate medical supplies, immunization, management of dehydration, and rehabilitation of health facilities.[8] Working with the US Office for Foreign Disaster Assistance (OFDA), CDC provided a critical link between the military and civilian NGOs working in the relief program.

Other health needs assessments were conducted in the early 1990s by CDC epidemiologists among Bhutanese refugees in Nepal (1992); Burmese refugees in Bangladesh (1992); Sudanese refugees in western Ethiopia (1992), where there was an outbreak of HIV infection and other sexually transmitted infections; and Somali refugees in Kenya (1992), where there was an outbreak of hepatitis E virus.

And Then ... on December 8, 1991, the Soviet Union Ceased to Exist

By New Year's Day of 1992, CDC epidemiologists had joined a Disaster Assistance and Response Team (DART) assembled by OFDA in Moscow. The assessment was wide-ranging and included food availability, medical facility capacity, and disease surveillance.[9] For a number of subsequent years, CDC continued to provide surveillance and outbreak investigation assistance in former Soviet republics, including Tajikistan and Armenia.[10]

The end of the Cold War and the breakup of the Soviet Union led to instability and conflicts across the globe. The number of armed, intrastate conflicts peaked during these years, reaching a high of 50 in 1992. Millions of Somalis were affected by famine amidst a vicious civil war fought by dozens of militia (1991–92). CDC assigned epidemiologists to UNICEF, where they conducted mortality and nutrition surveys and established surveillance in displaced persons camps.[11] This was one of the most dangerous missions ever undertaken by CDC and staff had to be protected by armed local militia called "technicals."

During 1993, CDC epidemiologists were mobilized through OFDA to the former Yugoslav republics of Serbia, Bosnia and Herzegovina, and Croatia. Public health needs assessments were conducted and disease surveillance established in Sarajevo and several Muslim enclaves in Bosnia along with expert advice on the water supply in Sarajevo.[12] Having witnessed the catastrophic impact of the war on public health, CDC discreetly employed advocacy for a US-led peace process.

Goma: The Big Test

In July 1994, around one million Rwandan refugees crossed a bridge into the small town of Goma in then-Zaire, now the Democratic Republic of Congo. Within days, the CDC director mobilized a dozen epidemiologists, who were attached to UNHCR, UNICEF, WHO and the International Federation of Red Cross and Red Crescent Societies. A devastating epidemic of cholera struck the refugee population that had dispersed into crowded, unplanned camps with inadequate sanitation and no access to clean water. During one week between July 25 and July 31, almost 30 thousand people died, only 10 percent in health facilities. The cholera outbreak was followed by a lethal outbreak of *shigella dysenteriae* Type 1 and by the end of the month after the arrival of the refugees, around 50 thousand had died. Other challenges included outbreaks of meningococcal meningitis and malaria.[13]

CDC worked with UNHCR, WHO and MSF to establish very basic disease surveillance and conduct population surveys in each of the three largest camps. Instituting outreach and assessing the quality of care was a critical role for CDC epidemiologists. Many aid workers were unfamiliar with oral rehydration; therefore, experts in cholera treatment were brought in from Bangladesh. A CDC epidemiologist intercepted a planeload of donated Gatorade that would have harmed children if used to treat dehydration.

Highlights of CDC Achievements up Until 1995

CDC has earned a reputation for timely, technically sound, and locally relevant assistance to populations affected by complex emergencies and has had a significant influence on what is now normative practice by aid agencies such as MSF in complex emergencies and inspired the formation of specialist agencies, such as Paris-based *Epicentre*.

CDC has made a number of evidence based recommendations to improve responses to humanitarian emergencies; for example, recommending a two-dose measles vaccination schedule in emergencies (at age 6 months and 9 months), which was adopted by UNHCR and WHO. CDC established a crude mortality rate threshold of one per 10,000 per day as the definition of a public health emergency, a threshold that is still used today. CDC led evidence-based advocacy for a minimum energy content of refugee food rations of 1,900 kilocalories per person per day plus recommended daily allowances of micronutrients. The minimum energy content was later raised to 2,100 kilocalories per day. CDC developed a widely adopted incidence threshold (15 per 100,000 per week for two consecutive weeks) for meningococcal meningitis to trigger mass vaccination. Recently developed serological tests were used to investigate an outbreak of hepatitis E among Somali refugees in Kenya.

Public health advocacy by CDC demonstrated to key agencies such as UNHCR and the World Food Programme and major donors the direct association between acute child malnutrition, inadequate food rations, and elevated child mortality. Following a review and analysis of methods used to measure mortality and nutritional status in Somalia in 1993, CDC highlighted the need to standardize methods and measurements in assessments of mortality, morbidity, and nutritional status.[14] CDC reports of inadequate clinical practices, such as rehydration, led to a global effort to develop minimum standards for humanitarian response programs, known as the Sphere Project. In 1992, MMWR published a special issue on recommendations for public health in complex emergencies.[15]

By the mid-1990s, compared with the situation in 1979, public health for refugees and internally displaced persons had evolved as a specialist field with its own tools, methods, indicators, policies, manuals, reference materials, and minimum standards. In 1993, CDC embarked on one of the first randomized controlled trials to be done in a refugee setting. Investigations of repeated cholera outbreaks in refugee camps in Malawi showed high rates of intrahousehold transmission. Four hundred Mozambican refugee households were systematically identified and followed over a 4-month period, one-fourth of the households were randomly assigned to exclusively use an improved container for water collection with a narrow neck. Analysis of water samples demonstrated that there was a 69% reduction in the geometric mean of fecal coliform levels in household water and 31% less diarrheal disease ($P = 0.06$) in children under 5 years of age among the group using the improved bucket.

The Legacy

The International Emergency and Refugee Health Branch (IERHB) was created in the late 1990s and was followed by the Emergency Response and Recovery Branch (ERRB) of CDC's Division of Global Health Protection, which has led the development of this book. When I visited CDC in late 2016, more than 20 years after I left the agency, CDC had evolved as a major global actor in the public health response to humanitarian emergencies. They have included complex, conflict-related emergencies, such as the mass displacement of Syrians, and natural disasters in fragile states, such as the 2010 earthquake and cholera epidemic in Haiti. Led by ERRB, the agency responded to 14 humanitarian emergencies between 2007 and 2016.[16] These responses included 62 discrete activities ranging across all elements of humanitarian assistance, including public health surveillance, epidemic investigation and control, water, sanitation, and hygiene (WASH), mental health, and nutrition, to name but a few.

The scale of CDC responses has continued to grow; for example, in 2016, in its first year of existence, ERRB's Global Rapid Response Team deployed more than two hundred CDC staff members to various humanitarian emergencies. Moreover, collaborations between CDC and a broad range of national and international humanitarian agencies have promoted standardization of approaches across the international humanitarian emergency response community and helped to improve the coordination of responses.

Among the many achievements of IERHB and ERRB, I would highlight the following:

- The first accurate estimate of the maternal mortality ratio in Afghanistan.
- Technical support to the first national measles immunization campaign in Afghanistan after the fall of the Taliban.
- Rapid assessments and surveys in Darfur, Sudan and refugee camps in Chad.
- Support for the Somalia communicable disease reporting surveillance system during a period of famine (2011–2014), designed to optimize early warning of outbreaks, by providing analysis and training; this system identified an outbreak of measles in 2011 and polio in 2013, enabling swift intervention.
- Estimating the prevalence of war-related mental health conditions in post-war Sri Lanka.
- Extensive assistance to Syrian refugees in Jordan, Turkey and Iraq, including needs assessments, surveillance, immunization campaigns, reproductive health, mental health, nutrition, tuberculosis, polio surveillance, cholera epidemic response in Iraq, and the establishment of an Early Warning and Response Network (EWARN) in northern Syria.

List of Abbreviations

MOH – Ministry of Health
MoHCDGEC – Ministry of Health, Community Development, Gender, Elderly and Children of Tanzania
MSF – Médecins Sans Frontières
NaDCC – sodium dichloroisocyanurate
NCDs – noncommunicable diseases
NFI – nonfood item
NGO – nongovernmental organizations
NIMS – National Incident Management System
NP – nasopharyngeal
NTP – National Tuberculosis Program
NTU – nephelometric turbidity units
OCT – outbreak control team
OCHA – United Nations Office of the Coordination of Humanitarian Affairs
ODI – Overseas Development Institute
ODS – Optional data set
OP – oropharyngeal
ORS – oral rehydration solution
OTP – outpatient therapeutic program
PEN – package of essential noncommunicable
PET – polyethylene terephthalate
PHAST – participatory hygiene and sanitation transformation
pLDH – plasmodium lactate dehydrogenase
PLHIV – persons living with HIV/AIDS
PLW – pregnant and lactating women
PoU – point-of-use
PCR – polymerase chain reaction
PFA – psychological first aid
PHO – public health officer
PTSD – posttraumatic stress disorder
RDT – rapid diagnostic test
ReSoMal – rehydration solution for malnutrition
RSV – respiratory syncytial virus
RUFs – ready-to-use foods
RUSF – ready-to-use supplementary food
RUTF – ready-to-use therapeutic food
SALT algorithm – Sort, Assess, Lifesaving therapy, Transport
SARS – severe acute respiratory syndrome
SC – stabilization center
SFP – supplementary feeding program
SODIS – solar disinfection
STEPS – WHO STEPwise Approach to Surveillance
TB – tuberculosis
TDS – total dissolved solids
tSFP – targeted supplementary feeding program
UDDT – urine-diversion dry toilet
UN – United Nations
UNHCR – Office of the United Nations High Commissioner for Refugees
UNICEF – United Nations Children's Fund
UNISDR – United Nations International Strategy for Disaster Reduction
UNRRA – United Nations Relief and Rehabilitation Administration
UNRWA – United Nations Relief and Works Agency
URTI – upper respiratory tract infection
USD – US Dollars
VIP – ventilated-improved pit
WASH – water, sanitation, and hygiene
WFP – World Food Programme
WHO – World Health Organization
WHOPES – WHO Pesticide Evaluation Scheme

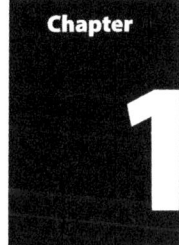

Section 1 — Humanitarian Emergencies

Chapter 1

Introduction to Humanitarian Emergencies

Mark Anderson and Michael Gerber

Introduction

> Disasters ... are all too often regarded as unusual events, not part of "normal life." In reality, however, the opposite is true. Disasters and emergencies are a fundamental part of normal life. They are consequences of the ways societies structure themselves, economically and socially; the ways that societies and states interact; and the ways that relationships between the decision makers are sustained.
> -United Nations Disaster Relief Organization (UNDRO, 1992)

Many of us perceive floods, epidemics, earthquakes, droughts, and wars as unusual events. But, the opposite is true. Rather than being rare events, disasters are common. Somewhere in the world, a disaster occurs almost daily. During the ten years between 2006–2015, there were 1,680 floods, 335 epidemics, 249 earthquakes, 179 landslides, 160 droughts, and 19 wars (Guha-Sapir et al., 2015; Pettersson and Wallensteen 2015). That is 262 disasters every year during that ten-year period.

Many of these events are small in scope, and the impact can be managed with local resources. However, some exceed the capacity of local governments, local public health systems, and local aid organizations. These are the disaster events that require international assistance. These are the events we hear about in the media: decades of war and economic hardship in Afghanistan, civil conflict and terrorism in Syria, earthquakes in Haiti, tsunamis in Indonesia, Ebola outbreaks in West Africa, and famine in Somalia. All of us would recognize the recent crises in Afghanistan, Syria, Haiti, Indonesia and West Africa as disasters. But, how do we define a disaster and distinguish humanitarian emergencies, the focus of this book, from other types of disasters?

Disasters

The United Nations Office for Disaster Risk Reduction (UNISDR) defines a disaster as (UNISDR 2009): "A serious disruption of the functioning of a society, causing widespread human, material, or environmental losses which exceed the ability of the affected society to cope using its own resources." There are two points in this definition worth emphasizing. First, a disaster is an event disruptive enough to affect the normal function of a community. In this case, the community might be limited to the town or village affected by a defined event such as a tornado. Or, it could be an entire nation affected by armed conflict. The second point worth emphasizing in this definition is that the event is significant enough that the affected society cannot cope with the impact using its own resources. In more developed countries, the support comes from national or local organizations. In less developed countries, international support is often required, and we call these events "humanitarian emergencies." Based on this definition, disasters and humanitarian emergencies do not occur every time a society is exposed to drought, tornadoes, wildfires, and even armed conflict (Abdallah and Burnham 2000).

The impact of disasters depends on the nature of the event and the vulnerability and preparedness of the population. Those countries prone to disasters are often highly vulnerable. Their vulnerability may be due to lack of resources, lack of preparedness, or both. These countries are often what many would consider "fragile states." They are limited by weak governance, poor social infrastructure, and environmental degradation. All of these factors contribute to their increased vulnerability and their inability to manage the shock and stress of a disaster.

Disasters are triggered by natural forces or human-made events. Some disasters occur without warning while others develop slowly, their full impact not being felt for years. With this in mind, disasters are classified into two major categories, natural and human-made disasters, and five subcategories: sudden impact disasters, slow onset hazards, industrial/

Table 1.1 Classification of disasters

Natural Disasters	Man-made Disasters
Sudden Impact – earthquakes, tropical storms, tsunamis, volcanic eruptions, etc.	**Industrial/Technological** – pollution, fires, spillages, explosions, etc.
Slow-Onset – drought, famine, pest infestation, deforestation, etc.	**Complex Emergencies** – wars, civil strife, armed aggression, etc.
Epidemic Diseases – water-borne, food-borne, vector-borne, etc.	

technological events, epidemics, and complex emergencies (Abdallah and Burnham 2000). This classification of disasters is shown in Table 1.1.

Natural disasters include events that occur suddenly, with little warning, such as earthquakes, floods, tropical storms, tsunamis, volcanic eruptions, and landslides. These are considered sudden onset disasters. Floods are the most common natural disaster and often result in widespread food shortages and population displacement. Earthquakes, although not as common, cause the most deaths and injuries.

Many natural disasters are slow in onset. This group includes droughts, famine, environmental degradation, deforestation, and pest infestation, such as locusts. Slow onset disasters are often the result of weather conditions, which can have profound effects on marginal communities. Because of poverty and overpopulation, these marginal communities have a limited capacity to cope with adverse conditions, such as drought. So, instead of being a hardship, slow onset events like drought become a disaster, leading to famine, population displacement, and sometimes, armed conflict.

Epidemics or disease outbreaks are natural phenomena that can evolve into disasters. The outbreak of Ebola in West Africa is an example of how a society's inability to contain an infectious disease can lead to a humanitarian emergency. Epidemic diseases can be waterborne, such as cholera; food-borne, such as dysentery; or, vectorborne, such as malaria. Some, like Ebola, are spread through person-to-person contact. Measles is an example of a common but vaccine-preventable disease that can have devastating effects on vulnerable communities. The overcrowding and poor sanitary conditions common in many marginal communities and in camps for displaced persons can promote measles outbreaks, causing many deaths.

Human-made disasters can be classified into two categories: industrial/technological disasters and complex emergencies. Pollution, chemical spills, explosions, and fires are examples of industrial/technological disasters. Inferior construction and inadequate safety procedures can trigger these events. The release of a toxic pesticide into the air of Bhopal, India caused thousands of deaths in 1984. The explosion of the Deepwater Horizon in 2010 released millions of gallons of oil into the Gulf of Mexico, resulting in a major environmental disaster. Sudden onset disasters, such as earthquakes and tsunamis, can often lead to industrial/technological disasters. An example is the destruction of the Fukushima Daiichi Nuclear Power Plant caused by an earthquake and tsunami in Japan in 2011.

Complex emergencies are the second type of human-made disaster. As their name implies, complex emergencies result from multiple factors. Many are associated with war, internal conflict, and terrorism (Abdallah and Burnham 2000). Population displacement is common in complex emergencies due to insecurity, food shortages, and destruction of services and infrastructure. We will examine the characteristics and impact of complex emergencies in more detail later in this chapter.

Humanitarian Emergencies

Any disaster, whether natural or human-made, can become a humanitarian emergency if international humanitarian assistance is needed to support the affected population. This is shown in Figure 1.1.

When international support is required to meet the basic needs of a population, including food, water, shelter, protection and other life-sustaining measures, it is a humanitarian emergency. For the purpose of this text, a humanitarian emergency may be defined as:

- A disaster requiring international support (humanitarian assistance) to meet the basic needs of the affected population

Examples of humanitarian emergencies include the famine in the Sahel region of Africa, where international humanitarian relief organizations established

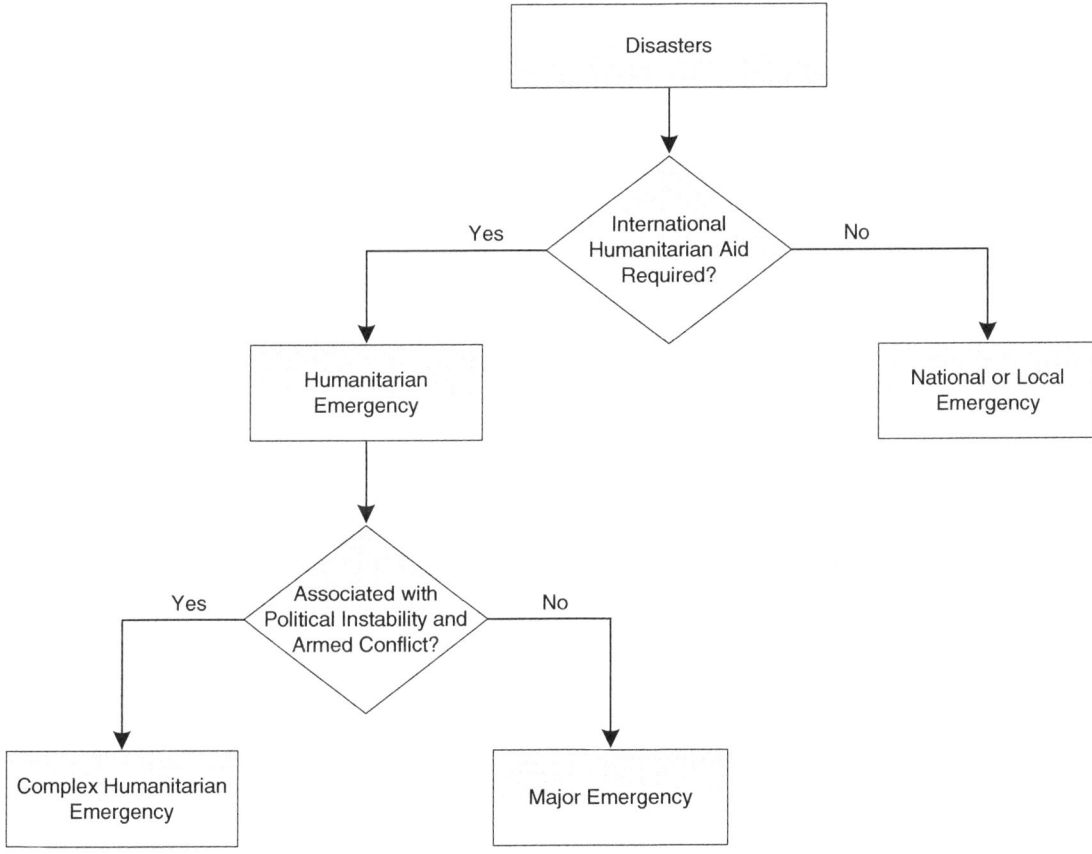

Figure 1.1 Disasters, humanitarian emergencies, and complex humanitarian emergencies

feeding programs and the earthquake in Haiti that required large-scale international assistance.

In a humanitarian emergency, local and national resources cannot meet the relief needs without international humanitarian aid/assistance. Often, the scope of the disaster response is beyond the capacity of any single humanitarian agency. Humanitarian emergencies can be divided into two general categories. The first is what the Inter-Agency Standing Committee (IASC) defines as a "major emergency" shown in Figure 1.1. For the IASC, a major emergency is "any situation where humanitarian needs are of a sufficiently large scale and complexity that significant external assistance and resources are required, and where a multi-sectoral response is needed with the engagement of a wide range of international humanitarian actors" (IASC 2007).

Major emergencies typically are not politically motivated, and there are no political or conflict-related restrictions to humanitarian access. However, there is a subgroup of humanitarian emergencies often associated with political instability and armed conflict; we call these "complex humanitarian emergencies" or "complex emergencies" as shown in Figure 1.1.

Phases of Humanitarian Emergencies

There are four commonly recognized phases of a humanitarian emergency. These phases are typically pictured as a continuum, with one phase leading into another. The reality is less clear. There is an ebb and flow within the emergency continuum, but it is still helpful to describe the unique aspects of these four phases, because recognizing the transition from one phase to another can help predict needs and plan resources. This continuum is also referred to as the Disaster Risk Management Cycle that is discussed briefly in Chapter 4.

Pre-emergency Phase

The first phase of the emergency continuum is the "preemergency phase." This is the period before disaster strikes when planning and preparedness should be emphasized. It is a time to assess the potential risks that a community may face and develop appropriate plans to respond to these risks. Stockpiling supplies, identifying shelters, planning evacuation routes, and developing incident management systems are some of the activities that should be undertaken during the preemergency phase. However, many resource-poor settings do not have the capacity for this type of planning and preparedness. As a result, many disaster events that occur in these settings evolve into humanitarian emergencies.

Acute Emergency Phase

The "Acute Emergency Phase" begins immediately after disaster strikes. This phase is often distinguished by population movement. During this phase, humanitarian organizations begin to respond, focusing on providing critical services such as food, water, sanitation, primary healthcare, and shelter. The priority during this phase is to keep the population alive (Abdallah and Burnham 2000).

Epidemiologists measure the severity of a humanitarian emergency by assessing the crude mortality rate (CMR) in the affected population. In an emergency setting, the CMR is expressed as the number of deaths per 10,000 persons per day. A doubling of the CMR from its baseline rate is considered the threshold for defining the acute emergency phase of a disaster. In the acute emergency phase, the CMR can be extraordinarily high. During the first months of the Rwandan crisis in 1994, as refugees streamed into what was then eastern Zaire, the CMR was 40 to 60 times the baseline rate for that population (Anon 1995).

Post-emergency Phase

As the population movement slows and the CMR returns to its baseline rate, a disaster enters what is called the "postemergency phase." During this phase, aid organizations turn their focus to providing more routine services and developing local capacity to support the needs of the affected population. Displaced populations begin to consider their long-term options, such as whether to return home, integrate into the local community, or relocate to a third country.

Recovery Phase

In the final phase, the "recovery phase," the focus shifts from emergency response to recovery and development. International relief organizations often leave during this phase. Development agencies take a more prominent role, and the responsibility for providing assistance is turned over to local authorities.

Population Displacement

Humanitarian emergencies, particularly complex emergencies, are often associated with population displacement. In a humanitarian emergency, people may be forced to move from their homes to find food, shelter or security. Those that must flee in the midst of a crisis are often the most vulnerable. They are often the poorest; those with sufficient income can leave early in a protracted crisis. In many humanitarian emergency situations, the majority of the displaced population are women, children, and the elderly. They are frequently malnourished and in poor health. Many are unaccompanied children or pregnant and lactating women. These characteristics contribute to many of the health issues discussed in this book and, as we will discuss in the following paragraphs, add to the "complexity" of complex emergencies.

When a person is displaced from his/her home, the journey from a place of insecurity can be the most taxing. The risk of death appears to be highest as displaced people travel to a place of safety. Reported crude mortality rates among Somali refugees in 2011 were more than twice as high during their journey than before they departed (CDC 2011). As mentioned, children and the elderly are at particular risk; most deaths among displaced populations occur in children less than five years of age. As shown in Figure 1.2 approximately 18 percent of Kurdish refugees in northern Iraq were under five years of age. However, 64 percent of all deaths were among this same age group (Anon 1991).

Most displaced persons are refugees or internally displaced persons (IDPs). Refugees flee their home out of fear of persecution for reasons of race, religion, nationality, membership in a particular social group, or political opinion. During their flight, refugees cross an international border seeking protection. Because they cross an international border, refugees are granted certain protections as defined by the Geneva Conventions and Added Protocols. Signatories of the Conventions must grant asylum to refugees within their territory. As described in Chapter 3, the United Nations High Commissioner for Refugees (UNHCR) is responsible for protecting the rights of refugees and

Chapter 1: Introduction to Humanitarian Emergencies

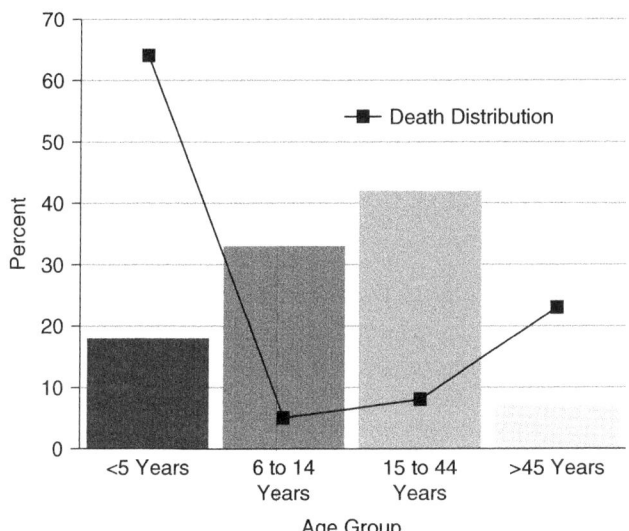

Figure 1.2 Age distribution of Kurdish refugee population (Anon 1991)

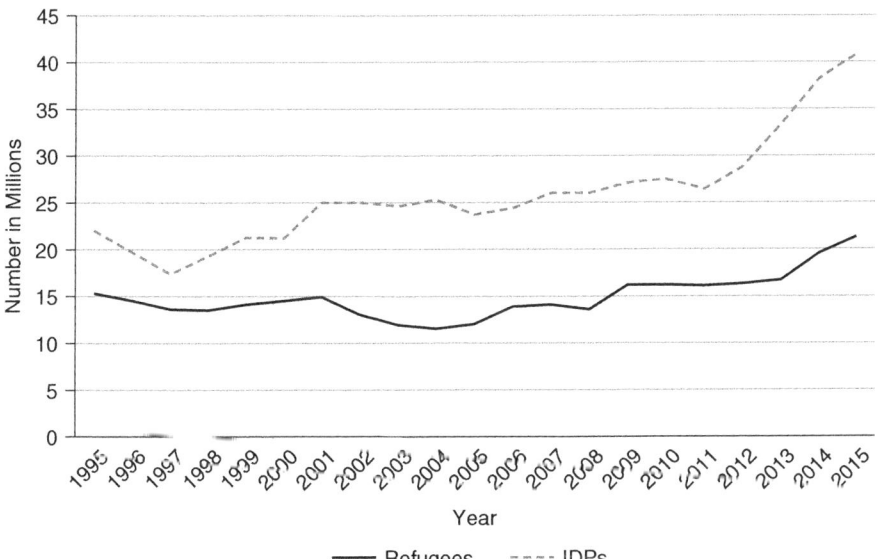

Figure 1.3 Number of refugees and IDP's – 1995–2015 (UNHCR 2016)

ensuring that they are treated according to internationally recognized standards. With the onset of the crisis in Syria, the number of refugees has increased dramatically in recent years as shown in Figure 1.3. In 2015, 21.3 million people were considered refugees; over half were under the age of 18 (UNHCR 2016).

By the end of 2015, an unprecedented 65.3 million people were forcibly displaced because of persecution, conflict, violence, or human rights violations. This is an increase of 5.8 million people from the previous year. If all the displaced persons in the world represented a single nation, it would be the 21st largest in the world (UNHCR 2016).

As shown in Figure 1.3, most of the displaced persons in the world are internally displaced (IDPs). There were 40.8 million IDPs in 2015. IDPs flee their homes for the same reasons as refugees, but they do not cross an international border, remaining instead within the boundaries of their country. Because of this, they do not have the same legal status as refugees and, until recently, were not provided the same level of protection and assistance as refugees. Since 2006, UNHCR has assumed more responsibility for IDPs

5

and is now assisting more IDPs than refugees (UNHCR 2016).

Complex Humanitarian Emergencies

Complex emergencies, sometimes called complex humanitarian emergencies, are a relatively recent concept in the humanitarian community. The term was introduced in the late 1980s to describe some of the humanitarian crises occurring in Africa. Through the 1990s, the term found common usage among various aid organizations, including the United Nations. Several influential academics also adopted and wrote about the term complex emergencies. In one such article called "Complex Emergencies and the Crisis of Developmentalism" complex emergencies are described (Duffield 1994): "For the UN, a complex emergency is a major humanitarian crisis of a multi-causal nature that requires a system-wide response. Commonly, a long-term combination of political, conflict and peacekeeping factors is also involved." Several aspects of this definition are important to highlight. First, a complex emergency (CE) is a humanitarian emergency caused by multiple factors. There is often a political context to complex emergencies, frequently armed conflict, war, and civil strife in particular. Finally, as in other humanitarian emergencies, a large-scale or "system-wide" humanitarian response is needed.

As we mentioned earlier in this chapter, complex emergencies are often viewed as "human-made" disasters. This distinction is attributed to the multi-causal nature of CEs, as opposed to natural disasters, which are often seen as having only one cause (Duffield 1994). The reality however, is not as simple; many natural disasters, such as droughts and floods, are complex events with multiple social and ecologic causes (Duffield 1994). And, CEs are not solely "human-made" events. Natural disasters can trigger the political instability that leads to armed conflict and CEs. Nearly 90 percent of the 30 largest CEs during the past decade were associated with a natural disaster (Spiegel et al. 2007).

What truly distinguishes complex emergencies from natural disasters is their "singular ability to erode or destroy the cultural, civil, political and economic integrity of established societies" (Duffield 1994). CEs are events where social, political, and economic systems are attacked. Even the humanitarian assistance provided in response to a CE may become a target of political misappropriation or direct violence. Complex emergencies are different from natural disasters. However, the distinction is due to the impact of a CE rather than what causes a CE (Duffield 1994).

In 1994, the Interagency Standing Committee (IASC), established in 1992 to coordinate humanitarian assistance among key UN and non-governmental organization (NGO) humanitarian partners, published a formal definition of the complex emergency. The IASC definition of complex emergency has since been recognized by the UN Office for the Coordination of Humanitarian Affairs (OCHA) and published in their Orientation Handbook on Complex Emergencies.

According to the OCHA Handbook, a complex emergency is defined as (OCHA 1999):

- A humanitarian crisis in a country, region or society where there is total or considerable breakdown of authority resulting from internal or external conflict and which requires an international response that goes beyond the mandate or capacity of any single agency and/or the ongoing United Nations country program.

According to the OCHA Handbook, complex emergencies share several characteristics, including:

- Extensive violence and loss of life; massive displacements of people; widespread damage to societies and economies;
- The need for large-scale, multifaceted humanitarian assistance;
- The hindrance or prevention of humanitarian assistance by political and military constraints;
- Significant security risks for humanitarian relief workers in some areas.

Complex Emergencies and Armed Conflict

The OCHA Handbook, as reflected in this quote from Sergio Vieira de Mello, then the UN Under-Secretary-General and Emergency Relief Coordinator, emphasizes the uniqueness of complex emergencies and highlights their connection with the changing nature of armed conflict (OCHA 1999):

> Contemporary armed conflict is seldom conducted on a clearly defined battlefield, by conventional armies confronting each other. Today's warfare often takes place in cities and villages, with civilians as the preferred targets, the propagation of

terror as the premeditated tactic, and the physical elimination or mass displacement of certain categories of populations as the overarching strategy. The acts of warring parties in recent conflicts in the former Yugoslavia, Sierra Leone and Afghanistan bear testimony to this. Breaches of human rights and humanitarian law, including mutilation, rape, forced displacement, denial of the right to food and medicines, diversion of aid, and attacks on medical personnel and hospitals are no longer inevitable by-products of war. They have become the means to achieve a strategic goal. As a result, even low intensity conflicts generate enormous human suffering. Humanitarian needs are disproportionate to the scale of military conflict. Meeting these needs has become more difficult, as the dividing line between soldiers and civilians has grown blurred.
- *Sergio Vieira de Mello, UN Under-Secretary General and Emergency Relief Coordinator, 1999*

Since 1946, there has been an overall increase in the number of internal armed conflict events each year. As shown in Figure 1.4, the number of events peaked in 1993. Between 1990 and 2015, there were 160 armed conflicts worldwide. Ninety-one percent of these conflicts were primarily or exclusively internal (Pettersson and Wallensteen 2015). This shift in the nature of armed conflict is tied to an overall increase in war-related injury among civilians. In recent years, the proportion of war-related deaths among civilians has ranged between 35% and 65% (Meddings 2001). Some authors put the number much higher, estimating that 90 percent of all conflict-related deaths occur among civilians (Ahlström and Nordquist 1991, OCHA 1999).

The political nature of internal armed conflict has also changed since the end of the Cold War. Politically driven conflict declined in East Asia and Latin America but increased in Africa, the Middle East, Eastern Europe, the Caucasus, and Central Asia. Between 1999 to 2015, nearly half (48.5%) of armed conflicts occurred in Africa and the Middle East. Armed conflicts are no longer driven by nationalist or socialist ideology. Instead, they are "resource wars that lack a clear social program" (Duffield 1994). Today, armed conflict is driven by social, economic, and ethnic grievances. The political, social, and economic factors associated with CEs can lead to profound suffering for the civilian populations affected.

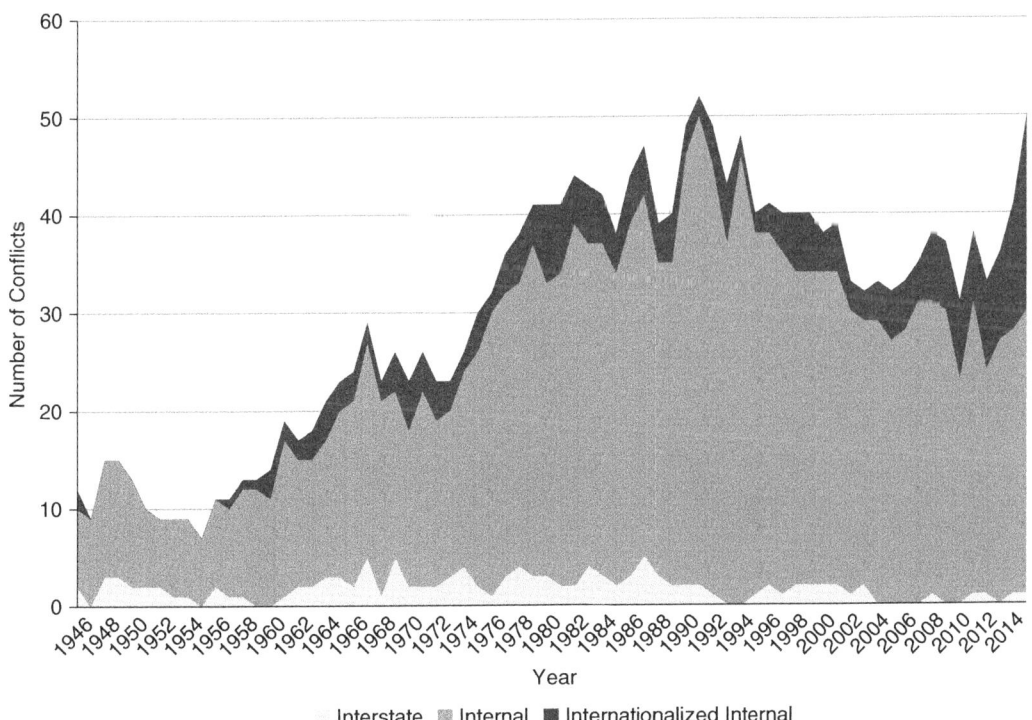

Figure 1.4 Active conflicts by type and year – 1946–2015 (Pettersson and Wallensteen 2015)

Although complex emergencies are often associated with armed conflict, their complexity can also be attributed to multiple factors that can trigger a CE. These factors can be political, economic, social or cultural, and any of them can initiate a chain of events that ultimately leads to a CE. For instance, political insecurity weakens already fragile states, driving many to civil conflict. As the conflict escalates, civilian populations are displaced from their homes in search of food, water, shelter, and security. The social fabric that holds communities together breaks down as more people are displaced. Community support systems are disrupted and vulnerable populations like children, adolescents, women, and the elderly suffer. Ethnic and religious factors may be exploited because of political instability and limited resources. Discrimination and ethnic hostilities may result in certain groups being denied services or targeted for violence; both are common factors leading to armed conflict. Overpopulation can be either a trigger or an outcome of the displacement common in CEs. More people competing for limited resources can worsen food deficits, raise prices on limited commodities, and lead to economic collapse, which further weakens a fragile government.

The point is that complex emergencies are often associated with a combination of factors, primarily (but not exclusively) armed conflict. Some of these factors may have developed quickly; others may have been developing for years. Some may have triggered the chain of events leading to a CE, while others may be outcomes that further exacerbate the situation. Regardless of the specific trigger or outcome, what truly distinguishes complex emergencies from other humanitarian emergencies is the human toll they exact.

Conclusion

The role of health professionals in humanitarian emergencies is to address this human toll, specifically to mitigate the impact on human health. Whether by addressing the direct threats of violent injury or the indirect threats of disease and malnutrition, the goal of public health is to reduce mortality and morbidity in humanitarian emergencies. And, that too is the purpose of this book.

References

Abdallah, S. and Burnham, G. (2000). *Public health guide for emergencies*, Johns Hopkins School of Hygiene and Public Health: Baltimore, MD.

Ahlström, C. and Nordquist, K. -Å. (1991). *Casualties of conflict: Report for the world campaign for the protection of victims of war*, Department of Peace and Conflict Research, Uppsala University: Uppsala, Sweden.

Anon. (1991). Public health consequences of acute displacement of Iraqi citizens—March-May 1991. *JAMA*, **266**, 633–634.

Anon. (1995). Public health impact of Rwandan refugee crisis: What happened in Goma, Zaire, in July, 1994? Goma Epidemiology Group. *Lancet*, **345**, 339–344.

Centers for Disease Control and Prevention. (2011). Notes from the field: mortality among refugees fleeing Somalia–Dadaab refugee camps, Kenya, July-August 2011. *MMWR Morbidity and Mortality weekly report*, **60**, 1133.

Duffield, M. (1994). Complex emergencies and the crisis of developmentalism. *IDS bulletin*, **25**.

Guha-Sapir, D., et al. (2015). EM-DAT: International disaster database. Catholic University of Louvain: Brussels. Retrieved from www.emdat.be (Accessed November 27, 2016).

IASC Task Team on the Cluster Approach. (2007). Operational guidance on designating sector/cluster leads in major new emergencies. Available at: www2.wpro.who.int/internet/files/eha/toolkit/web/Technical%20References/Cluster%20Approach/IASC%20Operational%20Guidance%20in%20Ongoing%20Emergencies.pdf (Accessed November 27, 2016).

Meddings, D. R. (2001). Civilians and war: A review and historical overview of the involvement of non-combatant populations in conflict situations. *Medicine, Conflict and Survival*, **17**, 6–16.

Office for the Coordination of Humanitarian Affairs (OCHA). (1999). *OCHA orientation handbook on complex emergencies*, OCHA. Available at: http://reliefweb.int/sites/reliefweb.int/files/resources/OCHA%C2%A0ORIENTATION%20HANDBOOK.pdf (Accessed July 12, 2017).

Pettersson, T. and Wallensteen, P. (2015). Armed conflicts, 1946–2014. *Journal of Peace Research*, **52**, 536–550.

Spiegel, P. B. et al. (2007). Occurrence and overlap of natural disasters, complex emergencies and epidemics during the past decade (1995–2004). *Conflict and Health*, **1**, 2.

United Nations Disaster Relief Organization (UNDRO). (1992). *An overview of disaster management*. 2nd edition. UNDP and UNDRO.

United Nations High Commissioner for Refugees (UNHCR). (2016). *Global trends: Forced displacement in 2015*, UNHCR. Available at: www.unhcr.org/en-us/statistics/unhcrstats/576408cd7/unhcr-global-trends-2015.html (Accessed July 12, 2017).

United Nations Offices for Disaster Risk Reduction (UNISDR). (2009) *UNISDR terminology on disaster risk reduction*. UNISDR: Geneva, Switzerland.

Chapter 2

History of Humanitarian Emergencies

Mark Anderson, Kristin Becknell, and Joanna Taliano

Introduction

In 1859, a young Swiss businessman named Henry Dunant traveled to the Italian city of Solferino. He arrived as a bloody battle for the town between the French and Austrian armies ended. What he witnessed there had a profound impact on his life and work and for many would mark the foundational moment in the development of the modern humanitarian movement.

Similar pivotal events characterize the history of humanitarianism, each event defining the evolution of the humanitarian movement, ultimately leading to the movement as we know it today. Some authors have suggested various schemes for dividing the history of humanitarian action. Barnett and Farré describe "ages of humanitarianism," starting with the period of "imperial humanitarianism," from the early nineteenth century through World War II, continuing with a period of "liberal humanitarianism" from the end of the Cold War to the present (Barnett and Farré 2011). Other authors identify the World Wars as distinct turning points in the history of the humanitarian movement. Davey, Borton, and Foley divide modern humanitarian history into four main periods: from the mid-nineteenth century until the end of the First World War in 1918; the "Wilsonian" period of the interwar years and the Second World War; the Cold War period; and the post–Cold War period (Davey et al. 2013).

This chapter provides a review of the history of humanitarian response and, in the process, describes several historical milestones, like the story of Dunant, that have been critical in the development of the field.

Prior to the Nineteenth Century

Natural disasters and armed conflict have occurred throughout human history, and writings from many ancient societies indicate that people have long been thinking about how to minimize their deleterious effects. However, organized efforts to support populations affected by these events are relatively recent phenomena (Rysaback-Smith 2015). Before the nineteenth century, humanitarian intervention was primarily based on religious belief and was often in response to famine, drought, and other natural disasters rather than war.

Many of the historical underpinnings of humanitarianism derive from religious tradition, and most early humanitarian efforts were conducted by religious organizations. Altruistic human behavior is a fundamental principle practiced in all major religions and philosophies and is, arguably, the guiding principle of humanitarianism as a whole (Walker and Maxwell 2014).

The religious concept of charitable giving also played a substantial role in early humanitarian movements. In early Christianity, for example, charitable giving was an individual responsibility; it was not until AD 325, when Roman emperor Constantine adopted Christianity as the state religion, that charity became an obligation of the church. The early Catholic Church was the dominant force behind organized charity until the Protestant Reformation over a thousand years later (Walker and Maxwell 2014). For Protestants, work and charity were closely related; all people were expected to work to support the community and communities were supposed to care for those in need.

The Islamic tradition of *zakat*, or charitable giving, outlines a duty to assist others and is one of the five pillars of Islam. In Muslim societies, *zakat* can include individual acts of charity or institutional welfare systems. *Zakat* in Muslim societies can include individual acts of charity or institutional welfare systems, and Islamic scholars describe *zakat* as the first formal social security system (Walker and Maxwell 2014). Another tradition in Islam, known as *waqf*, is a charitable mechanism to establish an endowment for the purchase of land for orphanages, schools, hospitals, and other buildings with a charitable purpose (Walker and Maxwell 2014).

Another factor in the early evolution of the humanitarian movement was the articulation of laws around the conduct of war. The ancient Greeks and Romans articulated laws on the acceptable conduct of war. In China, Sun Tzu outlined acceptable limits for how combatants should handle themselves during times of war in the *Art of War* (Davey et al. 2013). These principles, however, focused on the welfare of combatants, not on the care and well-being of those not directly involved in armed conflict. When these laws were articulated, those who suffered the indirect effects of armed conflict, including displacement, famine, and disease, were often left to fend for themselves.

One of the first recorded instances of mass population displacement occurred in seventeenth-century Europe when waves of Protestants fled religious persecution and violence in Catholic Europe to take refuge in Protestant England. The Protestants were being persecuted and killed in Catholic Europe and England intervened in support of the displaced. This event marked the first significant movement of people fleeing religious persecution and was the first time that the term "refugee" was used to describe the affected population (Walker and Maxwell 2014).

The eighteenth century saw one of the first international, government-sponsored, relief efforts, in response to an earthquake that destroyed the Portuguese capital of Lisbon in 1755 (Walker and Maxwell 2014). Both Spain and England sent humanitarian aid. This intervention introduced the concept of humanitarian action as an intrinsic property of "good nationhood," an idea that would gain importance in the coming century (Walker and Maxwell 2014).

The Nineteenth Century

The humanitarian movement, as we know it today, took root in the nineteenth century. As Walker and Maxwell state, "something changed around the middle of the nineteenth century which galvanized humanitarian action, by states and private individuals, from a handful of disconnected instances to a more organized series of thought through policies and activities with global connections" (Walker and Maxwell 2014). One driving factor behind this change was the interconnectedness that railways and the telegraph provided, facilitating trade, travel, and communication. Now, philanthropists and charitable organizations could support those in need anywhere in the world. Globalization, enhanced by trade and the growth of empires, fostered the development of the international humanitarian movement.

The motivation behind some nineteenth century relief efforts was not always altruistic in nature. Aid responses to the Indian famines of 1837 and 1866 and the Irish famine of 1845 to 1849 included public work programs to preserve British power. Some believe that the pragmatic concerns of maintaining political and social order in the colonies motivated the provision of aid more than any humanitarian imperative (Davey et al. 2013, Walker and Maxwell 2014), the goal being to control criminal behavior to ensure that the famine did not prompt thoughts of revolution.

Despite their origins in self-interest, the famine responses in India and Ireland, as well as the provision of cash assistance and other famine relief in colonial China in 1876–79, led to insights that would form the conceptual roots of humanitarian action (Davey et al. 2013). In India, for example, a government commission undertook the first organized study of the causes of famine and the appropriate responses. As a result of this assessment, and several subsequent famine assessments, the British developed the Indian Famine Codes (Walker and Maxwell 2014). The codes defined famine, outlined ways to measure it, identified early indicators of famine such as changes in market prices and population displacement, and recognized the role of free food distribution to support vulnerable populations (Davey et al. 2013).

In a sense, the colonies were an early testing ground for many of the techniques that would guide humanitarian response in subsequent years, such as famine relief and the provision of cash assistance (Davey et al. 2013).

At the same time that the British were implementing an organized approach to famine response in India, the humanitarian response to war was developing with the emergence of the Red Cross and Red Crescent Movement. The founding of the Movement by Henri Dunant marked a turning point in the humanitarian response to war and was, arguably, the most instrumental event in the history of humanitarian action.

Henri Dunant and the International Committee of the Red Cross (ICRC)

Henri Dunant lived in Geneva at a time when philanthropy was an activity open to young men. He grew up in a family of Seventh Day Adventists who were heavily engaged in charitable activities and taught their son the value of supporting those less fortunate. Dunant and several friends founded a charity called the League of Alms, which would expand internationally and evolve into the Young Men's Christian Association (YMCA) (Morgenstern 1979). His involvement in these ventures opened him to the possibilities of humanitarian action and guided his response to the carnage of Solferino.

On June 24, 1859, Dunant arrived in the northern Italian city of Solferino to witness the aftermath of a battle between the armies of the French/Sardinian Alliance and Austria. On the battlefield and in the city he found the dead and dying; approximately 40 thousand wounded and dying soldiers were left behind (Morgenstern 1979, Walker and Maxwell 2014). Dunant organized women in the surrounding villages to care for the wounded soldiers left on the battlefield. In doing so, he established the foundational principles of humanitarian intervention, such as negotiating access to the affected, providing care impartially, and maintaining neutrality. These principles, and his activities to organize civil society to provide volunteer relief, would eventually inform the ideals of the Red Cross movement and the modern concepts of humanitarian action.

After returning to Geneva, Dunant wrote of his experiences in an 1862 memoir called "A Memory of Solferino" (Dunant 1959). Here, he articulated the human costs of armed conflict and clarified the principles behind his intervention on the battlefield of Solferino, calling for a relief agency comprised of voluntary relief committees to assist soldiers in times of war. The popularity of Dunant's work increased public awareness of the heavy toll of war, which until this point had been a distant consideration for many.

The following year, the Geneva Society for Public Welfare established a committee to consider how to put Dunant's ideas into practice. This group of five men, called the International Committee for the Relief of the Wounded, organized an international conference in October 1863 that included representatives from 16 nations. The outcome of the conference was the establishment of what would become the International Committee of the Red Cross (ICRC) with recommendations that countries establish national committees to assist in the care of the wounded during times of war and, during peacetime, prepare materials for relief and training medical personnel for the eventuality of conflict. The conference also encouraged governments to support these relief committees and ensure the neutrality of medical personnel and facilities providing care for the wounded (Walker and Maxwell 2014).

Early in its existence, the ICRC worked internationally to promote the adoption of national relief societies or committees. These groups eventually became the national Red Cross and Red Crescent societies that we know today. In the US, for example, nurse Clara Barton founded the American Red Cross to institutionalize the values and activities that she had practiced during the American Civil War. The International Red Cross and Red Crescent Movement now includes over 190 national societies.

In 1864, twelve nations attended a diplomatic conference in Geneva that produced the first Geneva Convention, formally titled the *Geneva Convention for the Amelioration of the Condition of the Wounded in Armies in the Field*. The Convention outlined norms for the removal and care of wounded and ill combatants from the battlefield, regardless of their nationality, and for protecting aid workers during times of war (Brauman 2017). The ICRC also received a formal mandate to provide neutral assistance in the form of support and protection to civilian and military victims of war, becoming the first international aid organization (Palmieri 2012, Rysaback-Smith 2015). The 12 signatories committed to supporting the Convention in an attempt to civilize the conduct of war.

The Twentieth Century

While members of the International Red Cross Movement cemented their place as leading humanitarian actors during the nineteenth century, they would be profoundly tested by the events of two World Wars and a challenging interwar period during the first half of the twentieth century. The postwar period saw the founding of United Nations (UN) agencies that continue to play a leading role in humanitarian action today, as well as a shift of attention to humanitarian crises in developing countries, a proliferation of nongovernmental organizations (NGOs), and a growing emphasis on humanitarian response to civil wars, internally displaced persons and complex humanitarian emergencies.

The first real test for the newly formed Red Cross societies began with the outbreak of World War I in 1914. Although the scope and challenges of the conflict were unprecedented and financial and human resources were limited, the ICRC and national societies assisted tens of thousands of people during the war. They visited prisoners of war and their families, worked to repatriate the ill and the wounded, reunited families separated by the conflict, and served as a "watchdog" for the observance of the Geneva Conventions, which had been revised and expanded in 1906 (Davey et al. 2013).

When the conflict ended in 1918, members of the Red Cross Movement and the humanitarian community as a whole, started to address their roles outside of wartime. Lessons learned during the war were significant for the development of a truly global humanitarian relief effort (Davey et al. 2013). These experiences and the growing challenges faced by colonial populations, led to a more rigorous approach to the delivery of humanitarian aid, particularly in the areas of nutrition and public health.

The United States, having survived World War I relatively intact, was one of the few countries able to provide relief to Europe in the postwar years. Starting in 1914, the Commission for Relief to Belgium, led by Herbert Hoover, raised tens of millions of dollars in famine relief. The organization eventually became the American Relief Administration (ARA) with the broader mandate of providing relief across Europe and post-revolutionary Russia. The ARA's activities were instrumental in response to the Russian Povolzhye Famine of 1921–22, which eventually claimed over 5 million lives (Walker and Maxwell 2014).

League of Nations and League of Red Cross Societies

The Treaty of Versailles, signed in 1919, established the League of Nations, and brought several significant humanitarian reforms (Davey et al. 2013). Although the primary goal of the League of Nations was to prevent war, the organization also sought to address other issues, such as labor conditions and the treatment of colonial populations. The League established treaties and organizations that became essential to the humanitarian community's efforts to protect conflict-affected populations (Davey et al. 2013). The League created a succession of organizations and agreements to deal with new refugee situations. The International Relief Union (IRU), established by the League, was the first attempt to develop an intergovernmental structure explicitly to aid victims of disaster.

The interwar years also saw the establishment of the League of Red Cross Societies, comprised of Societies from France, Britain, Italy, Japan and the United States. Considered a humanitarian version of the League of Nations, the League of Red Cross Societies was an American-led effort to harness US resources in the reconstruction of Europe. The organizers hoped to remain independent of the ICRC and challenged the role and authority of the original Geneva-based committee. The ICRC and the new League of Red Cross Societies did cooperate on efforts to address the crisis in Russia, forming the International Committee for Russian Relief in 1921. The League of Red Cross Societies would eventually rename itself as the International Federation of Red Cross and Red Crescent Societies (IFRC) in 1991. Today, the IFRC is one of the largest humanitarian organizations in the world, with 190 members, focusing their work on natural disasters while the ICRC primarily operates in conflict settings (Walker and Maxwell 2014).

High Commissioner for Refugees

The League of Red Cross Societies was a key member of the IRU, but it was the ARA that was the backbone of the operation, itself feeding over ten million people a day and supporting over 120,000 employees in Russia. It was in this context that the League of Nations established the position of High Commissioner for Refugees (HCR).

In 1921, the League of Nations appointed Norwegian explorer Fridtjof Nansen to be the first High Commissioner for Refugees with the specific mandate of overseeing assistance to Russian refugees (Davey et al. 2013). Nansen worked tirelessly to repatriate nearly half a million Russian refugees. He expanded the activities of his office and negotiated international recognition of a travel document for refugees that became known as the "Nansen passport." Nansen's work was instrumental in the movement to ensure the rights of refugees (Davey et al. 2013). His efforts eventually led to the formation of the International Refugee Organization (IRO) and, its successor, the United Nations High Commissioner for Refugees (UNHCR), discussed below.

Save the Children Fund

While the ICRC supported those directly affected by armed conflict, namely soldiers, many saw a need to assist civilian populations as well. In 1919, Eglantyne Jebb and several colleagues established the Save the Children Fund (SCF) to provide relief to children and families affected by the ongoing blockades imposed on Germany and Austria-Hungary after the war. SCF became the first NGO solely dedicated to providing relief to civilian populations (Davey et al. 2013). SCF was distinct from the Red Cross movement because it did not rely on government recognition, funding, or law. The organization did its own fundraising and independently directed its own relief operations. Despite its early success, the organization quickly realized that the protection of vulnerable populations like children needed to be supported by laws. SCF worked hard to encourage the adoption of international legislation to protect children from abuse and armed conflict. Jebb worked to establish the *Declaration of the Rights of the Child*, which stated that all children have the right to relief. The Declaration was adopted by the League of Nations in 1924 and represents a milestone in humanitarian law.

During the interwar period, humanitarian response efforts expanded beyond Europe, advanced in part by the need for European powers to support and maintain order among colonial populations (Davey et al. 2013). Conflicts in China and the Middle East gained the attention of international relief organizations such as SCF. The response efforts of these organizations sometimes merged the political and imperial attitudes of the colonial powers, causing some to question their independence (Davey et al 2013).

Events of the 1930s posed new challenges to humanitarian response. Economic conditions led to a significant reduction in funds available for international relief operations (Davey et al. 2013). The rise of fascist regimes in Europe and the question of how to respond to their growing strength were especially vexing for the humanitarian community. The League of Nations itself could not respond effectively to the fascist movements in Germany, Italy, Spain, and Japan, with the outbreak of World War II being a vivid demonstration of its ineffectiveness (Davey et al. 2013).

World War II had profound and lasting effects on the humanitarian movement. The United Nations and its agencies came into existence; new international humanitarian laws were drafted and ratified, and many new NGOs were founded. Much of what we know today as the humanitarian system emerged from World War II and the Cold War that followed.

The growth of fascism in Europe proved to be a problem for the ICRC as well; although the organization was successful in negotiating access during the Spanish Civil War it was roundly condemned for its failure to respond the atrocities perpetrated by the Nazis and their allies during the war (Davey et al. 2013). The Geneva Conventions of the time, expanded again in 1929 to include prisoners of war, restricted the ICRC's actions because they were limited to international conflicts and did not cover civilian populations abused by their own governments. As a result, the ICRC had no mandate to protect those who were being forced into the concentration camps of Nazi Germany (Davey et al. 2013). The ICRC was heavily criticized for failing to condemn the Nazis and their allies and for being unable to protect their civilian victims effectively.

United Nations

In the wake of the war, US President Franklin Roosevelt and United Kingdom Prime Minister Winston Churchill envisioned the founding of three institutions, the United Nations, the International Monetary Fund, and the World Bank, as necessary to build a postwar world that was safe for capitalism by reducing the likelihood of global economic collapse and providing a mechanism to control the outbreak of armed conflict (Walker and Maxwell 2014). In 1944, delegates from 50 countries created the Charter of the United Nations. The Charter was ratified by the five permanent members of the UN later that year, and the first General Assembly was held in January 1946.

The new United Nations quickly set about drafting several frameworks focusing on the protection of human rights. In 1949, the Geneva Conventions were expanded to include civil or internal armed conflict and the protection of civilian populations (Davey et al. 2013).

International efforts to ensure the protection of civilians, including refugees, were greatly enhanced by the adoption of the Universal Declaration of Human Rights (UDHR) in 1948. The document described the minimum rights to which all people were entitled, which included the right to life, the right to protection from torture and ill-treatment, the right to a nationality, the right to freedom of movement, the right to leave any country, and the right not to be forcibly returned. The UDHR would inspire the development of several subsequent human rights treaties.

The 1951 Refugee Convention, drawn up in the wake of World War II, guarantees minimum standards for the treatment of refugees in their country of asylum. The Convention aimed to ensure that refugees are treated in the same way in all states party to it. The document was a legally binding treaty and represented a milestone in humanitarian law.

International Refugee Organization

At the end of the war, the UN established the United Nations Relief and Rehabilitation Administration (UNRRA) to assist in the repatriation of millions of displaced persons across Europe by providing aid, rehabilitation and resettlement assistance (Davey et al. 2013). UNRRA coordinated the work of voluntary relief agencies and hundreds of displaced persons camps in Germany and spent billions of dollars to rehabilitate the broken economies of Europe. By 1947, the organization faced financial crisis and criticism from the United States for repatriating nationals back to Eastern Europe, which was seen as strengthening Communist regimes. Consequently, the organization was disbanded and its responsibilities were transferred to the newly formed International Refugee Organization (IRO).

The UN established the IRO in 1946 to protect refugees, initially focusing on the 21 million people scattered throughout Europe after World War II (Davey et al. 2013; Walker and Maxwell 2014). The IRO's main objective at its inception was the repatriation of European refugees back to their home countries. From 1947 to 1952, the IRO repatriated 73,000 to their country of origin, resettled over one million refugees in third countries, and provided aid to 410,000 persons displaced within their own countries (OHCHR 2016). Because of Cold War politics, the operations of the IRO were both controversial and inadequately funded. As political tensions flared, the organization's focus turned from repatriation to resettlement. The IRO struggled financially during its lifespan; only 18 of the 54 UN member states contributed to the IRO's budget at a time when the costs of its operations were rapidly increasing, reaching $400 million by 1951 (OHCHR 2016).

The history of the IRO and its eventual evolution into the UNHCR was a function of the changing politics of the time. The United States was the primary funder of international relief efforts and saw the displacement of people fleeing Soviet-dominated countries as a political matter. This thinking influenced the IRO to broaden the definition of "refugee" to include individuals fleeing persecution, regardless of origin. The resulting increase in the number of people covered by IRO's mandate, the controversial nature of IRO's programs, ongoing funding challenges, and shifting postwar politics led to the organization's eventual replacement with the UNHCR (OHCHR 2016, Walker and Maxwell 2014).

United Nations High Commissioner for Refugees

In July 1951, the UN adopted the United Nations Convention Relating to the Status of Refugees. The Convention dealt only with refugees who left their home country before 1951 and in that way focused primarily on European populations. It did not apply to refugees in other regions such as Africa and Asia or those from Palestine. The Convention also formally established the UNHCR and its mandate for the protection of refugees. Initially, UNHCR served a coordination role, only later developing programs to support fundraising, operational protection and assistance. In 1967, the Convention was appended to remove the 1951 criteria for defining refugees, allowing UNHCR to assist refugee populations worldwide by removing criteria bound by time and place.

United Nations International Children's Emergency Fund

During the final meeting of UNRRA, concerns over the fate of Europe's war affected children were raised. It was proposed that the organization's remaining funds be used to create a program to support emergency aid for children. In December 1946, the UN General Assembly formally established the UN International Children's Emergency Fund (UNICEF). In 1953, the organization changed its name to the UN Children's Fund. The fund was initially seen as a short-term effort to provide food to children across Europe. In 1947, the organization set up its first committee to assist with fundraising in the United States; today more than 35 such committees support the organization's funding efforts.

Soon after its inception, UNICEF launched a campaign to vaccinate children across Europe against tuberculosis. This effort was the beginning of UNICEF's involvement in vaccination programs and public health and distinguished it from other UN agencies as being primarily an operational entity. Unlike other UN organizations, UNICEF established offices in the field and worked directly with government ministries and NGOs.

Since the 1950s, UNICEF has expanded its vaccination programs and evolved to support other important public health interventions. The organization has continued its nutrition programs and established itself in the areas of child protection and child development. Later in its history, UNICEF played an integral part in the eventual adoption of the new Convention on the Rights of the Child in 1989. The Convention has been ratified by 196 nations, making it the most accepted human rights convention on record.

World Food Programme

In October 1945, President Franklin Roosevelt convened an international conference on food and agriculture for the postwar era. One conference outcome was the establishment of the Food and Agricultural Organization (FAO). The organization outlined principles for using surplus food production to bolster global recovery and development. In 1961, the US led an effort to provide limited funds to support a food aid program that would focus on emergencies and pilot development projects. This proposal eventually resulted in the establishment of the World Food Programme (WFP). The new organization provided food aid to countries in Asia, Africa, southern Europe, and Latin America in order to stimulate land resettlement and reform and in support of special feeding programs. In the first three years of the program, WFP responded to 32 emergencies and administered 116 development projects (Walker and Maxwell 2014). Throughout the 1960s and 1970s, WFP continued to use food-for-work projects to promote social and economic development. In the late 1980s and early 1990s, WFP began to focus on providing food aid and food security exclusively in emergency situations (Walker and Maxwell 2014).

Food for Peace

The postwar period saw major changes in the delivery of humanitarian aid, often dictated by Cold War politics. These changes were particularly evident in the area of food aid, which came to be driven by surplus production rather than actual need. Instead of providing the means to increase local production, food aid programs often seemed to focus on finding uses for surplus agricultural production, particularly American wheat surpluses. In 1954, the United States established the Food for Peace program, which enabled US food aid to be used for development and relief purposes (Davey et al. 2013).

The years following World War II also saw a dramatic increase in the number of humanitarian agencies; nearly two hundred NGOs were created between 1945 and 1949 (Davey et al. 2013, Mackintosh 2000, Walker and Maxwell 2014). Most of these were based in the United States. The scope of these organizations shifted from focusing on Europeans to those in what was considered the "Third World," driven in part by decolonization and the waning power of the former empires (Walker and Maxwell 2014, Rysaback-Smith 2015, Mackintosh 2000). The process of decolonization created many newly independent nations, which would significantly impact the development of NGOs (Davey et al. 2013). The withdrawal of the colonial powers and the tensions of the Cold War left many of these new countries with limited resources. The NGOs were then left to fill the humanitarian gap determined by the geopolitical objectives of the West and the Soviet bloc nations.

The Cold War years were seen as a "fertile period" for the growth of the humanitarian movement (Davey et al. 2013, Rysaback-Smith 2015, Mackintosh 2000). During the 1960s, operating budgets for NGOs increased dramatically, fueling the development of even more organizations. Between 1960 and 1969, 289 new NGOs were created (Davey et al. 2013).

Republic of Biafra

Several pivotal events in the history of humanitarian action occurred between the late 1960s to the early 1980s. These included the Biafran War, the war in Vietnam, the genocide in Cambodia and the famine in Ethiopia and the Horn of Africa. The result was a consolidation of principles, practices, and personnel that would lead to expansion and professionalization within the field of humanitarian response. The Biafran War, in particular, marked a turning point in modern humanitarian action (Walker and Maxwell 2014).

In May 1967, the Republic of Biafra in the southeastern corner of Nigeria split from the rest of the country. The civil conflict that followed was bloody, with hundreds of thousands massacred or displaced. Because of Cold War politics, the UN resisted any suggestion that it intervene, maintaining that the Biafran secession was an internal issue for the Nigerian government to address (Davey et al. 2013).

The Nigerian government cut off Biafra's oil revenue and supply lines to instigate the fall of the revolutionary government. The human cost was profound, with widespread malnutrition and high mortality among the Biafran population; estimates of deaths from the famine ranged from several hundred thousand to over two million (Walker and Maxwell 2014).

In 1969, the Nigerian government banned ICRC from supplying humanitarian assistance to Biafra except on planes flying from Nigerian airports that were inspected before departure. The government eventually denied all daytime flights. ICRC, following its principles of neutrality, withdrew its operations and ceased humanitarian support. The departure of ICRC left a clear gap in humanitarian assistance; some claimed that 3,000 children were dying every day (Black 1992). The gap was quickly filled by a coalition of church agencies, working under the name Joint Church Aid, and several NGOs, including Oxfam and CARE (Davey et al. 2013).

The operation undertaken by Joint Church Aid was unique in terms of the scope of the relief supplied and its perseverance in the face of resistance from local authorities, resistance that included direct targeting by military forces. Of the 7,800 flights into Biafra, 5,310 were operated by Joint Church Aid, delivering 66,000 tons of relief supplies (Davey et al. 2013). Although the operation highlighted the ability of NGOs to provide assistance when the UN and ICRC could not, some have argued that the humanitarian aid provided through the airlift also prolonged the war and contributed to the deaths of nearly 200,000 people (Smillie 1995).

The response to the civil conflict in Biafra proved to be a formative experience in the humanitarian movement, introducing a new era of humanitarian action (Davey et al. 2013; Barnett and Farré 2011). The response to the suffering witnessed in Biafra was significant for the humanitarian community's outspoken condemnation of the conflict's effects and the use of the term "genocide" to describe the suffering (Brauman 2017). The practice of sending humanitarian workers into rebel areas without government authorization became a model for future response efforts. This tragic event was also instrumental in the development of a new generation of humanitarian workers who would go on to lead the field and form some of the most influential humanitarian agencies in history. These new organizations were "motivated as much by a sense of solidarity with the victims of crisis as by traditional humanitarian principles" (Walker and Maxwell 2014).

These new organizations were ready to move beyond the "Dunantist" philosophy of the ICRC, whose actions were thought to be limited by the organization's strict adherence to the principle of neutrality. Reacting to the criticism of the ICRC in Biafra, the new humanitarian agencies promoted a more interventionist approach to humanitarian response.

Concern and Médecins Sans Frontières

Two interventionist NGOs to come out of the aftermath of Biafra were Concern and Médecins Sans Frontières (MSF). Concern, later to become Concern Worldwide, was founded in 1968 in Ireland and would become a respected organization, addressing health, hunger, and humanitarian emergency response.

In the wake of Biafra, one of the ICRC's most outspoken critics was a former ICRC doctor named Bernard Kouchner. Infuriated by the human suffering he witnessed in Biafra and ICRC's failure to stand up to the Nigerian government, Kouchner and his colleagues committed to forming a new humanitarian organization, one that was dedicated to humanitarian principles but would not be silent in the face of atrocity. Médecins Sans Frontières was the result. Officially formed in 1971, this organization would become one of the most influential NGOs in modern history.

The 1970s saw another shift in humanitarian response with an increased focus on improving the lives of those forced to live in refugee camp settings. In these contexts, aid agencies were able to develop new skills and practices related to site planning, logistics, coordination, and camp management (Brauman 2017). The humanitarian response community also learned more about the factors leading to famine and other food crises. Many of these lessons were learned in response to the refugee crisis along the Thai/Cambodian border.

Between 1975 and 1979, the Cambodian genocide claimed between 1.5 and 2 million lives, and many others died of starvation and disease. Vietnam invaded Cambodia in late 1978, pushing the Khmer Rouge from power and initiating a refugee crisis as Cambodian refugees fled across the Thai border.

In response to the crisis, the UN named UNICEF its lead response agency. ICRC, hoping to avoid the problems it faced in Biafra, sought permission to lead an assessment inside Cambodia. A unique coalition of NGOs called the Coalition for Cambodia formed, raising an unprecedented $40 million to support their efforts (Walker and Maxwell 2014). The NGO consortium proved to be more nimble than the UN in responding to the crisis. The NGOs, free from the Cold War politics that limited the effectiveness of the UN response, provided support to the camp population and, eventually, were able to deliver relief within Cambodia itself. By doing so, the coalition was able to demonstrate how it was possible for NGOs to bypass the politics that had limited the UN system and ICRC (Walker and Maxwell 2014).

African Famines

Beginning in the 1970s, several large-scale famines in the Sahel and Horn regions of Africa focused the humanitarian community's attention on the continent and the need to respond more effectively to food crises (Davey et al. 2013).

In 1973, following years of drought, famine developed in the Sahel. Between 1973 and 1974, WFP and FAO supported a major response to the crisis. Although the response was massive, it was criticized for corruption, lack of coordination, and the potential harm caused to local markets (Davey et al. 2013). Like the Biafran War, the famine in the Sahel provided valuable lessons for the human community. As Walker and Maxwell note, "the manner in which the crisis was understood, in the pattern set by the response, had repercussions for decades" (Walker and Maxwell 2014).

A lack of high-quality information was partly to blame for the poor response in the Sahel. In the following years, Bengali Indian economist and philosopher Amartya Sen would promote the use of data in anticipating and responding to humanitarian emergencies. In looking at data from the famines of the 1970s, Sen was one of the first authors to define some of the risk factors that led to food shortages and eventually famine (Sen 1982). He was able to demonstrate that food crises have as much to do with a population's inability to access available food as they do with drought. In the Sahel, a decline in the value of labor, livestock, and other assets also reduced incomes among the affected populations (Walker and Maxwell 2014). These factors became collectively known as "entitlement failure" and were thought to be predictive of actual famine. Sen believed that by tracking how populations coped with declining food stocks, incomes, and other assets when dealing with drought and rising food prices, it would be possible to predict the onset of famine (Walker and Maxwell 2014). This work led to the development of the famine early warning systems we have today (Davey et al. 2013, Walker and Maxwell 2014).

In 1974, the FAO hosted the World Food Conference to address the experiences of the African famines. Outcomes of this meeting included the highlighting of the importance of planning for food crises and the establishment of WFP as a leader in this field (Davey et al. 2013).

The 1980s saw an easing of Cold War tensions that had limited the effectiveness of humanitarian response, particularly by the UN and ICRC. The period also saw renewed interest among the general public in the plight of those affected by humanitarian emergencies. This interest was stimulated by major crises that involved massive population displacement and, as a result, garnered intense media attention (Davey et al. 2013).

Perhaps no other recent event galvanized public support for those affected by humanitarian crises more than the famine in Ethiopia during the early 1980s. Dramatic television footage and photographs, and the sheer numbers of those impacted, with nearly one million dead and eight million affected, brought the world's attention to the human suffering caused by famine. It also became apparent that drought was not the only factor contributing to the crisis. There was evidence that the military used food shortages as weapon in its fight against opponents (De Waal 1991, Davey et al. 2013). These factors led to a massive international public response, culminating in the Band Aid initiatives led by the rock star Bob Geldof. The Live Aid concert raised over $140 million for famine relief and recovery programs. As a result, humanitarian organizations quickly realized the power of the media as a fundraising and advocacy tool.

In retrospect, it was apparent that the famine in Ethiopia was more than just a natural disaster. It was a crisis precipitated by both natural and human-made factors and was one of the first international events to be considered a "complex humanitarian emergency," a concept discussed in the previous chapter.

The 1990s were considered a time of great upheaval and growth in the humanitarian community (Walker and Maxwell 2014, Davey et al. 2013). The relaxation of tensions between the Cold War superpowers seemed to benefit humanitarian response, at least initially, leading to a globalization of humanitarianism. Western aid workers, for example, were able to respond to crises in the Soviet Union for the first time in more than 60 years (Davey et al. 2013). But the atmosphere of progress in the humanitarian sector did not last long. The humanitarian community was shaken by the emergence of a new type of warfare marked by extreme violence and high numbers of civilian deaths and displaced persons (Davey et al. 2013, Toole 1995).

Civil War

The 1990s saw a dramatic increase in civil or internal armed conflict. In 1993 for example, 43 of 47 active conflicts were civil wars (Toole 2000). These "new wars" were characterized by a breakdown of civil authority and the direct targeting of civilian populations by armed actors. As a result, the adverse effects of war became more extreme with high numbers of civilian casualties. Civilian populations were forced to flee their homes to escape the conflict but were often not able to cross into the relative safety of a neighboring country. As a result, these groups were considered "internally displaced persons" (IDPs) rather than refugees and did not receive the protections and benefits of refugee status, despite facing many of the same risks to their health and welfare. Three "new wars" in particular would have a profound impact on the humanitarian community and shape humanitarian response going forward: the Yugoslav Wars between 1991 and 2001, the civil war and famine in Somalia and, especially, the genocide and the refugee crisis in Rwanda.

The Yugoslav Wars of the 1990s were triggered by the collapse of Communist Yugoslavia and the rekindling of ethnic hostilities that had been held in check by its authoritarian leader Josip Broz Tito. As the wars escalated, the rest of Europe became increasingly concerned that conflict would move beyond the boundaries of the former Yugoslavia. As a result, many of the civilian victims of the wars were not able to cross an international border and were not covered under international laws pertaining to refugees. UNHCR, which led the humanitarian response in Bosnia, could only provide limited support to IDPs due to its legal mandate to protect refugees. Consequently, the organization's role became one of providing assistance rather than protection. UNHCR was able to maintain an airlift to the city of Sarajevo that provided food and other supplies during the siege of the city, while WFP delivered over a million tons of food aid (Walker and Maxwell 2014).

The Yugoslav Wars highlighted the need to develop mechanisms to protect civilian populations displaced internally. In an attempt to provide a semblance of protection for IDPs, the UN Security Council authorized the UN Protection Force for Yugoslavia (UNPROFOR). However, UNPROFOR's mandate was severely limited. They established "safe areas" but could not engage with the warring factions to provide any real protection to the civilian population. Nowhere was this more apparent than in UNPROFOR's lack of response to the massacre of eight thousand men and boys in the "safe area" of Srebrenica.

Once again, the wars in the former Yugoslavia led many in the humanitarian community to question the principles of neutrality and impartiality. Some felt that the humanitarian community's desire to ensure access to the affected population by maintaining neutrality may have made them passive participants in ethnic cleansing.

The subsequent conflict in the Serbian province of Kosovo ushered in a new concept in the sphere of humanitarian response that came to be known as "humanitarian warfare." In this case, NATO forces responded quickly to prevent a humanitarian crisis like that experienced in Bosnia. The response to the crisis in Kosovo demonstrated the gap between what donors were willing to provide in response to a crisis in Europe compared to ongoing crises in Africa, where similar events were occurring in Somalia and Rwanda.

The humanitarian response to the famine in Somalia marks what some have described as the end of "Pollyannaish" humanitarianism (Weiss 2005).

As in Ethiopia a decade earlier, the media played a significant role in influencing the scope of the humanitarian intervention. Images of local militias looting aid convoys, keeping food from the starving population, increased public pressure to respond more efficiently than what the humanitarian community could do alone. Military intervention was proposed by some NGOs to protect the convoys. In response, the UN approved a peacekeeping force to protect the convoys, but this force was too small to provide adequate protection. Under public pressure, President George H.W. Bush committed US troops, and Operation Restore Hope began in December 1992. The optimism of the effort was short-lived. In 1993, militias killed 24 Pakistani peacekeepers, leading to the US Army attack on Mogadishu in October of that year that left 18 US soldiers dead. Soon after this debacle, the United States withdrew its forces. In the end, this conflict provided the humanitarian community with an example of how, despite their best intentions, they became entangled in the crisis as participants instead of remaining neutral outsiders. These events damaged both US and UN credibility and discouraged the humanitarian community from further intervention in Somalia (Walker and Maxwell 2014, Davey et al. 2013). This hesitancy to intercede in complex emergencies would set the tone for years to come and influence the humanitarian response to the Rwandan genocide of 1994.

Rwanda

Many have argued that no event shaped modern humanitarian response more than the genocide in Rwanda (Davey et al. 2013, Walker and Maxwell 2014). Although it was the political failure of the international community to intervene that prolonged the genocide, the humanitarian response to the crisis was implicated in the aftermath. The result would be significant changes in the accountability and standards that define the appropriate response to emergencies.

Despite many warnings, the international community did not act in time to stop the widespread killing of the minority Tutsis and moderate Hutus by the Hutu extremists. In the three months that followed, nearly eight hundred thousand Tutsis and moderate Hutus were killed in Rwanda. After the fall of Kigali to the Rwandan Patriotic Front (RPF), nearly two million refugees fled to Tanzania and Zaire. More than a million refugees entered Zaire, making camp near the town of Goma. This setting lacked adequate food, water, and sanitation, which led to a major cholera outbreak that killed an estimated fifty thousand people in one month (Walker and Maxwell 2014). Nearly 100 NGOs descended on eastern Zaire and northwestern Tanzania to support the refugee crisis, containing the cholera outbreak within months. However, the former leaders of the genocide began to use the refugee camps as recruiting and staging grounds for attacks into Rwanda and the international community did little to intervene. As a result, several NGOs, including MSF and the International Rescue Committee (IRC), withdrew their operations. The unwillingness of the international community to regain control of the camps led to an assault on the camps in late 1996 by rebel forces, which forced the repatriation of refugees back into Rwanda and the extension of the Rwandan conflict into Zaire (Davey et al. 2013). It was stated that, "[t]he overwhelming conclusion was that humanitarian aid had been subverted to support those who had caused the crisis in the first place" (Walker and Maxwell 2014).

In the aftermath of the Rwandan crisis, the humanitarian community realized the need for a thorough evaluation of the response (Walker and Maxwell 2014; Davey et al. 2013). The Joint Evaluation of Emergency Assistance to Rwanda (JEEAR) assessed the response from a variety of perspectives, including explanations for the genocide, humanitarian aid and its effects and the recovery efforts. One of the key findings of the evaluation was the need to improve performance within the humanitarian sector through better standards and improved accountability. The results of the JEEAR evaluation led to significant changes in how the humanitarian community responds to emergencies, most notably the adoption of the Sphere Humanitarian Charter and its Minimum Standards for Disaster Response, which we will discuss below. The "Sphere Project" and the "Code of Conduct for the International Red Cross and Red Crescent Movement and Nongovernmental Organizations," released before the Rwandan genocide but not widely recognized until later, would "fundamentally shape the conduct of humanitarian practitioners" for years to come (Davey et al. 2013).

Complex Humanitarian Emergencies

Several significant themes emerged out of the events in the Balkans, Somalia, and Rwanda that would influence the humanitarian community in the coming years. First, the 1990s brought increasing attention to "complex emergencies," distinct from other emergencies in that they are characterized by multiple causes, involve multiple actors, and compel an international response (Calhoun 2008). The complex emergencies of the 1990s were often tied to the disintegration of the social, political, and economic order of affected societies, leading to massive population displacement. On defining complex emergencies, one author stated (Duffield 1994):

> So-called complex emergencies are essentially political in nature: they are protracted political crises resulting from sectarian or predatory indigenous responses to socioeconomic stress and marginalization. Unlike natural disasters, complex emergencies have a singular ability to erode or destroy the cultural, civil, political and economic integrity of established societies.

The displacement common to complex emergencies was increasingly internal, and numbers of IDPs grew rapidly throughout the world. Consequently, the challenges faced by IDPs became a major humanitarian issue at the end of the twentieth century.

The 1990s also saw growth in the importance of NGOs as governments and other large donors began to see these organizations as key players in providing humanitarian relief (Brauman 2017). As a result, donors became more interested in supporting humanitarian relief efforts, and aid agencies shifted their emphasis from development to relief. In 1976 no European Community emergency aid funding went to NGOs; by 1983, 40% did. (Davey et al. 2013).

Another shift that took place during the 1990s was the increasing use of the military in humanitarian interventions, typically in the form of peacekeeping operations. Between 1948 and 1988, the UN conducted only five peacekeeping operations; that number increased to 20 operations between 1989 and 1994. The increasing reliance on humanitarian military operations, as in the Balkans, Somalia, and Rwanda, created a debate within the humanitarian community. NGOs that saw their work in a more restrictive manner, valuing their independence, neutrality, and impartiality, saw the military contingents as parties to the conflict (Brauman 2017). These organizations, such as ICRC and MSF, saw groups that allied themselves with military partners as turning their backs on some of the fundamental principles of humanitarianism.

Inter-Agency Standing Committee

In what might be considered the most significant outcome of the 1990s, the humanitarian community undertook several initiatives to improve overall coordination and response. In 1992, the UN established the Inter-Agency Standing Committee (IASC), a global humanitarian forum that brings together the main operational relief agencies from the UN, the International Red Cross and Red Crescent Movement, the International Organization for Migration (IOM), and international NGOs. To improve humanitarian assistance, the IASC fulfills three main functions (IASC Task Team on the Cluster Approach 2016c):

- Produces system-wide policies, guidelines, and tools to harmonize and achieve better overall responses.
- Conducts operational activities to ensure coherent and timely emergency responses to major emergencies.
- Establishes consensus on common messages to advocate for respect for humanitarian principles and ensure support for humanitarian work.

Humanitarian Principles

During the 1990s, several organizations established principles to govern the delivery of humanitarian aid. In 1991, the UN General Assembly established three basic humanitarian principles, adding a fourth in 2004 (OCHA 2016). These included:

1. Humanity – Human suffering must be addressed wherever it is found. The purpose of humanitarian action is to protect life and health and ensure respect for human beings.
2. Neutrality – Humanitarian actors must not take sides in hostilities or engage in controversies of a political, racial, religious, or ideological nature.
3. Impartiality – Humanitarian action must be carried out on the basis of need alone, giving priority to the most urgent cases of distress and making no distinctions on the basis of nationality, race, gender, religious belief, class, or political opinions.
4. Independence – Humanitarian action must be autonomous from the political, economic, military, or other objectives that any actor may

hold with regard to areas where humanitarian action is being implemented.

Fundamental Principles

The Red Cross and Red Crescent Movement would outline seven Fundamental Principles, which would guide the work of the Red Cross and Red Crescent national societies, the ICRC and the IFRC (IFRC 2016). These principles included the four humanitarian principles adopted by the United Nations, with three additions (IFRC 2016):

1. Voluntary Service – it is a voluntary relief movement not prompted in any manner by desire for gain.
2. Unity – there can only be one Red Cross or one Red Crescent Society in any one country. It must be open to all. It must carry on its humanitarian work throughout its territory.
3. Universality – The International Red Cross and Red Crescent Movement, in which all Societies have equal status and share equal responsibilities and duties in helping each other, is worldwide.

These seven principles became the foundation of the Red Cross/NGO Code of Conduct for operations in disasters. Almost five hundred aid organizations signed on to the codes and committed to adhering to the humanitarian principles (OCHA 2016; IFRC and ICRC, 1994).

The Rwandan genocide was a catalyst for improving the quality and accountability of humanitarian aid. The experience of Rwanda led to the development of the humanitarian principles that defined standards for the provision of humanitarian assistance and affirmed the right of those affected by disaster to protection and high-quality humanitarian aid. In accordance with these principles, the humanitarian community undertook several initiatives to improve the accountability, quality, and performance of humanitarian response. These initiatives included the Active Learning Network for Accountability and Performance in Humanitarian Action (ALNAP), the Humanitarian Accountability Partnership (HAP), People in Aid, and the Sphere Project (Hilhorst 2002).

Sphere Project

One of the most recognized of these initiatives is the Sphere Project, initiated in 1997 to develop standards for the provision of humanitarian aid. The Project is a collaborative effort led by a group of humanitarian NGOs and partners in the International Red Cross and Red Crescent Movement. These minimum standards, collected in the Sphere Handbook, are a reflection of the UN's Humanitarian Principles and Red Cross/NGO Code of Conduct discussed earlier (Response 1998). The standards represent what the principles should look like in practice, ensuring rights to health, shelter and protection, food security and nutrition, and clean water and adequate sanitation, especially during humanitarian emergencies (Steering Committee for Humanitarian Response 2011, Buchanan-Smith 2015). The Sphere Standards were eventually adopted by all major humanitarian NGOs, governments, and donors. The Sphere Project is discussed in greater detail in Chapter 4.

The Twenty-First Century

At the start of the new century, a British politician, Clare Short, head of the UK's Department for International Development, posed the concept of a "new humanitarianism," defining a different type of humanitarian response that recognized the following:

- All aid is political, and that some of the ideals of classic humanitarianism were a little old-fashioned (none more so than the cherished classic ideal of neutrality);
- Human rights violations must be taken as seriously as shortfalls in meeting basic human needs;
- Humanitarian interventions and inputs sometimes cause as much harm as they do good, and humanitarianism needed to be accountable for both;
- Both the causes and symptoms must be addressed;
- Humanitarian response must be aligned with other objectives so that all resources could be brought to bear on the problem at hand. (Walker and Maxwell 2014)

Some organizations saw the new humanitarianism as a logical extension of the humanitarian principles outlined in the 1990s. However, some humanitarian agencies would reject the new humanitarianism, most notably MSF, which renounced the fifth principle of the new movement so as not to lose their independence. In many ways, the interventionist approach of organizations like MSF was on the rise at the turn of the century, while the more neutral approach of the

ICRC seemed to be in decline. But the interventionist approach and the whole concept of a "new humanitarianism" would be tested with the invasion of Afghanistan in 2001 and later, the invasion of Iraq in 2003.

In its fight against terror, the US government declared US-based humanitarian agencies as "force multipliers." This designation left many organizations facing a dilemma – they risked losing funding to support their activities unless they aligned themselves with the foreign policy of the US government. Conducting humanitarian activities in Afghanistan and Iraq meant taking sides in the conflict, which for many NGOs meant losing their hard-fought independence (Walker and Maxwell 2014). Some organizations, like MSF, rejected this approach and were very critical of those humanitarian agencies that did.

The early twenty-first century also saw the further refinement of efforts to reform the delivery of humanitarian aid. In 2005, after reviewing the humanitarian response to the crisis in Darfur, the IASC implemented the Humanitarian Reform (IASC Task Team on the Cluster Approach 2016a). The goal was to ensure sufficient response capacity, enhanced leadership, accountability, predictability, and strong partnerships. The Reform sought to improve humanitarian financing through the development of the Central Emergency Response Fund. To improve direction and coordination, the Reform proposed strengthening the Humanitarian Coordinator system and implementing a "cluster approach" to address the perceived gaps in humanitarian response. The cluster approach will be described elsewhere in this book.

Transformative Agenda

In 2010, the earthquake in Haiti and the flooding in Pakistan highlighted additional weaknesses in the international response system. To address these deficiencies, the IASC developed the Transformative Agenda, a set of concrete actions to transform the way the humanitarian community responds to emergencies. The Agenda includes recommendations to improve the efficiency and effectiveness of the humanitarian response system, through "stronger leadership, more effective coordination structures, and improved accountability" (IASC Task Team on the Cluster Approach 2016b).

Valerie Amos, Emergency Relief Coordinator and Chair of the Interagency Standing Committee stated, "In December 2011, the IASC adopted the Transformative Agenda. It focuses on three key areas: better leadership, improved accountability to all our stakeholders and improved coordination. The impact of these changes, which we are now introducing, will be more lives saved, faster."

The Transformative Agenda was designed to strengthen key humanitarian response actors, including the Humanitarian Coordinator, the Humanitarian Country Team, country clusters, and cluster lead agencies. The Agenda was unique because it marked the first time the IASC agreed on how to respond to major emergencies.

World Humanitarian Summit

In May 2016, over nine thousand participants from 173 member states came together in Istanbul for the first World Humanitarian Summit. The goal of the meeting was to outline reforms to make the humanitarian aid community, including the UN, NGOs, and donors, more responsive and effective. One of the Summit's major achievements was the "Grand Bargain" that included commitments to reform humanitarian financing by providing more cash-based assistance and acknowledging the relative advantages of national and local implementing partners. As part of the agreement, "donors would not simply give more but give better, by being more flexible, and aid organizations would reciprocate with greater transparency and cost consciousness" (High Level Panel on Humanitarian Financing 2016). Another significant achievement of the Summit was the "Global Partnership For Preparedness" that will assist 20 at-risk countries in reaching a basic level of preparedness for future emergencies by 2020 (IASC Task Team on the Cluster Approach 2016d; UN Secretary-General 2016).

Public Health Response

Increasing awareness of the public health impacts of humanitarian emergencies emerged in the early 1970s following natural disasters in Peru, Nicaragua, and Bangladesh (Noji and Toole 1997). Public health scientists began to see a role for epidemiology in studying the impact of emergencies on the health of populations by describing patterns in morbidity and mortality common to these events. In doing so, they highlighted the importance of data collection and analysis to guide effective response to humanitarian emergencies.

In 1973, the Centre for Research on the Epidemiology of Disasters (CRED) was established in Belgium with the goal of using epidemiologic data to understand how to prepare for disasters and how to respond more efficiently. Through analytic epidemiology, investigators at CRED and elsewhere defined potential risk and protective factors for fatal and non-fatal injuries in the context of natural disasters. The early work of these researchers helped influence the humanitarian community to recognize humanitarian emergencies as public health problems (Noji and Toole 1997).

An early focus for public health was to identify indicators for rapid needs assessments following natural disasters. In the 1990s, the World Health Organization (WHO) supported the development of protocols for rapid assessments in different disaster scenarios, including natural disasters, outbreaks, famine, and population displacement (Noji and Toole 1997). The early 1990s also saw the growth of university programs dedicated to conducting research and educating students on the public health consequences of natural disasters.

The end of the Cold War and the emergence of the "new wars" in the 1990s brought attention to the public health impact of armed conflict. These complex emergencies were associated with massive population displacement (Burkholder and Toole 1995). Studies documented excess mortality and morbidity caused by injury (direct consequences of war) and by disease, famine, and displacement (indirect consequences) among civilian populations in the context of war.

Epidemiologists found that death rates were significantly higher among displaced populations compared to rates in their home countries, sometimes 10–20 times higher (Toole and Waldman 1993). Toole showed that measles can be devastating in the crowded setting of a refugee camp, with mortality rates approaching 30% (Toole et al. 1989).

In 1992, CDC produced a summary of its findings on the public health consequences of humanitarian emergencies in "Famine-affected, refugee, and displaced populations: recommendations for public health issues." This document outlined the latest recommendations for preventing disease and death in refugee settings. MSF and Epicentre, an MSF partner organization, dedicated to research and training, also contributed to the growing body of public health literature on displaced populations. This work would help establish the practice of public health in humanitarian emergencies and identify public health priorities in refugee settings (Noji and Toole 1997).

The major public health priorities identified by these epidemiologists include malnutrition, measles, malaria, acute respiratory infections, and diarrheal disease. Addressing these conditions by ensuring access to adequate food, clean water, sanitation, shelter, and health care are the key interventions guiding the public health response to humanitarian emergencies and outline the scope of this book.

References

Anon. (1992). Famine-affected, refugee, and displaced populations: recommendations for public health issues. MMWR. *Morbidity and mortality weekly report: Recommendations and reports*, **41**, 1–76.

Barnett, M. N. and Farré, S. (2011). *Empire of humanity: A history of humanitarianism*. Ithaca, New York: Cornell University Press.

Black, M. (1992). *A cause for our times*. Oxford: Oxfam and Oxford University Press.

Brauman, R. (2017) War and humanitarian aid. Available at: www.msf-crash.org/drive/6722-rb-2017-war-and-humanitarian-aid-puf.pdf (Accessed on July 16, 2017).

Buchanan-Smith, M. (2015). How the Sphere Project came into being: a case study of policy making in the humanitarian-aid sector and the relative influence of research. Available at: www.odi.org/sites/odi.org.uk/files/odi-assets/publications-opinion-files/176.pdf (Accessed on July 16, 2017).

Burkholder, B. T. and Toole, M. J. (1995). Evolution of complex disasters. *The Lancet*, 346, 1012–1015.

Calhoun, C. (2008). The imperative to reduce suffering: Charity, progress, and emergencies in the field of humanitarian action, in M. N. Barnett and T. G. Weiss, eds., *Humanitarianism in Question*. Cornell University Press, pp. 73–97.

Davey, E., Borton, J., and Foley, M. (2013). *A history of the humanitarian system: Western origins and foundations*. Overseas Development Institute; London.

De Waal, A. (1991). *Evil days: 30 years of war and famine in Ethiopia*. New York: Human Rights Watch.

Duffield, M. (1994). Complex emergencies and the crisis of developmentalism. *IDS Bulletin*, **25**, 1–15.

Dunant, H. (1959). *A memory of Solferino*. Geneva: American Red Cross.

High Level Panel on Humanitarian Financing. (2016). *Too important to fail – addressing the humanitarian financing gap*. [online] Available at: www.un.org/news/WEB-1521765-E-OCHA-Report-on-Humanitarian-Financing.pdf (Accessed on July 16, 2017).

Hilhorst, D. (2002). Being good at doing good? Quality and accountability of humanitarian NGOs. *Disasters*, **26**, 193–212.

IASC Task Team on the Cluster Approach. (2016a). Action Plan for Implementing Humanitarian Reform. Available at: https://interagencystandingcommittee.org/system/files/legacy_files/Humanitarian%20Reform%2C%20Action%20Plan%2C%20Principals%2C%2020051212-25.pdf (Accessed on October 31, 2016).

IASC Task Team on the Cluster Approach. (2016b). Key Messages: The IASC Transformative Agenda. Available at: https://interagencystandingcommittee.org/system/files/legacy_files/KM%20and%20FAQ%20on%20Transformative%20Agenda%20final.docx (Accessed on October 15, 2016).

IASC Task Team on the Cluster Approach. (2016c). The Inter-Agency Standing Committee (IASC). Available at: https://interagencystandingcommittee.org/system/files/iasc_2-pager_v2015-06-18.pdf (Accessed October 15, 2016).

IASC Task Team on the Cluster Approach. (2016d). World Humanitarian Summit. Available at: https://interagencystandingcommittee.org/system/files/legacy_files/At%20a%20Glance%20EN.pdf (Accessed on October 15, 2016).

IFRC. (2016). The Seven Fundamental Principles (online). Available at: www.ifrc.org/who-we-are/vision-and-mission/the-seven-fundamental-principles/ (Accessed on October 10, 2016).

IFRC and ICRC. (1994). *Code of conduct for the International Red Cross and Red Crescent Movement and the non-governmental organizations (NGOs) in disaster relief*. International Federation of Red Cross and Red Crescent; Geneva, Switzerland.

Mackintosh, K. (2000). *The principles of humanitarian action in international humanitarian law. Study 4 in: The politics of principle: The principles of humanitarian action in practice*. Overseas Development Institute; London.

Morgenstern, S. (1979). Henri Dunant and the Red Cross. *Bulletin of the New York Academy of Medicine*, 55(10), 949–956.

Noji, E. K. and Toole, M. J. (1997). The historical development of public health responses to disasters. *Disasters*, 21(4), 366–376.

OCHA. (2016). OCHA on Message: Humanitarian Principles (online). Available at: https://docs.unocha.org/sites/dms/Documents/OOM-humanitarianprinciples_eng_June12.pdf (Accessed on October 10, 2016).

OHCHR. (2016). Fact Sheet No.20, Human Rights and Refugees (online). Available at: www.ohchr.org/Documents/Publications/FactSheet20en.pdf (Accessed on October 27, 2016).

Palmieri, D. (2012). An institution standing the test of time? A review of 150 years of the history of the International Committee of the Red Cross. *International Review of the Red Cross*, **94**(888), 1273–1298.

Rysaback-Smith, H. (2015). History and principles of humanitarian action. *Turkish journal of emergency medicine*, **15**(Suppl 1), 5–7.

Sen, A. (1982). *Poverty and famines: An essay on entitlement and deprivation*. Oxford: Oxford University Press.

Smillie, I. (1995). *The alms bazaar: Altruism under fire: Non-profit organizations and international development*. Ottawa: IDRC (International Development Research Centre).

Steering Committee for Humanitarian Response. (2011). *The Sphere Project: Humanitarian charter and minimum standards in humanitarian Response*, Bourton on Dunsmore, UK: Sphere Project.

Toole, M. J. (1995). Mass population displacement. A global public health challenge. *Infectious Disease Clinics of North America*, 9(2), 353–366.

Toole, M. J. (2000). Refugees and Migrants, in J. Whitman, ed., *Poverty, Development, Population Movements and Health*. London: Palgrave Macmillan UK, pp. 110–129.

Toole, M. J., Steketee, R. W., Waldman, R. J., and Nieburg, P. (1989). Measles prevention and control in emergency settings. *Bulletin of the World Health Organization*, 67(4), 381–388.

Toole, M. J. and Waldman, R. J. (1993). Refugees and displaced persons: War, hunger, and public health. *JAMA: The Journal of the American Medical Association*, 270(5), 600–605.

UN Secretary-General. (2016). Chair's Summary: Standing Up for Humanity: Committing to Action (online). Available at: https://consultations.worldhumanitariansummit.org/bitcache/5171492e71696bcf9d4c571c93dfc6dcd7f361ee?vid=581078&disposition=inline&op=view (Accessed on October 15, 2016).

Walker, P. and Maxwell D. G. (2014). *Shaping the humanitarian world*. London: Routledge.

Weiss, T. G. (2005). *Military-civilian interactions: Humanitarian crises and the responsibility to protect*. Lanham, Maryland: Rowman & Littlefield.

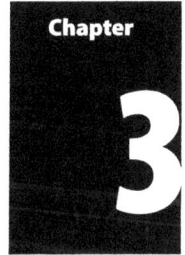

Chapter 3

Who's Who in Humanitarian Emergencies

Cyrus Shahpar and Thomas D. Kirsch

Introduction

The global community that responds to humanitarian emergencies and natural disasters includes thousands of organizations. Each humanitarian organization has particular resources, expertise, and a role in responding to humanitarian emergencies. Some provide aid and/or work directly with the affected population, while others provide indirect support, often in the form of coordination or funding.

Humanitarian organizations may be categorized by their size and the geographic scope of their work (local, national, or international), the scope of their practice (single sector or multisectoral), their target beneficiaries (the entire population or vulnerable populations, ages, and/or genders), and the timing of their activities (acute, recovery, or rehabilitation phases). Regardless of their mission or focus, humanitarian organizations should have clearly defined responsibilities and operate under established humanitarian principles.

The List

This chapter provides an overview of the types of humanitarian organizations, including a list with a brief description of the size and mission of each organization. The list is by no means comprehensive and focuses on larger global organizations with a long history of response and the capacity to deliver services for multiple events globally. The list includes primarily large humanitarian organizations that play a central role in response to humanitarian emergencies in the acute or recovery phases. Organizations chosen were members of the Interagency Standing Committee (IASC) Global Health Cluster and/or either the global Nutrition or WASH cluster in 2016. The list is intended to include examples of the different types of organizations and not intended to be comprehensive. Given these constraints, some important organizations are not listed.

The landscape of humanitarian organizations is dynamic, with new organizations frequently joining a field in which there is a continued need for additional capacity. The list is intended to provide the reader with a framework. Specific organizations may be discussed elsewhere in the text where relevant.

Resources

Some resources for updated information on humanitarian organizations operating in a particular country or emergency include:

- ReliefWeb
    - http://reliefweb.int/
- International Council on Voluntary Organizations
    - https://icvanetwork.org/our-members
- Humanitarian Accountability Project membership list
    - www.hapinternational.org/membership/members.aspx
- National Association of Independent Schools Relief Organizations for Natural Disasters List
    - www.nais.org/Articles/Pages/Relief-Organizations-for-Natural-Disasters-150850.aspx

Humanitarian Organizations

Types of humanitarian organizations include:

- United Nations (UN) Organizations
- The Red Cross and Red Crescent Movement
- Government Organizations
- Funding Organizations/Donors
- Nongovernment Organizations (NGOs). These can be further divided into the geographic scope of their activities (local, regional, global), their mission (secular, faith-based), their service focus (health, nutrition, WASH, etc.) and by other categories.
- Military and paramilitary humanitarian support

United Nations (UN) Organizations

The United Nations is recognized as the lead coordinating body for humanitarian strategy and response through the Inter-Agency Standing Committee (IASC) and Office for the Coordination of Humanitarian Affairs (OCHA). Other UN organizations provide relief, support, and assistance to countries affected by humanitarian emergencies and natural disasters.

United Nations Inter-Agency Standing Committee (IASC)

Founded 1992, HQ: Geneva, Switzerland

www.humanitarianinfo.org/iasc/

IASC is an interagency policy forum responsible for coordination, policy development, and decision-making involving the key UN and non-UN humanitarian partners. Members include UN operational agencies involved in humanitarian activities (OCHA, UNDP, UNICEF, UNHCR, WFP, FAO, WHO, UN-HABITAT). There is a standing invitation to ICRC, IFRC, IOM, OHCHR, UNFPA, the World Bank, and the Special Rapporteur on the Human Rights of IDPs as well as the NGO consortia, InterAction, International Council of Voluntary Agencies (ICVA), and the Steering Committee for Humanitarian Response (SCHR).

The IASC was established in June 1992 in response to a United Nations General Assembly Resolution on the strengthening of humanitarian assistance. Under the leadership of the Emergency Relief Coordinator, the IASC develops humanitarian policies, agrees on a clear division of responsibility for the various aspects of humanitarian assistance, identifies and addresses gaps in response, and advocates for effective application of humanitarian principles.

United Nations Office for the Coordination of Humanitarian Affairs (OCHA)

Founded 1998, HQ: Geneva, Switzerland and New York, United States

www.unocha.org/

OCHA is the part of the UN Secretariat responsible for coordinating international responses to emergencies. Their mission is to mobilize and coordinate humanitarian action in partnership with national and international actors in response to disasters and emergencies, as well as to advocate the rights of people in need, promote preparedness, prevention, and facilitate sustainable solutions. OCHA works in five main areas: coordination, policy, advocacy, information management, and humanitarian financing. The Office is led by the Emergency Relief Coordinator who acts as the lead of the Global Cluster during emergency responses. OCHA has more than two thousand staff working in over 50 countries and in regional and headquarters locations. OCHA maintains several coordination tools and services, including IRIN (a humanitarian news service) and ReliefWeb (a humanitarian information portal).

United Nations High Commissioner for Refugees (UNHCR)

Founded 1950, HQ: Geneva, Switzerland

www.unhcr.org

UNHCR leads and coordinates international action to protect and resolve the problems of refugees and stateless people. They are the lead agency for the Protection Cluster. Along with IFRC, they co-lead the Emergency Shelter Cluster and with IOM, co-lead the Camp Management and Coordination Cluster. UNHCR works to ensure the right to seek asylum and find safe refuge in another state, with the option to return home voluntarily, integrate locally, or resettle in a third country. UNHCR has the capacity to respond to a new emergency impacting up to five hundred thousand people and can mobilize more than three hundred trained personnel within 72 hours. The agency has also created emergency stockpiles of nonfood aid items in Copenhagen and Dubai to supplement local aid supplies in areas of need. In 2016, UNHCR had a staff of some 10,700 people in 128 countries.

United Nations Children's Fund (UNICEF)

Founded 1946, HQ: New York, United States

www.unicef.org/

UNICEF is mandated by the UN to advocate for the protection of children's rights, to help meet their basic needs, and to expand their opportunities to reach their full potential. They are the lead agency for the Nutrition Cluster and the Water, Sanitation and Hygiene Cluster and the co-lead, with Save the Children, for the Education Cluster. During emergencies, UNICEF provides resources to its partners to relieve the suffering of children and their caregivers. UNICEF's works in 192 countries through country programs and National Committees, with 85 percent of the organization's posts located in the field. The UNICEF Office of Emergency Programmes (EMOPS) is the focal point for emergency assistance, humanitarian policies, staff security, and support to UNICEF offices in the field, as well as strategic coordination with external humanitarian partners.

United Nations Population Fund (UNFPA)

Founded 1969, HQ: New York, United States

www.unfpa.org/

UNFPA is the lead UN agency focusing on reproductive health, gender equality and population and development strategies. In emergencies, the agency provides expertise on sexual and reproductive health, gender-based violence, and population data. Gender issues, particularly gender-based violence, often become more acute in humanitarian settings, so UNFPA humanitarian support targets vulnerable populations, mainly women, adolescents and young people. UNFPA works in about 150 countries.

World Health Organization (WHO)

Founded 1948, HQ: Geneva, Switzerland

www.who.int/

www.who.int/ihr/alert_and_response/outbreak-network/en/

WHO is the lead agency for the Health Cluster and acts to coordinate the international response to humanitarian health and public health emergencies. Its overall mission is to provide leadership on global health matters, shaping the health research agenda, setting norms and standards, articulating evidence-based policy options, providing technical support to countries and monitoring and assessing health trends. Through the Health Emergencies Programme, WHO supports countries to prepare for, respond to, and recover from emergencies with public health consequences. Over seven thousand people from more than 150 countries work for WHO offices in countries, territories, and areas, six regional offices, and its headquarters. In outbreaks, WHO coordinates international outbreak response using resources from the Global Outbreak Alert and Response Network (GOARN). This is a collaboration of international institutions and networks that pool human and technical resources for rapid identification, confirmation, and response to outbreaks of international importance.

World Food Programme (WFP)

Founded 1961, HQ: Rome, Italy

www.wfp.org/

WFP is the lead of the Emergency Telecommunications and the Logistics Clusters and the co-lead, with the Food and Agriculture Organization (FAO), of the Global Food Security Cluster. It is responsible for mobilizing food and funds for transport for refugee-feeding operations managed by UNHCR as its mandate is to combat global hunger through the distribution of food aid. WFP works with approximately three thousand NGOs to distribute its food and, after the emergency has passed, it uses food to help communities rebuild. WFP employs about 12,000 staff in over 80 country offices, 90 percent of whom work in the field delivering food and monitoring its use.

Food and Agriculture Organization of the United Nations (FAO)

Founded 1945, HQ: Rome, Italy

www.fao.org/

Humanitarian response is only part of the FAO mission to provide people with regular access to sufficient high-quality food to lead active, healthy lives. The main organizational goals are the eradication of hunger, food insecurity and malnutrition, the elimination of poverty, and the driving forward of economic and social progress for all, and the sustainable management and utilization of natural resources, including land, water, air, climate, and genetic resources. In emergencies, FAO is the co-lead of the Global Food Security Cluster with WFP and its work focuses on developing, protecting and restoring sustainable livelihoods. In 2015, FAO employed about 3,200 staff, 57 percent based at their headquarters in Rome, with the remainder in offices worldwide.

United Nations Development Programme (UNDP)

Founded 1949, HQ: New York, US

www.undp.org

In its capacity as the lead of the Early Recovery Cluster, UNDP works to eradicate poverty, and reduce inequalities and exclusion, by developing policies, leadership skills, partnering abilities, and institutional capabilities. Building resilience to sustain development results is a critical part of their mission. UNDP focuses on helping countries build solutions in three main areas including sustainable development, democratic governance and peacebuilding, and climate and disaster resilience. Under the 2030 Agenda for Sustainable Development UNDP is working to strengthen new frameworks for development, disaster risk reduction and climate change. UNDP works in nearly 170 countries and territories.

Office of the United Nations High Commissioner for Human Rights (OHCHR)

Founded in 1993, HQ: Geneva, Switzerland and New York, United States

www.ohchr.org

OHCHR's mandate is to promote and protect all human rights. The High Commissioner for Human Rights leads OHCHR and is the principal human rights official of the UN. According to their website, OHCHR's thematic priorities are "strengthening international human rights mechanisms; enhancing equality and countering discrimination; combating impunity and strengthening accountability and the rule of law; integrating human rights in development and in the economic sphere; widening the democratic space; and early warning and protection of human rights in situations of conflict, violence and insecurity." In 2013, the agency employed 1,085 staff in Geneva, New York and in 13 regional and country offices. In addition, there were over six hundred international human rights officers serving in UN peace missions or political offices.

International Red Cross and Red Crescent Movement

The International Red Cross and Red Crescent Movement's mission is to protect human life and health, prevent and alleviate suffering, and to work to ensure respect for all human beings. The movement's three distinct organizations that share common principles and objectives are:
- International Committee of the Red Cross (ICRC)
- International Federation of Red Cross and Red Crescent Societies (IFRC)
- National Red Cross and Red Crescent Societies.

The IFRC has over 180 National Societies members. National Societies work within their home country following the statutes of the Movement and the principles of international humanitarian law. In many countries, the National Societies are linked to the government (sometimes the national health care system) and provide additional services such as blood donation and emergency medical services.

International Committee of the Red Cross (ICRC)

Founded 1863, HQ: Geneva, Switzerland

www.icrc.org/

ICRC is an impartial, neutral, and independent organization whose exclusively humanitarian mission is to assist and protect the lives and dignity of victims of armed conflict and other situations of violence. The organization also acts to promote and strengthen humanitarian law and universal humanitarian principles. ICRC directs and coordinates the international activities conducted by the International Red Cross and Red Crescent Movement in armed conflicts and other situations of violence. ICRC's Health Unit provides people affected by conflict with access to basic preventive and curative health care that meets universally recognized standards. The organization has more than 12,000 staff in 80 countries around the globe. About 30 percent of the ICRC's operational activities are carried out in cooperation with country-level Red Cross National Societies.

International Federation of Red Cross and Red Crescent Societies (IFRC)

Founded 1919, HQ: Geneva, Switzerland

www.ifrc.org

The IFRC is the world's largest humanitarian organization, comprised of Red Cross and Red Crescent National Societies in 189 countries, a secretariat in Geneva, and more than 60 delegations strategically located to support activities around the world. The IFRC's work focuses on four core areas: promoting humanitarian values, disaster response, disaster preparedness, and health and community care. Through its National Societies, the organization carries out relief operations to assist victims of disasters, and combines this with development work to strengthen the capacities of its member National Societies.

Other IASC members

This includes non-UN and non–Red Cross and Red Crescent institutions that actively participate in the humanitarian cluster system at a global level and are standing invitees to the IASC.

International Organization for Migration (IOM)

Founded 1951, HQ Geneva, Switzerland

www.iom.int/

IOM is an intergovernmental organization with 162 member states that works in collaboration with governmental, intergovernmental and nongovernmental partners. The organization works to ensure the orderly and humane management of migration, to promote international cooperation on migration issues, to assist in the search for practical solutions to migration problems, and to provide humanitarian assistance to refugees and internally displaced people in need. IOM participates in coordinated humanitarian responses through interagency arrangements and provides migration services in other emergency or postcrisis situations. In 2016, the UN adopted a resolution approving IOM as a Related Organization of the UN, strengthening the relationship between the two organizations. IOM has over eight thousand operational staff in more than 150 countries worldwide.

InterAction

Founded 1984, HQ: Washington, DC, United States

www.interaction.org/

InterAction is an alliance of over 180 faith-based and secular NGOs based in the United States. Within the organization, the Humanitarian Policy and Practice Team supports InterAction members active in humanitarian response and advocacy. InterAction provides a forum for consultation, coordination and advocacy on emergency response. Focus areas include: humanitarian practice and policy, protection, prevention of sexual abuse and exploitation, NGO security, and shelter and settlements. InterAction also engages at various levels with United Nations agencies, the US government, NGO consortia, and individual international NGOs on crosscutting issues and specific country situations.

Governmental Organizations and Funding Agencies

Many national governments have organizations that participate in international humanitarian response and recovery. Today, participation in disaster and humanitarian response includes governments worldwide not only from Europe, North America, and Australia but also Asia, South America, Africa, and the Middle East. Participation by governmental organizations includes providing funding to other responders or implementing partners as well as providing direct technical assistance and service to humanitarian partners and affected populations.

Funding agencies (donors) are essential to humanitarian response and recovery. The majority of humanitarian funding comes from government donors rather than public donations or other private sources. The amount of donations and where they originate from and are delivered to can vary significantly from year to year. Up-to-date information on humanitarian funding can be found at the UN OCHA financial tracking service website at https://fts.unocha.org. Annual reports on global humanitarian funding are available at www.globalhumanitarianassistance.org.

In 2015, international humanitarian assistance increased for the third consecutive year to a total of US$28.0B, of which US$21.8B (79%) was from governments and European Union (EU) institutions and US$6.2B (21%) was from private donors. The top five donors by total funding provided in 2015 were the United States (US$6.4B), Turkey (US$3.2B), United Kingdom (US$2.8B), EU Institutions (US$2.0B), and Germany (US$1.5B). The largest increase in assistance in recent years came from governments in the Middle East and Sahara region, whose contributions reached US$2.4B in 2015, a nearly 500 percent increase from 2011. Multilateral development banks including the World Bank also reported direct and other crisis-related funding of US$2.6B in 2014.

The majority of international humanitarian assistance is directed initially to UN organizations followed by NGOs. The leading recipients of humanitarian assistance in 2015 were Syria (US$2.0B), South Sudan (US$1.5B), Iraq (US$1.2B), Palestine (US$1.2B), and Jordan (US$895M). Evidence of the variability in funding from year to year is apparent in Haiti, which was the leading recipient of funding in 2011 but fell by US$2.6B to US$533M in 2012. Domestic governments are also an increasingly important resource in response to crises, especially natural disasters, within their own borders. Overall only 63 percent of humanitarian assistance requirements were met in 2012.

Centers for Disease Control and Prevention (CDC)

Founded 1946, HQ: Atlanta, United States

www.cdc.gov/globalhealth

CDC is the United States health protection agency that works to save lives and protect people from health threats. The Emergency Response and Recovery Branch (ERRB) coordinates, supervises, and monitors CDC's work in international emergency settings and with displaced populations. ERRB applies public health and epidemiologic science to reduce the health impact of disasters and humanitarian emergencies. It also works to strengthen the recovery of health systems in these settings. Core activities of ERRB include rapid assessments, disease surveillance, outbreak response and control, operational research, program evaluation, training, and postemergency health systems reconstruction. ERRB consists of over 50 multidisciplinary staff working in partnership with other US government agencies, UN agencies, and NGOs.

Department for International Development (DFID)

Founded 1997, HQ: London, England and East Kilbride, Scotland

www.gov.uk/government/organisations/department-for-international-development

DFID is a United Kingdom government agency that works to end extreme poverty. The organization also leads the government's response to humanitarian emergencies in developing countries. DFID works with other UK government departments, international organizations such as the UN, aid agencies, and the governments of the countries affected to provide predictable, long-term financial support. In natural disasters and emergency conflict situations, DFID provides humanitarian aid resources and deploys staff to affected areas led by the Conflict Humanitarian Security and Emergency Operations Team, a contracted team of experts, advisers, and officers. DFID employs approximately 2,700 staff who work in offices in London, East Kilbride, and globally.

European Community Humanitarian Office (ECHO)

Founded 1992, HQ: Brussels, Belgium

http://ec.europa.eu/echo/

ECHO is an office of the EU and is one of the world's biggest donors of humanitarian aid. ECHO does not directly deliver services, but channels the aid through private organizations, the UN system and the Red Cross Movement. They carry out postemergency needs assessments to identify appropriate response services. After funding NGOs to provide services, they monitor the implementation of the EU-funded humanitarian projects. ECHO has more than three hundred people working in its headquarters in Brussels and more than four hundred in 44 field offices located in 38 countries around the world. In 2011, ECHO distributed €1.1 billion in humanitarian assistance. This provided assistance to 117 million of the world's most vulnerable people in over 91 countries outside the EU.

United States Agency for International Development (USAID)/Office of US Foreign Disaster Assistance (OFDA)

Founded 1961, HQ: Washington D.C., United States

www.usaid.gov

USAID is an independent US government agency with the mission to end extreme global poverty and promote the development of resilient, democratic societies that are able to realize their potential. Within USAID, the Office of US Foreign Disaster Assistance (OFDA) is responsible for leading and coordinating the US response to disasters overseas. The mandate of OFDA is saving lives, alleviating human suffering, and reducing the social and economic impact of disasters. OFDA can deploy a Disaster Assistance Response Team (DART) to coordinate and manage the US government response. In addition, OFDA funds implementing partners and other organizations and works in partnership with USAID functional and regional bureaus and other US government agencies. OFDA's main areas of work include emergency response, disaster risk reduction, and early recovery. OFDA responds to an average of 65 disasters in more than 50 countries every year. In FY 2017, USAID/OFDA provided a total of more than US$2 billion in humanitarian assistance to support life-saving interventions in various sectors across the globe. In addition to its headquarters in Washington, DC, OFDA has five regional offices and 22 field offices worldwide, as well as four commodities warehouses.

International Nongovernmental Organizations (NGOs)

International NGOs and their field staff typically comprise the majority of operational personnel during a humanitarian response. Many of the large international NGOs are based in the US and Western Europe and operate in multiple sectors around the world.

CARE International

Founded 1945, HQ: Geneva, Switzerland

www.care-international.org/

Cooperation for Assistance and Relief Everywhere (CARE) is a nonprofit international NGO that is a confederation of 13 National members and one Affiliate member organizations who work together to end poverty. Delivering relief in emergencies is one of the organizations core values with a focus on four humanitarian core sectors: shelter, WASH, food security, and sexual and reproductive health. CARE puts a special focus on girls and women when distributing food and emergency supplies. In 2015, CARE reached over 10 million people through its humanitarian response.

Concern Worldwide

Founded 1968, HQ: Dublin, Ireland

www.concern.net/

Concern Worldwide works to reduce poverty and suffering in the world's poorest countries, focusing on five core programs: livelihoods, health, education, HIV and AIDS, and emergencies. Approximately half of Concern's resources are devoted to emergency work which includes both response and disaster risk reduction. In acute response, their emergency unit consists of 14 staff with a rapid deployment unit that can be deployed at 24 hours' notice to respond to sudden emergencies. In many countries, they respond by supporting national charity partners. In 2012, Concern responded to 43 emergencies across 20 countries, directly reaching close to three million people.

HelpAge International

Founded 1983, HQ: London, United Kingdom

www.helpage.org/

HelpAge International is an international NGO that helps older people claim their rights, challenge discrimination and overcome poverty, so that they can lead dignified, secure, active, and healthy lives. In emergencies, the organization works to ensure that older people are included in immediate and long-term humanitarian relief efforts on the ground, and in humanitarian policies and guidelines. Their work in emergencies focuses on older people in the areas of relief distributions, healthcare, nutrition, livelihood support, protection, disaster risk reduction, advocacy, technical support, and capacity building. In 2015, HelpAge International directly responded to emergencies in 23 countries providing support to over 155,000 older people and their families.

International Center for Migration and Health and Development (ICMHD)

Founded 1995, HQ: Geneva, Switzerland

www.icmhd.ch

The International Centre for Migration, Health and Development is a nonprofit institution whose mandate is to work on research, training, and policy advocacy related to migration and health. The organization's work is predicated on the belief that by protecting the health and welfare of people on the move, the public health, social development, and human security of the larger society is also enhanced. ICMHD uses a multidisciplinary approach including public health, medicine, social sciences, law, medical geography, health economics, and political science.

International Medical Corps International (IMC)

Founded 1984, HQ: Los Angeles, United States and London, United Kingdom

https://internationalmedicalcorps.org/

International Medical Corps Worldwide is a global humanitarian alliance made up of two independent affiliate organizations, IMC and IMC UK. IMC acts to save lives and relieve suffering through health care training and relief and development programs. Its mission is to improve the quality of life through health interventions and related activities that build local capacity in underserved communities worldwide. In emergencies, IMC seeks to be operational within 48 hours from the decision to deploy. Their emergency response teams provide emergency health care, nutrition, water, and sanitation, and other health services. In 2012, IMC staff worked in 35 countries to treat over three million patients including over one million children.

International Rescue Committee (IRC)

Founded 1933, HQ: New York, United States

www.rescue.org/

IRC is an international humanitarian NGO that offers emergency and long-term aid to refugees and those displaced by war, persecution, or natural disaster. Their services include emergency response, health care, water and sanitation, child and youth protection and education, reducing gender-based violence, post-conflict development, local capacity building, and supporting civil society. They also have resettlement offices in the United States to assist new refugee arrivals. In emergencies, IRC strives to arrive on the scene within 72 hours with urgently needed supplies and expertise that protect people caught in the midst of chaos. It also maintains an Emergency Response Team of specialists with expertise in key areas necessary to assess critical survival needs and mount an effective response to sudden or protracted emergencies. The team includes coordinators, logisticians, doctors, and water and sanitation experts. It also includes specialists who focus on human rights protection, the special needs of children in crisis, the prevention of sexual violence, and aid for rape survivors. In 2015, IRC operated in over 40 countries and 29 US cities and provided 23 million people with aid.

Islamic Relief Worldwide (IRW)

Founded 1984, HQ: Birmingham, United Kingdom

www.islamic-relief.com/

IRW is a faith-based independent international relief and development NGO. The organization's aims are protecting life and dignity, empowering communities, campaigning for change, and strengthening the Islamic relief family. IRW promotes sustainable economic and social development by working with local communities to eradicate poverty, illiteracy, and disease. They also respond to disasters and emergencies, focusing on the basic necessities of food, water, shelter, and medical treatment. After the emergency phase, IRW assesses possibilities of rehabilitation and long-term development. The organization works in over 40 countries through national offices and partners.

Medair International

Founded 1989, HQ: Ecublens, Switzerland

http://relief.medair.org/

Medair is a Christian faith-based international humanitarian NGO providing relief in some of the world's most remote and devastated places. Core activities focus on health, nutrition, WASH, and shelter. In disasters and humanitarian emergencies Medair rapidly deploys to provide shelter and household items, safe drinking water and sanitation, safe demolition, and emergency health care. To safeguard against future disasters, they help families rebuild their homes back better than before using strong building materials and disaster-resilient construction methods. In 2013, Medair had over seven hundred employees who worked in 11 countries to directly provide services to over 1.2 million beneficiaries.

Médecins Sans Frontières (MSF)

Founded 1971, HQ: Geneva, Switzerland

www.msf.org/

MSF is an international, independent, medical humanitarian NGO that delivers emergency aid to people affected by armed conflict, epidemics, natural disasters, and exclusion from healthcare. Services offered include rehabilitating and running hospitals and clinics, basic healthcare, surgery, maternal care, infection control, immunization campaigns, nutrition, and mental health. When necessary, they provide WASH services and distribute relief. MSF consists of 23 independent associations attached to five operational directorates located in Amsterdam, Barcelona-Athens, Brussels, Geneva, and Paris. Common policies are coordinated by the International Council in Geneva, Switzerland. In emergencies, MSF staff offer basic healthcare, perform surgery, fight epidemics, rehabilitation and running of hospitals and clinics, carrying out vaccination campaigns, operating nutrition centers, and providing mental healthcare. In 2015, MSF provided over eight million outpatient consultations in over 69 countries. In 1999, MSF was awarded the Nobel Peace Prize.

Save the Children

Founded 1919, HQ: London, United Kingdom

www.savethechildren.net/

Save the Children is an international NGO that is comprised of Save the Children International and 30 member organizations. They work to improve the lives of children through the provision of education, health care, psycho-social support and economic opportunities, and by providing emergency aid in natural disasters and humanitarian emergencies. In 2015 Save the Children responded to 99 humanitarian crises in 53 countries around the world, directly reaching 13.8 million people including 7.1 million children. In July 2013, Merlin joined Save the Children to create a global humanitarian force that can provide faster and more cost-effective support in a humanitarian crisis. Save the Children currently serves as co-lead (with UNICEF) for the IASC education cluster.

Terre des Hommes International Federation

Founded 1960, HQ: Geneva, Switzerland

www.terredeshommes.org/

Terre des Hommes International Federation is a network of ten national organizations in Europe and Canada working for the rights of children and to promote equitable development. In emergencies, they provide services from the distribution of first aid items to WASH services. Beyond immediate logistic and material aid, the organization also has technical expertise in the protection, care, and psychosocial support of victims of natural disasters and conflicts. In 2013, Terre des Hommes supported 840 development and humanitarian aid projects to improve the living conditions of the most underprivileged children, their families and communities in 64 countries.

World Association for Disaster and Emergency Management (WADEM)

Founded 1976, HQ: Madison, Wisconsin, United States

www.wadem.org/

WADEM is a nonoperational, nongovernmental, multidisciplinary organization whose mission is the global improvement of pre-hospital and emergency health care, public health, and disaster health and preparedness. The organization fosters international collaboration in the application of knowledge gained from data collected through qualitative and quantitative research to develop strategies aimed at promoting all aspects of human health, decreasing susceptibility, and increasing resilience to future health disasters and emergencies. It produces its own international, peer-reviewed journal, Prehospital and Disaster Medicine, sponsors biennial World Congresses, and supports regional conferences of its affiliated societies and partner organizations.

World Vision International

Founded 1950, HQ: Middlesex, United Kingdom

www.wvi.org/

World Vision is an independent global Christian faith-based organization that provides emergency relief, education, health care, economic development, and promotion of justice. During emergencies they provide food, shelter, and medical care to victims of natural or man-made disasters. Many of these relief projects focus on children and the transition into development activities. In 2015, World Vision assisted 12 million people in almost one hundred countries.

Local and National Humanitarian Partners

Local and national humanitarian partners are an essential component of humanitarian aid delivery and end-stage program implementation. Most successful programs engage these partners that are most adept at incorporating the cultural context of the emergency to effectively respond to emergencies. This includes both local NGOs and host government emergency response agencies. Host governments are also responsible for the security and safety of, assistance to, and law and order among refugees and internally displaced people in their territory, though in emergencies they may rely on international partners to support them.

Military and Paramilitary Humanitarian Support

In emergencies, many countries provide military or paramilitary support to affected states. These resources can rapidly deploy unique assets in difficult settings and are an important component of overall humanitarian response, especially in the acute emergency phase. In large emergencies, military actors often work in the same areas as civilian organizations and effective coordination and dialogue is needed to ensure that both groups operate effectively. This often includes training on both military and civilian humanitarian policies and principles. This coordination or coexistence of activities is often facilitated by the OCHA United Nations Humanitarian Civil-Military Coordination (UN-CMCoord). This group facilitates dialogue and interaction between civilian and military actors, which is essential for protecting and promoting the humanitarian principles, avoiding competition, minimizing inconsistency and, when appropriate, pursuing common goals. They also develop specific guidance on this coordination in natural disasters and complex emergencies.

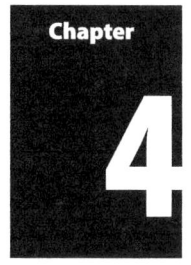

Chapter 4: Response to Humanitarian Emergencies

David A. Townes, Andre Griekspoor, Peter Mala, Ian Norton, and Anthony D. Redmond

Introduction

The scale, scope, timing, and duration of the response to a humanitarian emergency depends upon many factors including the type of disaster, the region, country, or location, the local capacity to respond, the international capacity and willingness to respond, and the willingness of the affected country or population to accept assistance. These factors are influenced by the political context both within and outside the affected country.

Disasters may be categorized as natural or man-made and rapid/sudden onset or slow onset, all of which may lead to humanitarian emergencies necessitating a humanitarian response. The type of disaster or emergency will influence the response both in terms of the type of interventions needed and the timing and duration of the response. For example, the response to a rapid/sudden onset natural disaster such as an earthquake will differ significantly from the response to a slow onset natural disaster such as a drought and subsequent famine. Depending on the disaster, a large-scale response involving many international and local stakeholders over an extended period of time may be required.

Rapid Onset Natural Disasters

The timing of the response to rapid/sudden onset natural disasters generally needs to be more rapid than for slow onset disasters due to the different injury and trauma profiles of these disasters and their evolution over time. In rapid onset, natural disasters such as earthquakes, most of the deaths and injuries occur during the first few hours or days. Following the 1995 earthquake in Kobe, Japan, of the 6,435 people who died, it is estimated that 71 percent died within 14 minutes of the earthquake and another 10 percent within 6 hours (Benjamin et al. 2011). In the hours and days after an earthquake, there will likely be a need for urban search and rescue (USAR), trauma and orthopedic surgery, in addition to routine medical and surgical interventions and services. The first 24–48 hours after the disaster is when appropriate interventions can have the greatest impact on survival from trauma related morbidity and mortality.

Slow Onset Natural Disasters

In contrast, during a slow onset natural disaster such as a famine, the initial needs are more likely to be delivery of food, treatment of malnutrition, and provision of sufficient water, sanitation, and hygiene. In some settings, it may be that service delivery is not affected, but barriers to access result in need. This may include lack of purchasing power due to loss of livelihood or insecurity. In this context, interventions are likely to be needed over extended periods of time from months to years. An example of a slow onset natural disaster is the famine in the Horn of Africa after the drought of 2011–12.

Complex Humanitarian Emergencies (CHE)

Some humanitarian emergencies cannot be simply categorized as natural, rapid/sudden onset or slow onset, or man-made. As discussed in Chapter 1, often major humanitarian emergencies are influenced by multiple factors including political, economic, civil unrest, or conflict, leading to the displacement of the population. These emergencies, often referred to as complex humanitarian emergencies (CHE) require a large-scale, system wide, coordinated humanitarian response. The famine in the Horn of Africa, while a slow onset natural disaster, became a complex humanitarian emergency, created by a combination of natural and man-made factors, including drought, with crop failure and armed combat, resulting in displacement of large numbers of people. Another example of a complex humanitarian emergency is the civil war in Syria that began in 2011.

Response to CHE is often the most complicated and challenging, requiring a multifaceted response. Initial needs may include treatment for injuries sustained from armed combat, management of both acute and chronic illness, delivery of food, treatment of malnutrition, and provision of sufficient water, sanitation, and hygiene. CHE are a particularly dynamic environment, and these interventions may be required at different times and in different quantities over the duration of the response, which may be months, years, or decades, depending on the context.

Displaced Populations

In all types of disasters there is potential for displacement of the affected population. Depending on the situation, some of those displaced may remain in their home country as internally displaced persons (IDPs), while others may cross an international border to become refugees. While many of the health needs of IDPs and refugees are similar, access to IDPs may be restricted and more difficult than for refugees depending on the context. IDPs may be more likely to sustain injuries related to armed combat given their proximity to the fighting compared with refugees.

Some refugees and IDPs may be living in spontaneous or makeshift camps with little or no public health or healthcare services while others may be living in more formalized camps or settlements with on-site services. Still others may be living within the host community. This may be in a rural or urban setting. All of these factors must be considered for an effective response.

Humanitarian Principles

The humanitarian relief community has adopted humanitarian principles that originally grew out of the International Federation of the Red Cross and Red Crescent Movement (Burkle 2006). The humanitarian principles are:

Humanity

Human suffering must be addressed wherever it is found. The purpose of humanitarian action is to protect life and health and ensure respect for human beings.

Neutrality

Humanitarian actors must not take sides in hostilities or engage in controversies of a political, racial, religious, or ideological nature.

Impartiality

Humanitarian action must be carried out on the basis of need alone, giving priority to the most urgent cases of distress and making no distinctions on the basis of nationality, race, gender, religious belief, class, or political opinion.

Independence

Humanitarian action must be autonomous from the political, economic, military, or other objectives that any actor may hold with regard to areas where humanitarian action is being implemented.

Delivery of health aid for humanitarian emergencies must adhere to these principles as they provide the foundation for humanitarian assistance and are essential for an effective response. This includes both external entities as well as the host government that is obligated to provide for their populations, including providing access to humanitarian assistance.

Humanitarian Professionalism

Humanitarian aid workers are often volunteers who sometimes lack sufficient training and experience. There is a need for a diversity of high-quality training programs for those interested in the field, including training for health professionals on public health issues pertinent to humanitarian emergencies (Brennan and Nandy 2001).

In response, there has been significant growth in training opportunities in an effort to increase professionalism within the field (Burkle 1995). This includes a number of initiatives such as Enhancing Learning and Research in Humanitarian Action (ELRHA), which has a stated objective of working with others to improve humanitarian outcomes through partnership, research, and innovation (ELRHA 2017).

The required skill set is broad, including a basic understanding of food security and nutrition, water and sanitation, rapid assessment, infectious disease surveillance, epidemic management, immunization, communicable disease control, and maternal and child health care. This range of skills is unlikely to be covered in most schools of medicine, public health, nursing, or engineering. In addition to a basic understanding, these skills need to be applied to austere and potentially dangerous environments.

Myths and Realities

There are some common myths about responding to humanitarian emergencies (Noji and Toole 1997). These include:

- *Myth:* Foreign medical volunteers with any kind of medical background are needed.
- *Reality:* The local population and the national health services will likely provide immediate life-saving needs, and only medical skills that are unavailable or insufficient in the country may be needed. Improperly trained staff and inadequately supported medical teams will not prove useful. Emergency medical teams (EMTs) that respond should do so only on request or invitation by the host government and must adhere to standards for such teams.
- *Myth:* Any kind of international assistance is needed.
- *Reality:* A response not based on a good needs-assessment will likely only contribute to the problem. Most initial needs are met by local governments and agencies, not by foreign assistance. Assistance not directed at filling clear needs often results in an influx of unnecessary, useless, and culturally inappropriate items, including unusable clothing and other commodities, outdated drugs, ineffective vaccines, and unsustainable equipment. After the 1988 Armenian earthquake, it took 50 people six months to inventory the drugs sent to Armenia in the first few weeks after the earthquake. Further, transporting items that might be sourced locally, such as bottled water, may displace other items in the supply pipeline that cannot be obtained locally. This influx of inappropriate commodities and personnel has been labeled "the second disaster."
- *Myth:* Epidemics and plagues are inevitable after every disaster.
- *Reality:* Large scale, spontaneous epidemics are generally uncommon after disasters; however, outbreaks do occur, such as the cholera outbreak after the earthquake in Haiti, although the exact cause of this outbreak and the contribution of the earthquake remain unclear. Disasters may affect transmission of endemic diseases and may have an impact on noncommunicable diseases.
- *Myth:* Dead bodies and dead animals will lead to outbreak of disease and need to be disposed of immediately.
- *Reality:* Dead bodies do not generally cause disease or outbreaks of disease (Morgan et al. 2009). Body disposal should be done as soon as possible but in alignment with local customs and cultural practices. There are exceptions however, including the Ebola outbreak in West Africa in 2104. Generally, the key to disease outbreak prevention often involves interventions, such as providing adequate water and sanitation, immunizations to prevent measles and other vaccine preventable diseases, or long-lasting insecticide-treated bed nets (LLINs) to prevent malaria depending on the context.

Local Response and International Assistance

There are some general principles applicable to the response to most humanitarian emergencies and complex humanitarian emergencies whether caused by natural disasters, man-made disasters, or a combination of factors.

Local Response

The initial response to most humanitarian emergencies is local, with members of the affected community themselves providing relief and assistance in the immediate period after the emergency. For example, after an earthquake, many of the survivors are removed from the rubble by their neighbors and countrymen long before international USAR teams are on the ground. Food and water, while potentially in limited supply and uncertain quality, are initially provided from local sources. Similarly, shelter is often created from locally available materials or existing structures.

This initial local response may be spontaneous and ad hoc or it may be more formal and systematic depending on the affected area's level of disaster preparedness, capacity, and the level that the health infrastructure remains intact. In situations where there has been predisaster planning, there may be a more organized response including trained first responders, prepositioned supplies, and surge capacity of the healthcare and public health system.

Part of this initial, local response may also include the National Red Cross and Red Crescent Societies, nongovernmental organizations (NGOs), United Nations (UN) organizations, and/or foreign governmental agencies or similar organizations already working in the area in other capacities. During the initial response, they may refocus their human resources, commodities, and technical expertise from their ongoing programs to the response to the emergency.

In many resource poor and/or disaster prone countries, the initial response to a humanitarian emergency is often a combination of spontaneous, ad hoc, and more formally organized local efforts in combination with redirected efforts of international organizations with an on-the-ground presence in the country when the disaster occurred.

International Assistance

When the needs exceed the local response capacity to a humanitarian emergency, international humanitarian assistance is often required. Humanitarian assistance may be offered prior to being requested, but it is ultimately only on request by the government of the affected country, assuming the government is recognized and functioning, that humanitarian assistance is delivered.

There are exceptions to this where humanitarian assistance has been delivered without the request of the host government, such as in Syria, but the political, legal, and ethical background for this action is beyond the scope of this text. The context for such action is commonly a complex humanitarian emergency where there is no recognized government or the government is incapacitated, overwhelmed, or ineffective. In these situations, humanitarian assistance often comes in the form of cross-border or cross-line delivery of needed commodities.

As previously discussed, immediately after a disaster, organizations already working in the country may redirect their resources towards humanitarian assistance. These organizations are often the first to bring in additional international assistance in the form of human resources, technical assistance, and commodities directed at humanitarian assistance in an attempt to meet the need. These organizations have the advantage of already working in country, which gives them invaluable familiarity and operational experience, and a relationship with and by the local population. A potential disadvantage is that these organizations may not have sufficient experience or expertise in humanitarian response, as they may have had a focus on development in the country prior to the disaster. One of the challenges for these organizations is switching from development to humanitarian assistance, including potentially temporarily stopping or repurposing their normal programs.

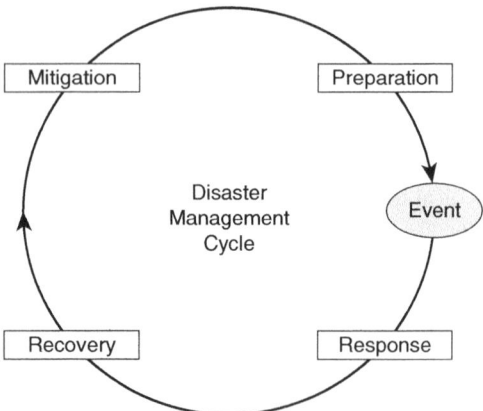

Figure 4.1 The disaster response cycle

Disaster Risk Management Cycle

The response to most humanitarian emergencies is a progression from the "emergency phase to the post-emergency phase" (MSF 1997). This response cycle has also been described more recently as a progression from "relief to recovery" or "emergency response to development" and called the humanitarian program cycle or the disaster risk management cycle. A simple example is shown in Figure 4.1.

Early on in the response cycle, a needs assessment is completed followed by implementation of programs based on the needs identified. Once implemented, monitoring and evaluation of these programs helps determine their effectiveness and impact as well as identify evolving and changing needs. As the initial needs are met, there is a transition from the emergency phase to the postemergency phase, including shifting focus to development and local capacity, including disaster risk reduction (DRR). The timeline of the disaster response cycle will vary significantly depending on the context.

The initial response from the international humanitarian after rapid onset natural disasters, such as earthquakes and typhoons, needs to be fast with a rapid scale-up of capacity. The initial response to slow onset disasters such as famine, as well as complex humanitarian emergencies such as armed conflict, may be a more gradual scale-up of capacity. In many of these situations, the response and scale up may be delayed for days, weeks, or months for a variety of logistical, economic, and political reasons.

The timeline from needs assessment to effective program implementation and transition to recovery or development varies tremendously depending on the situation. Ideally, the full progression may take several months to several years; although more commonly, it takes decades, especially in protracted humanitarian emergencies. Completion of this progression is faster and more successful in natural disasters compared with armed conflict, where the progression from the emergency phase to the postemergency phase is often delayed or never realized.

Frequently, there is unclear delineation between the emergency phase and the postemergency phase and the progression from emergency response and relief to recovery and development. Setbacks and movement backwards in the relief cycle are common, especially in complex humanitarian emergencies.

During the emergency phase, priorities include immediate life-saving interventions directed at reducing excess mortality and alleviating suffering. Once a certain degree of stability has been achieved, there is a shift to the postemergency phase. In this stage, the situation is still considered labile, at risk of deterioration, but with excessive mortality under control. It is during this phase that new priorities are established, programs evaluated, and priorities redirected towards recovery and development. In situations with displaced populations, including refugees, the postemergency phase also includes programs directed at their repatriation and resettlement.

Response Priorities

It is important that humanitarian relief organizations and other stakeholders have a common understanding of the health priorities of the initial response to humanitarian emergencies.

The top ten priorities of intervention for controlling the mortality rate among people displaced by humanitarian emergencies are shown in Table 4.1 (MSF 1997).

Other sources have since proposed that priorities to reduce mortality and morbidity include protection from violence, including sexual and gender based violence (SGBV); provision of adequate food rations, clean water and sanitation; diarrheal disease control; measles immunization; maternal and child health care; management of common infectious diseases

Table 4.1 Top ten priorities for controlling the mortality rate among people displaced by humanitarian emergencies

1. Initial assessment
2. Measles immunization (immunization against other vaccine preventable diseases depending on context)
3. Water and sanitation
4. Food and nutrition
5. Shelter and site planning
6. Health care in the emergency phase (including restoring capacity for service delivery to ensure continuity of care and treatment)
7. Control of communicable diseases and epidemics
8. Public health surveillance
9. Humanitarian resources and training
10. Coordination

Source: Adapted from *Refugee health: An approach to emergency situations*, 1997, Médecins Sans Frontières (MSF).

with epidemic potential; and selective feeding programs (Toole and Waldman 1997). These priorities very closely echo those proposed by MSF.

Humanitarian priorities have been further refined through the development of standards, guidelines, and tools. These include the Sphere Project, outlining minimum standards in disaster response, and various clinical guidelines for the management of specific disorders including cholera, meningococcal meningitis, fever, and malnutrition to name a few. Examples of public health tools include the Early Warning and Response Network (EWARN) by the World Health Organization (WHO) and the Cholera Toolkit by the United Nations Children's Fund (UNICEF).

The first nine priorities listed in Table 4.1 are discussed elsewhere in the text. The tenth priority, *Coordination*, is discussed in in this chapter.

Sphere Project

The Sphere Project began in 1997 by a group of NGOs and the International Red Cross and Red Crescent Movement with the aim to improve the quality and accountability of disaster response.

The Sphere Project is based on two core beliefs:

- That those affected by disaster or conflict have a right to life with dignity and, therefore, a right to assistance
- That all possible steps should be taken to alleviate human suffering arising out of disaster or conflict

In support of these core beliefs, the Sphere Project Handbook includes a set of minimum standards in key life-saving sectors such as water supply, sanitation and hygiene promotion, food security and nutrition, shelter, settlement and nonfood items, and health action.

These standards are evidence-based and/or represent sector-wide consensus. For each standard, key actions, key indicators, and guidance notes are included. These minimum standards must be met during a humanitarian response for the affected populations to survive and recover in stable conditions and with dignity. Affected populations were included in the development of these standards.

The Sphere Handbook

The Sphere Handbook, available at www.spherehandbook.org, first published in 2000, is designed for planning, implementation, monitoring, and evaluation during a humanitarian response. It is generally well accepted by the humanitarian community as a whole and is one of the most widely recognized set of standards for humanitarian response.

The format of the Handbook for each standard begins with a general statement followed by key actions, key indicators, and guidance notes.

First, the minimum standard is stated. This tends to be qualitative including specific minimum levels to be attained in humanitarian response. Next, practical key actions to attain the minimum standard are suggested, followed by a set of key indicators. The key indicators reflect whether or not a minimum standard has been attained. The key indicators relate to the minimum standard, not to the key action.

Finally, guidance notes are included with context-specific considerations when aiming at reaching the key actions and key indicators. They provide guidance on practical challenges, benchmarks, prioritizing and cross-cutting themes. They may also include critical issues relating to standards, controversies, and knowledge gaps. They do not prescribe how to implement a specific activity.

An example is shown in Figure 4.2.

The technical minimum standards chapters may contain appendices including such information as assessment checklists, formulas, tables, and examples of report forms.

Often, standards described in one sector need to be addressed in conjunction with standards described in others. As a result, chapters in the Handbook are interconnected and contain numerous cross-references.

Public Health and Healthcare/Clinical Response

Implementation of programs designed to provide public health and healthcare/clinical services in response to a humanitarian emergency should be based on health needs, risks to health, and analysis of the national response capacity to deliver services. Ideally, this should be determined through performance of a needs assessment and in situations where this is unrealistic, based on anticipation of need utilizing experiences from similar past humanitarian emergencies. Needs assessments are discussed in Chapter 7.

Historically, the major causes of morbidity and mortality in persons displaced by a humanitarian including diarrheal disease, acute respiratory infection, malaria, measles, neonatal causes, and malnutrition. Malnutrition may be an independent cause of morbidity and mortality or exacerbate other causes. It may not be reported as an independent cause of death (Toole and Waldman 1997). Malnutrition is discussed in Chapter 25.

Increasingly, morbidity and mortality has been attributed to other etiologies including HIV/AIDS (Chapter 23), tuberculosis (Chapter 29), chronic and noncommunicable diseases (NCDs) (Chapter 31), violence and injury (Chapter 30). Injury and NCD have become increasingly recognized as contributors to morbidity and mortality particularly in middle-income countries, with a large burden of NCDs at baseline, with large numbers of war-related injuries due to armed conflict. Syria is an example.

Health programs implemented during a humanitarian emergency should be directed at common causes of morbidity and mortality to address specific gaps in services and needs. These needs are often at both the individual and community level and include both public health and healthcare. There is obvious overlap in the public health and healthcare response and many organizations work in both areas concurrently. Too often, however, the public health and healthcare/clinical response organizations are not well integrated.

Water supply standard 1: Access and water quantity: All people have safe and equitable access to a sufficient quantity of water for drinking, cooking and personal and domestic hygiene. Public water points are sufficiently close to households to enable use of the minimum water requirement.

- **Key actions**
  - Identify appropriate water sources for the situation, taking into consideration the quantity and environmental impact on the sources
  - Prioritize and provide water to meet the requirements of the affected population

- **Key indicators**
  - Average water use for drinking, cooking, and personal hygiene in any household is at least 15 liters per person per day (l/p/d)
  - The maximum distance from any household to the nearest water point is 500 meters
  - Queueing time at a water source is no more than 30 minutes

- **Guideline notes**

1. Water sources selection: The following factors should be considered in water source selection: availability, proximity, and sustainability of sufficient quantity of water; whether treatment is needed; and its feasibility, including the existence of any social, political, or legal factors concerning the source. Generally, groundwater sources and/or gravity-flow supplies from springs are preferable, as they require less treatment and no pumping. In disasters, a combination of approaches and sources is often required in the initial phase. All sources need to be regularly monitored to avoid overexploitation.

2. Needs: The quantities of water needed for domestic use is context-based, and may vary according to the climate, the sanitation facilities available, people's habits, their religious and cultural practices, the food they cook, the clothes they wear, and so on. Water consumption generally increases the nearer the water source is to the dwelling. Where possible, 15 l/p/d can be exceeded to conform to local standards where that standard is higher.

3. Measurement: Household surveys, observation, and community discussion groups are more effective methods of collecting data on water use and consumption than the measurement of water pumped into the pipeline network or the operation of hand pumps.

4. Quantity/coverage: In a disaster, and until minimum standards for both water quantity and quality are met, the priority is to provide equitable access to an adequate quantity of water even if it is of intermediate quality. Disaster-affected people are significantly more vulnerable to disease; therefore, water access and quantity indicators should be reached even if they are higher than the norms of the affected or host population. Particular attention should be paid to ensure the need for extra water for people with specific health conditions, such as HIV and AIDS, and to meet the water requirement for livestock and crops in drought situations. To avoid hostility, it is recommended that water and sanitation coverage address the needs of both host and affected populations equally.

5. Maximum numbers of people per water source: The number of people per source depends on the yield and availability of water at each source. These guidelines assume that the water point is accessible for approximately eight hours a day only and water supply is constant during that time. If access is greater than this, people can collect more than the 15 liters/day minimum requirement. These targets must be used with caution, as reaching them does not necessarily guarantee a minimum quantity of water or equitable access.

6. Queueing time: Excessive queueing times are indicators of insufficient water availability due to either an inadequate number of water points or inadequate yields at water sources. The potential negative results of excessive queueing times are reduced per capita water consumption, increased consumption from unprotected surface sources, and reduced time for other essential survival tasks for those who collect water.

7. Access and equity: Even if a sufficient quantity of water is available to meet minimum needs, additional measures are needed to ensure equitable access for all groups. Water points should be located in areas that are accessible to all, regardless of, for example, gender or ethnicity. Some hand pumps and water carrying containers may need to be designed or adapted for use by people living with HIV and AIDS, older people, persons with disabilities, and children. In situations where water is rationed or pumped at given times, this should be planned in consultation with the users, including women beneficiaries.

Figure 4.2 Example of minimum standard, key actions, key indicators, and guidance for water supply
Source: Water supply standard 1: Access and water quantity. In: The Sphere Project. Available at: www.spherehandbook.org/en/water-supply-standard-1-access-and-water-quantity/

Public Health

Organizations involved in the "public health" response might provide support to the host government and affected community, including supporting public health infrastructure, performing needs assessments, providing technical assistance, and implementing programs in areas such as water, sanitation and hygiene, nutrition, protection, reproductive health, communicable disease surveillance, outbreak detection and response, community mobilization and education, immunization, and other prevention methods, such as long-lasting insecticide treated bed net (LLIN) use for prevention of malaria. Many of these programs are directed at the community level. These organizations tend to be a mix of UN, international, and governmental organizations, as well as NGOs.

Healthcare/Clinical Response

Organizations involved in the healthcare or clinical response might provide immediate lifesaving interventions as well as preventive, primary care, and reproductive health services. These services tend to be focused on the individual. Organizations are often NGOs, joined more recently by government-based emergency medical teams that provide direct patient care to the affected population.

Whether providing public health services, healthcare/clinical services, or both, an organization should be experienced in humanitarian emergency response with staff who are culturally aware, including having the ability to communicate in the local language and be completely self-reliant (Babcock, et al. 2012).

As part of the healthcare/clinical response, medical teams may work relatively independently or in direct support of national staff and/or at an existing facility. Depending on the timing and the context, the focus might be to treat injury and illness directly related to the emergency and/or restore the full range of health services for the community. It is critical that responding medical teams understand the needs depending on the context and deploy with personnel, equipment, and supplies to meet those needs.

In the response to some prior humanitarian emergencies, the deployment of teams was not always in line with the needs, resulting in a mismatch between the capacities and capabilities of the teams deployed and the needs on the ground. For example, in the response to the Haiti earthquake and the Pakistan floods of 2010, many experts have stated that the deployment of medical teams to each emergency was not sufficiently based on need and teams varied significantly in terms of capacities, capabilities, competencies, and adherence to professional standards.

Emergency Medical Teams (EMT) Initiative

Experiences including the international responses to the humanitarian emergencies in Haiti and Pakistan led to the development of the WHO Emergency Medical Team Initiative (initially the Foreign Medical Teams Initiative). Often-cited problems with the clinical response to humanitarian emergencies include lack of informed consent, lack of appropriate follow-up, and poor documentation/medical records. As healthcare providers must practice with ethical and professional standards, they should only provide care and services and perform procedures for which they are qualified and regularly perform at home and should request informed consent, respecting the right of patients to refuse care even when their life is at stake. Providers must consider what is appropriate for the setting, which may be different than in their home country, and how realistic appropriate aftercare and follow-up are in the context (Benjamin et al. 2011).

In response to these challenges, the Foreign Medical Teams (FMT) Working Group was established within the Global Health Cluster, under the guidance of WHO. Since 2011, the FMT Working Group has developed guidance, procedures, and minimum standards for FMT to ensure better consistency and predictability in the response capacity and help direct receiving countries to identify FMTs that are able to meet and adhere to minimal standards. The first edition of a classification system and minimum standards for FMTs providing trauma and surgical care in the first month following a rapid/sudden onset disaster has been completed and successfully implemented in the response to Typhoon Haiyan. The Initiative has been renamed the Emergency Medical Teams (EMT) Initiative to better reflect the focus on building and supporting local capacity with an emphasis on national emergency medical teams trained and equipped to respond within their own counties. These teams may also respond internationally, both within and outside their own region, depending on need (WHO 2016).

Coordination

Coordination is critical to an effective response and has been the focus of much of the effort by the humanitarian community in trying to improve the international response to humanitarian emergencies.

For an international humanitarian response to be most effective, there needs to be coordination between the host government and the major humanitarian relief organizations including the UN, international organizations, such as the International Federation of the Red Cross and Red Crescent Societies (IFRC), foreign governments, and NGOs.

Insufficient coordination among the main organizations that respond to humanitarian emergencies is often cited as one of the major obstacles to an effective response. This is not surprising given the diversity of these organizations and the challenges inherent to the context in which they operate.

Recognition of insufficient coordination has led to several important developments intended to improve effectiveness of the overall humanitarian response. Among these are establishment of the Office for the Coordination of Humanitarian Affairs (OCHA) in 1991 and the United Nations Disaster Assessment and Coordination (UNDAC) System in 1993, introduction of the Cluster Approach in 2005, adoption of the Hyogo Framework for Action in 2005, the Transformative Agenda in 2010, and the WHO Emergency Response Framework in 2013.

United Nations Office for the Coordination of Humanitarian Affairs (OCHA)

In December 1991, the UN General Assembly adopted resolution 46/182 designed to strengthen the UN response to complex emergencies and natural disasters, while improving the overall effectiveness of humanitarian operations in the field. Establishing the Department of Humanitarian Affairs (DHA) followed in 1992 to promote greater collaboration by UN agencies responding to emergencies. The resolution also created the high-level position of Emergency Relief Coordinator (ERC), the Inter-Agency Standing Committee (IASC), the Consolidated Appeals Process, and the Central Emergency Revolving Fund. The members of the IASC are discussed in Chapter 3 (Burkle 2006, Lautze et al. 2004).

In 1998, the DHA was reorganized into the Office for the Coordination of Humanitarian Affairs (OCHA) that now directs the UN response to humanitarian emergencies. The core functions of OCHA include advocacy, coordination, financing, information management, and policy (Burkle 2006, Lautze et al. 2004).

While the ultimate authority for the coordination of the relief effort rests with the government of the affected or host country, the responsibility often falls to OCHA. In this capacity, OCHA is responsible for making sure there is consensus and understanding of the response priorities among the main relief organizations.

When there is a disaster, the UN Resident Coordinator (RC) who is usually the most senior UN official in the affected country, is often appointed by the ERC to serve as the Humanitarian Coordinator (HC) representing OCHA. In this capacity, the HC is responsible for leading and coordinating the efforts of humanitarian relief organizations, both UN and non-UN. In addition to the HC, there is a humanitarian country team (HCT) that includes representatives of IASC members, NGOs, and the Red Cross and Red Crescent Movement.

United Nations Disaster Assessment and Coordination (UNDAC) System

Upon request of the UN RC, HC or the host government, OCHA may deploy resources as part of the UNDAC System created in 1993 as part of the international response system for rapid/sudden onset disasters. It is designed to support the UN and the government of a disaster-affected country during the initial phase of the emergency. UNDAC includes specialists from over 60 countries, international agencies, and NGOs. An UNDAC team can deploy within 48 hours to a disaster anywhere in the world upon the request of the RC or HC or by the host government.

Among its responsibilities, UNDAC assists in the coordination of incoming international relief organizations at the country level and/or at the site of the emergency. This may include establishing an on-site Reception/Departure Center and Operations Coordination Center (OSOCC).

International Search and Rescue Advisory Group (INSARAG)

In the specific case of an earthquake requiring USAR, the UNDAC team sets up the OSOCC to help coordinate USAR teams. International USAR teams collectively make up the International Search and Rescue Advisory Group (INSARAG). Established in 1991 by

SAR teams that responded to the 1988 earthquake in Armenia, INSARAG is a network of disaster-prone and disaster-responding countries and organizations dedicated to USAR. INSARAG develops and promotes internationally accepted standards and procedures for operation, coordination, and cooperation between international USAR teams at the disaster site.

The UN serves as the INSARAG secretariat through the Field Coordination Support Section (FCSS) within OCHA's Emergency Services Branch (ESB). In this role, they facilitate participation and coordination of ISARAG member organizations.

The EMT initiative has followed the example of INSARAG and applied it to the first wave of clinical care teams and field hospitals. Agreements between WHO and OCHA mean that EMTs are now coordinated using the "Virtual-OSOCC" in the first hours of a major disaster and medical teams document their arrival using the same Reception Departure Center (RDC) system as Search and Rescue teams. While the OSOCC can be used for EMT coordination, the EMT Coordination Cell (EMT-CC) is best placed directly inside the government's Health Emergency Operations Center, as was done in Nepal in 2015 and Ecuador in 2016. This allows the Ministry of Health (MoH) to deploy its own national EMTs first, and then request, register, license, and task arriving international EMTs to where they are needed most.

Cluster Approach

In response to the humanitarian crisis in Darfur in 2004 and the Indian Ocean tsunami in 2004/2005, the UN ERC commissioned the Humanitarian Response Review (HRR) with the goal to improve the effectiveness and timeliness of humanitarian response to emergencies (Humphries 2013).

The four major recommendations of the HRR included:

- Improving humanitarian leadership through the Humanitarian Coordination System
- Better coordination of humanitarian action through the Cluster Approach
- Promote faster, more predictable, and equitable funding through improved financing, including the Central Emergency Response Fund (CERF)
- More effective partnership among all humanitarian actors through the Principles of Partnership implemented in 2007

The Cluster Approach was first established in 2005 by the IASC as part of the UN Humanitarian Reform process to ensure predictable leadership in the main areas of humanitarian response and strengthen system-wide coordination (WHO 2007). Clusters or sectors are groups of humanitarian organizations, both UN and non-UN, working in each of the main areas of humanitarian action. They are designated by the IASC and given the responsibility for coordination within their sector with clearly outlined accountability. The cluster approach aims to "improve the predictability, timeliness, and effectiveness of humanitarian response and pave the way for recovery" (WHO 2007).

Clusters are not intended to substitute for national capacity. Instead they provide support for national authorities and capacity as outlined in the 2011 IASC Guidance Note on Working with National Authorities that discusses that wherever possible, international humanitarian actors should organize to support or complement existing national response mechanisms rather than create parallel systems that may actually weaken or undermine national efforts (IASC, 2011). When appropriate, as early as possible, government or other national counterparts should be encouraged to co-chair cluster meetings with the Cluster Lead Agency.

The Cluster Approach was first applied following the 2005 earthquake in Pakistan. Initially there were nine clusters but this was subsequently increased to 11. Each cluster is assigned an agency to serve as the cluster lead. The clusters and their corresponding lead agencies are shown in Figure 4.3.

The cluster coordinator for each cluster provides leadership and facilitates cluster activities in alignment with the overall operational response plan. This includes identifying and preventing gaps and duplications in the response and coordinating with other clusters, especially in relation to intercluster activities and crosscutting issues. The cluster serves as a partner for the host government and has a role in sharing information and resources among responding agencies.

The core functions of a cluster at country level are to:

- Support service delivery by:
  - Providing a platform that ensures service delivery is driven by the Strategic Response Plan and strategic priorities
  - Developing mechanisms to eliminate duplication of service delivery

- Inform the HC/HCT's strategic decision-making by:
  - Preparing needs assessments and analysis of gaps (across and within sectors, using information management tools as needed)
  - Identifying and finding solutions for (emerging) gaps, obstacles, duplication, and crosscutting issues
  - Formulating priorities on the basis of analysis
- Plan and develop strategy by:
  - Developing sectoral plans, objectives, and indicators that directly support realization of the response's strategic priorities
  - Applying and adhering to common standards and guidelines
  - Clarifying funding requirements, helping to set priorities, and agreeing upon cluster contributions to the HC's overall humanitarian funding proposals
- Monitor and evaluate performance by:
  - Monitoring and reporting on activities and needs
  - Measuring performance against the cluster strategy and agreed results
  - Recommending corrective action where necessary
- Build national capacity in preparedness and contingency planning
- Promote advocacy by:
  - Identifying concerns that contribute to HC and HCT messaging and action
  - Undertaking advocacy on behalf of the cluster, cluster members, and affected people

The Cluster Approach is structured at both the global and country level with a lead agency for each cluster at each level.

Global Level

The aim of the cluster approach at the global level is to strengthen system-wide preparedness and technical capacity to respond to humanitarian emergencies by ensuring predictable leadership and accountability in all the main sectors or areas of humanitarian response (IASC, 2011). At the global level, the clusters are led primarily by UN agencies, international NGO, or IFRC and are continuously active.

At the global level, the cluster lead reports to the UN ERC. The cluster leads are shown in Figure 4.3. The Global Health Cluster, led by WHO, directs activities and program related to health. Other clusters may have an interdisciplinary relationship with the health cluster, including the Protection Cluster led by the United Nations High Commissioner for Refugees (UNHCR), the Nutrition Cluster led by UNICEF, the Food Security Cluster led by World Food Program (WFP) and the Food and Agriculture Organization (FAO), the Water, Sanitation and Hygiene Cluster led by UNICEF, and the Camp Coordination and Management Cluster led by UNHCR and the International Organization for Migration (IOM).

The Health Cluster includes over 30 partners, under the direction of WHO, engaged in development of guidance, training, tools for assessment and information management, and facilitating surge capacity within the health cluster. WHO is also a member of the nutrition; water, sanitation, and hygiene; shelter; and protection clusters to help promote intercluster coordination.

Country Level

At the country level, the aim is to "strengthen humanitarian response by demanding high standards of predictability, accountability, and partnership in all sectors or areas of activity" (IASC 2011). The country level clusters are normally activated only in response to a specific humanitarian emergency. There are exceptions where a cluster is activated outside of a specific humanitarian emergency, but these are uncommon. An example of this is the continuous activation of the Health Cluster in Nepal.

The criteria for cluster activation at the country level are met when (IASC 2015):

- Response and coordination gaps exist due to a sharp deterioration or significant change in the humanitarian situation
- Existing national response or coordination capacity is unable to meet needs in a manner that respects humanitarian principles due to the scale of need, the number of actors involved, adoption of a more complex multisectoral approach, or other constraints on the ability to respond or apply humanitarian principles

At the country level, clusters are established in-country in response to a specific humanitarian emergency. The HC, with the support of OCHA, is

Section 1: Humanitarian Emergencies

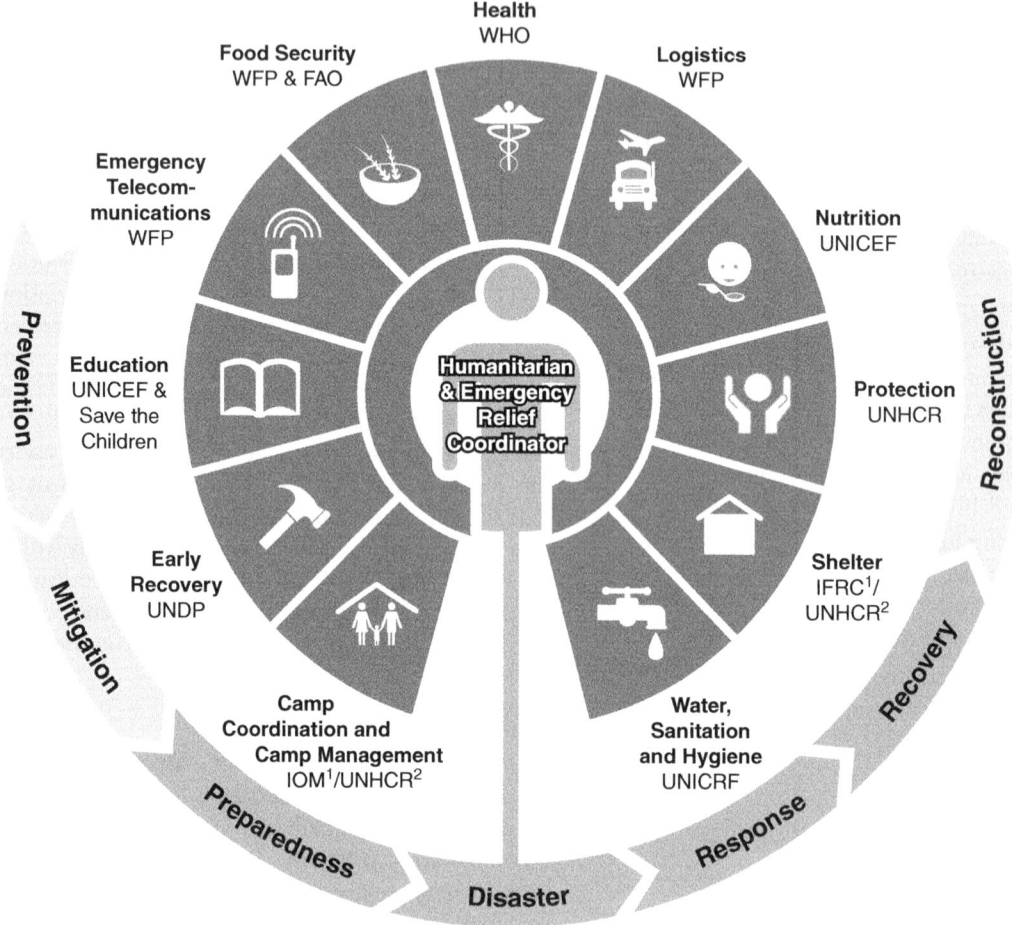

Figure 4.3 Clusters and corresponding lead agencies. Image provided courtesy of the UN Office for the Coordination of Humanitarian Affairs. Source: www.humanitarianresponse.info/clusters/space/page/what-cluster.

responsible for the overall humanitarian response at the country level and reports to the ERC. At the country level, the global lead agency is usually also the country lead agency, unless decided otherwise. Any IASC member may serve as the cluster lead. It does not need to be a UN or international agency. Often this role is filled by a NGO with significant experience in international humanitarian response. The country level cluster leads are accountable to the HC and member of the HCT.

The cluster lead agency is responsible for appointing a person, with appropriate experience, skills, and training, to be the cluster or sector coordinator. In this role, the cluster lead has the responsibility to ensure that those responding to the humanitarian emergency build on local capacities and maintain appropriate links and communication with the local or host government and authorities, civil societies, and other stakeholders.

Depending on the particular context and need, not all of the 11 clusters are activated for every emergency. In some situations clusters may be combined, for example, health and nutrition into the Health and Nutrition Cluster.

Once activated, most of the clusters hold regular meetings, often weekly, as a way to exchange ideas, resources, and information, reaffirm priorities, and share experiences and expertise. Ideally a representative of each organization involved in that particular aspect of the response attends the cluster meetings; however, there is no mandate for attendance. For example, attendance at the health cluster meeting might include organizations involved in direct clinical care, public health response, including health system strengthening, disease surveillance, outbreak prevention and response, immunizations and organizations involved in related sectors, such as water, sanitation and hygiene, nutrition, and protection.

Criticism and Challenges

The UN implemented the Cluster Approach in an attempt to increase and improve coordination among humanitarian actors and improve coherence in humanitarian response. While there are many experts who agree that the cluster approach has increased the effectiveness of humanitarian action, it is not without critics, especially within the NGO community, who have questioned the overall effectiveness (Humphries 2013).

Criticisms include gaps in predictable leadership due to high turnover rates and insufficient training and experience of cluster coordinators. Some NGOs feel that the Cluster Approach impedes the humanitarian principles of independence, impartiality, and neutrality and at times, includes a lack of impartiality of cluster lead agencies. Another criticism is that the cluster system has failed to create an appropriate sense of NGO ownership and involvement, resulting in many NGOs not feeling they are equal partners with the UN in the cluster. This extends to the process of deciding which organizations are invited. Some critics feel the cluster system is too "UN-centric" with a lack of NGO input and is nothing more than the UN trying to take control away from the NGOs. Additionally, the Cluster Approach has been criticized for not having a sufficient mechanism to ensure and enhance accountability to the affected population and reaches its limits in situations of large scale, complex humanitarian emergencies (Humphries 2013). Finally, the Cluster Approach has been criticized for being too focused on process and not results.

While some of these criticisms of the Cluster Approach are likely justified, prior to implementation, response to humanitarian emergencies was generally viewed as lacking sufficient coordination to be maximally effective. There were countless organizations involved with different missions, mandates, agendas, capabilities, and capacities as well as differing views of the best approach to the response. The Cluster Approach was designed to fill gaps and prevent overlap and ensure organizations work together to achieve a common objective.

The purpose of this was to result in a more coherent, effective, and efficient response.

The need to promote operational effectiveness and efficiency through improved coordination seemed a good place to start. A centralized, hierarchical structure was generally preferred by government and intergovernmental agencies; one based on a less centralized approach was favored by many NGOs, who felt that diversity of effort and approach would ensure success. The Cluster Approach was a compromise of these two philosophies (Humphries 2013).

There are some inherent operational challenges of the Cluster Approach at the country level. As critics have pointed out, this includes an insufficient supply of individuals with appropriate training and experience to serve as the cluster lead. Further, there may be inconsistencies in leadership due to frequent turnover. For representatives of member organizations, it may be challenging to attend the cluster meetings as they may require a great deal of staff time in terms of planning, travel, and attendance. Member organization representatives may experience meeting overload, especially if they are required to attend multiple cluster meetings.

Additional operational challenges include meetings not being held in the local language and being held in the capital city often far from where the member organization is working, requiring lengthy travel that takes them away from other activities and may be dangerous, depending on the situation. Further, smaller, less experienced and national NGOs may not be familiar with the cluster system and not know meetings are being held. This is especially concerning given organizations with less experience in humanitarian assistance are potentially likely to benefit the most from attendance. NGOs should register with the MoH or similar entity within the host government; however, in reality, this is inconsistent.

The benefits of the Cluster Approach seem to outweigh the costs, and no coordination is not an option. However, there are still challenges, justified criticisms, and room for greater involvement, ownership and improvement.

Humanitarian Relief Organizations

The major organizations that respond to humanitarian emergencies in a public health or healthcare capacity include UN organizations, such as WHO,

United Nations Population Fund (UNFPA), UNICEF, UNHCR, the International Organization for Migration (IOM), and the World Food Program (WFP), international organizations such as IFRC, NGOs such as Save the Children and MSF, faith based organizations, and governmental organizations, such as the European Community Humanitarian Office (ECHO), and the United States Office of Foreign Disaster Assistance (OFDA). In addition, military forces are often involved in the response to large-scale humanitarian emergencies.

These are just a few examples and not intended to be a comprehensive list. Numerous similar organizations also work in the areas of coordination, program implementation, technical assistance, and financial support. Many organizations work in multiple areas during a humanitarian response. Chapter 3 includes a more comprehensive discussion of these organizations.

Humanitarian assistance organizations frequently have criteria delineating when and in what capacity they will respond. This is often complicated as it involves a combination of mandate and mission, capacity and capability, and political will.

United Nations (UN) Organizations

There are many UN organizations involved in public health and healthcare response to humanitarian emergencies. WHO has a leadership role and is extensively involved in many aspects of the public health and healthcare response to humanitarian emergencies. In addition to leading the Global Health Cluster and country health clusters, WHO provides technical guidelines and training on a wide variety of public health and healthcare topics, including clinical management of a wide variety of injury and illness, infectious disease prevention, communicable disease surveillance and outbreak response, and best practices in a wide variety of topics, including reproductive health, mental health, laboratory, pharmaceuticals, and medical supplies and equipment. In addition, WHO personnel may be deployed as part of the UNDAC team. There are several other UN agencies that are involved in the health or health related aspects of a humanitarian response, namely UNICEF, UNFPA, and UNHCR.

The International Organization for Migration (IOM) was established in 1951 to resettle those displaced across Europe by World War II. In September 2016, IOM joined the UN and now serves as the leading UN organization in the field of migration. In the context of emergencies, IOM activities focus on "relief, return, reintegration, capacity-building and protection of the rights of affected populations."

WHO Emergency Response Framework

As the Global Health Cluster Lead, WHO plays an essential role in supporting Member States and partners to prepare for, respond to, and recover from humanitarian emergencies in which there are public health consequences. The Emergency Response Framework was adopted by WHO in 2013 as an internal framework to clarify its roles and responsibilities and provide a common approach for its work in emergencies. Among its components include setting out WHO's core commitments in emergency response, which are those actions WHO is committed to delivering to minimize mortality and life-threatening morbidity by leading a coordinated and effective health sector response; outlining during emergency response WHO's four critical functions of leadership, information, technical expertise, and core services; outlining WHO's emergency response procedures; and verifying three essential emergency policies to optimize WHO's response effectiveness of surge policy, the health emergency leader policy, and the no-regrets policy (Burkle 2006, IASC 2011).

Nongovernmental Organizations (NGOs)

There are countless NGOs involved in the health response to humanitarian emergencies. Some are large, multinational organizations, international NGOs (INGOs) with extensive experience in humanitarian assistance, while others may be smaller, less experienced organizations. Some may be local organizations that started in response to a specific disaster. Many of these NGOs focus on direct provision of healthcare services. Others operate public health programs or provide technical assistance. Several INGOs, including Epicentre, have a focus on health research and epidemiology in the humanitarian response setting.

Examples of INGOs that work in healthcare, public health, and related areas in humanitarian response include MSF, International Medical Corps (IMC), Save the Children, International Rescue Committee

(IRC), World Vision, Action Contre la Faim/Action Against Hunger (AAH), CARE, the Mentor Initiative, and Mercy Corps (MC), just to name a few. In large scale crises, there may be more than two hundred medical partners registered under the health cluster.

Sources of funding of NGOs include governments, foundations, and donations from both public and private entities. Many NGOs rely extensively on volunteers for their workforce.

International Organizations

The International Federation of the Red Cross and Red Crescent Movement is the world's largest humanitarian network. It is made up of nearly 100 million members and volunteers. The three main components include IFRC, the International Committee of the Red Cross (ICRC) and 189 Red Cross and Red Crescent Societies worldwide.

IFRC was formed in 1919 in Paris in the aftermath of World War I. Under the direction of the Secretariat in Geneva, Switzerland, it carries out relief operations for victims of disasters with a focus on the four main areas of promoting humanitarian values, disaster response, disaster preparedness, and health and community care.

IFRC works in a wide variety of disciplines related to humanitarian response, including health. Within the health response, IFRC activities include emergency response and first aid, prevention and health promotion, epidemic control, psychosocial care, community empowerment, and addressing stigma.

Government Agencies

Government agencies from all over the world are involved in response to humanitarian emergencies. Involvement may include acting as a donor for implementing partners, providing lifesaving commodities, conducting needs assessments, deploying personnel to provide technical assistance, or deploying medical teams through the EMT Initiative. Six examples are in the sections that follow.

The United Kingdom's Department for International Development (DFID)

DFID, also referred to as UKaid, leads the United Kingdom's work in the areas of relief and development. Its response to humanitarian emergencies is led by the Conflict Humanitarian and Security Department (CHASE), and key similar government agencies are involved in a variety of capacities. As a donor, DFID provides predictable, long-term financial support to humanitarian partners, including UN agencies and NGOs. DFID also provides commodities, human resources, and technical assistance.

The European Community Humanitarian Office (ECHO)

ECHO is responsible for humanitarian assistance from the European Commission. As the world's largest collective donor of humanitarian aid, ECHO projects have the common objective to alleviate suffering of the affected population. They work with over two hundred organizations, including UN agencies, IOM, IFRC/ICRC, and NGOs providing funding and human resources. ECHO also performs needs assessments as well as monitoring and evaluation of ECHO funded programs.

The Australian Government's Department of Foreign Affairs and Trade (Australian Aid)

Australian Aid leads and coordinates Australia's disaster risk reduction, preparedness, and response activities in developing countries. Similar to other agencies, during a humanitarian response, this might include funding of implementing partners, direct delivery of commodities, and providing technical assistance and other human resources.

The Office of US Foreign Disaster Assistance (OFDA)

OFDA is responsible for leading and coordinating response to disasters overseas for the United States government (USG). OFDA is within the Bureau for Democracy, Conflict and Humanitarian Assistance (DCHA) at the United States Agency for International Development (USAID). Some of OFDA's response capacity includes providing funding to implementing partners responding to humanitarian emergencies, maintaining a stockpile of emergency relief commodities with logistical and operational capacities to deliver them rapidly, and deploying Disaster Assistance Response Teams (DART) to coordinate, manage and optimize the USG response.

The US Centers for Disease Control and Prevention (CDC)

CDC responds to humanitarian emergencies at the request of the USG, the government of the affected country, or a UN agency. Many of the individuals with extensive experience and expertise in response to humanitarian emergencies work in the Emergency Response and Recovery Branch (ERRB) within the Center for Global Health. Much of the work is in the form of technical assistance, training, monitoring and evaluation, and operational research. Areas of expertise include epidemiology, needs assessments, nutrition, reproductive health, mental health, water, sanitation and hygiene, infectious diseases including malaria and tuberculosis, disease surveillance, outbreak detection and response, training, and development of standards and guidelines in a variety of areas.

Military Forces

In many large-scale humanitarian emergencies, an integral part of the response may include military forces, such as UN peacekeeping forces or troops from countries responding to the disaster.

The UN does not have its own military force. Rather, it depends on Member States, the 122 countries that contribute military and police personnel. As of March 2014, there were over 100,000 personnel both military and civilians working in the field as UN peacekeepers. During a response to a humanitarian emergency they offer protection for the delivery of humanitarian aid.

Countries responding to humanitarian emergencies may include their military as part of the response. This is especially likely in large-scale emergencies that require the unique capabilities of the military not found elsewhere, such as security, medical evacuation, communications, transportation, logistics, heavy lifting, transportation, and shelter (Burkle 1995, Burkle et al. 1995).

As NGOs and military forces have different mandates, guidance has been provided for how they need to work together to be most effective (IASC 2011). The global health cluster (GHC) provides guidance to country-level health clusters on how to apply IASC civil-military coordination principles to humanitarian health operations. Trends and challenges in humanitarian civil-military coordination have also been described (Metcalfe et al. 2012).

Transformative Agenda

Two concurrent large-scale humanitarian emergencies in 2010, the earthquake in Haiti and the floods in Pakistan, brought to attention shortcomings of the multilateral humanitarian response model. In response, the IASC set forth to improve the humanitarian response model, in part, through implementation of the Transformative Agenda. The major objectives of the Transformative Agenda include establishing a mechanism to deploy strong experienced senior humanitarian leaders, strengthening of leadership capacities and rapid deployment of humanitarian leadership, improving strategic planning, enhancing accountability of the HC, and streamlining coordination mechanisms.

Enhanced accountability of the HC includes that relief organizations responding to humanitarian emergencies must be accountable to the donor (commonly referred to as upward accountability), to the other cluster members (referred to as lateral accountability), and most importantly, to the affected population (referred to as downward accountability). Organizations may find these are in conflict at times.

Hyogo Framework for Action

The Hyogo Framework for Action is intended to mitigate the impact of disasters through improved risk reduction. It was established to reduce the impact of disasters and make risk reduction an essential component of development policies and programs (UNISDR 2007). In 2005, over 168 governments pledged to implement the three strategic goals to integrate disaster risk reduction into sustainable development policies and planning; to develop and strengthen institutions, mechanisms, and capacities to build resilience to hazards; and to systematically incorporate risk reduction approaches into the implementation of emergency preparedness, response, and recovery programs. While not specifically intended to improve the effectiveness of the response, it is a likely outcome if the three strategic goals of the Framework are achieved.

Conclusion

As we look to the past and the future, there are some important trends that have impacted the response to recent humanitarian emergencies and are likely to continue to impact responses in the near future.

There has been a shift of displaced persons, both IDPs and refugees, from rural to urban. Today, it is estimated that at least half of the world's refugees live in urban settings (UNHCR 2017). Due to the increase in internal as opposed to interstate wars, there has also been a shift from refugees to IDPs (UNHCR 2012).

Many of the programmatic interventions utilized in humanitarian response are based on refugees living in camp settings. Additional work needs to examine the effectiveness of these programs directed at IDPs and displaced persons living in urban settings and to develop new programs when these programs are not effective.

More than ever before, humanitarian emergencies occur in countries where NCDs and chronic illness are significant contributors to morbidity and mortality. NCDs are now recognized as a real and growing threat to population health and development in humanitarian disasters and emergencies (Demaio et al. 2013). The humanitarian community as a whole has not developed sufficient guidelines and standards for the evaluation and management of NCDs in response to humanitarian emergencies although work in this area is underway.

Some recent disease outbreaks in the setting of humanitarian emergencies have highlighted the importance of ensuring a rapid response to increase the likelihood of controlling public health threats at their source, and thereby enhancing global health security.

Finally, it has been recognized that in several recent humanitarian emergencies, the transition from emergency response to development has been ineffective and expensive. No matter what the initial response, as humanitarian emergencies become protracted, there will be the need to rebuild both the public health and healthcare infrastructure. This should be acknowledged by both the emergency response and development communities and incorporated into how they view their role in humanitarian emergencies. In part, an emphasis on DRR, disaster preparedness and mitigation, resilience, as well as better coordination between emergency response and development stakeholders is essential.

There is no single response model that is effective for every type of humanitarian emergency. Every humanitarian emergency is different. While there are many common characteristics of an effective response, the response should reflect the specific situation and be based on specific needs.

References

Babcock, C., Theodosis, C., Bills, C., Kim, J., Kinet, M., Turner, M., Millis, M., Olopade, O., and Olopade, C. (2012). The academic health center in complex humanitarian emergencies: Lessons learned from the 2010 Haiti earthquake. *Acad Med*, **87**:1609–1615.

Benjamin, E., Bassily-Marcu, A. M., Babu, E., Silver, L., and Marin, M. (2011). Principles and Practices of Disaster Relief: Lessons from Haiti. *Mt Sinai J Med*, **78**:306–318.

Brennan, R. J. and Nandy, R. (2001). Complex humanitarian emergencies: A major global health challenge. *Emergency Medicine*, **13**:2, 147–156.

Burkle, F. M. (2006). Complex humanitarian emergencies: A review of epidemiological and response models. *J Postgrad Med*, **52**:2, 110–115.

Burkle, F. M. (1995a). Complex humanitarian emergencies I: Concept and participants. *Prehospital and Disaster Medicine*, **10**:1, 36–42.

Burkle, F. M. (1995b). Complex humanitarian emergencies II: Medical liaison and training. *Prehospital and Disaster Medicine*, **10**:1, 43–47.

Burkle, F. M., McGrady, K. A. W., Newett, S., Nelson, J. J., Dworken, J. T., Lyerly, W. H., Natsios, A. S., and Lillibridge, S. R. (1995). Complex humanitarian emergencies III: Measures of effectiveness. *Prehospital and Disaster Medicine*, **10**:1, 48–56.

Demaio, A., Jamieson, J., Horn, R., de Courten, M., and Tellier, S. (2013). Non-communicable diseases in emergencies: A call to action. *PLOS Currents* – Disasters.

Enhancing Learning and Research for Humanitarian Assistance (ELRHA). Improving humanitarian outcomes through partnership, research, and innovation. Available at: www.elrha.org/about/our-work/. Accessed March 1, 2017.

Humphries, V. (2013). Improving humanitarian coordination: Common challenges and lessons learned from the cluster approach. *The Journal of Humanitarian Assistance*. Available at: https://sites.tufts.edu/jha/archives/1976. (Accessed March 10, 2017).

Inter-Agency Standing Committee (IASC). (2011a). Operational guidance for cluster lead agencies on working with national authorities. Available at: www.humanitarianresponse.info/system/files/documents/files/IASC%20Guidance%20on%20Working%20with%20National%20Authorities_July2011.pdf. (Accessed March 10, 2017).

Inter-Agency Standing Committee (IASC). (2011b). Global health cluster – Civil-military coordination during humanitarian health action. Provisional version. Available at: www.who.int/hac/global_health_cluster/about/policy_strategy/ghc_position_paper_civil_military_coord_2_feb2011.pdf (Accessed December 15, 2015).

Inter-Agency Standing Committee (IASC). (2015). Reference module for cluster coordination at the country level. Available at: www.who.int/health-cluster/about/cluster-system/cluster-coordination-reference-module-2015.pdf (Accessed March 13, 2017).

Lautze, S., Leaning, J., Raven-Roberts, A., Kent, R., and Mazurana, D. (2004). Assistance, protection, and governance networks in complex emergencies. *Lancet*, **364**:2134–2141.

Médecins Sans Frontières (MSF). (1997). *Refugee health: An approach to emergency situations*, London: Macmillan.

Metcalfe, V., Haysom, S., and Gordon, S. (2012). Trends and challenges in humanitarian civil–military coordination: A review of the literature. Humanitarian Policy Group. Available at: www.odi.org/publications/6584-civilian-military-humanitarian-response (Accessed November 11, 2015).

Morgan, O., Tidball-Binz, M., and van Alphen, D., eds. (2009). *Management of dead bodies after disasters: a field manual for first responders*. Washington, DC: Pan American Health Organization (PAHO).

Noji, E. K. and Toole, M. J. (1997). The historical development of public health response to disasters. *Disasters*, **21**:4, 366–376.

The Sphere Project. (2014). Available at: www.spherehandbook.org. (Accessed March 1, 2017).

Toole, M. J. and Waldman, R. J. (1997). The public health aspects of complex humanitarian emergencies and refugee situations. *Annu Rev Public Health*, **18**:283–312.

United Nations High Commissioner for Referees (UNHCR). Urban refugees. Available at: www.unhcr.org/en-us/urban-refugees.html (Accessed March 13, 2017).

United Nations Office for Disaster Risk Reduction (UNISDR). Hyogo Framework for Action (HFA). Available at: www.unisdr.org/we/coordinate/hfa (Accessed December 10, 2015).

United Nations Refugee Agency (UNHCR). (2012). The state of the world's refugees – In search of solidarity. Available at: www.unhcr.org/4fc5ceca9.pdf (Accessed October 25, 2016).

World Health Organization (WHO). (2007). Humanitarian health action: The cluster approach, Annex 7. Available at: ww.who.int/hac/techguidance/tools/manuals/who_field_handbook/annex_7/en/. (Accessed March 3, 2017).

World Health Organization (WHO). (2016). Emergency Medical Teams-World Health Organization EMT Initiative. Available at: www.who.int/hac/techguidance/preparedness/emergency_medical_teams/en/. (Accessed March 10, 2017).

Chapter 5

Epidemiology

Christine Dubray and Debarati Guha-Sapir

Introduction

Since the famines of 1984 in the Sahel region of Africa, there has been increased use of epidemiology in the setting of humanitarian emergencies, including both natural disasters and civil conflicts. Generally, epidemiology is used to describe a problem through numbers, rates, risk ratios, and other techniques such as prevalence and incidence. In humanitarian emergencies, epidemiology is used to identify and define health risks, suggest the most efficient response options, and monitor performance of the public health response.

This trend reflects a growing demand from donors, governments, military, and humanitarian groups for credible information to support the planning and evaluation of health inputs in war (McDonnell et al. 2004). In the last two decades, professional interest in expanding capacity for epidemiological analyses in the setting of humanitarian emergencies has significantly increased.

The use of key epidemiological indicators in humanitarian emergencies is essential to estimate the health needs of affected populations. Epidemiological methods are used to understand the scope and severity of humanitarian emergencies, including the health effects and the factors that contribute to these effects.

This chapter provides an overview of the use and application of epidemiology in humanitarian emergencies. It will also cover findings of studies on the main causes of morbidity and mortality, highlighting some of the differences between different types of emergencies. Other essential indicators used during humanitarian emergencies are discussed in chapters dedicated to specific topics including, for example, nutrition, surveys, water, sanitation, and hygiene (WASH), and vaccine preventable diseases.

Background

Many of the quantitative techniques used in humanitarian emergencies today are derived from epidemiology and related disciplines including demography or biostatistics. Epidemiological principles are now used widely in humanitarian emergencies for rapid health assessments, population surveys, outbreak investigations, program assessments, surveillance, and monitoring and evaluation.

In the early 1970s, the primary focus of epidemiology in humanitarian emergencies included outbreak investigation and risk factor analyses of mortality and morbidity. Today, the scope and use of epidemiologic techniques has widened considerably including setting priorities and resource allocation. Epidemiologic techniques such as rapid assessments may be used to describe the scope of a disease or health condition in the affected community and determine the damage and remaining capacity of the health system/infrastructure. Similarly, population surveys are central to calculate rates and risks. Given the constraints of human and material resources, choosing the most effective health interventions among many competing ones is a common and critical task of health managers. Epidemiological techniques can help inform these decisions.

In the setting of humanitarian emergencies, some common uses of epidemiology include:

- Identify the priority health problems in the affected community and determine interventions
- Determine the extent of disease within a community
- Identify the causes and risk factors of disease
- Determine the extent of damage and the capacity of the local health system/infrastructure
- Monitor health trends of the community
- Evaluate the impact of health programs (The Johns Hopkins Bloomberg School of Public Health and the International Federation of the Red Cross and Red Crescent Societies 2008).

Epidemiological Indicators

Indicators are measures that reflect the state of a population in terms of relevant parameters such as health or socioeconomic status. Indicators may be measured through surveys or from existing health information system. They might be quantitative or qualitative in nature. In humanitarian emergencies, indicators are useful for providing baseline measurements as well as measuring and describing the effects of a disaster on a population. During and after the response, these measurements help evaluate the effectiveness and outcome of the response. Indicators discussed in this chapter include mortality and morbidity indicators. A list of key indicators used during humanitarian emergencies is shown in Table 5.1.

Table 5.1 Surveillance indicators and sources of information

Type of Surveillance	Indicators	Source of Information
Demographic	• Total population • Population structure (age, sex) • Rate of migration (new arrivals, departures) • Identification of vulnerable groups • Births	• Registration records • Population census • Community health worker reports • Volunteers
Mortality	• Crude mortality rate (CMR) • Age-specific mortality rate (<5, >5) • Cause-specific mortality • Case fatality ratio (CFR)	• Hospital death registers • Religious leaders • Community reporters (including community health workers) • Burial shroud distribution • Burial contractors • Graveyards • Camp administration
Morbidity	• Incidence rate (new cases) • Prevalence (total existing cases) • Age-/sex-specific morbidity • Proportional morbidity	• Outpatient and admission records • Laboratories • Feeding center(s) records • Community health worker records
Nutrition	• Global malnutrition prevalence • Severe malnutrition prevalence • Weight gain/loss in maternal and child health (MCH) clinics • Prevalence of micronutrient deficiency disorders • Incidence of low birthweight • Average daily ration	• Nutrition surveys • MCH clinic records • Feeding center records • Birth registers • Camp administration
Program process	• Shelter coverage (link with incidence of acute respiratory infection [ARI]) • Feeding center enrollment and attendance • WASH (water quantity, quality, access, and monitor diarrhea incidence) • Immunization coverage • Reproductive health (antenatal care attendance, deliveries, family planning uptake, STI/HIV prevalence) • Outpatient and inpatient attendance • ORS distribution • Community-based mental health care	• Facility records • Immunization surveys • Other surveys (WASH, RH) • Traditional birth attendant records

Source: The Johns Hopkins and International Federation of Red Cross and Red Crescent Societies Public Health Guide for Emergencies, 2nd Edition, Geneva, 2008.

Affected Populations

The number of persons affected by humanitarian emergencies varies widely depending on the nature of the disaster (natural disasters vs. man-made/conflict), the location, and the duration. Similarly, the economic impact may vary considerably. It is important to determine who the affected population is, not only to target aid but also to provide a denominator for epidemiological measurements. For example, the civilian population affected by conflict can be divided into three categories: refugees, internally displaced people (IDPs), and conflict-affected residents (CAR) (Guha-Sapir and Dubus 2013).

Before 1990 and the end of the Cold War, the largest share of conflict-affected populations left the country and became refugees. At that time, they numbered around 40 to 50 million and some had a right to United Nations High Commissioner for Refugees (UNHCR) protection. Today, the number of refugees has declined to less than 20 million.

Those unable to cross an international border into a neighboring country, often settling in inhospitable conditions within their own country, are internally displaced persons (IDPs). They move, often en masse, to seek refuge away from conflict affected areas while remaining within national borders. Compared with refugees, access to IDPs is often compromised, as most do not live in camps and they are often located closer to conflict areas, and may be dispersed over large areas of regions. This impedes their access to health and other services, including vaccination programs and food distribution, making them more vulnerable to diseases.

Those unable to leave, live on as conflict-affected residents, and in many conflicts, represent the biggest share of the total victims. No estimates exist regarding how many people currently live in areas affected by conflict. Methodological problems in making such estimations are undoubtedly daunting, but this lack of population estimates may exclude these communities from adequate consideration in regular development programming. Conflict-affected residents experience the very worst conditions of nutrition and health, rivalling or surpassing those in the poorest areas of their own country (Guha-Sapir and D'Aoust 2011).

The definitions of the different affected populations are:

- **Internally displaced persons (IDPs)**: persons or groups of persons who have been forced or obliged to flee or to leave their homes or places of habitual residence, in particular as a result of or in order to avoid the effects or armed conflict, situations of generalized violence, violations of human rights or natural or human-made disasters, and who have not crossed in internationally recognized state border (UNHCR 2007).
- A **refugee**: any person who owing to a well-founded fear of being persecuted for reasons of race, religion, nationality, membership of a particular social group, or political opinion, is outside the country of his/her nationality, and is unable to or, owing to such fear, unwilling to avail himself/herself of the protection of that country (UNHCR 2010)
- **Conflict-affected residents**: the people affected by conflict who, for any reason, did not flee or leave their homes or places of habitual residence (Centre for Research on the Epidemiology of Disasters 2013)

Number of Persons Affected

Natural Disasters

The Centre for Research on the Epidemiology of Disasters (CRED)(Centre for Research on the Epidemiology of Disasters 2014a) has maintained an Emergency Events Database (EM-DAT) (Centre for Research on the Epidemiology of Disasters 2014c) since 1988 that collects core data on the occurrence and effect of mass disasters. The database focuses on natural and technological disasters. To be included in the database, at least one of the following criteria must be fulfilled:

- Ten or more people reported killed
- One hundred or more people affected
- A declaration of a state of emergency
- A call for international assistance

EM-DAT provides information on number of country-level disasters, countries affected, people killed, people affected, as well as the economic damages.

The number of people affected by disasters will be determined, to a large extent by the nature, scale, and location of these disasters. This is illustrated by the data collected by EM-DAT for the years 2004 and 2013. In 2004, 94 percent of all recorded deaths (241,400) from natural disasters were due to the Indian Ocean tsunami. In comparison, the year 2013 was characterized by the absence of natural disasters with large human impact. Overall, 334 country level

Section 1: Humanitarian Emergencies

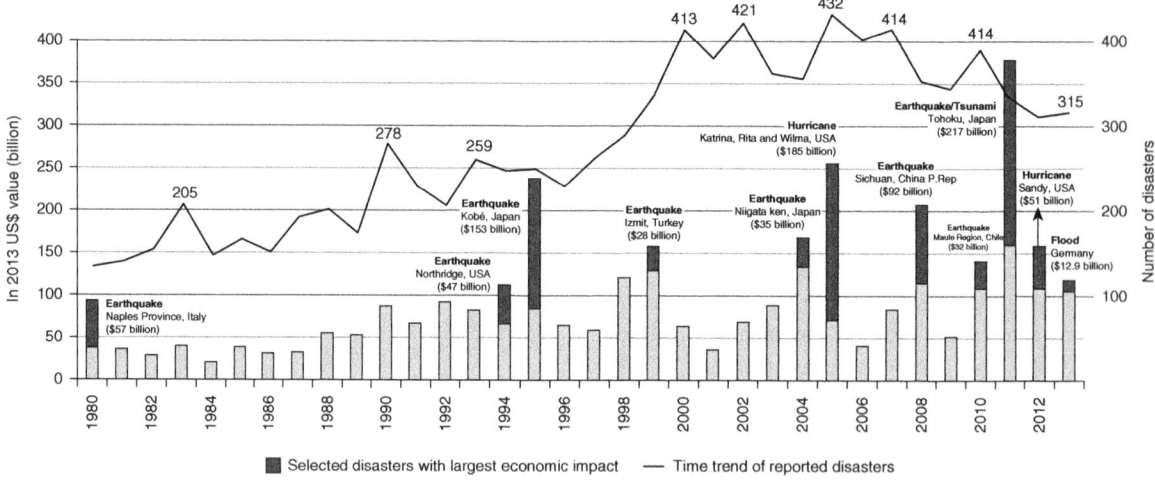

Figure 5.1 The annual occurrence and reported economic damages from disasters 1980–2013 (Centre for Research on the Epidemiology of Disasters, CREDCrunch, 35)

disasters were recorded in EM-DAT, 22,616 people were killed as a result of these disasters, and 96 million persons were affected. The total economic damages were estimated to be US$118B dollars.

The annual occurrence and reported economic damages from disasters during 1980–2013 are shown in Figure 5.1 (Centre for Research on the Epidemiology of Disasters 2014d). This graph illustrates that the economic impact caused by disasters are not related to the number of persons affected and vice versa. For example, the economic damage caused by the earthquake/tsunami that occurred in Japan in 2011 was estimated at $217 billion and the estimated number of persons affected was 368,820. In contrast, the estimated number of persons affected by the earthquake/tsunami that occurred in Indonesia in 2004 was 532,898 but the estimated economic damages were estimated at $4.4 billion, or 50 times less than the estimated economic damages for the earthquake/tsunami in Japan.

An analysis of the earthquakes in Haiti and Chile that happened only few months apart in 2010 also shows that the number of persons affected and the economic impact can vary dramatically even between apparently similar natural disasters. In Haiti, the magnitude of the earthquake was 7.0 and the epicenter was in Leogane, 25 km west of the densely-populated Port-au-Prince area, with a population of approximately 3 million. Approximately 230,000 persons died, 3.7 million were affected, and estimated damage was $8 billion dollars. In Chile, the magnitude of the earthquake was 8.8 and affected the Maule region with an estimated population of 1 million. Less than 600 persons died, 2.6 million persons were affected, and estimated damage was $32 billion dollars (CRED 2014a). These events are shown in Figure 5.1.

Conflicts

Civil conflicts may involve an entire country or region or be limited to selected areas while the rest of the country or region experiences relative stability. Health and population data for conflict-affected areas is scarce. Different sources of information can be consulted to estimate the number of people affected by conflict, but because of the difficulty in accessing recent data, most of these sources contain data that are not up to date.

The Office of the United Nations High Commissioner for Refugees (UNHCR) website (UNHCR 2014) provides information on the number of refugees and IDPs to whom UNHCR extends protection and or assistance. The Internal Displacement Monitoring Centre (IDMC) monitors and analyzes information on internal displacement. Data are broken down between displacement induced by conflict and violence and by natural disaster. The website also provides data on the proportion of IDPs protected or assisted by UNCHR. The estimated number of IDPs in 2012 due to conflict and violence was 28.8 million, and of those 17.7 million (61%) were protected/assisted by UNHCR (Internal Displacement

Monitoring Centre 2014). In 2013, it was estimated that in Syria alone more than 6.5 million persons were internally displaced and 2.1 million persons were refugees (Internal Displacement Monitoring Centre, 2014).

In 2013, the CRED published *People Affected by Conflict: Humanitarian Need in Number* (Centre for Research on the Epidemiology of Disasters 2013) in which a new methodology was described to estimate the number of conflict-affected residents. This document described that in 2012, the proportion of national population affected by conflicts ranged from 1 percent in Burundi to 92 percent in Libya. In Libya, 5.4 million people were conflict-affected residents, which represented 99 percent of the people affected by the conflict. In Syria, where 74 percent of the population was affected by the conflict in 2012, 4.2 million people were IDPs (25%), 0.5 million were refugees (3%) and 11.9 million were conflict-affected residents (72%). It is essential to understand the type of population(s) affected and the type of displacement (IDPs, refugees protected by UNCHCR, or local residents) since most of the assistance will be mediated by the type of population targeted. These results are shown in Figure 5.2.

ReliefWeb, a specialized digital service of the United Nations Office for the Coordination of Humanitarian Affairs (OCHA), also provides humanitarian actors with reliable and timely humanitarian information on global crises and disasters so they can make informed decisions and plan effective assistance (ReliefWeb 2014).

Mortality and Morbidity

When providing health assistance during a humanitarian emergency, information is needed to determine if the health of the population is improving or not, and whether the implemented program adequately addresses the burden of disease. Systematic measurement, analysis, and programmatic use of essential health indicators including mortality rate, prevalence of malnutrition, and coverage of essential services such as vaccination are described in various manuals and policy documents, however they are scarcely available (Checchi 2010). These indicators are important to quantify the magnitude of the crisis and monitor the effectiveness of health programs and other relief efforts, including providing important data on the impact on health, and are used to advocate for action. This section includes an explanation of mortality and morbidity indicators, an overview of the causes of mortality and morbidity, and a description of various initiatives and manuals that provide useful guidelines and information for responders to humanitarian emergencies.

Mortality Indicators

The rate of civilian deaths in humanitarian emergencies is the most used indicator to assess the urgency for humanitarian assistance. Most deaths during humanitarian emergencies are due to preventable causes, especially increased rates of infectious diseases, malnutrition, and violent trauma. Non-communicable diseases are also thought to contribute to mortality during humanitarian emergencies, especially in urban settings and middle-income countries. Mortality rates within vulnerable populations, such as children less than five years of age, may be earlier indicators of the decline in the overall health of a population.

Information on the cause of mortality can help target limited resources and be used to advocate for additional resources. Data on mortality rates collected over time can monitor the impact of events, such as armed conflict or natural disaster, as well as the effect of specific interventions such as childhood vaccination (Cairns et al. 2009). Conversely, mortality can be considered as a late indicator: by the time the mortality rates spike, the conditions are likely to be serious and redress can be difficult or impossible (Guha-Sapir and D'Aoust 2011).

Mortality rates are often developed from demographic principles and are commonly used to indicate disease severity, health system performance, or the impact of violent events. However, the various rates and nomenclature are frequently confused. Rates derived from calculations for a virtual birth cohort that is followed over time indicate the probability of dying before a certain age and include the true population at risk of dying. Mortality rates, therefore, are often expressed per 1,000 live births. This calculation method is commonly used for infant mortality rates and was recently introduced for other age groups. Mortality rates used during humanitarian emergencies, on the other hand, are not based on a virtual birth cohort but use a midterm population count as the denominator. This does not represent the true population at risk, because the number changes within the period considered, due to migration, births, and deaths. Death rates are expressed per 1,000 or 10,000 population per day, month, or year.

Section 1: Humanitarian Emergencies

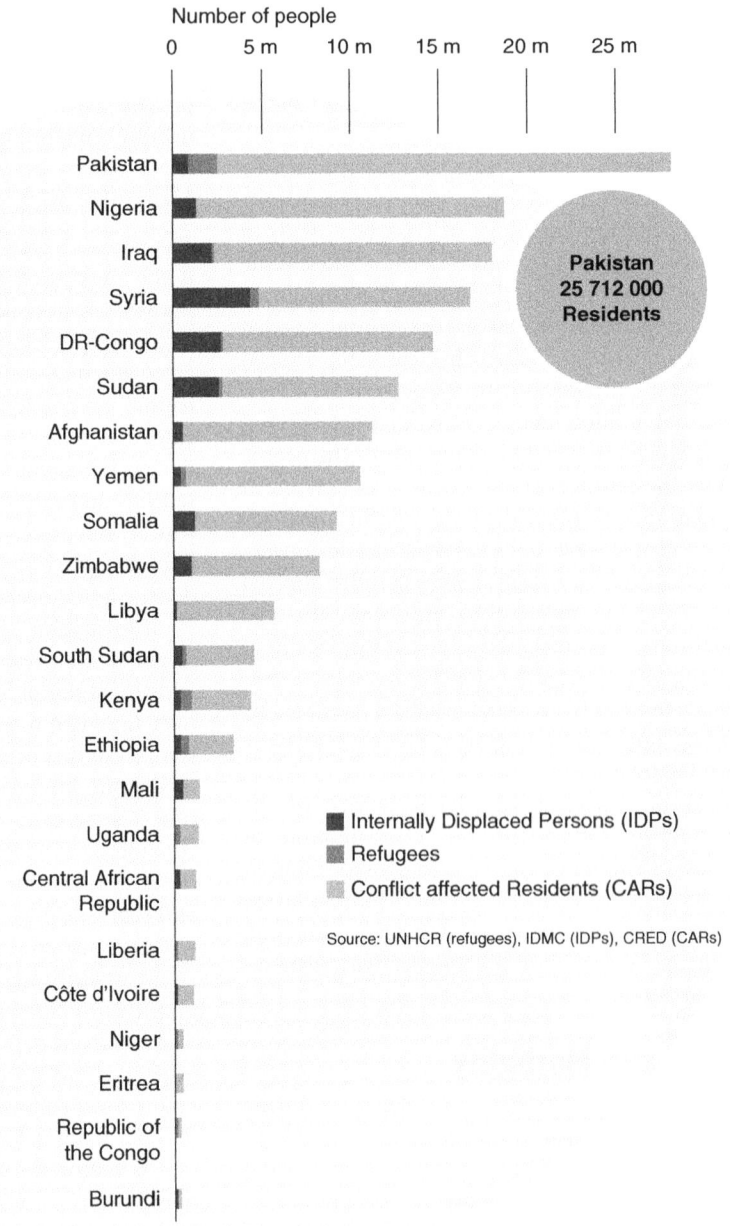

Figure 5.2 Number of people affected by conflict (PAC) by country in 2012. (c) EM-DAT: The Emergency Events Database – Université catholique de Louvain (UCL) – CRED, D. Guha-Sapir – www.emdat.be, Brussels, Belgium.

During humanitarian emergencies, mortality rates may be estimated from hospital and burial records, community-based reporting systems through surveillance, or retrospective population surveys. Mortality surveys conducted during humanitarian emergencies rarely cover the entire affected population and mapping information coverage in real time to draw attention to the regions where information is lacking or outdated is important to coordinate efforts to gather data (Checchi 2010). In addition, most surveys take place in relatively secure zones, and it is possible that the most affected communities are in areas inaccessible to those performing the surveys. However, secure zones might also act as a magnet for the most severely affected members of the population, especially where humanitarian assistance has been deployed. In either case, it is difficult to extrapolate the findings of mortality surveys conducted in specific locations to broader populations, especially those in conflict-affected areas (Toole and Waldman 1997).

Although consensus has slowly developed on the methodology to accurately measure mortality indicators, errors in the application of the survey methodology and analysis have persisted. In a study that aimed to identify common methodological weaknesses in mortality surveys and to provide practical recommendations for improvement, only 3.2 percent of crude mortality rate surveys met the criteria for quality (Prudhon and Spiegel 2007). It is therefore important to develop initiatives that help establish a range of standards and indicators to inform the planning, coordination, monitoring, and evaluation of humanitarian response. Measurement of mortality indicators through prospective community surveillance could provide real-time information for action, but it is prone to under-reporting. A surveillance system should build upon the existing health information system (HIS) whenever possible. In some disasters, a new or parallel HIS may be required. This is determined by an assessment of the performance and adequacy of the existing HIS and the information needs for the current emergency. During the response, data on mortality should include, but not be limited to, deaths recorded by health facilities including under-five deaths, proportional mortality, and cause-specific mortality (The Sphere Project 2011).

The Network Paper, *Interpreting and using mortality data in humanitarian Emergencies: A primer for nonepidemiologists,* describes the key indicators used to measure mortality rates and how to assess, interpret, and use mortality reports (Checchi and Roberts 2005). The paper also discusses the politics of mortality figures. The SMART (Standardized Monitoring and Assessment of Relief and Transitions) Methodology is an inter-agency initiative launched in 2002 by a network of organizations and humanitarian practitioners (SMART 2014). It looks to reform and harmonize assessments of, and responses to emergencies, including surveillance. The SMART Methodology website provides guidelines and training on mortality and nutritional survey methods that balances simplicity and technical soundness. The Complex Emergency Database (CE-DAT), a database of mortality and malnutrition rates, is managed by the CRED and was created in 2003 as an outcome of SMART (Centre for Research on the Epidemiology of Disasters 2014b). Nutrition indicators are discussed in Chapter 12.

The most frequently used indicators for population mortality include (Checchi and Roberts 2005):

- The **mortality rate**: number of deaths occurring in a given population at risk during a specified time period. In emergencies, this is usually expressed as deaths per 10,000 persons per day. Alternatively, it may be expressed as deaths per 1,000 persons per month or per year.
- The **crude mortality rate (CMR)**: the mortality rate among all groups due to all causes. The **emergency threshold** is considered to be ≥1 per 10,000 per day with an assumed baseline of 0.5 per 10,000 per day.

$$\text{CMR} = \frac{\text{Total deaths during the time period}}{\text{Mid} - \text{period population at risk} \times \text{duration of time peroid}} \times 10,000$$

- The **under-five (U5) mortality rate**: the number of deaths occurring in a given population of children under five years old during a specified time period. The emergency threshold is considered to be ≥2 per 10,000 per day with an assumed baseline of 1 per 10,000 per day.

$$\text{U5MR} = \frac{\text{Total deaths of U5 during the time period}}{\text{Mid} - \text{period U5 population at risk} \times \text{duration of time peroid}} \times 10,000$$

- The **cause-specific mortality rate**: the mortality rate due to a specific disease (e.g. cholera) or phenomenon (e.g. violence).

Morbidity Indicators

Morbidity rates or incidence rates refer to the number of new cases of illness or injury, occurring in a given population at risk, during a specified period of time (Sphere Project Glossary). Morbidity rates, especially the incidence of infectious diseases, are essential for prioritizing health interventions and detecting epidemics, and are considered a leading indicator (vs. a late indicator) as they allow a better understanding of cause of death and type of intervention needed (Brennan and Nandy 2001).

Morbidity indicators can be calculated retrospectively through survey methods or analysis of medical records, or, ideally, through passive or active prospective surveillance. During emergencies, a specialized surveillance system such as the early warning and response network (EWARN) is used for detecting and responding to disease outbreaks. The ministry of health usually sets it up with support from WHO and other partners. Additional objectives of these systems are to monitor trends of diseases and clinical activities (WHO 2010). Surveillance is discussed in detail in Chapter 9. Even when a surveillance system is implemented, incidence rates can be difficult or impossible to calculate as the total population of interest may be unknown or subject to substantial and rapid change, as often happens during displacement (Polonsky et al. 2013). Even when the total population is known, measuring morbidity rates can be challenging in light of frequent movement of the population, such as daily new arrivals in a refugee camp.

The most frequently used indicators for population morbidity include:

- The **incidence rate**: the number of new cases of a disease that occur during a specified period of time in a population at risk of developing the disease.

$$\frac{\text{Number of new cases of a disease in a time period}}{\text{Population at risk of developing the disease} \times \text{Number of months in the time period}} \times 1,000 = \text{New cases}/1,000 \text{ persons/month}$$

- The **attack rate**: often used as a synonym for cumulative incidence during an outbreak. It is the risk of getting the disease during a specified time period, such as the duration of an outbreak.

Causes of Mortality and Morbidity

The primary goal in responding to humanitarian emergencies is to prevent and reduce excess mortality and morbidity. This includes aiming to maintain or reduce the CMR and U5MR at or less than double the baseline rate documented for the population prior to the disaster. Different types of disaster are associated with differing scales and patterns of mortality and morbidity, and the health needs of an affected population will vary according to the type and extent of the disaster (The Sphere Project 2011).

Even for a specific type of disaster, morbidity and mortality may vary significantly depending on the context. The estimated public health impacts of selected disasters are shown in Table 5.2 (*Sphere Handbook* 2011).

In the case of rapid onset natural disasters such as earthquakes and hurricanes, most death and injuries occur during the first few hours and secondary public health effects are related to displacement of the affected population, destruction of public utilities, and disruption of basic health services and infrastructure. Long-term public health consequences can be due to crop destruction or prolonged population displacement in unsanitary camps or settlements. Outbreaks of communicable diseases are rare following natural disasters in industrialized countries; however, outbreaks of diarrheal diseases and hepatitis have occurred following some natural disasters in developing countries (Toole and Waldman 1997).

Table 5.2 Public health impact of selected disasters (*Sphere Handbook* 2011)

Effect	Complex emergencies	Earthquakes	High winds	Floods	Flash floods/tsunamis
Deaths	Many	Many	Few	Few	Many
Severe injuries	Varies	Many	Moderate	Few	Few
Increased risk of communicable diseases	High	Varies*	Small	Varies*	Varies*
Food scarcity	Common	Rare	Rare	Varies	Common
Major population displacements	Common	Rare (may occur in heavily damaged urban areas)	Rare (may occur in heavily damaged urban areas)	Common	Varies

* Dependent on the postdisaster displacement and living conditions of the population.

In conflict-affected settings, 60–90 percent of deaths have been attributed to four major infectious causes:
- Acute respiratory infections
- Diarrhea
- Measles
- Malaria (where endemic)

Acute malnutrition exacerbates these diseases, especially in children under 5 years of age. When outbreaks occur, they are generally associated with risk factors such as population displacement, overcrowding, inadequate shelter, insufficient and unsafe water, and inadequate sanitation (*The Sphere Project* 2011).

Infectious Diseases

The 2010 earthquake in Haiti killed approximately 230,000 people in a matter of minutes, injured over 300,000, and destroyed numerous health care facilities. In some areas, 70 percent of homes were destroyed or damaged (United Nations Office for the Coordination of Humanitarian Affairs 2011). With a population of over 3 million in the affected areas, this equates to a mortality rate of approximately 72 deaths per 1,000 (Doocy et al. 2013a). A surveillance system implemented shortly after the earthquake identified ARIs, acute watery diarrhea, and malaria/fever of unknown origin as the predominant causes of morbidity. The CMR and the U5MR were generally below the emergency thresholds for Latin America and the Caribbean (<0.3 deaths per 10,000 person-days for both CDR and U5MR) during the period of surveillance. In October 2010, 10 months after the earthquake, a *Vibrio cholerae* outbreak was detected in Haiti. A disease that had been absent from the country for a century, the transmission of *Vibrio cholerae* among the Haitian population was facilitated by factors such as overcrowding, poverty, poor nutrition, inadequate water, and sanitation infrastructure and a strained health infrastructure. The National Cholera Surveillance System (NCSS), established after the beginning of the outbreak, identified more than 600,000 cases of infection and 7,436 deaths over a 22-month period. The cumulative attack rate was 5.1 percent at the end of the first year and 6.1 percent at the end of the second year. The departmental cumulative case fatality rate at the 2-year mark ranged from 0.6 percent to 4.6 percent (Barzilay et al. 2013).

Measles can be particularly deadly among displaced, vulnerable populations. Crowded living conditions, low vaccination coverage, and malnutrition in refugee camps and settlements can lead to or increase the likelihood of measles outbreaks with severe morbidity and mortality. In 2011, a large measles outbreak occurred in Dadaab, Kenya among refugees fleeing famine and conflict in Somalia. The massive influx of vulnerable refugees combined with ongoing measles virus transmission in the region led to an explosive measles outbreak in the congested camps. According to unpublished data from the UNHCR, 1,366 measles cases and 32 measles deaths were reported between June and November 2011. Cases and deaths were mostly among refugees who arrived in 2011. Gastrointestinal, respiratory, and neurological complications and acute malnutrition were commonly diagnosed in children hospitalized for measles. The CFR among children who were hospitalized in Dadaab during the 2011 measles outbreak was 4.6 percent (Mahamud et al. 2013).

Injury, Noncommunicable Diseases, and Mental Illness

Although surveillance systems tend to focus on diseases with epidemic potential, injuries, mental health conditions, and chronic diseases can also account for a large proportion of health-related needs in humanitarian emergencies. The proportion of the population affected by these conditions will vary according to context and location such as urban or rural and industrialized or developing countries. For example, in Haiti after the 2010 earthquake, approximately two-thirds of conditions recorded by the surveillance system were not included in the list of diseases under surveillance and were listed under "other." These were primarily mental health conditions, physical injuries sustained during the earthquake, and typical chronic conditions such as cardiovascular disease and diabetes (Polonsky et al. 2013).

After the 2004 Indian Ocean tsunami, medical-treatment facilities were established to respond to the health need of the population. The pattern of diseases was assessed in one such facility, an International Red Cross Committee (ICRC) field hospital in Banda Aceh, Indonesia. The most frequently seen conditions were respiratory diseases (21%), chronic diseases such as diabetes and hypertension (17%), trauma and injury (10%), and mental health problems (10%). There was an increase of chronic disease in the first week of the study that could be attributed to the complete absence of health services in the previous two weeks, causing an interruption of treatment and resulting in patients seeking care as soon as the field hospital opened (Guha-Sapir et al. 2007).

A study to identify health-related needs of residents returning home after Hurricane Katrina struck the Gulf Coast of the United States in 2005 showed that 56 percent of households contained one or more members with chronic health conditions and 50 percent of adults exhibited high levels of emotional distress, indicating a potential need for mental health services (CDC 2006).

Mental health and psychosocial problems occur in all humanitarian emergencies. The horrors, losses, uncertainties and numerous other stressors associated with conflict and other disasters place people at increased risk of diverse social, behavioral, psychological, and psychiatric problems. Mental health and psychosocial support involves multisectoral, coordinated implementation including a cross-cluster or cross-sectoral working group (*The Sphere Project* 2011).

One study in Haiti illustrates the importance of collecting data related to mental health conditions in order to appropriately address these conditions among the affected population during the emergency and reconstruction phase of the disaster. The study documented the association between earthquake-related experiences and the risk for posttraumatic stress disorder (PTSD) and major depressive disorder (MDD) 2–4 months following the 2010 Haiti earthquake. The study uncovered an extraordinary burden of traumatic events and stressors experienced by the population after the earthquake. The prevalence of PTSD and MDD two months after the event among the 1,315 respondents, were 24.6 percent and 28.3 percent respectively. Further, the impact of selected pre- and postearthquake factors on PTSD and MDD was stronger for individuals who had a prior history of violent trauma. Finally, experiences associated with MDD and PTSD differed, at least marginally significantly, between men and women (Cerda et al. 2013).

Injury is usually the major cause of excess mortality and morbidity following acute onset natural disasters such as earthquakes. Many acute onset natural disasters are mass casualty events, meaning there are more victims than locally available resources can manage using standard procedures. A review of earthquakes between 1980 and 2009 describes the impact of earthquakes in terms of mortality, injury, and displacement (Doocy et al. 2013b). Injuries were reported for 420 earthquakes with an estimated total of 995,219 reported injuries (range: 845,345–1,145,093). Using the highest reported number for the event there were an average of 3,499 (median = 100, range 1–374,171) injuries per earthquake. The primary cause of earthquake related mortality was building collapse most frequently leading to soft tissue injuries, fractures, and crush injuries/syndrome. Risk factors for earthquake-related death and injury included very young and very old age, poor socioeconomic status, being indoors, and being in a poorly constructed building during the time of the event. Earthquake losses are likely to increase in future years due to population growth in high-risk seismic areas and in the case of low- and medium development areas, inadequate construction quality.

The health effects of Non-communicable diseases should not be forgotten when planning to respond to humanitarian emergencies. The potential ways in which excess morbidity and mortality related to non-communicable diseases (NCDs) might occur during humanitarian emergencies have been described (Demaio et al. 2013). First, persons with NCDs are more vulnerable in humanitarian emergencies as they are likely less able to cope without access to adequate nutrition, medications, and close follow-up. Second, there may be acute exacerbations and complications of NCDs because consistent access to health systems, medications, and providers may not be possible during and following an emergency. Third, humanitarian emergencies can result in long-term implications for persons with NCDs. Suboptimal management of NCDs during and after a humanitarian emergency can lead to social and health ramifications. Finally, the impact of NCDs and humanitarian emergencies is reflected in the fact that developing countries are often disproportionately burdened with both NCDs and disasters in comparison to higher income countries. This may be exacerbated by the increase in urbanization and growing slum-populations. Common examples of NCDs that need particular attention during humanitarian emergencies are diabetes, renal failure requiring dialysis, and chronic respiratory and cardiac diseases.

Flooding is now the most common type of disaster worldwide, and flash flooding, usually associated with

Chapter 5: Epidemiology

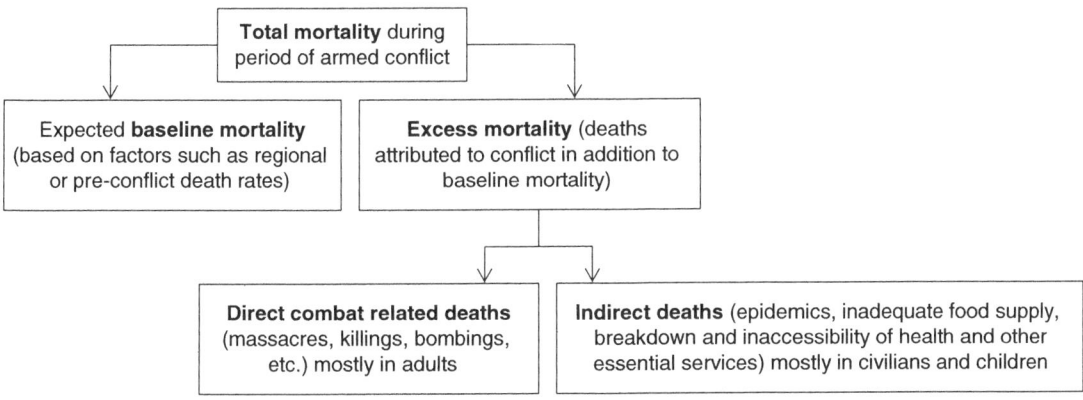

Figure 5.3 The direct and indirect health consequences of armed conflict. (c) Centre for Research on the Epidemiology of Disasters – CRED (2013) People affected by conflict: Humanitarian needs in numbers. CRED: Brussels.

tropical storms, is the leading cause of weather-related deaths in the United States (Diaz 2004).

Nonfatal injuries together with exacerbation of chronic illness are the leading causes of morbidity among affected residents immediately following floods (Alderman et al. 2012). In the aftermath of Hurricane Katrina, an active injury and illness surveillance system was established in functioning hospitals and medical clinics. From September 8 to October 14, 2005, injury-related visits represented 29 percent (7,543/26,192) of the total visits to medical treatment facilities. Common mechanisms of injury were cut/pierce/stab (20%), fall (20%), struck by/against/crush (11%), bite/sting (9%), and motor-vehicle crash (8%) (Sullivent et al. 2006). During major disasters, prospective surveillance systems that document morbidity associated with injuries and other frequent health-related problems in a timely manner help initiate health-targeted prevention activities and communication campaigns.

The changing demographics of armed conflict have shifted the burden of losses from combatants to civilian populations. The health consequences of armed conflict, described as both direct and indirect, are shown in Figure 5.3. Direct health consequences include violent death, injury, disability, psychological trauma, and sexual violence. Indirect health consequences of armed conflict are attributed to social disruption and the collapse of health systems and services. These include increased rates of infectious diseases, malnutrition, and complications of chronic disease. It is important to note that both the direct and indirect health consequences occur in every conflict. Different patterns of morbidity and mortality can be discerned between humanitarian emergencies in the developing world and in Europe (Brennan and Nandy 2001).

Data from the CE-DAT database were used in an analysis of retrospective mortality surveys that were done in Darfur between February 2003 and December 2008 (Degomme and Guha-Sapir 2010). The analysis examined the association of all age, child (≤5 years), and cause-specific mortality with variables such as the proportion of internally displaced people in the surveyed population, the conflict phase, and the location (one of three states in Darfur). The model was used to retrospectively predict patterns in mortality rates and excess number of deaths for the entire affected population in Darfur. The estimated number of excess deaths during the study period was about 300,000. With a higher baseline, there would be about 90,000 fewer excess deaths. Mortality rates decreased after peaking near the end of 2003 to early 2004 when the CMR was eight to ten times higher than expected and almost four times higher than the emergency level of one death per 10,000 people per day. Although during the peak of displacement and attacks in 2004, mortality was mainly attributed to violence, 80 percent of the 300,000 estimated deaths were due to disease during the entire period from 2004–2008. These results are in agreement with studies of other conflicts in which initial mortality peaks were often related to a period of intense violence and subsequently a high number of violence related deaths, but the main causes of mortality during the stabilization period were diseases such as diarrhea rather than violence. The study also found that surveys of populations with large proportions of IDPs had higher mortality rates than did those consisting of only nondisplaced individuals.

Characteristics of Humanitarian Emergencies

The World Health Organization defines a complex humanitarian emergency as a humanitarian crisis in a country, region, or society where there is total or considerable breakdown of authority resulting from internal or external conflict and which requires an international response that goes beyond the mandate or capacity of any single and/or ongoing UN country program (WHO 2014). Those suffering the consequences of the violence are primarily civilians (50%–90%) and especially vulnerable populations including children, women, the elderly, and the disabled (Burkle 2006).

In general, armed conflicts have decreased globally but advances in small-arms technology and struggles over natural resources make conflict resolution challenging and civilians bear the burden. Families are forced to move from their homes to escape internecine violence. Refugees cross national borders and are legally entitled to assistance in United Nations–managed camps. Increasingly since the mid-1980s, people have been unable to cross international frontiers and so remain internally displaced (Leaning and Guha-Sapir 2013). Conflict and post-conflict environments are often characterized by fragile ceasefires and continuing conflict with varying levels of intensity, susceptibility to reversals, and opportunity. It is estimated that 40 percent of countries emerging from conflict experience conflict again within a decade. In Africa, this percentage rises to 60 percent (Garfield et al. 2012).

The majority of humanitarian assistance is directed at the recovery and rehabilitation of basic public health infrastructure required both by civilian and military-aid providers under mandates of international humanitarian law. Traditionally, humanitarian assistance has been primarily focused on refugee and IDPs populations, most often in rural settings. In the last two decades, however, rural populations, especially in Asia and Africa, have moved to urban areas, seeking security and social services. Urban public health infrastructure demands are more complex and have not kept up with the growing and increasingly dense urban populations. Consequently, humanitarian assistance is moving to urban centers. It has now become a challenge for humanitarian actors to support the type and complexity of public health infrastructure recovery required in urban settings (Burkle 2006).

Three models for conflict-affected countries have been proposed (Burkle 2006):

Developing countries

Conflict-affected developing countries are primarily seen in Africa and Asia. They are characterized by acute-onset severe malnutrition, outbreaks of communicable diseases, and a failure of basic public health infrastructure including water, sanitation, food, shelter, and fuel. Studies confirm that most deaths are from preventable diseases, such as measles, diarrhea, acute respiratory illnesses, and malnutrition (Coghlan et al. 2006). Although these diseases are common to many developing countries, the deteriorating public health conditions and malnutrition eventually lead to poor immunity and micronutrient-deficiency diseases. The epidemiological pattern will result in overall high crude death rates, with the majority coming from under-five deaths. Additional age and gender-specific death rates will further define the nature and extent of vulnerability.

Smoldering or chronic countries

Smoldering or chronic countries are those that have been in conflict for many years such as the Democratic Republic of Congo. These countries share a history of many years of violence, social and political unrest, poor maintenance of basic public health infrastructure, little access to health and education, and a below-sustenance-level economy. The baseline health profile includes chronic malnutrition and stunted growth. In these countries women lack access to basic reproductive health services such as safe birthing practices and tetanus immunizations, leading to high maternal and infant mortality rates. There are few indigenous health-care providers, and NGO programs often represent the only public health infrastructure available. The health profile deteriorates even further when armed conflicts increase or when the country is hit by a natural disaster like the earthquake that struck Haiti in January 2010 after years of social and political unrest. Though this epidemiological model reveals priorities in emergency relief and critical development, the international aid response tends to focus on emergency relief with little emphasis placed on long-term development. Death rates are typically higher in the under-five population, but adult populations can also suffer high death rates when fleeing rebel forces, as was seen at the beginning of the conflict in Darfur (Depoortere et al. 2004).

Developed countries

Conflict in developed countries such as the former Yugoslavia, Iraq, and Chechnya are characterized by high rates of advanced weapon-related deaths. These humanitarian emergencies occur in relatively healthy populations with preconflict health profiles similar to that seen in Western industrialized countries. With increasing violence, populations flee; however, elderly populations often resist displacement from their ancestral homes despite the surrounding violence, often suffering complications of untreated chronic diseases such as diabetes, heart disease, high blood pressure, and under-nutrition. Epidemics, common to the developing and chronic smoldering country models, are rarely seen. Even with a deteriorating public health infrastructure, the educated population in developed countries is aware of the need for basic hygiene and handwashing. In this model, high crude death rates will be expected as adults die from war-related injuries. In addition, rape and psychological trauma are common consequences of ethnic cleansing. There will be comparatively low death rates among children under the age of five if public health protections remain intact. The longer a complex emergency is allowed to continue in a developed country, the more severe the effects on public health infrastructure and access. The health profiles begin to deteriorate and can mirror those characteristically seen in the developing and chronic smoldering country models.

Conclusion

Field epidemiology in crisis settings is central for evidence-based decision-making and monitoring progress of interventions. The methods used are largely standard epidemiological methods with new adaptations to account for transient populations and insecure settings. The use of epidemiological methods may differ between armed conflict and natural disasters as the challenges and problems and nature of response can be substantially different. While conflicts are characterized by mass displacement, violence, and breakdown of health structures, natural disaster settings present different constraints. Examples from both contexts are presented in this chapter. Specialized training of field staff in the uses of epidemiology has expanded and courses for different types of health personnel at different levels of competence are increasingly available. However, training opportunities in the affected regions are still limited and more involvement of national institutes is required. One challenge that remains is the need for development of better approaches for assessing morbidity and cause of death in these settings. These are indisputably difficult challenges to resolve but are nonetheless central to improving effectiveness and sustainability of the humanitarian interventions.

Notes from the Field

Darfur (2004)

An epidemiological study of the effect of armed incursions on mortality was carried out in Darfur in 2004 to provide a basis for appropriate assistance to IDPs (Depoortere et al. 2004). The surveys took place among 215,400 IDPs in four sites of West Darfur. The mortality recall period covered both the predisplacement and postdisplacement period in three sites. Heads of households described the family structure and provided dates, causes, and places of deaths. The mortality rates, expressed as deaths per 10,000 per day, before displacement in the three sites where this information was available were 5.9 (95% CI 2.2–14.9), 9.5 (6.4–14.0), and 7.3 (3.2–15.7), clearly above the emergency threshold. Violence caused 68%–93% of these deaths. People who were killed were mostly adult men, but included women and children. U5MR for that period in the three sites were 2.8 (95% CI 0.9–7.8), 2.1 (1.0–4.2) and 1.5 (0.1–10.3). Most households fled because of direct village attacks. This study is a good illustration of how field epidemiology can help orient and evaluate relief programs, as well as how it can provide key testimony about past events.

Rwanda (1994)

In July 1994, hundreds of thousands of people fleeing Rwanda crossed the border into Zaire (now the Democratic Republic of Congo) at Goma. In a week, epidemics of cholera and shigellosis spread in this population. A mortality survey in Katale, a camp located 80 km north of Goma, found an extraordinary high mortality rate among the refugee populations (Paquet and van Soest 1994). A mortality household cluster survey was carried out in the camps. A total of 344 deaths were reported by the heads of the 594 households examined that represented 8.3 percent (95% CI 7.1–9.5) of the initial population of 4,163. Over the 20 days of the recall period, this corresponded to an average CMR of 41.3 per 10,000 daily, which is 40 times the emergency threshold. U5MR was extremely high as well, 40.4 per 10,000 daily over the same period. Cholera, dysentery, or other diarrheal diseases were associated with 90 percent of the deaths. The survey also identified that 16 percent of the households did not include a male adult and 47 percent did not have any distributed material for shelter.

Haiti (2010)

An examination of the rapid establishment of an IDP surveillance system (IDPSS) after the 2010 earthquake in Haiti highlights the complexity of collecting morbidity data during large complex emergencies (CDC 2010). The primary challenges of implementing IDPSS were communication difficulties with an ever-changing group of NGO partners and limitations to the utility of IDPSS data because of lack of reliable camp population denominator estimates. The hundreds of IDP camps that were established spontaneously in Port-au-Prince further complicated IDPSS data collection. A cluster approach was used to coordinate the Haiti humanitarian response, and the IDPSS experience reinforced the need to improve local communication and coordination strategies. It also showed the need to develop and distribute easily adaptable standard surveillance tools, develop an interdisciplinary strategy for an early and reliable population census, and develop communication strategies using locally available internet and cellular networks during humanitarian emergencies.

References

Alderman, K., Turner, L. R., and Tong, S. (2012). Floods and human health: A systematic review. *Environ Int*, **47**, 37–47.

Barzilay, E. J., Schaad, N., Magloire, R., Mung, K. S., Boncy, J., Dahourou, G. A., Mintz, E. D., Steenland, M. W., Vertefeuille, J. F., and Tappero, J. W. (2013). Cholera surveillance during the Haiti epidemic–the first 2 years. *N Engl J Med*, **368**(7), 599–609.

Brennan, R. J. and Nandy, R. (2001a). Complex humanitarian emergencies: A major global health challenge. *Emerg Med (Fremantle)*, **13**(2), 147–156.

Brennan, R. J. and Nandy, R. (2001). Complex humanitarian emergencies: A major global health challenge. *Emerg Med*, **13**(2), 147–156.

Burkle, F. M. (2006). Complex humanitarian emergencies: A review of epidemiological and response models. *J Postgrad Med*, **52**(2), 110–115.

Cairns, K. L., Woodruff, B. A., Myatt, M., Bartlett, L., Goldberg, H., and Roberts, L. (2009). Cross-sectional survey methods to assess retrospectively mortality in humanitarian emergencies. *Disasters*, **33**(4), 503–521.

CDC. (2006). Assessment of health-related needs after Hurricanes Katrina and Rita–Orleans and Jefferson Parishes, New Orleans area, Louisiana, October 17–22, 2005. *MMWR Morb Mortal Wkly Rep*, **55**(2), 38–41.

CDC. (2010). Rapid establishment of an internally displaced persons disease surveillance system after an earthquake – Haiti, 2010. *MMWR Morb Mortal Wkly Rep*, **59**(30), 939–45.

Centre for Research on the Epidemiology of Disasters. (2013). People affected by conflict: humanitarian needs in number.

Centre for Research on the Epidemiology of Disasters. (2014a). Available at: www.cred.be/ (Accessed July 20, 2014).

Centre for Research on the Epidemiology of Disasters. (2014b). Complex Emergency Database, Available at: http://cedat.be/ (Accessed July 24, 2014).

Centre for Research on the Epidemiology of Disasters. (2014c). Emergency Events Database, Available at: www.emdat.be/ (Accessed July 18, 2014).

Centre for Research on the Epidemiology of Disasters. (2014d). Natural disasters in 2013. CRED Crunch, (35), Available at: http://cred.be/sites/default/files/CredCrunch35.pdf (Accessed July 18, 2014).

Cerda, M., Paczkowski, M., Galea, S., Nemethy, K., Pean, C., and Desvarieux, M. (2013). Psychopathology in the aftermath of the Haiti earthquake: A population-based study of posttraumatic stress disorder and major depression. *Depress Anxiety*, **30**(5), 413–424.

Checchi, F. (2010). Estimating the number of civilian deaths from armed conflicts. *Lancet*, **375**(9711), 255–257.

Checchi, F. and Roberts, L. (2005). Interpreting and using mortality data in humanitarian emergencies. *Humanitarian Practice Network*, 52.

Coghlan, B., Brennan, R. J., Ngoy, P., Dofara, D., Otto, B., Clements, M., and Stewart, T. (2006). Mortality in the Democratic Republic of Congo: A nationwide survey. *Lancet*, **367**(9504), 44–51.

Degomme, O. and Guha-Sapir, D. (2010). Patterns of mortality rates in Darfur conflict. *Lancet*, **375**(9711), 294–300.

Demaio, A., Jamieson, J., Horn, R., de Courten, M., and Tellier, S. (2013). Non-communicable diseases in emergencies: a call to action. *PLoS Curr*, 5.

Depoortere, E., Checchi, F., Broillet, F., Gerstl, S., Minetti, A., Gayraud, O., Briet, V., Pahl, J., Defourny, I., Tatay, M., and Brown, V. (2004). Violence and mortality in West Darfur, Sudan (2003–04): Epidemiological evidence from four surveys. *Lancet*, 364(9442), 1315–1320.

Diaz, J. H. (2004). The public health impact of hurricanes and major flooding. *J La State Med Soc*, 156(3), 145–150.

Doocy, S., Cherewick, M., and Kirsch, T. (2013a). Mortality following the Haitian earthquake of 2010: a stratified cluster survey. *Popul Health Metr*, 11(1), 5.

Doocy, S., Daniels, A., Packer, C., Dick, A., and Kirsch, T. D. (2013b). The human impact of earthquakes: a historical review of events 1980–2009 and systematic literature review. *PLoS Curr*, 5.

Garfield, R. M., Polonsky, J., and Burkle, F. M., Jr. (2012). Changes in size of populations and level of conflict since World War II: implications for health and health services. *Disaster Med Public Health Prep*, 6(3), 241–246.

Guha-Sapir, D. and D'Aoust, O. (2011). *Demographic and Health Consequences of Civil Conflict*. Washington, DC: World Bank.

Guha-Sapir, D. and Dubus, B. (2013). Epidemiology of natural disasters and civil conflicts.

Guha-Sapir, D., van Panhuis, W. G., and Lagoutte, J. (2007). Short communication: patterns of chronic and acute diseases after natural disasters – a study from the International Committee of the Red Cross field hospital in Banda Aceh after the 2004 Indian Ocean tsunami. *Trop Med Int Health*, 12(11), 1338–1341.

The Internal Displacement Monitoring Center. (2014). Database Available at: www.internal-displacement.org/global-figures#conflict (Accessed July 20, 2014).

Leaning, J. and Guha-Sapir, D. (2013). Natural disasters, armed conflict, and public health. *N Engl J Med*, 369(19), 1836–1842.

Mahamud, A., Burton, A., Hassan, M., Ahmed, J. A., Wagacha, J. B., Spiegel, P., Haskew, C., Eidex, R. B., Shetty, S., Cookson, S., Navarro-Colorado, C., and Goodson, J. L. (2013). Risk factors for measles mortality among hospitalized Somali refugees displaced by famine, Kenya, 2011. *Clin Infect Dis*, 57(8), e160–e166.

McDonnell, S. M., Bolton, P., Sunderland, N., Bellows, B., White, M., and Noji, E. (2004). The role of the applied epidemiologist in armed conflict. *Emerg Themes Epidemiol*, 1(1), 4.

Paquet, C. and van Soest, M. (1994). Mortality and malnutrition among Rwandan refugees in Zaire. *Lancet*, 344 (8925), 823–824.

Polonsky, J., Luquero, F., Francois, G., Rousseau, C., Caleo, G., Ciglenecki, I., Delacre, C., Siddiqui, M. R., Terzian, M., Verhenne, L., Porten, K., and Checchi, F. (2013). Public health surveillance after the 2010 Haiti earthquake: The experience of Medecins Sans Frontieres. *PLoS Curr*, 5.

Prudhon, C. and Spiegel, P. B. (2007). A review of methodology and analysis of nutrition and mortality surveys conducted in humanitarian emergencies from October 1993 to April 2004. *Emerg Themes Epidemiol*, 4, 10.

ReliefWeb. (2014). Available at: http://reliefweb.int/ (Accessed July 20, 2014).

Sullivent, E. E., 3rd, West, C. A., Noe, R. S., Thomas, K. E., Wallace, L. J., and Leeb, R. T. (2006). Nonfatal injuries following Hurricane Katrina–New Orleans, Louisiana, 2005. *J Safety Res*, 37(2), 213–217.

The Johns Hopkins Bloomberg School of Public Health and the International Federation of the Red Cross and Red Crescent Societies. (2008). The Johns Hopkins and International Federation of Red Cross and Red Crescent Societies Public Health Guide for Emergencies, Available at: http://pdf.usaid.gov/pdf_docs/PNACU086.pdf (Accessed July 7, 2017).

The Sphere Project. (2011). The Sphere Project: Humanitarian charter and minimum standards in humanitarian response, Available at: www.sphereproject.org/ (Accessed July 19, 2014).

Toole, M. J. and Waldman, R. J. (1997). The public health aspects of complex emergencies and refugee situations. *Annu Rev Public Health*, 18, 283–312.

UNHCR. (2007). Handbook for the protection of internally displaced persons, Available at: www.unhcr.org/4c2355229.html (Accessed July 7,2017).

UNHCR. (2010). Convention and protocol relating to the status of refugees, Available: www.unhcr.org/3b66c2aa10.html (Accessed July 19, 2014).

UNHCR. (2014). Available at: www.unhcr.org/cgi-bin/texis/vtx/home (Accessed July 20, 2014).

United Nations Office for the Coordination of Humanitarian Affairs. (2011). Haiti, one year later, Available at: www.unocha.org/country/issues-in-depth/haiti-one-year-later (Accessed July 7, 2017).

World Health Organization. (2010). Early warning surveillance and response in emergencies: WHO technical workshop, December 2009. *Wkly Epidemiol Rec*, 85(14/15), 129–136.

World Health Organization. (2014). African Programme for Onchocerciasis Control: progress report, 2013–2014. *Wkly Epidemiol Rec*, 89(49), 551–560.

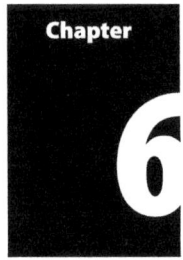

Chapter 6

Ethics

Barbara Tomczyk and Aun Lor

Introduction

In discussions of emergency preparedness, attention is often focused exclusively on moral dilemmas and "tragic choices" (i.e., public choices involving life and death situations that pit irreconcilable values against one another) that arise during the response phase when time is scarce, decisions are pressing, essential resources must be rationed, and individual interests may be subordinated to the public interest. Reflection on ethics will not provide clear-cut rules or directives in such situations. This does not mean that ordinary morality becomes irrelevant during emergency responses; it does mean that acting ethically and making ethically justified decisions will depend largely on specific and concrete circumstances that cannot be fully specified in advance. The best contribution of ethics is to inform advance planning and organization of emergency response so as to minimize the number of tragic choices that must be made. *(Jennings and Arras 2008)*

Public health principles and practice in humanitarian emergencies should be guided by ethical norms and guidelines in order to protect the dignity, rights, and welfare of the affected population. An ethical orientation based on relevant goals, principles, and frameworks is an essential component to guide decision making to benefit those who are in greatest need during a humanitarian emergency. Difficult decisions are made on a regular basis in the practice of public health and emergency response. However, the process for decision-making that supports ethical choices may not always be clearly articulated. There are various examples that can illustrate how ethical dilemmas arise during a humanitarian emergency. Some examples include how to distribute scarce resources to those most in need, how to prevent excess morbidity and mortality in hard to reach and insecure areas, and how to maintain high quality health care services in protracted crises (Hunt et al. 2012).

The field of public health research has made substantial contributions to humanitarian emergencies over the past several decades (Williams 2001). The field will continue to grow building more robust methods and scientific tools to increase the understanding of the distribution of health and illness and the physical, biological, behavioral, social, and environmental determinants among populations in humanitarian settings (Williams 2001). Progress in disease prevention in humanitarian emergencies has been developed through the use of data collection, analysis, and dissemination during and after the emergency. It is important however, that new investigational options should not divert attention or resources from the public health measures that are the main priority in humanitarian emergencies. When research is necessary, it should only be conducted by or supervised by qualified and experienced investigators who are trained in the ethical principles of conducting research (Black 2003). Any data collection activity should lead to public health action that will ultimately benefit the population.

The investigator has a primary duty to protect the rights and welfare of research subjects and to ensure scientific integrity of the research. Protection of research subjects is provided through careful planning and implementation of the research protocol. The ethical oversight of a research study by an Institutional Review Board (IRB) should help to make the process as transparent as possible and make the results of the research publicly available as soon as possible and avoid unnecessary bureaucratic obstacles (CFR 2015). Investigators will need to include participation of the affected community early on in the research process in order to ensure that their input is obtained. In addition, researchers should not create false expectations among the community especially since they are largely dependent on external aid for their survival. In ethical terms, these populations are vulnerable due to their displacement status, and therefore guidelines to evaluate the scientific and ethical merits of the study should be applied (Berry and Reddy 2010).

This chapter addresses some of the ethical issues, dilemmas, principles, processes, and requirements that arise during humanitarian emergencies and the planning that must precede such situations in order "to minimize the number of tragic choices that must be made" (Jennings and Arras 2008). This chapter presents a practical guide, as opposed to a philosophical discussion, for addressing ethical issues related to conducting data collection and responding in humanitarian emergencies.

Research Ethics

Two ongoing debates in public health are whether conducting research during a humanitarian emergency can be ethically justified, and whether biomedical research ethical principles can be applied to public health research (NRC 2002). While these debates are unlikely to be resolved in the foreseeable future, humanitarian actors must anticipate and address issues related to research ethics during a humanitarian emergency. Researchers must take into considerations the ethical principles as outlined in national and international guidelines and regulations, as well as local law, culture, and customs when preparing their research protocols for the IRB or Ethics Review Committee (ERC) for approval.

Historically, the primary aim of research is to develop new and/or generalizable knowledge that can be applied to individuals in other settings and not to benefit individual participants. Under this circumstance, researchers have ethical obligations to protect participants from potential risks associated with research. There are a number of important research ethical norms/guidelines including:

- The Nuremberg Code (Thieren and Mauron 2007)
- The US Code of Federal Regulations, Title 45, Part 46, Protection of Human Subjects (The Common Rule) (DHHS 1979, 1991, 2009)
- The Belmont Report developed by the National Commission for the Protection of Human Subjects of Biomedical and Behavioural Research (DHHS 1979)
- Ethics and Epidemiology: International Guidelines (CIOMS 1991)
- World Health Organization (WHO) Guidelines for Good Clinical Practice (GPC 1995)
- Consultation on Applied Health Research Priorities in Complex Emergencies (ALNAP, 1997)
- The Helsinki Principles (WMA 2013)
- The International Ethical Guidelines for Biomedical Research Involving Human Subjects developed by the Council for International Organizations of Medical Sciences (CIOMS 2002)

These guidelines highlight some unique issues and problems typical of research conducted in humanitarian emergencies, but those are embedded in the documents and not easily accessible. Of these, the first significant contribution to the ethics of research on health interventions in humanitarian emergencies is found in the 1997 ALNAP report.

Worldwide, medical research on human subjects is dependent on ethical review by an IRB or ERC. People affected by humanitarian emergencies might fall outside the reach of any regular IRB. It is the duty of relief agencies that take care of populations affected by humanitarian emergencies to make sure those research proposals that include human subjects are properly reviewed and approved by a qualified IRB or ERC. The United Nations High Commissioner for Refugees protects the rights of refugees as outlined in the Convention and Protocol Relating to the Statute of Refugees, but these do not apply to other displaced persons (UN Convention 1951). Internally displaced persons (IDPs) who have not crossed an international border have the same basic rights and freedoms enjoyed by other persons in their country and those rights must also be respected (UN 2004). IDPs are entitled to special protection under international humanitarian and local laws, and member states are obligated to provide assistance for individuals under their jurisdictions. Therefore, when conducting research among refugees or internally displaced populations, ethical conduct related to their status as a refugee or displacement status as research subjects is conferred by the Nuremberg Code, the Helsinki Declaration, the guidelines of the Council for International Organizations of Medical Sciences (CIOMS), and WHO Guidelines for Good Clinical Practice (GPC). It is important to review these documents prior to conducting research in order to understand the unique human subjects issues to ensure ethical research practices.

Three fundamental principles for the ethical conduct of biomedical research that includes research in humanitarian emergencies (The Belmont Report 1979) are in the following sections.

Respect for Persons

The principle of respect for persons is related to the principle of autonomy and that individuals with diminished autonomy are given additional protection when they are recruited as research participants. Autonomy entails researchers providing sufficient information about the risks and benefits in order for individuals to make informed decision on whether to participate in the research. Respect for persons is implemented through an informed consent process that can be written or oral in some circumstances. Under the Common Rule, eight required elements of informed consent are needed before an IRB will approve a research protocol.

Beneficence

While these were developed for biomedical research ethics, public health research must also follow these same principles. Beneficence means that the researcher must go beyond personal obligation to protect participants from harm. Though paternalistic, it has long been accepted as one of the fundamental principles in research. According to the Belmont Report, "Two general rules have been formulated as complementary expressions of beneficent actions in this sense: (1) do not harm; and (2) maximize possible benefits, and minimize possible harms."

Justice

The principle of justice means both risks and benefits of research are to be fairly distributed. Research must be inclusive during participant recruitment, unless they can justify excluding certain segments of the population, for example, the conflict-affected population that is inaccessible due to security issues. This principle also calls for additional protection for vulnerable populations such as children, pregnant women, and prisoners, who may not be able to provide free and informed consent.

The Ethics of Humanitarianism

Under urgent and stressful conditions that are common in humanitarian emergencies, public health responders have to make tough choices to save lives among populations affected. The humanitarian imperative and its moral obligation to provide aid wherever it is needed to those who need it most is built on the four fundamental principles of humanity, neutrality, impartiality, and independence. These are shown in Table 6.1 (Humanitarian Principles 1965). Neutrality and impartiality are generally mentioned together or are often used interchangeably. However, they are distinct and should be regarded as partially overlapping principles rather than the same principle. These principles are considered to be the most essential to humanitarian ethical action and are endorsed by the UN General Assembly as guidelines for the UN Office for the Coordination of Humanitarian Affairs (UNOCHA) as well as by hundreds of nongovernmental organizations (NGOs).

The Code of Conduct for The International Red Cross and Red Crescent Movement and NGOs in Disaster Relief was developed and agreed upon in the summer of 1994. These are shown in Table 6.1 (IFRC, 1995). The Code of Conduct continues to be used by the International Federation to monitor its own standards of relief delivery and to encourage other agencies to set similar standards. Governments and donor organizations may also use the code to evaluate the conduct of those agencies with which they work. Humanitarian emergency-affected communities have a right to expect that those who assist them abide by these standards. More than 492 organizations have signed the Code of Conduct. A related, important operational guideline is The Sphere Project Humanitarian Charter and Minimum Standards in Humanitarian Response that focuses on how to improve the quality of humanitarian assistance and the accountability of humanitarian actors to their constituents, donors and affected populations (Sphere Project 2014). The Sphere Project is discussed in detail in Chapter 4.

Humanitarian principles provide the fundamental foundations for humanitarian action. The principles of humanitarian action serve as the governing rules for humanitarian agency operations and interactions in situations of crisis and are ultimately about protecting a community. Successful response to humanitarian emergencies must rely on a sense of justice and concern for others in need.

Challenges and Controversies

Conducting Research in Emergencies

Ideally, research should be ethically undertaken that will result in information that will provide well-

Table 6.1 The principles of humanitarian action and principles of conduct for the International Red Cross and Red Crescent Movement and NGOs in disaster response programs (Humanitarian Principles 1965 and IFRC 2015)

The Principles of Humanitarian Action	Principles/Code of Conduct for the International Red Cross and Red Crescent Movement and NGOs in Disaster Response Programs
• *Humanity*: "Human suffering must be addressed wherever it is found. The purpose of humanitarian action is to protect life and health and ensure respect for human beings." More than any other principle, humanity is rooted in a philosophy of altruistic charity. • *Impartiality*: "Humanitarian action must be carried out on the basis of need alone, giving priority to the most urgent cases of distress and making no distinctions on the basis of nationality, race, gender, religious belief, class or political opinions." • *Neutrality*: "Humanitarian actors must not take sides in hostilities or engage in controversies of a political, racial, religious or ideological nature." • *(Operational) Independence*: "Humanitarian action must be autonomous from the political, economic, military or other objectives that any actor may hold with regard to areas where humanitarian action is being implemented."	• The humanitarian imperative comes first. • Aid is given regardless of the race, creed or nationality of the recipients and without adverse distinction of any kind. • Aid priorities are calculated on the basis of need alone. • Aid will not be used to further a particular political or religious standpoint. • We shall endeavor not to act as instruments of government foreign policy. • We shall respect culture and custom. • We shall attempt to build disaster response on local capacities. • Ways shall be found to involve program beneficiaries in the management of relief aid. • Relief aid must strive to reduce future vulnerabilities to disaster as well as meeting basic needs. • We hold ourselves accountable to both those we seek to assist and those from whom we accept resources. • In our information, publicity and advertising activities, we shall recognize disaster victims as dignified human beings, not hopeless objects.

coordinated and high quality support to meet the unique needs of the population, assure that humanitarian responses occur efficiently and effectively, and make evidence-based decisions to continually improve and monitor program outcomes. To accomplish this, priority must be given to applied health research, such as descriptive epidemiology studies to define the problem, intervention studies that develop an effective approach, operational research that looks at how to deliver the intervention, and health services research that examines how effective the system can manage the various interventions. When research is conducted in these settings the project should have appropriate ethical oversight and review. Appropriate ethical oversight in the context of a humanitarian emergency does not necessarily involve an IRB but responsibility for conducting systematic data collection should be guided by ethical principles of the researchers and the agencies that are collaborating on the project. A study must be scientifically rigorous and high impact to enhance the outcome on the affected population.

Research should improve the capacity to identify, deal with or monitor major health problems. Besides looking at the impact on morbidity, mortality, and psychological well-being of individuals, one should consider whether research findings could promptly and effectively benefit populations. For example, it is important to consider how much of a change is attributed to a specific intervention or humanitarian aid program. Researchers need to be careful not to mistakenly attribute too much to external assistance and to underestimate the endogenous or internal pathological factors contributing to the response. Many factors contribute to poor health outcomes in humanitarian emergencies, and both the gaps in response and the pathology and disease risks of the population need to be taken into account. Understanding the complex interplay between exogenous and endogenous factors is crucial in addressing the urgent health needs of the population. However, in general, during humanitarian emergencies, no agents, such as drugs or vaccines, should be tested that have not been proven safe elsewhere.

Research is needed to accurately document the characteristics of the emergency and to evaluate the effectiveness of the relief interventions. Research studies can be carried out during or after an emergency but regardless of the timing it is vital to consider the ethics of conducting research in humanitarian emergencies and to apply guidelines to ensure that research is ethically sound. The most important question before moving forward with research is to define the purpose and how the data will be used for public health action. Good intentions for conducting research should be aligned with addressing key information gaps and not solely on the interest of the researcher (Lee 2012). A plan must be in place to put research results to good use to address the ethical dilemma of using data for action.

In general, ethical guidelines on conducting research in humanitarian emergencies are relatively ad hoc and unregulated. Therefore, any research conducted should help to develop affordable and feasible interventions producing information that is practical and useful for program managers and field workers. Research projects should not overburden relief operations nor deprive populations of resources normally allocated in relief programs. The period of early response to a humanitarian emergency may not be the best time to conduct a large survey that will utilize vehicles and medical staff that are needed for emergency transport or treating patients. When data collection is needed in humanitarian emergencies, careful consideration needs to be placed on the time and resources needed to conduct the research and the benefits it will bring to the affected population. For example, needs assessments are important so that responding agencies can plan their operations and programs and/or analyze how effective their interventions have been. Research projects such as those looking at the effects of the aide program on the political economy for example, may not directly benefit the population and should not be considered an immediate priority. Regardless, data collection activities should convey to the affected communities the benefits and limitations of research, no false expectations should be raised, and cultural as well as ethical norms should be respected (Giffin 2001).

The *Code of Ethics for Emergency Nurses* provides a helpful list of issues to draw on for researchers to consider before embarking on a public health investigation and include the following (Code of Ethics for Emergency Nurses 2004):

- The researcher should ensure that he/she conducts research with compassion and respect for individuals and communities.
- The researcher should maintain the highest sense of scientific rigor and competency.
- The researcher should ensure that victims of emergency situation's welfare are not further jeopardized because of the research.
- The rights to privacy and confidentiality of subjects have to be respected.
- Research should not hamper relief efforts but rather facilitate the delivery of the same.
- Where appropriate, collaborations with other researchers and agencies should be encouraged in order to enhance care.
- Research in emergency situations should be carried out only when similar data cannot be obtained otherwise.
- Research should be responsive to the needs of the victims of the emergency.
- Only research that does not hinder or obstruct effective and appropriate interventions should be carried out.

Ethical Considerations for Decision-Making

Health professionals and other responders are traditionally guided by their professional codes of ethics within their respective disciplines (Schwartz 2012). Due to unfamiliar ethical challenges, those responding to humanitarian emergencies must pay careful attention to the complex social, cultural, and human rights factors associated with the chaotic nature of disasters that create a challenging operating environment. Preparing and responding to any humanitarian emergency requires multidisciplinary collaboration and coordination of efforts among responding partners to address the enormous ethical challenges involving highly vulnerable populations. Among these challenges include:

- Allocating scarce resources
- Obtaining free and informed consent from individuals with diminished autonomy for research and nonresearch activities
- Making decisions with incomplete information
- Addressing the gap between what should be done and what can be done
- Addressing sensitive cultural, religious, and social issues
- Understanding the political, legal, economic, and security issues

Applying ethical and legal principles to response to humanitarian emergencies requires a concerted effort by all agencies and individuals working on the issue. Aid in the form of food, water, or shelter can have a great economic value, and this can give considerable power to governments or armed actors that are able to influence where, how, and to whom it is provided. The distribution of aid requires additional resources to ensure that humanitarian aid does not end up in the hands of conflicting parties instead of reaching the beneficiaries. It can be challenging and dangerous to allocate resources to those who need it most. For example, if monitoring activities are not set up early on it can lead to major frustration within the community. In order to avoid any possible misunderstandings, it is critical to explain to the population that humanitarian aid has to be provided to the most vulnerable populations as a priority.

Assistance has to be given in priority to those who need it most, but negative consequences may occur if the humanitarian needs of one community are clearly more important than those of another and agencies did not consider rolling out activities for each of them in order to prevent social fragmentation, conflict, and reprisals.

Another challenge is that the displaced population may have a deteriorating effect on the living conditions of the host community. The host population may have helped the displaced population with water, food, and shelter that affect the well-being of the local population. If tensions already exist between two communities, bringing humanitarian assistance to the most vulnerable community could increase existing tensions and make agencies seem partial. In this case, providing humanitarian aid to all communities would not only be needed to prevent dissent, but would also come as a legitimate response to new or evolving humanitarian needs of the host population. As many responders may be unaccustomed to decision-making from a population perspective based on ethical principles, it is crucial that individual providers be aware of these issues.

Research Gaps

There are known gaps in research in humanitarian emergencies that the global community should acknowledge and build upon (Ford 2008). Partnerships between the academic community, NGOs, and international agencies should expand and open possibilities for multi-disciplinary research. Dissemination of findings, if done in conjunction with the community, will lead to improved outcomes. Another area of research that is needed is on quality of care studies to establish best practices in different emergency settings. Standard, validated tools for the initial assessment of public health problems are also needed. Research into technology and methods for collecting data on population size, women of reproductive age, and mortality is especially urgent with regard to mobile and dispersed populations. Lastly, program monitoring and evaluation should take into account the extent to which the needs of populations are effectively met including the most vulnerable populations.

Research versus Nonresearch

A fundamental problem inherent in public health is the question of what activities constitute research. During a humanitarian emergency, this question may not come across as critically important, but it must be considered in advance to ensure regulatory and ethical compliance for research that is funded by certain entities including the United States government. As an example, the United States federal regulatory definition of research is "a systematic investigation, including research development, testing and evaluation, designed to develop or contribute to generalizable knowledge," but this definition has been a source of confusion in public health (CFR 2009). Traditional public health activities such as surveillance, outbreak investigations, and program evaluations have not been considered as research (MacQueen 2004).

According to Beauchamp, "First, it uses the notion of research to define the term 'research,' creating problems of circular definition. Second, it does not define any of the several important terms (the key conceptual conditions) used in the definition, such as 'systematic investigation,' 'testing' and 'generalizable knowledge,' and these terms can be understood in several ways. Third, the definition is vague and overly broad because it is not clearly confined to biomedical research, clinical research and behavioral research – or even to *scientific research*, more generally. Its scope is left unclear. Fourth, and perhaps most importantly, it does not preclude 'research' from having a very close tie to 'practice'" (Beauchamp 2011).

When a research activity is warranted, there are two guidance documents that are available to assist researchers in determining whether an activity constitutes human subjects research. A report, commissioned by the Council of State and Territorial Epidemiologist (CSTE) in 2001, was developed to assist states and local health departments in the United States in making distinctions between public health research and practice (Hodge 2007). Also, the Centers for Disease Control and Prevention (CDC) has its own "Policy on Distinguishing Public Health

Research and Public Health Practice" that offers an interpretation of the regulatory definition of research (CDC 1997). According to CDC, "The purpose of research is to generate new or generalizable knowledge. The purpose of nonresearch in public health is to prevent or control disease, injury and improve health, or to improve a public health program or service." Table 6.2 summarizes CDC's interpretation and provides examples of when a public health activity, such as surveillance, emergency response, or program evaluation, might be considered research.

A best practice is to anticipate the possibility of conducting research in this context before a public health emergency arises. Several important predeployment steps are the following:

- Consult with appropriate individual(s), including but not limited to IRB/ERC member(s) on whether the activity is human subjects research that requires ethical approval.
- Prepare generic protocols that could be quickly adapted for submission to the IRB/ERC (Schopper 2009).
- Ensure that all relevant personnel take appropriate ethics training and obtain certification that permits them to conduct human subject's research.
- Ensure that appropriate IRB approval(s), including local approvals when appropriate, have been obtained before initiating research activities.
- When possible, designate different personnel who are emergency responders and those whose activities will be focused on research (Ford et al. 2009).

Conclusion

Public health principles and practice in humanitarian emergencies should be guided by ethical norms and guidelines in order to protect the dignity, rights, and

Table 6.2 Assessing research versus nonresearch

	Research	Practice (nonresearch)
Concepts		
Definition	"…systematic investigation, including research development, testing, and evaluation, designed to develop or contribute to generalizable knowledge." (ref. 45 CFR 46)	May use scientific methods to identify and control a health problem with benefits for the study participants or their communities.
Primary Purpose	To generate new or generalizable knowledge (information that can be applied in other settings).	To benefit study participants or the communities from which they come.
Methodology	• Scientific principles and methods used • Hypothesis testing/generating • Knowledge is generalizable	• Scientific principles and methods may be used • Hypothesis testing/generating • Knowledge may be generalizable
Examples	•	•
Surveillance Projects	• Requested data are broad in scope (and may involve as yet unproven risk factors) • Comparison of different surveillance approaches • Hypothesis testing • Subsequent studies planned using cases identified	• Regular, ongoing collection and analyses to measure occurrence of health problem • Scope of data is health condition or disease, demographics, and known risk factors • Invokes public health mechanisms to prevent or control disease or injury
Emergency Response	• Samples stored for future use • Additional analyses performed beyond immediate problem • Investigational drugs tested	• Solves an immediate health problem • No testing of methods or interventions
Program Evaluation	• Test an untried intervention • Systematic comparison of standard and nonstandard interventions	• Assess success of established intervention • Evaluation information used for feedback into program (management)

welfare of the affected population. This applies both to the delivery of services as well as data collection and research. Traditionally, the primary aim of research is to develop new and/or generalizable knowledge that can be applied to individuals in other settings, and not to benefit individual participants. In the setting of humanitarian emergencies, research should be ethically undertaken that will result in information that will provide well-coordinated and high quality support to meet the unique needs of the population, assure that humanitarian responses occur efficiently and effectively, and make evidence-based decisions to continually improve and monitor program outcomes. Research that is scientifically robust and uses ethical guidelines/norms as a tool and process can help to improve the intended benefits and minimize the risks to the population affected by humanitarian emergencies.

Applying ethical and legal principles to response to humanitarian emergencies requires a concerted effort by all agencies and individuals working on the issue. The humanitarian imperative and its moral obligation to provide aid wherever it is needed to those who need it most is built on the four fundamental principles of humanity, neutrality, impartiality, and independence.

Notes from the Field

Afghanistan (2002)

Spin Boldak, meaning "white desert," is a border town in the southern Kandahar province of Afghanistan and the headquarters of Spin Boldak District. Despite rainfall across parts of Afghanistan, the majority of the area remained gripped in the throes and aftermath of a four-year drought that resulted in heavy losses of seeds, tools, and traction animals, and in dry aquifers. Most families were facing acute food insecurity and food assistance was required to save lives. In addition, conflict in years preceding 2002 years took its toll on the people in the area. Many families had their houses destroyed and livestock and assets looted. Blockades hampered labor and trade routes, while minefields have caused the loss of agricultural lands. Poor sanitation, inadequate health facilities, and shortage of medications and supplies are also a major problem.

Nonetheless, large numbers of returnees and displaced families continued to return to the area as a result of political stability and a cessation of fighting throughout Kandahar. In 2002, waves of IDPs arrived at camps and, at times, overwhelmed the infrastructure. The arrival of over twenty thousand IDPs at camp facilities built to house much smaller populations were extremely difficult to deal with. Because of the conflict, the inclement weather, and poor and dangerous roads, vitally needed supplies such as food, water, nonfood items, and health care were in short supply. Even when supplies were available, transport was a major issue. For example, a large shipment of charcoal was delayed for months and then arrived at the beginning of the warm season. Blankets were delivered and placed into storage but were not distributed. Camp management was constantly in a crisis mode trying to make do with too few supplies for too many people.

Children in Afghanistan face many risks that contribute to high rates of morbidity and mortality. Afghanistan's infant mortality rate (IMR) remains among the highest in the world and more than 15 percent of children die before reaching their first birthday. The infant mortality rate was estimated at 257 deaths per 1,000 live births in 2006 (Viswanathan 2010), and the neonatal mortality rate at 60 per 1,000 live births in 2004 (UNICEF 2006). The harsh conditions in the IDP camps presented specific threats and vulnerabilities to newborn health that needed to be considered by camp management and health partners.

The temperature fell to zero degrees Fahrenheit and wind chill registered −10 below. The IDPs had little more than tents to shield from the cold and wind. Reports started coming in that a high number of deaths among newborns was occurring. A team of health staff raced to the camps to investigate the deaths and the UN distributed blankets. The investigation concluded that all of the children were ill prior to dying and that the cold weather may have contributed but was not the main cause of death. The investigation resulted in the following:

- Established a health working group to address the multiple needs of the IDPs
- Conducted assessments in water and sanitation, housing, and food insecurity
- Established mortality data collection in the camps
- Produced guidelines on data sharing and use
- Conducted assessments of health services in the camps

Despite the rapid investigation conducted by the health partners, lessons learned were that newborn health needed to be considered early on in a response. The results of the investigation were shared with the community leaders, but they were furious and believed the deaths were attributable to lack of blankets, clothing, and charcoal to warm the children in the cold weather. It is difficult to have a loss of life in these situations especially when it is preventable. In this setting, the investigation did highlight the underlying causes that needed to be addressed. However, the situation for newborns in Spin Boldak was especially dangerous and precautions should have been implemented earlier to prevent newborn mortality.

Conducting a rapid investigation in this setting was appropriate to document the direct and indirect causes of neonatal mortality. The investigation was determined to be nonresearch by the Ministry of Health, Kandahar, because the main intent was to prevent or control neonatal mortality and improve the public health program. The investigation was conducted to identify, characterize, and solve the causes of neonatal mortality that was an immediate health problem. The knowledge gained from the activity directly benefited the neonatal community. It is important to note, however, an emergency response investigation might have a research component if, for example, samples are stored for future use or additional analyses are conducted beyond those needed to solve the immediate health problem.

This situation highlights that tough decisions by the humanitarian agencies were made not because there was a right or wrong answer but because choices had to be made. Ethical principles and guidelines can be used early on in a humanitarian emergency to help explore some of these tough choices and provide a transparent process that is helpful in humanitarian emergencies were there are numerous shifting priorities. In this situation the investigation did not block relief efforts but facilitated the delivery of blankets and charcoal, albeit too late. Neonatal mortality data had not been previously collected in the camps, so the investigation was necessary to document the incidence and underlying causes. Lastly, the findings were used to improve the overall needs of the IDPs in the emergency.

References

Beauchamp, T., Bowie, N., and Arnold, D. (2011). Mythinkinglab – Standalone Access Card – For Ethical Theory and Business. Available at: www.amazon.ca/Mythinkinglab-Standalone-Access-Ethical-Business/dp/020524713X (Accessed on April 15, 2015).

Bengo, J., Masiye, F., and Muula, A. (2008). Ethical challenges in conducting research in humanitarian crisis situations. *Malawi Medical Journal June* 20(2): 46–49. Available at: www.ncbi.nlm.nih.gov/pmc/articles/PMC3345669. (Accessed on March 31, 2015).

Berry, K. and Reddy, S. (2010). Safety with dignity: Integrating community-based protection into humanitarian programming. Humanitarian Practice Network. Network Paper Number 68.

Black, R. (2003). Ethical codes in humanitarian emergencies: From practice to research? *Disasters* 27(2), 95–108.

Centers for Disease Control and Prevention. (2010). Distinguishing public health research and public health Nonresearch. Available at:www.cdc.gov/od/science/integrity/docs/cdc-policy-distinguishing-public-health-research-nonresearch.pdf (Accessed on June 13, 2014).

Code of Federal Regulations (CFR). (2009). 46.102, Title 45, Public Welfare Department of Health and Human Services, Part 46, Protection of Human Subjects. Available at: www.hhs.gov/ohrp/humansubjects/guidance/45cfr46.html#46.102 (Accessed on April 17, 2015).

Code of Federal Regulations (CFR). (2015). Title 21. US Department of Health and Human Services. Available at: www.accessdata.fda.gov/scripts/cdrh/cfdocs/cfcfr/CFRSearch.cfm?CFRPart=56 (Accessed on March 18, 2015).

Consultation on Applied Health Research Priorities in Complex Emergencies. (1997). Available at: www.alnap.org/resource/2643 (Accessed on March 1, 2015).

Council for International Organization in Medical Science. (2008). Ethics and epidemiology: International guidelines. Available at: www.ufrgs.br/bioetica/cioms2008.pdf (Accessed on March 1, 2015).

Council for International Organizations of Medical Sciences (CIOMS). 2002. International ethical guidelines for biomedical research involving human subjects. Available at: www.cioms.ch/publications/layout_guide2002.pdf (Accessed on May 30, 2014).

Department of Health and Human Services. (1979). The Belmont Report: Ethical principles and guidelines for the protection of human subjects of research.
The National Commission for the Protection of Human Subjects of Biomedical and Behavioral Research. Available at: www.hhs.gov/ohrp/humansubjects/guidelines/belmont.html (Accessed on May 23, 2014).

Department of Health and Human Services. (1979, 1991, 2009). Code of Federal Regulations (45CFR46). Available at www.hhs.gov/ohrp/humansubjects/guidelines/45cfr46.html#46.102 (Accessed on May 30, 2014).

Emergency Nurses Association: Code of Ethics for Emergency Nurses. (2004). Available at: www.emergency.net/ethics.htm (Accessed on June 20, 2014).

Ford, N., Mills, E.J., Zachariah, R., and Upshur, R. (2009). Ethics of conducting research in conflict settings. *Conflict and Health*, **3** (7). Available at: http://conflictandhealth.com/content/3/1/7 (Accessed on June 13, 2014).

Giffin, G. (2001). Bioethics Research: Universal Ethics – A Foundation for Global Dialogue

Hodge, J. G. and Gostin, L. O. (2004) Public health practice vs. research: A report for public health practitioners including cases and guidelines for making distinctions. Council of State and Territorial Epidemiologists. Available at: www.vdh.virginia.gov/OFHS/policy/documents/2012/irb/pdf/Public%20Health%20Practice%20versus%20Research.pdf (Accessed on June 13, 2014).

Humanitarian charter and minimum standards in humanitarian response sphere project. (2011). Available at: www.sphereproject.org/handbook (Accessed on March 2, 2015).

Humanitarian Principles. (1965). The fundamental principles of the International Red Cross and Red Crescent Movement, proclaimed in Vienna in 1965 by the 20th International Conference of the Red Cross and Red Crescent Movement. Available at: United Nations resolution 46/182: www.un.org/documents/ga/res/46/a46r182.htm (Accessed on March 15, 2015)

Hunt, M., Sinding. C., and Schwartz, L. (2012). Tragic choices in humanitarian health work. *Journal of Clinical Ethics* **23**. (**4**), 333–44.

International Federation of the Red Cross and Red Crescent Society (IFRC). (2015). Promoting the Fundamental Principles and Humanitarian Values. Available at: www.ifrc.org/en/who-we-are/vision-and-mission/principles-and-values (Accessed on March 1, 2015).

Jennings, B. and Arras, J (2008). Ethical guidance for public health emergency preparedness and response: Highlighting Ethics and values in a vital public health service. Available at: www.cdc.gov/od/science/integrity/phethics/docs/White_Paper_Final_for_Website_2012_4_6_12_final_for_web_508_compliant.pdf (Accessed on May 22, 2014).

Lee, L. (2012). Public health ethics theory: Review and path to convergence. *Journal of Law, Medicine & Ethics*. Available at: http://onlinelibrary.wiley.com/doi/10.1111/j.1748-720X.2012.00648.x/abstract. (Accessed on January 10, 2015).

MacQueen, K. M. and Buehler, J. W. (2004). Ethics, practice, and research in public health. *American Journal of Public Health* **94** (6), 928–931.

National Research Council (NRC). (2002). *Research ethics in complex humanitarian emergencies.* Summary of a Workshop. Washington, DC: National Academy Press. 2001. Available at: www.bioethics.org.au/Resources/Online%20Articles/Opinion%20Pieces/1302%20Universal%20ethics%20a%20foundation%20for%20global%20dialogue.pdf (Accessed on February 19, 2015).

Schopper, D., Upshur, R., Matthys, A., et al. (2009). Research ethics review in humanitarian contexts: The experiences of the independent ethics review board of medecins sans frontieres. *PLoS Med* **6**(7): e1000115 Available at: http://journals.plos.org/plosmedicine/article?id=10.1371/journal.pmed.1000115 (Accessed on March 3, 2015).

Schwartz, L., Hunt, M., Sinding, C., et al. (2012). Models for humanitarian health care ethics. *Public Health Ethics*, 5 (1), 81–90.

The Belmont Report. (1979). Available at: www.hhs.gov/ohrp/humansubjects/guidance/belmont.html. (Accessed on March 1, 2015).

The code of conduct for the International Red Cross and Red Crescent Movement and NGOs in Disaster Relief. (1995). Available at: www.ifrc.org/Docs/idrl/I259EN.pdf (Accessed on March 1, 2015).

The Sphere Project. (2014). Available at: www.spherehandbook.org. (Accessed March 1, 2017).

Thieren, M., and Mauron, A. (2007). Nuremberg code turns 60. Bulletin of the WHO 85 (8):569–648 Available at: www.who.int/bulletin/volumes/85/8/07-045443/en (Accessed on April 17, 2015).

United Nations. (2004). guiding principles on internal displacement. Available at www.unhcr.org/43ce1cff2.html (Accessed on May 22, 2014).

United Nations Children's Fund. (2006). State of the world's children. Available at: www.unicef.org/infobycountry/afghanistan_statistics.html (Accessed on March 31, 2015)

United Nations Convention on Refugees. (1951). Available at: www.unhcr.org/pages/49da0e466.html (Accessed on March 2, 2015)

Viswanathan, K., Becker, S., Hansen, P. M., et al. (2010). Infant and under-five mortality in Afghanistan: current estimates and limitations. Available at: www.who.int/bulletin/volumes/88/8/09-068957/en (Accessed on March 31, 2015).

Williams, H. A. and Bloland, P. B. (2001). A practical discussion of applied public health research in the context of complex emergencies: Examples from malaria control in refugee camps. *National Association for the Practice of Anthropology Bulletin*. 21(1), 70–88. Available at: http://onlinelibrary.wiley.com/doi/10.1525/napa.2001.21.1.70/pdf (Accessed on January 5, 2015)

Williams, H. A. and Waldman, R. (2001). Public health in complex emergencies: toward a more integrated science. *National Association for the Practice of Anthropology Bulletin* 21(1), 89–111. www.researchgate.net/publication/229445382_Public_Health_in_Complex_Emergencies_Toward_a_More_Integrated_Science (Accessed on March 15, 2015).

World Health Organization expert committee on selection and use of essential medicines. (1995). Technical Report Series no 850 Annex 3. Available at: http://apps.who.int/medicinedocs/en/d/Jwhozip13e. (Accessed on March 1, 2015).

World Medical Association. (2013). Declaration of Helsinki-Ethical principles for medical research involving human subjects. Available at: www.wma.net/en/30publications/10policies/b3/index.html (Accessed on May 30, 2014).

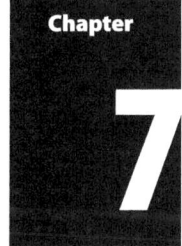

Section 2 Public Health Principles

Chapter 7

Needs Assessments

Richard Garfield, Johan von Schreeb, Anneli Eriksson, and Patrice Chataigner

Introduction

The response to humanitarian emergencies should be guided by field-based information on the magnitude and severity of the emergency and be driven by the needs of those affected. Assistance should be prioritized for those experiencing imminent threats to life, subsistence, and physical security. Further, an effective response must evolve to reflect these needs of the affected population as they change over time. In practice, it is frequently unclear what are the greatest needs and how best to respond. Thus, how needs are defined, identified, and prioritized has profound implications for those affected by humanitarian emergencies. Needs assessments, as they are discussed in this chapter, are field-based data collection and analysis exercises used to define, identify, and prioritize needs in the setting of humanitarian emergencies.

Needs assessments are intended to provide an understanding of the disaster and analysis of threats to life, dignity, health, and livelihoods to determine, in consultation with the relevant authorities, if an external response is required and the nature of the response (The Sphere Project 2011). Needs assessments require a process of obtaining and analyzing original information from affected people to determine the current status and service needs of a defined population and/or geographic area (NOAA 2015). A variety of methods and groups are involved in the collection, analysis, and presentation of this information.

To be most effective, needs assessments must collect and analyze information from many people and in many areas to make sound recommendations. They must, however, do so very rapidly and repeatedly if they are to be relevant to the rapidly evolving situation common to humanitarian emergencies. This balance between adequacy of information for making inferences and timeliness to influence what is done characterizes a continual challenge in needs assessments during humanitarian emergencies. *Good enough information* in a timely manner is a basic tenet of a needs assessment.

Objectives

There are multiple potential objectives of a needs assessment. These include:

Inform Operational, Strategic, and Response Decisions

- Identify and locate affected groups requiring immediate assistance
- Determine local capacities and humanitarian constraints
- Determine whether or not to intervene
- Provide baseline data
- Determine the nature and scale of the intervention
- Design program strategies to best deliver goods and services
- Identify further information needs

Influence Response Decisions

- Secure resources from donors and establish a basis for support of proposed efforts
- Prioritize needs
- Influence policy
- Establish and strengthen partnerships

Justify Response Decisions and Appeal for Funds

- Provide evidence for justification of allocation of resources
- Provide initial measures for response evaluation

In practice, however, a needs assessment cannot be all things to all interested parties. With so many potential objectives, lack of consensus over priorities is inevitable. The overall, fundamental goal of a needs assessment in this context is to provide adequate information to enable better-informed decision-making in response to humanitarian emergencies.

Common Needs Assessment

In the setting of humanitarian emergencies, needs assessments may be referred to as common needs assessments (CNA), defined as a "time-bound, multi-sectoral, multistakeholder process of collecting, analyzing and interpreting data to assess needs and inform decisions on humanitarian and early recovery responses" (Garfield et al. 2011). Ideally, this is an interagency, intersectoral, process to help develop a better joint understanding of the needs, capabilities, and appropriate response.

It should include both the collection of new or original information from affected individuals and communities and the collation of secondary information from relevant sources created prior to the disaster for analysis and priority setting.

Examples include the CAN performed in Myanmar after Cyclone Nargis that showed that some communities were much worse off than others, and they were often not the areas that had received assistance. In Haiti, a postearthquake CNA showed that the greatest short-term need was for food. In Pakistan following floods, a CNA demonstrated that though food was in short supply, what people most wanted were shovels and other agricultural tools. In Syria, several CNA found that medicines and food were not in short supply except in areas that were being besieged. In each of these examples, a CAN helped identify the population in need, the urgency of their need, and what commodities or services are needed most.

It takes time and resources to conduct needs assessments, and even when funds and experienced assessors are available, in the past, results have not always been useful or timely. If managed poorly, the needs assessment process itself may create a need for more coordination between agencies, rather than making coordination easier as intended.

Many of the components of needs assessments in humanitarian emergencies differ from standard public health survey methodologies performed in more stable settings. A comparison of methodologies of needs assessment done in humanitarian emergencies and common public health surveys done in stable settings is presented in Table 7.1.

Due to the fluid nature of humanitarian emergencies, identifying variations from one group or place to another and monitoring changing conditions by repeated small samples will provide more relevant information than seeking a large representative sample for a one-time survey.

Qualities and challenges of a good needs assessment are shown in Table 7.2.

A needs assessment often has to cover a large geographic area but cannot depend on a large sample size. In fact, representative sampling is seldom possible in an emergency setting, so statistical generalizability with the information collected is limited. Only qualitative and tentative inferences can be made from these descriptive data but when field-based information is scarce in an emergency or disaster, such limited information is far better than planning based only on past experience and assumptions.

Key to valid interpretation is specification of a period, or stage for which it is considered valid. As conditions evolve rapidly, information should be organized to reflect changes over a defined period of time. Analysts should not try to predict the future with precision or in detail; rather, they should highlight areas of major vulnerability or concern in the short term and highlight areas for which further information is needed.

Many agencies, lacking broad-based data from the field, instead report on "worst case" scenarios. It is far more useful to characterize common conditions and major priorities, while describing the variations among groups found.

According to the Inter Agency Standing Committee (IASC) Needs Assessment Task Force, "Accurate information about the ground reality in a post emergency situation should be the foundation on which decision-making for a coordinated and effective response is based" (IASC 2009). In the setting of humanitarian emergencies, this should be interpreted with caution however, as this idea may reinforce a mistaken focus of attention on large representative surveys using methods appropriate to a stable residential population rather than the collection of information from multiple sources, including precrisis information for comparisons, and focusing on the context and analysis of all this information to get a dynamic picture of what is being done and what is needed next.

Chapter 7: Needs Assessments

Table 7.1 Comparison of needs assessment and common public health survey methodologies

Component	Common Public Health Survey	Needs Assessment
Population sampled	Representative sample of entire population	Samples of most affected population from accessible areas
Sample size	Typically 600–2,000 individual households	Typically 10–30 sites, but to be determined in practice depending on logistical conditions and when observers decide they have an overall picture
Sampling method	Cluster, systematic or random	Purposive
Data collection means/tools	Questionnaire and biological measures among individuals and their household members	Observation, key Informants in communities, possibly individual interviews, social media and "big data"
Analysis	Statistical	Iterative, interactive and evolving
Use of historical data	Usually mentioned only in introduction to report	Source of most of the information used in the first weeks
Comparisons over time	Typically every 12–24 months	Every 4–8 weeks as conditions change rapidly
Generalizability	Statistically valid methods used	Qualitative methods used
Uncertainty	Calculated statistically	Often qualitative or not presented
Cost[1]	Typically $200,000–$500,000 (US)	Typically under $50,000 (US)
Time it takes to carry out	6 months	1 month

Table 7.2 Qualities and challenges of a needs assessment

Quality	Challenge
Timeliness	Agreement between agencies and collection and interpretation of data may take a lot of time
Relevance	Agencies may have mandates that may not be key to act on in an emergency
Coverage	Focus should be on those most affected but some high-need groups may still be missed
Validity	Additional aide may expect if answering "correctly" Conditions change rapidly, and what was recorded two weeks ago is no longer true when the data is released
Transparency	Frequent reports of "representative" samples may in fact be convenience samples
Continuity	Trying to get all questions into one assessment inhibits efforts to repeat data collection
Cost-effectiveness	Large samples in remote locations can cost up to $200,000 (US) per survey

Donors typically make initial funding decisions within ten days of a sudden-onset emergency and make major allocations within six weeks (Humanitarian Response 2015a). These funding decisions are often based, at least in part, on information from the very NGOs and UN organization that seek funding. In the absence of timely, relevant, unbiased information, donors may make decisions based on press reports, sometimes referred to as the "CNN effect." Needs assessments are thus important for donors and responders to make better-informed decisions to support the most effective response.

Information

Good Enough Information

Given the overall lack of information and general uncertainty, especially early on in a humanitarian emergency, even a relatively small amount of good information or data, or "good enough" information, may significantly reduce the degree of uncertainty.

In deciding what information to collect and how to analyze available information, several questions need to be considered:

- What are the risks the population is facing in short-, medium-, and long-term perspective?
- Are current needs new or mainly the result of problems that have evolved over a long period?
- Are the conditions of the whole group of main interest, or are special vulnerable groups the main concern?
- Will more questions or interviews with more people in more places provide a fuller picture of conditions?
- Community participation in designing and analyzing the data may be ideal, but utility requires that the process finish within days or weeks. There are some widely used, robust, comparable indicators used to assess humanitarian conditions. Should these be the main focus, or does the unique context of this event require original terms and measures?
- Is the assessment designed as an initial assessment for which there will be ongoing monitoring, or is this a one-time assessment?
- Is it possible to create a representative sample among the affected population, or is Purposive sampling more efficient at this time?
- Should the assessment depend mainly on community leaders, local officials, or people in their homes to identify needs?

In addition, it is important to gather context-specific information including:

- Information on drivers of the crisis that led to the emergency
- Capacities, resources, and the response of affected people
- Vulnerabilities and vulnerable groups within the population
- Access and limitations to access for those assisting the affected population

Good enough information is tentative and identifies major trends, issues, and conditions, as well as identifying those that are not major issues or conditions. As conditions are changing so rapidly, good enough information does not attempt to identify conditions as if they were static. It should provide an objective and transparent basis to summarize the main issues, including priority geographic areas, people most in need, and the things they need most.

Identifying a standard set of indicators, observation categories, and survey questions has proved impossible, as each situation is different, necessitating development or adaptation for the specific context.

Accuracy vs. Precision

Public health surveys typically seek to establish precise information in a stable environment, from representative household samples in order to generalize to a larger population. In the setting of a humanitarian emergency, many people may be displaced from their homes, so what might be a representative sample prior to the disaster, such as household samples, may not be at all representative and in fact exclude most affected individuals.

In contrast to stable settings, in performing needs assessments during a humanitarian emergency, it is accuracy rather than precision, that is key. The situation is often changing rapidly and excess precision may give a false sense of accuracy as the situation may have changed by the time the data is reported.

Increases in both precision and accuracy in the methods used for data collection from the field are associated with an increase in the time and cost. This relationship is shown in Figure 7.1 (unpublished work, Chatagnier, 2015).

Original and Secondary Data

Original data may be gathered through direct observation. This can be used to help determine what people have, what they have lost, and if they are able to perform basic needs such as washing and preparing food. In addition, it may include what affected individuals say they need most to recover. This qualitative information may provide direction to areas where further data collection may be necessary.

Some of the information needed for decision-making is available from secondary sources, thus limiting the need for time spent on original data collection. Secondary data may be used to predict the needs of the affected population based on the type of disaster. For example, past experience has shown the differences in the risks and needs of a population affected by floods compared with earthquakes. Secondary data may also be used to predict the areas of a region with the greatest vulnerabilities prior to the disaster, often areas that are

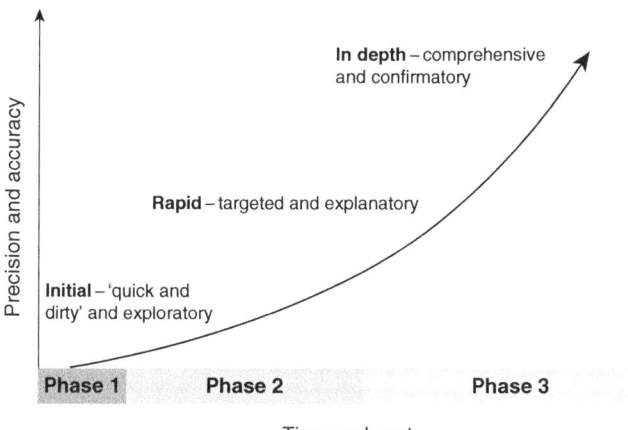

Figure 7.1 The relationship between precision and accuracy and time and cost

remote and disadvantaged. Secondary data may also give information on the likely level of coping capacity at national, regional, and individual level, linked to socioeconomic situation, and health needs related to the predisaster burden of disease.

Tools

Initial Rapid Assessment (IRA)

With humanitarian reform of the UN and the establishment of the cluster system starting in 2005, the global clusters in health, nutrition, and WASH together created the Initial Rapid Assessment (IRA) to help organize and facilitate needs assessments. The intent was to provide a basic survey form for use in a wide variety of emergencies, to avoid the need to invent a new survey tool each time. After more than a year of discussion among the three clusters, an IRA form was released. Its implementation was limited as few countries found it directly applicable for a variety of reasons, including that local conditions were often different, the desired form was either shorter or longer, and local organizations often wanted to include additional questions. It became clear that one size did not fit all, as was originally hoped.

The Health and Nutrition Tracking Service

The Health and Nutrition Tracking Service (HNTS), an independent interagency initiative hosted by the World Health Organization (WHO), revised the IRA form and provided guidance for its use in an attempt to meet the different needs of users. The United Nations IASC Needs Assessment Task Force, coordinated by the World Food Program (WFP) and the Office for Coordination of Humanitarian Affairs (OCHA), empowered OCHA to hire staff and lead this effort. This resulted in the development of the Multicluster/sector Initial Rapid Assessment (MIRA) discussed below.

Several UN organizations, notably WHO and WFP, have their own specialized survey and assessment tools to use in emergencies, as do many NGOs.

Phases Specific Assessment Tools

In the setting of a rapid onset emergency, the needs of the affected population progress through predictable phases. The order of these phases is generally maintained from one emergency to another; however, the timing of the transition from one phase to another is more variable.

The information to be gathered in a needs assessment during a humanitarian emergency is time sensitive. To be useful, phase specific assessment tools should be used. Examples are shown in Figure 7.2 (MIRA, 2015).

During the first phase, beginning in the days immediately after the disaster, typically, only observational data may be available. During the second phase, a field-based assessment of the magnitude and impact of the disaster, including the major needs and response capacity, can be made using key informants and focus groups. This should be completed during the second or third week after the disaster. Finally, during the third phase, more in-depth, sector-specific

Section 2: Public Health Principles

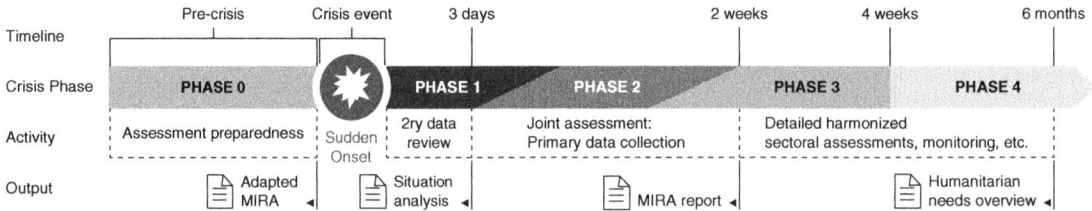

Figure 7.2 Phases of an emergency and phase-specific assessment tools

assessments using household interviews and repeated multisector recovery monitoring can be carried out.

The demarcation between the phases may not be clear. The information most useful during phase 1 may be very different than what is useful during phases 2 or 3. Part of the challenge is flexibility to decide what is the most useful information in a rapidly changing environment.

Multicluster/Sector Initial Rapid Assessment (MIRA)

As part of the effort to improve the utility and applicability of the IRA form and provide guidance for the use, OCHA led an effort that included The Assessment Capacities Project (ACAPS) to develop Operational Guidance for Coordinated Assessments in Humanitarian Crises (IASC 2012). This effort has since trained UN staff in many countries and led to the creation of the manual for Multicluster/Sector Initial Rapid Assessment (MIRA). Criticisms of the MIRA and challenges with its implementation have resulted in two subsequent revisions.

While guiding how information should be collected, the MIRA does not attempt to prescribe what information should be collected. There was enough disagreement between the different agencies involved on the content needed in a field-based assessment to prevent prescribing the information to be collected. Rather, the ability to adapt existing tools to unique situations should be prioritized, as a one-size-fits-all approach has been shown to work poorly.

A revised version of the MIRA Guidance was released in January 2015. It purports to reflect, "a common vision of what is methodologically sound and realistically feasible in the highly challenging environment in which emergency humanitarian needs assessments take place." To do so, it included the main areas of wide agreement and thus is shorter than previous consensus documents (IASC 2015).

The MIRA provides an evidence base for strategic response planning but cannot deliver statistically representative data on humanitarian needs. The MIRA builds on an analytical framework that includes the geographic scope and scale of the current crisis, the severity of its impact, the level of the current response and gaps in it, and operational constraints on responders. An excerpt from the MIRA document is shown in Figure 7.3 (Humanitarian Response 2015b).

The Assessment Capacities Project (ACAPS)

The Assessment Capacities Project (ACAPS), initially established in 2009 as a consortium of three NGOs (Norwegian Refugee Council, Save the Children, and Action Contre la Faim), is dedicated to improving the assessment of humanitarian needs in complex emergencies and crises. The membership has grown since that time. ACAPS was a critical contributor to the development of the MIRA. In addition, as part of their work, criteria were developed to assess the quality of needs assessments performed in emergency settings.

In 2015, ACAPS undertook a review of needs assessments undertaken after disasters or during humanitarian emergencies from 2000–2015. Needs assessment reports were retrieved from public domain sources including ReliefWeb, Humanitarian Response, One Response, OCHA, and NGO forums, and combined with information from other sources. The investigators estimated collection of at least 70 percent of all coordinated needs assessments undertaken between 2000 and 2010 and 95 percent of coordinated assessments undertaken between 2011 and 2015 (ACAPS 2015a).

Chapter 7: Needs Assessments

Crisis impact		Operational environment	
The crisis impact themes are directly related to the identification of sectoral humanitarian needs, vulnerabilities and risks, and an assessment of their severity as well as their immediate causes. • Assessing the crisis impact entails assessing the crisis drivers and their consequences in terms of number and type of group affected. • It also requires understanding the conditions of the affected population and qualifying the severity of the crisis at the sector level.		The operational environment themes are used to identify the degree to which the population in need is assisted. • Understanding the operational environment entails estimating the capacity to meet the needs of the affected population in the different sectors of interest, and the resulting gaps in response that need to be addressed. • It also requires assessing the degree to which humanitarian access is granted and how this impacts planning and delivery of goods and services (operational constraints).	
Scope and scale of the crisis	**Conditions of affected population**	**Capacities to respond**	**Humanitarian access**
Drivers are a factor or a set of factors that (can) trigger or expose to suffering or life-threatening conditions. They are differentiated by effects, from primary to secondary, such as a hurricane causing floods (primary effect), triggering population displacement (secondary effects) and subsequent loss of livelihood. Underlying factors are contextual elements that exacerbate the crisis, such as pre-existing food insecurity, lack of governance capacity, hazard-prone conditions, gender inequalities, social discrimination, remoteness.	Understanding the condition and status of the population calls for the assessment of the humanitarian outcomes in each key sector/cluster, and the existing vulnerabilities and risks resulting directly or indirectly from the crisis. The immediate causes of identified issues should be assessed in order to tackle their root causes (degree of accessibility, availability, awareness, quality and usability of goods and services). Finally, physical disruption of key infrastructures and losses needs to be estimated, as well as the losses directly and indirectly caused by the crisis.	Capacities and responses (planned or ongoing) refer to the ability of main stakeholders involved in the humanitarian response to meet the population needs. It is measured at different levels (national and international capacity, coping mechanisms of the affected population).	Assessing humanitarian access entails estimating the degree to which people in need are able to reach and be reached by humanitarian aid. It covers the access of relief actors to the affected population, the access of the affected population to markets and assistance, and security and physical constraints affecting both humanitarian actors and the affected population.
Humanitarian profile	**Severity of the crisis**	**Gaps in response**	**Operational constraints**
The analytical output of this theme is the geographical scope and scale of the crisis, including the estimate of the number and type of affected groups.	The analytical output of this theme is the severity of the crisis, including an estimate of the number of people in need at each sector level.	The analytical outputs of this theme are the gaps in response, including an estimate of the number of people whose needs cannot be fulfilled with the current level of response or capacity.	The analytical output of this theme is the identification of the operational constraints, including an estimate of the people in need unable to receive regular assistance.

In analyzing the impact of the crisis and of the operational environment as parallel and complementary themes, the MIRA analytical framework derives an analysis of unmet needs and key humanitarian priorities.

Figure 7.3 Excerpt from MIRA

In total, 109 needs assessment reports were identified: 55 were undertaken for sudden onset disasters and 54 for other types of crises such as conflict, displacement, or food insecurity. The results are shown in Figure 7.4 (ACAPS 2015a).

The number of common needs assessments carried out by year has generally increased over the last decade and a half. While most CNAs were carried out in sudden onset emergencies, over time an increased proportion of all assessments have been for chronic or complex emergencies. (Data for 2015 is not complete in the figure.)

Each of the needs assessment identified was reviewed for according to criteria of quality outlined in the 2012 ACAPS review of flash appeals (ACAPS 2015b). These criteria are shown in Table 7.3.

Quality scores were calculated for specific sections of the report demonstrating that in the past several years, improvements have been realized across all

Table 7.3 Needs assessment review criteria based on 2012 ACAPS review of flash appeals

Metadata	Methodology	Summary	Sector Information
• Year • Country • Disaster type • Report name • Coordination type • Number of sectors covered • Lead agency name and type • Disaster date • Report date • Use of secondary data • Support received • Questionnaire and report number of pages • Preparedness	• Objectives • Sampling strategy • Sample size and locations • Data collection techniques • Limitations • Date of field assessment • Questionnaire attached	• Disaster overview • Area background information • Total affected pop • Recommendations for coordination • Cross cutting issues • Operational constraints • Key findings • Key priorities • Key recommendations • Most affected groups, areas and sectors	• Precrisis information • Total affected pop • SADD • Group and area disaggregated data • Key findings • Key priorities identified by communities and assessment teams • Key recommendations • Ongoing response • Cross-cutting issues • Constraints

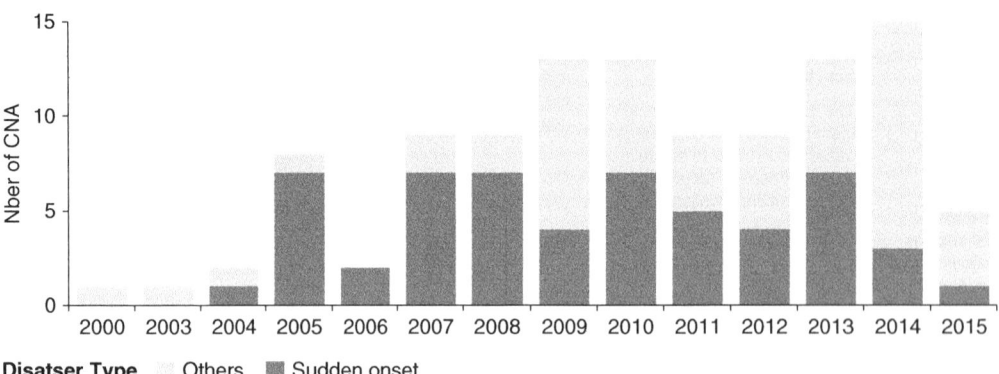

Figure 7.4 Number of needs assessment reports per year from 2000–2015 (ACAPS 2015a)

report sections with more systematic and consistent results. Quality, on average, has increased in CNA reports for both sudden onset disasters and other types of crises. The average quality scores for needs assessment reports are shown in Figure 7.5.

In addition, reports have become more concise and more often have included data comparing current conditions to historical data. Those with training in assessments did not notably improve the quality of reports but they did, importantly, shorten the time period needed to create the report (ACAPS 2015b). Countries with needs assessment preparedness covered at least as many information areas, and did so in about half the time when compared with common needs assessments without prior training.

Challenges

Broadly, challenges in performing needs assessments in the setting of humanitarian emergencies include balancing collection of information that is both adequate and timely, developing needs assessment tools that are both generally applicable and flexible, converting collected information into humanitarian action, and responding to the ever-changing situation.

One of the challenges in performing a needs assessment is identifying the key groups and variables before any information is collected. It is often necessary to depend on qualitative information through observation, conversation, and from historical data to get a wider, overall view. The combination of qualitative information with quantitative data from measurable indicators provides an overall picture that best represents the true state of the population at the time of the assessment. In deciding what information to collect and how to collect it, it is important to balance precision, accuracy, time, and cost.

Assessors performing needs assessments in humanitarian emergencies may not know who is making

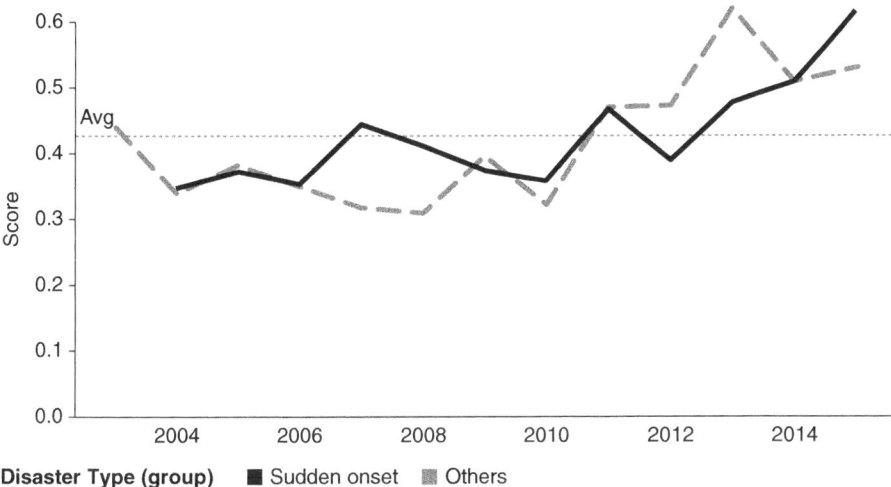

Figure 7.5 Average quality scores for needs assessment reports by type from 2000 to 2015 (ACAPS 2015b)

the key decisions or what options those decisions makers have. It is important to be watchful that the issues focused on are not too old or not yet relevant when the decisions are made. Some assessors may come from a background in formal research in stable settings with well-established households and months to gather information. In contrast, a needs assessment performed during an emergency is by definition in an unstable setting where the population is not in well-established households and the information is needed in weeks rather than months.

A study in 2003 found that "needs assessment, as currently practiced is inadequate to provide the information upon which to base genuinely impartial responses" (Darcy 2003). The main critique was the lack of established methods and inadequate transparency in how results were reached. It was also noted that too little priority was given to the process of needs assessments throughout the course of an emergency, recommending instead that initial needs assessments be a first step toward ongoing monitoring through the months and years of recovery. Finally, it was noted that agency approaches were too closely aligned to the front-end fund-raising process and needs assessment results were not considered sufficiently independent and objective.

Similarly, in 2009, the United Nations Interagency Needs Assessment Task Force found (IASC 2009):

- Lack of essential baseline information required at the onset of a humanitarian emergency
- Significant overlap in data collection between different initiatives
- Need for a core set of indicators for consistency and comparability
- Need for better sharing of lessons learned and best practices on needs assessments and their design
- Insufficient contingency planning and use of precrisis information as the basis for the needs assessment

Information Overload

People carrying out needs assessments are often under pressure to collect far more information than is realistic or useful at the time decisions will be made. This happens because questionnaires typically are produced through wide consultation among interested organizations, each with an agenda that goes beyond the initial needs assessment. Too often, data collection from affected areas is not appropriately grounded in precrisis information, leaving insufficient understanding of the information collected. In one survey, for example, people were asked if they had soap in their home following a disaster. Data was summarized and analyzed without understanding whether they typically had soap in their home prior to the disaster.

Further, when too much data is produced with too little analysis, it is challenging to make sense of it all to direct actions. The rapid rise in data collected and reports created during humanitarian emergencies in the past decade has led, at times, to information overload. For example, in 2010 there was an average of 216 reports per disaster while in 2014 the average

Section 2: Public Health Principles

Examples of indicators to measure input, output, and outcomes

	Input Indicators Describe	**Output Indicators Describe**	**Outcome Indicators Describe**
Health	The human/material resources available for the provision of health services	The level of health services provided to the population	Health status of the population
	e.g. number of health facilities	*e.g. number of consultations*	*e.g. prevalence of a disease*
Nutrition	The human/material resources available for the prevention and/or correction of malnutrition	The services provided for the prevention and/or correction of malnutrition	The nutritional status of the population
		e.g. number of children enrolled in therapeutic feeding programs	*e.g. prevalence of severe acute malnutrition (SAM)*
Food security	Production, distribution and availability of food	The level of commodities and services provided to improve people's access to food	The population's access to food
	e,g. availability of food on the local markets	*e.g. quantity of food distributed*	*e.g. percentage of households by duration of staple foods*
Water, sanitation and hygiene	The infrastructure, facilities and services available	The quantities delivered	The population's access to water and to sanitation facilities
	e.g. number of hand pumps for water	*e.g. number of liters/person/day*	*e.g. % of households by time to collect water*

Source: NATF, Operational Guidance on Coordinated Assessments in Emergencies, July 23, 2009, p. 18.

Figure 7.6 Examples of input indicators, output indicators, and outcome indicators

---

number of reports per disaster had grown to 795 (ReliefWeb 2015).

Despite this rapid rise in the sheer volume of data collected during humanitarian emergencies, a great deal of progress has been made since the findings of the IASC in 2009, and by 2015 more realistic goals and agreement on methods for information collection have greatly improved the utility of needs assessments (personal communication, Garfield 2015).

Indicators

There remains no agreement on a common set of indicators across the major sectors necessary to inform needs assessment design and subsequent monitoring and evaluation efforts. The Health, Nutrition, Food Security, and WASH sectors have attempted to develop a stable set of core information needs. These are shown in Figure 7.6. Even the tools to develop survey instruments or track information from secondary sources over time are limited, resulting in a need to "reinvent the wheel" each time. Identifying key indicators for different stages and contexts across a wide variety of humanitarian crisis remains a major task.

Notes from the Field

Myanmar (2008)

The cyclone in Myanmar in 2008 had winds of greater than 100 mph and flooding 25 miles inland, resulting in more than two hundred thousand deaths. Prior to the disaster, little was known about the affected region where government had long restricted international access and communications. Initially government tried to restrict humanitarian assistance; ultimately a large-scale representative sample survey attempted to reach all affected areas. So successful was this effort that three follow-up surveys using similar methods were carried out over the following two years of recovery, keeping access open and international assistance flowing. Many believe this experience helped bring the country out of isolation and take steps toward wider citizen participation.

Pakistan (2008)

The 2008 earthquake in Pakistan led to the formation of an ongoing national team to do postdisaster needs assessments. This effort led to a much clearer picture of damages and needs than had been available when a massive earthquake struck Pakistan three years earlier. As a result, the international community saw its assistance funds used more effectively and supported via UNICEF the maintenance of this team, which refined its approach and has served in many national disasters since.

Haiti (2010)

The 2010 earthquake in Haiti was the first major disaster to affect a country's capital city. There was an effort to recreate the comprehensive geographic approach that had been used in Myanmar. The effort was far less successful on Haiti than it had been in Myanmar (Stoianova 2015, Rencoret 2015). This was a result, in part, of far too many organizations taking part, leading to unnecessary inquiry in many unaffected parts of the country. This contributed to the information from the assessment not being available until months after it was needed.

Pakistan (2010)

Floods affected more than half of the landmass of Pakistan in 2010. Teams utilized a uniform approach across the country performing interviews of people already recovering while downstream flooding was just starting. Methodologically, it was an advance to identify high and low affected areas for comparison, rather than trying to reach all communities of interest. This was possible, in part, because survey teams had become skilled in this practice in the prior three years.

Syria (2013)

Ongoing, repeated assessments were needed in Syria, where humanitarian conditions deteriorated in the setting of several years of warfare. Geographic access was severely limited when the first assessment was organized. Only teams of locals, organized across the borders, were able to go in and triangulate the responses of mayors and other local authorities in about half of the targeted areas. In subsequent rounds over the following years, additional communities in hard-to-reach areas were covered and trends over time were identified.

Conclusion

In the coming years, demands for timely field-based information on humanitarian conditions will continue to increase rapidly. Even more rapid will be the increase in data of many types, especially those using electronic means of communication and remote sensing. This will manifest in the availability of ever more systems, figures, colors, and datapoints. It also will require hearing more from victims and beneficiaries themselves, to identify what they want and need most as conditions involve (Semrau et al. 2015).

In 2015, a report produced for the World Humanitarian Summit called for the development of mechanisms to verify and improve the quality and credibility of needs assessments (Lovon and Austion 2016). The summit subsequently resulted in a commitment to create a single, joint common-needs analysis for future major humanitarian emergencies. Clarity on those mechanisms still does not exist. The idea that only one assessment would be created demonstrates potential shortsightedness of how needs assessments are actually used. No single assessment could at the same time be widely inclusive and rapid. Disagreement between UN organizations to lead this effort shows that we are neither organizationally or methodologically yet ready to fulfil many aspirations that exist for needs assessments.

Further progress will depend on improved precrisis decisions on what information to collect, the methods used to collect the information, and development of analytical and communications skill. The demand for ever better and faster access to information creates an opportunity to make these improvements. Unless the opportunity is managed well, this rising level of information will not translate into better decisions and deeper shared situation awareness. That depends on identifying the data needed for a particular phase, associating it with information from the past and tracking its evolution, and putting it in a wider context of the social, political, and economic context of affected populations. Unfortunately, it is easier to expand the amount of data than improve its analysis or dissemination.

References

ACAPS. (2015a). A review of needs assessments undertaken after disasters or during humanitarian emergencies from 2000–2015, ACAPS, unpublished.

ACAPS. (2015b). ACAPS 2012 Review of flash appeals. Available at www.acaps.org (Accessed December 31, 2015).

Darcy, J., Hofman, C. A. (2003). *According to need? Needs assessment and decision-making in the humanitarian sector.* ODI: London, September 2003. Available at www.odi.org/sites/odi.org.uk/files/odi-assets/publications-opinion-files/285.pdf (Accessed December 31, 2015).

Garfield, R., Blake, C., Chatainger, P., Walton-Ellery, S. (2011). *Common needs assessments and humanitarian action.* HPN network paper 69. ODI: London: 2011. Available at www.odihpn.org/documents/networkpaper069.pdf (Accessed December 31, 2015).

Humanitarian Response. (2015a). Available at www.humanitarianresponse.info/en/programme-cycle/space/resource-mobilization-overview (Accessed December 31, 2015).

Humanitarian Response. (2015b). Available at www.humanitarianresponse.info/en/programme-cycle/space/document/multi-sector-initial-rapid-assessment-guidance-revision-july-2015 (Accessed December 31, 2015).

IASC needs assessment task force, operational guidance for coordinated assessments in humanitarian crises. (2009). Draft version For Needs Assessment Task Force, Geneva, 23 July 2009.

IASC operational guidance on coordinated assessments in humanitarian crises, NATF, 2012. (2012). Available at www.humanitarianrepsoonse.info/programmecycle/space/document/operational-guidance coordinated-assessments-humanitarian-crises-0 (Accessed December 31, 2015).

Initial Rapid Assessment (IRA) tool. (2009). Available at http://washcluster.net/resources/iasc-initial-rapid-assessment-tool-ira-2009/and www.who.int/hac/network/global_health_cluster/ira_guidance_note_june2009.pdf (Accessed December 31, 2015).

Lovon, M., and Austion, L. (2016). *OCHA coordinated assessment support section review of coordinated assessment and joint analysis processes and outputs.* Geneva: OCHA, 2016.

NOAA. (2015). Available at http://coast.noaa.gov/needsassessment/# (Accessed December 31, 2015).

ReliefWeb. (2015). Available at www.reliefweb.int (Accessed December 31, 2015).

Rencoret, N., Stoddard, A., Haver, K., Taylor, G., and Harvey, P. (2010). Alnap: London, 2010. Haiti earthquake response, context analysis, pp. 25–27. Available at www.alnap.org/pool/files/haiti-context-analysis-final.pdf (Accessed December 31, 2015).

Semrau, M., Petragallo, S., Griekspoor, A., de Radigues, X., and van Ommeren, M. One innovative example is the HESPER scale. The HESPER Scale: a tool to assess perceived needs in humanitarian emergencies. Available at www.odihpn.org/the-humanitarian-space/news/announcements/blog-articles/the-hesper-scale-a-tool-to-assess-perceived-needs-in-humanitarian-emergencies (Accessed December 31, 2015).

Stoianova, V. Donor funding in Haiti, Assessing humanitarian needs after the 2010 Haiti earthquake. Available at www.globalhumanitarianassistance.org/report/haiti-funding-according-to-needs (Accessed December 31, 2015).

The Sphere Project. (2011). Available at www.sphereproject.org/handbook/ (Accessed December 31, 2015).

Chapter 8

Surveys

Oleg O. Bilukha, Olivier Degomme, and Eva Leidman

Introduction

Field surveys are a standard, widely used method of measuring key nutrition and health indicators in humanitarian emergencies. In the absence of vital registration systems, often inadequate or completely destroyed in the setting of humanitarian emergencies, key data are obtained through surveys. Surveys provide information needed to understand the challenges of a disaster, document trends, allocate resources, design appropriate response interventions, and evaluate the effectiveness of public health programs.

This chapter describes surveys and provides a general overview of field survey methods. Some of the key challenges of implementing surveys in the context of humanitarian emergencies as well as the efforts and methods aimed at ensuring quality data despite these challenges are highlighted.

Surveys

Surveys usually collect data from a representative population sample. Surveys often use random sampling procedures to gather population representative data. Representative sampling allows for collection of information about a large group of people by assessing only a representative subset, or sample, of them. In rare occasions, surveys may collect information from all eligible subjects in the target population, this is referred to as an exhaustive survey or census.

Surveys are cross-sectional. Data are collected at one specific point of time. Survey data provide a snapshot image of the population. The results represent the situation on the day(s) of the survey or during the recall period as in the case of mortality surveys.

Surveys primarily collect quantitative data. Quantitative data includes any information that can be expressed as a number or quantified. Surveys may include measurements such as anthropometry or water quality tests, observations such as the presence and type of latrines or quantity and volume of water storage containers, or questions asked to respondents that can be answered with discrete responses. Information that can be presented on a nominal scale, such as gender or ethnicity, may also be collected. A structured questionnaire is usually used to collect data.

Surveys collect data at the household or individual level. Surveys randomly select households or individuals, for instance women of reproductive age or children under five, and collect their individual information. The entity on which information is collected, often the household or individual, is referred to as a survey subject. The type of survey subject is determined by the goals and objectives of the survey.

These defining characteristics of surveys translate into important strengths that make surveys a key tool for collecting information in humanitarian emergencies. For instance, the representative sampling design may allow the results to be generalized to the entire target population. As stated previously, information about the population at large, through a representative view of all affected, can be very useful in understanding the magnitude of an emergency, documenting trends, allocating resources, designing appropriate response interventions, and evaluating the effectiveness of activities.

The cross-sectional design means data collection for surveys is completed during a relatively short time period. Compared to methods that require ongoing data collection, such as surveillance, surveys are relatively easy to implement and supervise. Surveillance is discussed in Chapter 9. With a dedicated team and adequate resources, a few well-trained survey teams can collect enough information in a few days or weeks to give robust information on the status of the affected population. It is feasible to provide rigorous training to a limited number of enumerator teams, followed by close supervision during the period of data collection. By comparison, ensuring continuous quality for longitudinal data collection methods requires ongoing supervision, periodic retraining and quality control over months or years.

Analysis of quantitative data allows for quality checks that may not be possible with qualitative data. Individual or household level data provides more detailed information than data collected at the community level. Survey results can, for example, demonstrate differences in key outcomes by demographic groups such as age, sex, or geography or identify correlations between indicators at individual or household level. This kind of analysis is not feasible with data collected at the community level.

An important strength of surveys as a means of data collection is the existence of standard methods and guidance. Field survey methodologies are well documented in manuals and simple tools including those from the World Food Programme (WFP) and Centers for Disease Control and Prevention (CDC), Save the Children, and the SMART Methodology (Save the Children 2004, SMART Methodology 2012, WFP and CDC 2005). There are "how to" guides that clearly outline the process of undertaking a survey and analyzing data in language easily understood by field practitioners. In addition, there are several free software packages available for analyzing survey data.

One of the main reasons that surveys have become a key assessment method in humanitarian emergencies is that they are the standard method for measuring several key indicators used to benchmark the severity of the humanitarian emergency. High-quality representative surveys are often the best available source for many key nutrition, health, water and sanitation, and mortality indicators (Spiegel et al. 2004).

Due to these strengths, surveys are used prolifically; however, surveys are just one of several methods used to collect data in humanitarian emergencies. The other key methods are rapid assessments and surveillance, discussed in Chapters 7 and 9 respectively. The following are some key features that distinguish these methods.

Rapid Assessments

Both rapid assessments and surveys are cross-sectional. They both collect data at one specific point of time. Data collected represent the situation on the day(s) of the assessment.

Compared with surveys, rapid assessment methodology is simplified to ensure feasibility and efficiency during the immediate aftermath of a disaster. For instance, rapid assessments may only visit a few sites, for example, villages, camps, or towns. Site selection is often not random, but instead determined by factors including access and logistical feasibility. This is in contrast to survey methods which require visiting at least 25 or more randomly selected sites (Binkin et al. 1992). The simplified methods used in rapid assessments are designed to ensure that they can be carried out during the first two weeks following a disaster. In this initial period, information is greatly needed, but the context is often chaotic. Surveys, because of more demanding logistic requirements, are generally done at least three to four weeks, or later, after the onset of a disaster.

Rapid assessment methods often require fewer teams and fewer resources. Visiting fewer sites requires fewer assessment teams, or fewer days of work per team, compared to surveys. Logistic requirements such as transportation and lodging may be less demanding. Streamlining logistic and human resources may decrease costs.

Rapid assessments usually gather information at the community rather than individual or household level. Information is collected from key informants such as community leaders or health workers or small focus groups, about the community as a whole rather than about individual persons or households. Community-level data collection requires less time than household assessments used in surveys, where teams visit hundreds of families door-to-door.

Rapid assessment methods are less structured. Survey methods are globally standardized. By comparison, the methods of rapid assessments may vary in different contexts. Rapid assessment guidelines give flexibility in determining the procedures used to collect data. Data collection generally includes a combination of direct observation, key informant interviews, and focus group discussions. Often a checklist or a semistructured questionnaire is developed to aid data collection.

Rapid assessments collect qualitative data that require only basic analysis. The direct observation and focus group methods are best suited for collecting qualitative data, descriptions, or ranking of key problems and needs for example. These data are best suited for simple descriptive analysis. Systematic debriefings of field teams may be sufficient

(Inter-Agency Standing Committee 2012). In contrast to surveys, advanced quantitative analysis of the data is not necessary or feasible given the type of data collected. Field teams can generally interpret rapid assessment results without statistical training. This is important to produce recommendations for rapid, evidence-based programming during the initial phase of the response to a humanitarian emergency.

Surveillance

Surveillance systems collect longitudinal rather than cross-sectional data. Health facilities or community workers collect data continuously and report findings routinely.

Surveillance can capture incident cases and monitor trends in real time. Continuous data collection enables capture of new cases as they appear. Therefore, surveillance data is more suitable to measuring incidence, a measure of the frequency with which new cases of illness, injury, death, birth, or other health condition or vital event occur in the population. The cross-sectional design of surveys is less conducive to capturing incidence; however, surveys are better suited to measure prevalence.

Like surveys, surveillance collects data at the level of the individual. In surveillance, while individual data may be collected, more often only aggregate data are reported by sites to the central level. For example, clinicians may record diagnosis for all children in a clinic register and then tally the aggregate numbers diagnosed with reportable conditions such as the number of measles cases this week. Often only the aggregates are reported, disaggregated by basic demographics, such as gender and age.

Primarily health professionals collect surveillance data as part of routine activities. Examples include data collection by a nurse at a health center, a nutritionist at a feeding center, or a coroner at a morgue, in contrast to data collection by dedicated enumerators in surveys. Linking data collection with routine activities at surveillance sites helps ensure ongoing, systematic reporting. This is a key distinction from surveys and rapid assessments that generally hire and train staff specifically for the duration of the assessment.

Surveillance systems usually collect fewer indicators than do surveys. To reduce the burden of ongoing data collection, surveillance systems generally collect limited information. Unlike survey enumerators, routine health staff often do not have the time to administer lengthy questionnaires without detracting from their primary duties. Surveillance systems designed for humanitarian emergencies generally collect only a few key figures such as number of diagnosed cases of a few priority diseases (WHO 2012). Many of these priority diseases are infectious diseases with epidemic potential.

Surveillance is usually designed to achieve universal coverage. Surveillance systems aim to capture all cases of notifiable conditions, whereas surveys that are sampling a subset of the population register a representative sample of cases but by definition, cannot capture all cases, unless the survey is exhaustive.

Existing surveillance systems are often disrupted in humanitarian emergencies. It therefore may be necessary to put in place a simplified surveillance system to function during the immediate response until normal data collection can resume. This can be achieved in some, but not all settings. Where it is too difficult to set up continuous data collection, periodic, repeated surveys might be used to monitor trends. For example, in some emergency settings, systems have been put in place that conduct periodic surveys every three to six months to track trends in acute malnutrition. Repeated surveys do not allow for real-time continuous appraisal but enable limited periodic monitoring of trends (Bilukha et al. 2012).

Key characteristics of different assessment methods discussed above are summarized in Table 8.1.

Key Indicators Measured in Field Surveys

When a physician evaluates a patient, he or she may decide to obtain some lab tests in order to help assess the type and severity of the illness or disease and determine what therapy may be required. Specifically, if the results of these tests are beyond the normal parameters or outside the reference range, this may indicate the nature and severity of the illness and help the physician in reaching a diagnosis and treatment plan.

In a very similar way, epidemiologists conduct surveys in order to assess the type and severity of a humanitarian emergency and identify major public health problems. Two indicators commonly measured during humanitarian emergencies through surveys are nutrition and mortality. Both of these

Table 8.1 Comparison of assessment methods commonly used in humanitarian emergencies

	Rapid Assessment	Survey	Surveillance
Objective	Rapid appraisal	Medium-term appraisal	Continuous appraisal
Data Collection	Cross-sectional	Cross-sectional	Longitudinal
Data Type	Mostly qualitative	Quantitative	Quantitative
Method	Usually convenience sample of sites	Random representative sample	Universal capture of cases seen at surveillance sites
Survey Subject	Community level	Household/individual level	Individual level, often aggregate data
Data Collectors	Dedicated assessment staff (enumerators)	Dedicated assessment staff (enumerators)	Routine health staff

indicators provide a good indication of the overall health status of the surveyed population. In that sense, nutrition and mortality indicators may be considered "routine surveys" in humanitarian emergencies. Just like the physician comparing a patient's lab result with reference values, epidemiologists compare the nutrition and mortality figures in the population against expected values and conclude whether or not the situation warrants intervention and/or further investigation.

Being cross-sectional, surveys are a good tool for measuring health conditions present in the population at the time of the survey. Nutrition surveys are a typical example. Prevalence studies comprise an important share of these surveys and may be used not only to measure the current situation but also may measure a time period in the past. A retrospective mortality survey is a typical example of a retrospective survey. Retrospective surveys may be limited by events in the past being forgotten or omitted, resulting in recall bias.

Nutrition Indicators

In humanitarian emergencies, nutrition surveys measure the level of malnutrition in a population. Most of the time, this is done using anthropometric measurements such as length or height, weight, and sometimes the mid-upper arm circumference (MUAC). Anthropometry is generally collected on children aged 6 to 59 months as they are considered to be among those most vulnerable to fluctuations in daily dietary intake plus environmental and health conditions and therefore serve as a good proxy for the nutrition status of the general population.

In humanitarian emergencies, it is important to evaluate fluctuations of the population's nutritional status. Different nutritional indicators reflect different types of malnutrition. For example, an indicator that reflects acute malnutrition is weight-for-height (W/H) of the surveyed children. For each child, weight is compared against a reference range accounting for the child's height and sex (WHO Multicentre Growth Reference Group 2006) to calculate a z-score. Children who have z-scores that are below two standard deviations below the reference mean (−2 z-scores) are considered malnourished or "wasted." Children below −3 z-scores are considered to have severe acute malnutrition (SAM). These data are then aggregated into a population level indicator, global acute malnutrition (GAM), which is defined as the percentage of malnourished children among all children 6 to 59 months. Also included in this indicator are children that have bilateral pitting edema, assessed by pressing the thumb on the foot, independent of the z-score calculation, since this is indicative of severe malnutrition.

In addition to weight-for-height, z-scores, and the presence of bilateral pitting edema, acute malnutrition may also be assessed by measuring a child's MUAC by applying a standardized measuring tape around the child's left upper arm. Utilizing this method, SAM is the percentage of children 6 to 59 months with a MUAC below 115 mm (11.5 cm). Moderate acute malnutrition is the percentage of children 6 to 59 months with a MUAC between 115 mm and 125 mm (Global Nutrition Cluster 2011). Because MUAC cutoffs in humanitarian emergencies are the same for all children between six and 59 months of age, the prevalence of low MUAC is age dependent, generally higher for younger children than for older children (Gernaat et al. 1996). MUAC is often used as admission criterion for feeding programs since estimating the population prevalence of children with low MUAC can be used to predict expected overall program admission. However, weight-for-height remains the primary indicator of acute malnutrition measured in nutrition surveys.

In order to evaluate the severity of a humanitarian emergency, standard emergency threshold for GAM and SAM have been established against which survey results are compared. For GAM, 15 percent is commonly used as the emergency threshold; however, in the presence of aggravating factors such as a measles epidemic, the emergency threshold is lowered to 10 percent (WHO 2000).

Nutrition and malnutrition are discussed in greater detail in Chapters 12 and 25.

Mortality Indicators

In addition to nutrition, the other key indicator in humanitarian emergencies is the mortality rate. Although vital registration systems are the best way to measure mortality, in humanitarian emergencies these systems are often disrupted or do not exist. Pending the establishment of a registration system, surveys are a valuable tool to quantify and monitor mortality rates in the affected population. In these surveys, data are collected on demographic composition of households in a sample over a specified period in the past. This time period that can vary from a few weeks to several years is called the recall period. The duration of the recall period depends on several factors, but generally, longer recall periods reduce the required sample size at the cost of increasing the risk for a recall bias. Recall periods in emergency settings usually range from three to six months.

The household census method is used to collect data on vital events within households such as deaths and births. While there are variants of this method, in general, the aim is to obtain an enumeration of deaths, births, departures, and arrivals in the household during the recall period (Cairns et al. 2009). Mortality rate is calculated as the total number of deaths divided by the number of persons in the sampled households during the recall period. This calculated indicator reflects the total mortality in the population and is called the crude mortality rate (CMR), typically expressed during humanitarian emergencies in "deaths per 10,000 people per day."

In addition to CMR, it is often important to know the level of mortality among children under five years of age, called the under-five mortality rate (U5MR). It is obtained from the same data as CMR, but only includes children less than five years of age in both the numerator (deaths) and denominator (population size).

Since mortality *rates* include a time parameter, they are measures of incidence, as opposed to nutrition indicators that are measures of prevalence.

To evaluate the severity of a humanitarian emergency utilizing mortality indicators, the Sphere Project suggests emergency thresholds using baseline mortality levels seen in the absence of crisis (The Sphere Project 2011). The emergency threshold for CMR or U5MR is reached when they exceed twice the baseline CMR or U5MR respectively. Since baseline mortality rates vary by region, so do the emergency thresholds. When baseline rates are unknown, absolute emergency thresholds for CMR and U5MR of 1 death/10,000/day for CMR and 2 under-five deaths/10,000/day for U5MR are utilized. The Sphere Project is discussed in greater detail in Chapter 4.

Additional Indicators

Surveys often collect information on other indicators in addition to nutrition and mortality. In many cases, these indicators are added to nutrition surveys rather than collected using separate dedicated surveys. An example of indicators often included with nutrition surveys is a group of indicators assessing the population's food security. This may be helpful in understanding the causes of malnutrition in a population. Typically, information collected on food security indicators includes types of foods available to the households, their sources, the household's purchasing power, access to food assistance, coping strategies, and dietary diversity. In addition, indicators on infant and young child feeding practices (IYCF) provide insights on breastfeeding practices and types of foods consumed by young children aged zero to 23 months.

Additional examples of indicators commonly added to nutrition surveys in humanitarian emergencies include measles vaccination coverage, usually measured in children aged nine to 59 months, vitamin A coverage, and the occurrence of illnesses in the past two weeks, both commonly measured in children aged 6 to 59 months.

In some situations, information on additional indicators requires a separate survey or a complete module to be added to the existing survey questionnaire. Information on water, sanitation, and hygiene (WASH) indicators such as access to safe water sources, quantity of water available per person, and practices of excreta disposal are examples. Surveys with a focus on mental health or reproductive health are additional examples. These surveys may collect data from different types of survey subjects than those commonly assessed in nutrition and mortality surveys. For instance, surveys on reproductive health typically assess women of reproductive age. These surveys may require advanced or specialized interviewing skills, as they may include more sensitive questions or may be too lengthy to include in routine surveys.

It may be tempting to include additional survey questions to meet the needs of different sectors. It is important to balance this need to collect additional information with the reality that every addition results in a longer questionnaire and thus a longer interview, increasing the time needed for data collection and increasing the likelihood of respondent or interviewer fatigue. The result may be more information but of considerably poorer quality. Therefore, one should aim to limit questions to those indicators that are most relevant for the programming of key emergency interventions. Further, including questions that are not standardized nor been validated previously is not recommended (Watson et al. 2011).

Conducting Field Surveys

The process of conducting a survey may be divided into three parts including planning, data collection, and analysis and reporting:

Planning

Planning is done before data collection. It includes several broad tasks that have to be completed, often concurrently rather than sequentially.

- Formulating the goals and objectives of the survey, determining what indicators to measure, creating a survey instrument or questionnaire, development of survey protocol, and obtaining human subjects clearance
- Determining sampling strategy, getting population data, calculating sample size, and carrying out sampling
- Recruitment, training and testing survey teams, preparing equipment, supplies, and logistics including transportation and lodging

Data Collection

Data collection is performed in the field.

- Data collection requires properly trained survey teams who understand the survey and are provided the logistical and financial support to undertake the survey.
- Survey teams should be supervised on-site rather than remotely.

Analysis and Reporting

Analysis and reporting is normally done after the data collection is completed. It includes several tasks that have to be completed sequentially.

- Data entry
- Data cleaning and quality checks
- Data analysis
- Report writing
- Dissemination of the results
- Follow-up on recommendations articulated in the report

Steps in Performing a Survey

The process of conducting a survey presents many challenges and requires several considerations.

The basic steps of performing a survey are shown in Figure 8.1 and outlined in greater detail below:

Determine Whether a Survey is Needed and Logistically Feasible

Prior to undertaking a survey, it is important to determine whether a survey is needed and logistically feasible. A survey is a resource-intensive exercise and requires advanced epidemiological expertise as well as availability of qualified enumerators, equipment, and supplies, means of transport, and funds. Therefore, the goals and objectives of the survey have to be clearly justified, even more so in emergency settings where surveys compete for resources with other, often lifesaving, activities. To justify the survey, one must be able to clearly articulate why measuring given indicators in a given time frame is vital to key public health programs and demonstrate that critical data are

Chapter 8: Surveys

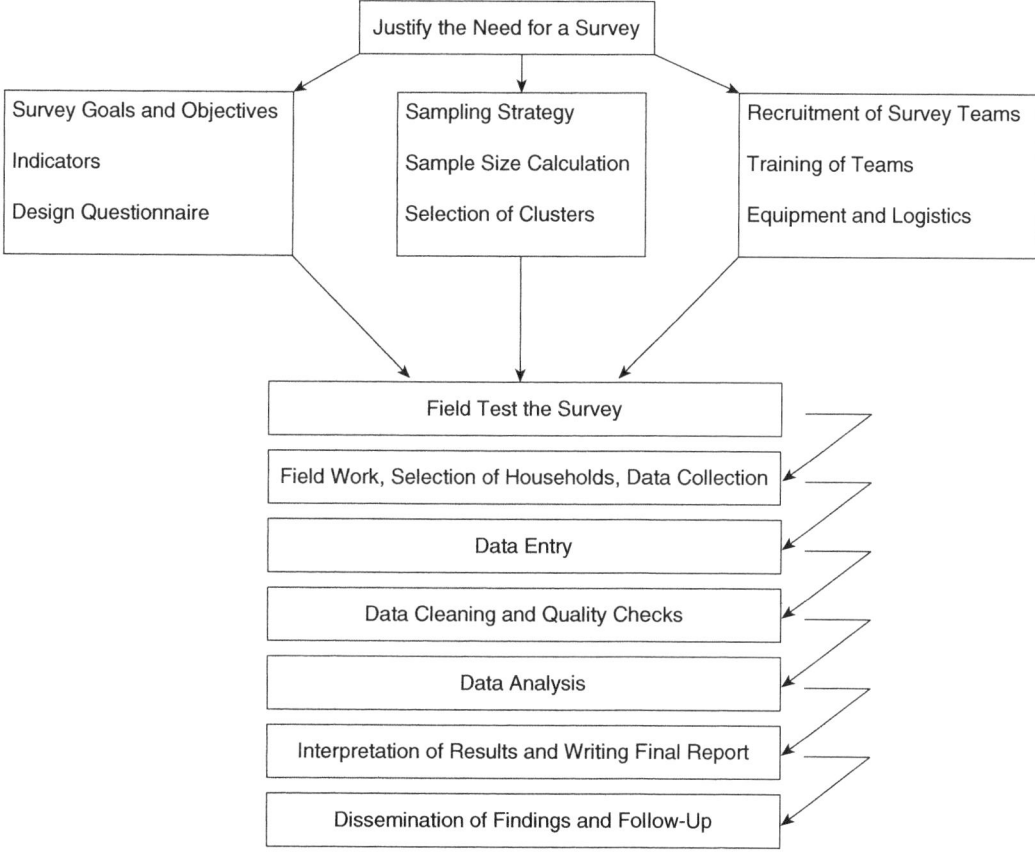

Figure 8.1 Steps in performing a survey

not already available from other sources such as surveillance, rapid assessments, or preemergency sources. Often preemergency surveys conducted in the same area can be used for some indicators, since many indicators may not be affected, or affected very little, by the emergency.

Formulate the Goals and Objectives of the Survey

In articulating what to measure in the survey, the goal is a broad statement of what the survey is about, for example: "To determine nutritional status, morbidity, and mortality in a refugee camp X." followed by formulating detailed, concrete objectives. Each objective specifies the indicator or group of indicators to be measured (e.g., anthropometry, anemia, access to safe water and sanitation facilities, infant feeding practices, etc.) and defines the population group in which each of these outcomes is to be measured (e.g., children 6 to 59 months, women of reproductive age, or households)

Goals and objectives have to be discussed and agreed upon with the major stakeholders that will use survey results to inform their programming decisions. The number of objectives, and hence things to measure, should be kept to a minimum. Each objective has to be justified by describing what key programming decisions will be informed by measuring given indicators.

Formulate Survey Questions and Create Survey Questionnaire

The importance of this step is often underappreciated. To be able to collect valid, reliable, and useful data, the questions have to be formulated clearly, succinctly, and in the language understandable to those being interviewed. Care should be taken such that the questions are formulated in a neutral, nonleading way, that they are not too complex, not too sensitive, and ask about matters that can be reasonably remembered by the respondent. Objectives formulated in the previous step should guide what questions or measurements need to be included in the survey.

The formatting of a questionnaire is also very important and at times, neglected. The questionnaire should be in sufficiently large font for the interviewers to read, the questions must be clearly aligned with the answer options, and sufficient space should be given to record answers. Answer options should be clearly and consistently coded. For example, all answer options "Yes" use code 1, all "No" use code 2, and all "Unknown" use code 88. If the survey is initially written in one language and the subsequent interviews are conducted in another language, then the questionnaire should be translated by one translator from the first language to the second language and then translated back to the first language by another, independent translator, not familiar with the original, first language version. This allows for verification of whether the translation is appropriate and the meaning of all questions preserved. The "final" version of the questionnaire has to be tested during the field test, as described below.

Determine Sampling Strategy and Collect Population Data

As described previously, surveys usually measure a sample or a small subset of the target population, since the populations are usually large and it is not feasible to measure every eligible subject. Therefore, one needs to decide on the general sampling strategy. If the population is concentrated in a small geographically compact area such as a town or a refugee camp, and a list of households is available, one can use a simple or systematic sampling method. If the population is dispersed in numerous villages, towns, or spontaneous settlements, and no listing of households is available, it is often not feasible to visit all of them. In these situations a cluster sampling method may be used.

To be able to conduct sampling, one first needs to collect population data. For example, if the plan is to randomly select households in a refugee camp, an up-to-date list of all households in the camp is needed. If the plan is to conduct cluster sampling, a list of all villages, towns, and spontaneous settlements from the survey area and the population size of each settlement is needed. Collecting accurate population data and creating complete up-to-date lists of households or settlements is extremely important but often very difficult in the setting of humanitarian emergencies. Such a list describing the population in the survey area is called a sampling frame. It is important that the list be both complete and accurate. For instance, if newly arrived refugee households were not included on the refugee camp list, these households would have no chance of being selected as survey participants. Similarly, if the census data is outdated, there may be current villages, towns, or settlements that did not exist when the census was taken. These households would have no chance of being selected as survey participants. Exclusion of households because they are not included in the listing of households may result in bias of the survey results.

Carry Out Sampling

The simplest approach to sampling is appropriately called the simple (random) sampling method. In this method, individuals or households are randomly selected from a list of all eligible individuals or households similar to a lottery. The probability of being selected is exactly the same for every individual or household on the list. It is therefore critical that the list is available and is both exhaustive and updated when using this method. In reality, such a list is seldom available in humanitarian emergencies. In these contexts surveyors may use several methods.

- Field staff enumerating all households and/or eligible individuals can generate a list. Once the list is completed, sampling may be carried out as described above.
- If the households or living units are arranged in an orderly manner, which may be the case in certain settlements or refugee camps, the systematic sampling method may be used. In this method, instead of using the "lottery" approach, field staff will define a path that runs exactly once along each eligible household or living unit. They will then move along that path and select households or living units using a predefined interval called the sampling interval. The sampling interval means that after visiting a selected household or living unit, a certain number of households or living units must be passed or skipped before the next household or living unit is selected, visited, and sampled. The sampling interval is calculated by

dividing the total number of eligible households or living units by the required sample size. For example, if a sample of five hundred households or living units were needed to recruit from a sample of five thousand eligible houses, the sampling interval would be 5,000/500 = 10. If the sampling interval is ten, once a household or living unit is surveyed, the next nine households or living units along the path would be skipped and the 10th household or sampling unit would be surveyed. This process would continue until the entire sample of five hundred households or living units were surveyed.

- If neither of the above approaches is feasible, the *EPI (Expanded Program on Immunization) method* may be utilized. As the name infers, the EPI method was first developed and implemented in the context of that program. Classically, this method consists of going to the center of the village, spinning a bottle or pen, walking in the direction indicated until the border of the village is reached and a random house along that path selected. Subsequently, all other houses to be selected will be those adjacent to this first, randomly selected house. While this approach has its merits, it has important drawbacks including difficulty precisely locating the center and border of the village and an unequal probability of selection for houses located in the central, more densely populated part of the village, versus those located on the outskirts ultimately resulting in a sampling bias (Turner et al. 1996). In addition, this method gives significant control to survey teams, making it less reproducible and sensitive to the diligence of the survey team.

While these methods may select a representative sample they can be very costly and time if there are hundreds of dispersed settlements in the survey area. Another approach consists of randomly selecting a limited number of settlements at the first stage of sampling and subsequently sampling only in those selected settlements. This approach is called a two-stage cluster sampling method. In addition to being more logistically efficient, it has the advantage of not requiring precise individual or household population lists of the whole survey area.

In the first stage, the selection of clusters, a list of all settlements, called primary sampling units (PSU), in the survey area, is required as well as their estimated population. From this list of PSUs, a predefined number of clusters are selected randomly, taking into account the population size of each PSU. This means that PSUs with larger population have a proportionally higher probability of being selected. This sampling is called probability-proportional-to-size (PPS). PPS ensures that the probability of being selected remains equal for every individual household or living unit in survey area.

In the second stage of sampling, households or living units are selected within clusters. This is done using simple, systematic or EPI method sampling. If the selected clusters are very large, an alternative approach is first to divide the cluster along administrative or natural boundaries into segments small enough to be reasonably enumerated or mapped, a process called segmentation, and then randomly selecting one of the segments.

One of the key characteristics of surveys is that data are collected from a sample representative of the total population. Flawed sampling, resulting in selection of a nonrepresentative sample, may lead to selection bias. Nonrepresentative samples may result from situations in which some settlements are located in inaccessible areas, selected households not being present at the time of the survey, the list of PSUs being incomplete, or the boundaries of villages being incorrectly determined, thus denying some household or living units a chance of being selected. If it is expected that some areas will be inaccessible, it is recommended to decide a priori to exclude these from the sampling frame. This implies that the findings of the survey may not be representative of excluded areas. An example of sampling bias is where all members of a household or living unit have died, making it impossible to collect retrospective information, such as mortality data, from that household. This particular type of bias is called survival bias.

Calculate the Sample Size

In the design of a field survey, a major decision concerns the sample size. A small sample size will result in a less costly and more rapid survey but with a tradeoff of lower precision. This will result in a larger range of uncertainty or confidence interval (CI). For instance, a GAM prevalence of 19% with a 95% CI ranging from 4% to 34% means that there is 95% chance that the GAM truly lies between 4% and 34% . In reality, this result may not be very useful as 4% is an acceptable GAM level while 34% is famine level. Thus, this level of precision is not sufficient for the result to be meaningfully interpreted or to decide what interventions may be required in a given situation. To prevent this problem, larger sample sizes could have been used to give more precise findings but at a higher cost and time investment. It is therefore essential to determine the best sample size to achieve the right balance between precision, cost, and time.

The following equation can be used to calculate the minimum required sample size for a survey estimate to attain the desired precision:

$$N = \frac{t^2 * (p) * (1-p) * \mathit{deff}}{\mathit{precision}^2}$$

- *N*: The minimum required sample size.
- *t*: A constant; equal to 1.96 for simple random surveys. For cluster surveys, *t* will be slightly higher (e.g., 2.045 for surveys with 30 clusters).
- *p*: The expected prevalence of the indicator of interest, based on contextual and/or historical information and expert judgment. For instance, based on a previous survey that reported a GAM of 20 percent as well as observations that the nutritional situation has improved since that survey, it may be reasonable to conclude the expected prevalence of GAM to be approximately 15 percent.
- *precision*: This is the required precision. The fact that the precision is squared in the denominator means that even small increases in precision, requiring a narrower CI, will result in exponential increases in sample size. Required precision depends on several factors including the type of indicator, the type of decisions to be made based on the results, and the expected prevalence of the indicator. In emergency nutrition surveys, for example, precision of +/− 3%–5%, depending on prevalence, around the estimate, is usually sufficient for meaningfully interpreting the results.
- *deff*: This is design effect which is a kind of "statistical penalty" for using methods other than simple random sampling such as cluster sampling. For simple random samples the design effect equals one. For other types of sampling the design effect may be higher than one. This is due in part to the fact that people who live near each other may be more likely to have similar characteristics than people living apart from each other. If there is little difference between different settlements, or low heterogeneity, this factor will not have an important effect, but when there are considerable differences between settlements, or high heterogeneity, this effect will not be negligible. In the former situation the design effect will be close to one, while in the latter, it may be higher, depending on the magnitude of the differences or degree of heterogeneity. For anthropometry indicators in nutrition surveys, the design effect tends to be low (around 1.5) in most settings (Kaiser et al. 2006).

Higher design effects may be seen in contexts with localized epidemics, pockets of violence, or low access to foodstuffs, or where public health interventions targeted only a part of the surveyed area. For example, if one village was attacked and sustained high levels of mortality while another village was unharmed, of the numbers of deaths between these villages will be high. In such a situation, a high design effect should be assumed for mortality surveys.

As an example, for a cluster survey with an expected prevalence of GAM of 15 percent, a required precision of 4 percent, and a design effect of 1.5, the minimum required sample size is calculated as:

$$N = \frac{2.045^2 * 0.15 * (1-0.15) * 1.5}{0.04^2} = 500$$

This means that for this survey, 500 children aged 6 to 59 months need to be measured in order to ensure an acceptable precision. However, surveyors typically do not sample children but rather households. There are several reasons for this. First, it is often easier to create lists of households rather than individuals. Second, it ensures that for surveys with household level indicators, such as mortality, all eligible households, not just those with children, are surveyed. Third, households are a common unit for comparing the sample size needed for different indicators that have different survey subjects. For example, nutrition indicators calculate number of children 6 to 59 months, but mortality indicators calculate number of all people irrespective of age.

Therefore, to perform this survey, it is important to estimate how many households will be required to survey five hundred children. This can be accomplished by using demographical data on household composition for the area to be surveyed. For instance, if the average number of children per household is 0.8, then 500/0.8 or 625 households will be needed to reach the required number of children.

In certain situations, some households may be absent or refuse to participate in the survey. Rather than replacing these missing households in the field, it is recommended to increase the original sample size at the planning stage to account for expected nonresponse. For instance, if 5 percent nonresponse is expected, one should increase the above sample size according to the following formula:

$$\frac{625}{1.00-0.05} = 658$$

Finally, for a cluster survey one needs to decide how many clusters will be selected. It is recommended that at least 25 clusters be selected. Most emergency nutrition surveys use 30 to 35 clusters (Binkin et al. 1992). The decision of how many clusters to use should be informed by field realities such as distance between clusters and time required for each interview. In the above example, if 30 clusters were selected, surveyors would need to visit 22 households in each cluster to achieve the planned sample size of 658. If, however, teams cannot reasonably visit the required number of households in a day, it is preferable to increase the number of clusters instead of having them try to visit 22 households in a day, as this may result in rushed field work and low quality data.

Recruit and Train Survey Teams

One of the fist logistic tasks for a survey manager is recruiting enumerators for survey teams. Enumerators should be literate, fluent in the language(s) of the interviews, motivated, flexible, and available for the duration of the survey. Ideally they should have a relevant professional background; however, this is not critical. They must be trained to clearly understand the survey goals, objectives, logistics, and other details of how fieldwork will be organized. During the training, enumerator teams should review the survey questionnaire, learn the household selection process, practice techniques for measurements such as measuring height and weight or MUAC, learn how to fill out the questionnaires, and if applicable, how to enter data on a mobile device. Trainings usually last from three to five days, depending on the survey's complexity.

The importance of rigorous training is often underestimated. Simply handing questionnaires to enumerators without proper training will result in the survey not being administered consistently. Ideally, the questionnaire should be reviewed in detail with the teams to explain the essence of each question and underlying indicator, and the teams should role-play to learn how to correctly ask each question. Another critical component of the training is household selection. Teams should review the definition of "household" used in the survey. This may, for instance, be people living under the same roof or people eating from the same cooking pot. Teams should discuss how to apply the definition to different family situations relevant to the survey setting, for instance, polygamous families or compounds, and review other special circumstances particular to the survey, such as measurement guidelines for children with disabilities or sampling procedures in cases where houses are absent or abandoned.

Some surveys require additional instruction on correct techniques for measurement of certain indicators. In nutrition surveys, for example, training should include practicing anthropometric measurements followed by a standardization test, in which enumerators demonstrate their skills by measuring at least ten healthy children twice. The anthropometry training and standardization test are repeated until teams are proficient. In settings where children will likely not have birth certificates, survey teams are trained to determine age using a local events calendar that includes significant, memorable events such as local holidays, seasons, or commonly known historic events from the last five years.

Rigorous training and preparation is necessary to minimize bias. As discussed previously, bias can result from errors in the measurement of any parameter. For example, improperly calibrated scales used to weigh children resulting in invalid z-scores, improperly used MUAC tapes, poorly translated questionnaires, or expired chlorine tests for water quality can all cause measurement bias. Bias can also result from mistakes in selection of the sample. Using outdated census data, for example, would introduce selection bias. Bias may be difficult to detect, and, if present, can affect the accuracy and thus interpretability of survey results. Rigorous training of teams and close supervision in the field are the best methods to prevent bias.

Secure Equipment, Materials, and Plan Logistics

Survey managers are responsible for identifying what equipment and materials (such as height boards or water tests) need to be ordered, what is already available, and what can be sourced in-country. Surveys require high-quality equipment in good working condition. Detailed lists of recommended survey equipment are available in the WFP/CDC survey manual (World Food Programme [WFP] and Centers for Disease Control and Prevention (CDC) [2005]). Once the survey dates and location have been determined, a plan for logistics such as security, lodging, transportation, and remuneration for enumerators should be developed. In insecure settings, security officers should be consulted to ensure teams are safe during data collection.

Field-Test the Survey

The field test is a full-day exercise that takes place after the training but before beginning the actual survey. During the field test teams practice all steps of data collection, including selecting households, interviewing respondents, and recording data. The field test provides the survey manager an opportunity to observe the enumerators' skills in household selection, measurement techniques, interviews, and data recording. In addition, the feasibility of the sampling method, including the time it takes to select households and to conduct the interview, can be reviewed.

Collect Data in the Field

Ideally, teams should be well trained and motivated before being deployed to the field. Once in the field there will be limited control over the data collection process. How long teams will be in the field depends on sample size, number and distance between clusters, and survey complexity. Field supervisors are responsible for detecting and correcting problems in the field and communicating updates regularly to the survey manager. One method to identify and address data quality problems early is having teams enter data every evening. In this way, it may be possible to identify problems such as measurement rounding, and then correct the problem, for example, by instructing the teams to take more accurate measurements.

Check Data Quality

Prior to analyzing the data, a critical step is checking the quality of data. If the data quality is poor, the results have little meaning. Quality analysis begins with detecting data entry mistakes. This can be done with random checks, comparing the records in the database with the paper questionnaires, or data can be entered twice and software can be used to compare the inputs, a method called double data entry. The next step is looking at the percentage of survey subjects with missing data for each indicator, a measure of data completeness. A high proportion of missing data is problematic and may suggest that the data on a given indicator is not representative. If age and sex are collected, it is possible to check whether the sample is balanced by comparing the proportion of males and females or various age groups in the survey sample to that in the population.

For some indicators, more advanced checks are possible. For example, with anthropometry data, looking at whether weight and height measurements are rounded, generally to the nearest centimeter or kilogram, is an important data quality check. In settings where people do not know their exact birthdates, it is common for age to be rounded to the nearest six- or 12-month interval, a practice known as age heaping. In such circumstances, if teams were rounding age, the data should include more children who are exactly two years old than those 23 or 25 months old.

It is also possible to identify outliers, for example, in nutrition surveys, values of weight for height, or height for age so extreme that they are biologically and statistically unlikely. As the distribution of z-scores is expected to approximate a normal bell shaped curve, several tests of normality can be performed. If the survey includes mortality data, it is possible to look at how many deaths and births were recorded in each household and in each cluster. In stable situations, births and deaths are generally randomly distributed across clusters. If there is a pattern, such as nearly half of all deaths occurring in one cluster, it is useful to investigate whether the pattern can be explained by, for instance, violence or an epidemic, or if it is likely poor data quality.

Performing a quality analysis of the data disaggregated by survey team is also useful. Large differences in the results among teams may indicate problems in how the teams asked questions or interpreted or recorded the answers.

Analyze Data and Write a Report

After the quality analysis has been completed and the data set cleaned and validated, the next step is data analysis. Preliminary results should be disseminated in a timely fashion, ideally within a week from the completion of data entry. Approvals from the sponsoring organization or the local government are often needed before an official report can be released; however, this should not delay sharing preliminary results for key indicators.

A standard report includes an introduction with basic information about the context, the population surveyed, and the survey objectives. This is followed by an explanation of methods, results, discussion, and recommendations. For results to be interpreted, methods have to be presented in sufficient detail to allow readers to understand the sampling strategy and how the survey was conducted. For each indicator, results must include the estimate, confidence interval, and sample size for the indicator to indicate nonresponse, and, if applicable, the range used for exclusion of outliers. Software packages that perform automatic analysis of survey data, such as Emergency Nutrition Assessments (ENA) for SMART, are useful tools as they ensure analysis is accurate and minimum reporting standards are met (ENA for SMART 2011). Finally, in the discussion, it is useful to interpret the results in context, with consideration of global thresholds, previous assessments, seasonal variations, and survey limitations. Recognizing that a survey is justified only if it informs key public health programs, the report should provide guidance on how results should inform programing.

Disseminate Findings and Follow-up

Because a survey's purpose is to guide programmatic actions, the findings are only useful if accompanied by specific and actionable recommendations, and those recommendations are effectively communicated to decision-makers. Therefore, once the full survey report is drafted, the results should be shared with key stakeholders, including government agencies, NGOs, donors, researchers, and journalists. A one- or two page executive summary or press release may also be disseminated to reach a broader audience. It can also be useful to convene a meeting of major stakeholders to discuss the survey's implications for programming and funding.

Several initiatives have been dedicated to centralizing survey data in repositories including the Complex Emergency Database (CE-DAT) hosted by the Centre for Research on the Epidemiology of Disasters (CRED) and the Nutrition Survey Results Database hosted by the United Nations System Standing Committee on Nutrition (United Nations Standing Committee on Nutrition 2009). This has included the development of analytical tools and resulted in several publications (Degomme and Guha-Sapir 2007, CE-DAT 2009). The main objective of these initiatives was to make survey results accessible to a wide range of stakeholders and encourage evidence-based decision-making. While most of these are no longer updated, having a central survey repository remains an interest of many agencies and researches that collect and use survey data.

Common Challenges Collecting Data in Emergency Contexts

There are many challenges in surveying populations during humanitarian emergencies, which are often insecure and inaccessible, compared with nonemergency settings, which are more likely to be calm and stable. Natural disasters and armed conflicts destroy infrastructure such as roads and bridges, thus restricting movement of survey teams. During conflict, armed groups may set up checkpoints or use force to restrict survey team access to the population. Often, these insecure and inaccessible areas are where information from surveys is most needed.

Compared to stable settings, there may also be many urgent, conflicting priorities. In humanitarian emergencies, where personnel and resources are often severely limited, there is a trade-off between allocating time and resources to assessments including surveys or to the provision of critical humanitarian assistance. Qualified staff may not be available to participate in assessments if they are engaged in other potentially lifesaving activities.

In addition to these inherent challenges, in humanitarian emergencies there are other challenges that are common but can be avoided or mitigated. These challenges have impacted the quality and interpretability of assessments in many past humanitarian emergencies.

Lack of Technical Expertise

It is not uncommon to have survey field staff managed by clinicians with no formal training in public health or epidemiology. Organizations often do not prioritize on the job training in management of surveys for these professionals, understanding it to be both expensive and time consuming, especially given the high turnover in these positions. Training for survey field staff is also often inadequate. Errors in field surveys have been shown to be related to the shortage of properly trained staff with the specific knowledge of how to design and manage surveys (Spiegel et al. 2004).

Poor Adherence to Standard Methodologies

Several meta-analyses from the 1990s and 2000s have shown that field surveys in the past were often of low quality (Prudhon and Spiegel 2007, Spiegel et al. 2004). These analyses found that nutrition surveys regularly failed to include enough children for sufficient precision, selected clusters without consideration for population size, included only one child per household instead of all eligible children, used incorrect measurement techniques for anthropometry, and misinterpreted survey results. The quality of the survey implementation varied significantly by organization.

No Standard Method to Evaluate Data Quality

Statistical tests can be used to determine the quality of survey data and the plausibility of the results produced; however, survey managers may not routinely use these tests to review the quality of field surveys. They often do not have experience with statistical analysis or access to free, user-friendly statistical software. Even when survey managers do review the plausibility of the data, in the absence of global quality standards or set of standard tests it proves difficult to compare the quality across surveys.

Survey Reports Incomplete and Untimely

Reports are not always written, and when drafted the reports were often unstructured and incomplete. Many reports do not include sufficient detail on survey methods to allow for proper interpretation of the results. This includes not reporting confidence intervals or documenting the sampling method. Many field reports fail checks of internal consistency and completeness (Degomme and Guha-Sapir 2007, Prudhon and Spiegel 2007). In addition, reports are often not disseminated for months following data collection. One reason cited for this delay is the reliance on global headquarters staff to analyze data. Given that the shelf life of survey findings in emergency situations is extremely short, to be most useful, survey data needs to be shared within weeks, or ideally, days after completion of data collection.

Additional Variables Not Standardized

Variables added to assess other sectors, such as food security, morbidity, or water and sanitation, are often not standardized. No consensus exists regarding how many variables could be reasonably added to a survey without affecting the quality of the data collected. Additionally, the same indicator may be measured using different questions by different organizations. As a result, indicators are not comparable across surveys and provide little utility because of limited interpretability (Watson et al. 2011).

All of these challenges are avoidable and impact the quality and utility of the data collected. For example, if a survey fails to achieve a large enough sample size, the survey will not have sufficient precision. Results will be difficult to interpret. If, however, the sample size is overestimated, time and resources will be spent unnecessarily. Properly trained professionals are needed to correctly design a survey, including calculating sample size. Errors in selecting eligible households affect the representativeness of the sample. If the sample selected is not representative, then the survey results cannot be generalized to the target population and the ultimate goal of assessment is not achieved. If measurements are not accurate, the survey results are likely to be biased and the resulting estimates may not be valid. If survey reports are incomplete, there is a lack of information necessary to determine whether the results are valid. This may lead to inappropriate use for programming and allocating resources. If it takes several months for the survey report to be produced and released, the survey does not serve its primary function of informing humanitarian action in a timely manner. By the time results are released, the data may be outdated and not useful for programming.

Innovations to Improve Field Surveys

In recent years, the international community has made major strides in improving the quality and utility of the data collected by field surveys in humanitarian emergencies. Many innovations and improvements have been achieved as part of the Standardized Monitoring and Assessment of Relief and Transitions (SMART) Initiative (SMART Methodology 2012). SMART is the method for assessing nutrition and mortality with surveys in humanitarian emergencies. Representatives from many NGOs, UN organizations, research institutes, and donor agencies participated in developing the standardized survey guidance.

The initiative has improved quality through rigorous training, improved survey guidance, and user-friendly software. The software, Emergency Nutrition Assessments (ENA) for SMART, provides a package of tools that can be used to simplify each phase of the survey process (ENA for SMART 2011). The software assists in completing many survey tasks, making adherence to recommended methods more automatic.

Recent innovations and advances to improve the quality of surveys in humanitarian emergencies, many of which are part of the SMART Initiative, are listed below.

Building Capacity of Survey Professionals

One of the most impactful activities of the initiative was developing a training course for field professionals (generally NGO staff and survey consultants) who design, plan and implement surveys. The curriculum is an advanced field methods course, which emphasizes the technical components of survey design and data analysis. The course is taught several times a year in regions prone to emergencies. A pool of experts involved in the SMART initiative teach the course so that individual organizations are not as burdened with building staff capacity. Subject matter experts update the curriculum on an ongoing basis in response to new research and feedback from practitioners. Training materials are free and available in several languages. To supplement the regular trainings, a team of global technical specialists are deployed ad hoc to the field to train local staff and oversee the implementation of surveys in emergency settings as needed.

A separate curriculum, a simplified version of the survey manager training, has been developed to train enumerators directly involved in collecting survey data or supervising survey teams. The enumerator training emphasizes random selection of households and proper anthropometry measurement. The training is provided prior to implementing a survey. Slide decks, sample agendas, and teaching guides exist for each module.

Improving Quality of Survey Planning

Survey managers often find steps of the survey design process complicated, particularly calculating sample size and performing the procedure of cluster selection. The initiative has developed several tools to simplify these procedures. The sample size calculator in the ENA software helps survey managers determine the number of households needed to achieve adequate precision. The survey manual provides clear guidance on how to determine the appropriate values for parameters, such as expected design effect and desired precision, needed to calculate sample size. The calculator then computes sample size automatically.

For cluster surveys, additional planning tools exist to aid the two stages of sampling. For the first stage of sampling, a software application randomly selects clusters. The survey manager provides a list of the settlements in the survey area, the population of each settlement, and the total number of clusters desired, usually from 30 to 35. The software automatically assigns the clusters using the PPS method. For the second stage of sampling, a sampling decision tree helps determine the most appropriate method for selecting subjects within each cluster based on the geography of the area, the size of the settlement, and availability of household lists.

Properly Training Field Teams

To help ensure that survey teams meet the minimum standards of anthropometry measurements, the SMART initiative developed standard guidance for how survey managers should organize a Standardization Test. In addition, the measurements taken during the Standardization Test can be automatically analyzed using the ENA software. The software compares the team's first and second measurements of the same child to assess precision. This analysis allow for a numeric, objective measure of surveyor quality that can be compared across settings.

Standardizing Assessment of Data Quality

One of the major innovations of the initiative is developing an automated quality analysis. The ENA software program performs a series of statistical tests, together called the plausibility check, that assess the representativeness of the sample in terms of age and sex distributions and provide a comprehensive analysis of the quality of anthropometry measurements. The software produces a standard, comprehensive, and transparent report of the data quality.

The report makes it simple for survey managers to compare the quality of surveys across organizations and countries. This analysis provides information as to what deficiencies or mistakes may have taken place during the data collection. For example, if survey teams were rounding anthropometry measurements or there were difficulties with estimating correct age of the children, these mistakes can be taken into account and prevented as much as possible in future surveys. Analysis by individual team provides information on each team's performance.

There are additional tools that use field survey reports, rather than raw data as in plausibility check, to review all aspects of the survey methods. Two algorithms, one for nutrition surveys and one for mortality surveys, have been proposed that allocate points for errors, such as incorrect sampling design, measurement errors, response biases, and analysis errors (Prudhon et al. 2011).

Automating Data Analysis

Analysis of the survey results, like the data quality check, is automated such that standard table shells are populated with results, with the push of a button. Automatic analysis eliminates errors common in manual data analysis. The automatic analysis in ENA software is available for anthropometry and mortality indicators. Other variables need to be analyzed separately.

Automating Report Generation

The populated result tables generated in ENA are embedded within a full, standard report template that outlines the appropriate structure of a field report. Each section of the template prompts survey managers to provide sufficient information to interpret the data, in accordance to the Completeness Checklist. The Completeness Checklist, developed by CRED and the CE-DAT Expert Group, outlines the minimum essential information for survey reports (CE-DAT Expert Group 2010).

With these advances, as soon as data are entered and quality of data verified, preliminary results for anthropometry and mortality indicators are instantly available, permitting organizations to release preliminary findings within a day or two of finishing data collection and entry. This advancement is a key advantage, particularly in humanitarian emergencies where data is particularly time-sensitive.

Standardizing Additional Variables

To standardize additional indicators included in nutrition surveys, several organizations are developing standard modules for specific sectors such as food security and water and sanitation. Such modules generally include a set of appropriate indicators for each sector, typically limited to six to ten key indicators, measured with a standardized set of questions. Standardization improves comparability, eliminates the need for field practitioners to reinvent survey questionnaires for each assessment, and is conducive to creating common algorithms for data analysis. As an example, the United Nations High Commission for Refugees (UNHCR) has developed the Standardized Expanded Nutrition Survey (SENS) modules for surveys conducted in refugee settings (United Nations High Commissioner for Refugees 2014). SENS includes six modules including anemia, infant and young child feeding, food security, water sanitation and hygiene, mosquito bed net coverage as well as anthropometry and health. The decisions to include specific modules are based on local context and information needs. For example, in the settings where malaria is not endemic and there is no bed net distribution, the mosquito bed net coverage module would be irrelevant.

Use of Mobile Technology

In addition to the innovations described, the proliferation of mobile technology may serve to further improve the quality of field surveys. Mobile phones and tablets, used increasingly for digital data collection in the field, provide several benefits over paper data collection, including eliminating the need for data entry after the survey, automating skip patterns, restricting ranges for answers, and prompting enumerators to remeasure implausible values in the field. Mobile tools can collect additional useful data such as global positioning system (GPS) coordinates and record timestamps, which may provide additional opportunities for assessing how randomly households were selected and how much time data collection required. Mobile technologies, however, also introduce new challenges. Mobile devices can be prohibitively expensive, often require advance expertise to program questionnaires, have limited battery life, and necessitate additional enumerator training on their use, among other challenges. Efforts to capitalize on the benefits and minimize the limitations are ongoing.

In spite of all of these advances, some methodological challenges remain. For example, some variables are difficult to measure with sufficient precision in field surveys because they require much larger sample sizes than those feasible in humanitarian emergencies and increasing sample size is costly and logistically challenging.

Some examples of such indicators are in the next section.

Indicators Measured in a Small Subset of the Population

Many indicators measured for infant and young child feeding (IYCF) are measured in very narrow age ranges, for example, children six to eight months of age for introduction of complementary foods and zero to five months of age for exclusive breastfeeding. In a typical field nutrition survey with approximately 400–600 children aged 6 to 59 months, we would expect to find fewer than 60 children under six months of age and even fewer six to eight months old. This is too few to achieve meaningful precision.

Indicators Measuring Rare Events

A similar challenge exists when measuring relatively rare events, such as deaths among children under five years of age or maternal deaths. The more rare the event, the greater the sample size needed to capture the event with sufficient precision. The World Health Organization estimates that achieving sufficient precision for maternal mortality may require surveying as many as 200,000 households (WHO and UNICEF 1997). This is an impossibly large number, particularly in the setting of a humanitarian emergency.

Indicators Assessing Coverage

Indicators of coverage of selective feeding programs for malnourished children assess the proportion of children enrolled in feeding programs among those eligible, which includes all acutely malnourished children. The denominator of these indicators, only those acutely malnourished, is a relatively small subset of the population sampled for nutrition surveys, and generally insufficient to achieve reasonable precision. The notable exception is in the case of blanket nutrition programs, for which all children in the population are eligible. In this case, the whole survey sample can serve as denominator for estimating coverage, thus providing sufficient sample size to achieve meaningful precision.

Conclusion

Surveys are a powerful tool in the setting of humanitarian emergencies, and can provide an accurate and precise representative snapshot of the key public health indicators of the population. However, certain advanced expertise as well as careful planning, training, and supervision are required in order to collect appropriate accurate, complete, and representative, quality data. Standardized methods, guidance, training programs, and software packages are available to aid field practitioners in this task.

References

Bilukha, O., Prudhon, C., Moloney, G., Hailey, P., and Doledec, D. (2012). Measuring anthropometric indicators through nutrition surveillance in humanitarian settings: options, issues, and ways forward. *Food Nutr Bull*, **33**(2), 169–176.

Binkin, N., Sullivan, K., Staehling, N., and Nieburg, P. (1992). Rapid nutrition surveys: How many clusters are enough? *Disasters*, **16**(2), 97–103.

Cairns, K. L., Woodruff, B. A., Myatt, M., Bartlett, L., Goldberg, H., and Roberts, L. (2009). Cross-sectional survey methods to assess retrospectively mortality in humanitarian emergencies. *Disasters*, **33**(4), 503–521.

CE-DAT. (2009). CE-DAT Complex Emergency Database (online). Available at: http://cedat.be/ (Accessed on June 30, 2017).

CE-DAT Expert Group. (2010). CE-DAT Completeness checklist (online). Available at: http://cedat.be/sites/default/files/completeness%20checklist%20form%20170610_0.pdf (Accessed on June 30, 2017).

Degomme, O. and Guha-Sapir, D. (2007). Mortality and nutrition surveys by non-governmental organisations. Perspectives from the CE-DAT database. *Emerg Themes Epidemiol*, **4**, 11.

ENA for SMART. (2011). ENA for SMART – Software for Emergency Nutrition Assessment (online). Available at: www.nutrisurvey.net/ena/ena.html (Accessed on June 30, 2017).

Gernaat, H. B., Dechering, W. H., and Voorhoeve, H. W. (1996). Absolute values or Z scores of mid-upper arm circumference to identify wasting? Evaluation in a community as well as a clinical sample of under fives from Nchelenge, Zambia. *J Trop Pediatr*, **42**(1), 27–33.

Global Nutrition Cluster. (2011). Harmonised Training Package (online). Available at: www.nutritioncluster.net/training-topics/harmonized-training-package (Accessed on June 30, 2017).

Inter-Agency Standing Committee. (2012). Multi-Cluster /Sector Initial Rapid Assessment (MIRA). *Inter-Agency Standing Committee*, Geneva, Switzerland.

Kaiser, R., Woodruff, B. A., Bilukha, O., Spiegel, P. B., and Salama, P. (2006). Using design effects from previous cluster surveys to guide sample size calculation in emergency settings. *Disasters*, **30**(2), 199–211.

Prudhon, C., de Radigues, X., Dale, N., and Checchi, F. (2011). An algorithm to assess methodological quality of nutrition and mortality cross-sectional surveys: development and application to surveys conducted in Darfur, Sudan. *Popul Health Metr*, **9**(1), 57.

Prudhon, C. and Spiegel, P. B. (2007). A review of methodology and analysis of nutrition and mortality surveys conducted in humanitarian emergencies from October 1993 to April 2004. *Emerg Themes Epidemiol*, **4**, 10.

Save the Children. (2004). *Emergency nutrition assessment: Guidelines for field workers*. Save the Children: London.

SMART Methodology. (2012). Standardized monitoring and assessment of relief and transitions (online). Available : http://smartmethodology.org/ (Accessed on June 30, 2017).

Spiegel, P., Salama, P., and Maloney, S. (2004). Quality of malnutrition assessment surveys conducted during famine in Ethiopia. *JAMA*, **292**, 613–618.

The Sphere Project. (2011). The Sphere Project: Humanitarian charter and minimum standards in humanitarian response (online). Available at: www.spherehandbook.org/ (Accessed on July 6, 2017).

Turner, A. G., Magnani, R. J., and Shuaib, M. (1996). A not quite as quick but much cleaner alternative to the Expanded Programme on Immunization (EPI) Cluster Survey design. *Int J Epidemiol*, **25**(1), 198–203.

United Nations High Commissioner for Refugees. (2014). UNHCR standardised expanded nutrition survey (SENS) (online). Available at: www.sens.unhcr.org/ (Accessed on June 30, 2017).

United Nations Standing Committee on Nutrition. (2009). Nutrition information in crisis situations (online). Available at: www.unscn.org/web/archives_resources/files/NICS_No_1.pdf (Accessed on June 30, 2017).

Watson, F., Negussie, B., Dolan, C., Shoham, J., and Hall, A. (2011). Quality and potential use of data collected during nutrition surveys: an analysis of surveys in Ethiopia. *Int Health*, **3**(2), 85–90.

WHO Multicentre Growth Reference Group. (2006). *WHO child growth standards: Length/height-for-age, weight-for-age, weight-for-length, weight-for-height and body mass index-for-age: Methods and development*. World Health Organization; Geneva, Switzerland.

World Food Programme and Centers for Disease Control and Prevention. (2005). *A manual: measuring and interpreting malnutrition and mortality*. World Food Programme: Rome, Italy.

World Health Organization. (2000). *The management of nutrition in major emergencies*. World Health Organization: Geneva, Switzerland.

World Health Organization. (2012). *Outbreak surveillance and response in humanitarian emergencies: WHO guidelines for EWARN implementation*. World Health Organization: Geneva, Switzerland.

World Health Organization and United Nations Children's Fund. (1997). *The sisterhood method for estimating maternal mortality: Guidance notes for potential users*. World Health Organization: Geneva, Switzerland.

Chapter 9

Surveillance

Farah Husain and Peter Mala

Introduction

Public health surveillance comprises a wide range of health conditions including communicable and noncommunicable diseases. This chapter provides an overview of key epidemiological principles for monitoring communicable diseases during humanitarian emergencies. It also provides lessons learned from systems implemented in previous emergencies.

Public health surveillance is the monitoring of health events among a population. Surveillance data are used to describe and monitor the health status of a population in order to plan, implement, and evaluate public health programs. It is defined as "The ongoing systematic collection, analysis, and interpretation of health data, essential to the planning, implementation, and evaluation of public health practice, closely integrated with the timely dissemination of these data to those who need to know" (Thacker and Berkelman 1988). If any parts of this definition are not adhered to, then the data collected from the surveillance system are unreliable and the system, ultimately, is ineffective.

Disease surveillance during emergencies is critical and one of the top ten public health priorities (Refugee Health 1997). Population displacement, overcrowding, inadequate food, water, and sanitation, and a disrupted health infrastructure can increase the risk of rapid spread of communicable disease and lead to increased mortality, particularly from outbreak-prone diseases.

Morbidity and mortality rates are usually highest immediately following an emergency when resources are scarce, systems are nonfunctional and populations are at highest risk for disease (Toole and Waldmann 1990). There are several examples that illustrate these trends from past humanitarian emergencies. In 1994, after the influx of eight hundred thousand Rwandans into the Democratic Republic of Congo, the case fatality ratio (CFR) during a cholera and shigellosis epidemic reached 48 percent in one day (Siddique et al. 1995). In 1998, two thousand deaths caused by relapsing fever took six months to investigate during the ongoing civil war in South Sudan (Gayer et al. 2007), and from 2000 to 2001, over one thousand cases of measles were identified among Burundi refugees living in Tanzanian camps (Kamugisha et al. 2003). Although such explosive outbreaks are rare, failure to promptly identify them can result in unnecessary deaths that can be prevented with simple public health measures.

National public health surveillance systems collect information on a vast number of diseases to track the health of its population. These systems usually consist of four main components:

- Immediately notifiable diseases
- Communicable diseases
- Noncommunicable diseases
- Other program indicators

During an emergency, conditions of biggest threat are the immediately notifiable ones as they have the potential to spread quickly and result in high morbidity and mortality. These include diseases such as cholera, shigellosis, and measles. Early detection and control of these diseases requires a robust alert-and-response or early warning mechanism. In theory, all public health surveillance systems should have an early warning component that can allow for the rapid control of outbreaks, but in humanitarian emergencies, routine surveillance may underperform or be too cumbersome to effectively address the needs of the affected population. This is especially true for countries where national surveillance systems are already underresourced and barely functional prior to the emergency.

The primary goal of communicable disease surveillance during humanitarian emergencies is to rapidly detect and respond to epidemic-prone diseases.

Additional uses for surveillance data in emergencies are to:

- Estimate the magnitude of the problem
- Assess the main health priorities of the affected population
- Determine changing needs of the emergency
- Plan and guide programs
- Advocate for resources and policies

Key Principles

Given the challenging operational environment and the need for quick information, only data that are useful and will be acted upon in the field should be collected. Timely and accurate data are essential for an effective response, and thus, are often prioritized at the expense of other more detailed information. In order to ensure prompt detection and rapid response, a few key guidelines have been developed when implementing a surveillance system in emergencies.

Implement Early

A surveillance system should be set up as soon as possible following a humanitarian emergency and implemented in conjunction with the initial rapid assessment.

Minimize Indicators

Collect information on the minimum number of indicators necessary. Oftentimes, the only source of quantitative information available during the early phases of an emergency is surveillance data. It is common to want to collect as much information as possible. However, it's also important to focus resources on collecting essential information that will help achieve the system objective of detection and responding to epidemic-prone diseases. Identified outbreaks will require detailed information that should be captured in line lists, but this level of detail is not necessary in the absence of an ongoing outbreak. There are many aspects of health events that are "nice to know," but the list must be narrowed down by assigning priority by asking, "What is essential to know?" Each element of collected data should have a clearly demonstrated use.

Limiting data collection to a few indicators necessary for public health action will prevent the commonly held view that surveillance is merely the reporting of disease (Teutsch and Churchill 2000). This may be accomplished in several ways, one of which is to limit data collection to two age categories. During the emergency phase, it is recommended to collect data on 0–4 years (vulnerable, high-risk group) and $\geq$ 5 years. Additional age information may be useful for programmatic purposes but will not influence response efforts during the early stage of an emergency. This will not only reduce data aggregation burden but will also facilitate data analysis at the field level where immediate action and response should take place. A surveillance system during emergencies should be "lightweight" so it can be implemented quickly and "nimble" so it can respond to emerging health problems or changes in program activities. A system with few indicators will be simple and flexible enough for easy roll out, easy adaptability to the changing needs of the emergency and more likely to be used by health partners.

Prioritize Health Events

Prioritize eight to ten health events under surveillance. During the emergency phase, data collection should only cover health problems that have the potential to spread rapidly, produce the highest mortality and morbidity, and can be effectively prevented or treated. Acute diarrhea results in high morbidity especially among children and those living in overcrowded, resource-poor settings. Many of these cases are due to viral gastroenteritis that is ubiquitous globally; thus very little is done with this information in the emergency setting. Suspected cholera or shigellosis, however, is a specific type of diarrhea that spreads quickly, affects both children and adults and can result in high CFR. Similarly, influenza-like illness (ILI) becomes a catchall for any respiratory infection ranging from the common cold to severe forms of influenza. Numerous cases are generated every week, but most cases are not of immediate threat. In fact, the influenza virus does not cause most cases of ILI or upper respiratory infections at all (Centers for Disease Control and Prevention [CDC] 2001). Severe acute respiratory illnesses (SARI) or lower respiratory tract infections, to which the population has no immunity, result in severe disease and should be distinguished from mild or moderate health events. Daily aggregation of many cases of nonspecific diarrhea or common respiratory conditions can tax the health staff and the health system, compromise data quality, and the overall utility of the system.

Determine which health events to select by achieving a consensus on the diseases under surveillance by all key stakeholders of the system. This involves a systematic assessment of disease risk within the geographic area and population under surveillance, and therefore, will be different in different settings. Some inclusion criteria are the frequency of occurrence, the severity of the disease, the resources needed to treat the disease, its preventability, communicability, the public interest in the disease, and whether the disease is targeted for global elimination or eradication. Health-related events that affect many persons or require large expenditures of resources, such as cholera or measles, are high priority events. However, health-related events that affect few persons might also be important, especially if the events cluster in time and place, or result in high mortality, as in the case of Ebola. In other instances, public concerns might focus attention on a particular health-related event, creating or heightening the importance of an event, for example, SARS. Diseases that are now rare because of successful control measures might be perceived as unimportant, but their level of importance should be assessed in selected health facilities or for their potential to reemerge. Polio is an example of such a disease.

Some common priority health events include:

- Cholera
- Shigellosis
- Measles
- Poliomyelitis
- Meningitis
- Viral hemorrhagic fever (Ebola, Dengue)
- Acute Jaundice syndrome (Hepatitis)

For more information on priority conditions see *Outbreak surveillance and response in humanitarian emergencies: WHO guidelines for EWARN implementation* (WHO 2012).

Use Syndromic Surveillance

The system should be based on syndromic surveillance with the exception of diseases that have readily available rapid diagnostic tests (RDT) such as malaria. Diagnosis using clinical signs and symptoms rather than laboratory confirmation is commonly used in public health surveillance, particularly when identifying an unrecognized or emerging disease. Surveillance of disease syndromes is preferred during emergencies when diagnostic tests or functioning laboratories are not readily available. Furthermore, health workers may also be affected by the emergency resulting in limited human resources, and staff of varying clinical skills such as community health workers may be responsible for diagnosing cases. There is loss in specificity when using syndromic surveillance, but the increase in sensitivity allows for early detection of possible outbreaks.

Establish Separate Mortality Surveillance

Most deaths occur at home and within the community, not at the outpatient health facility where many surveillance systems are implemented. If the early warning emergency surveillance system is implemented at the health-facility level, mortality should not be included. Instead, consider establishing separate mortality surveillance that includes additional data sources outside the health facility such as burial grounds, community health workers, traditional healers or religious leaders.

Coordinate Roles and Responsibilities

There should be one overall coordinating body, but inclusion of all relevant health partners (Refugee Health 1997). Responsibility for organizing and supervising the surveillance system should be clearly assigned to one responsible party or agency, but close coordination between all partners is essential. Usually, this is the Ministry of Health (MoH) with support from the WHO. The United Nations High Commissioner for Refugees (UNHCR) oversees response efforts including surveillance for refugees through its implementing partners. In settings where there is no functioning MoH or UN presence, a coordinating body must be identified and recognized by health partners to initiate and oversee surveillance during the emergency.

Identify an Exit Strategy

Ensure there is an exit strategy right from the beginning. Successful transition from early warning surveillance in emergencies to routine surveillance remains a challenge, especially in settings where preexisting surveillance was dysfunctional or in settings that experience recurrent crises. Identifying different

Section 2: Public Health Principles

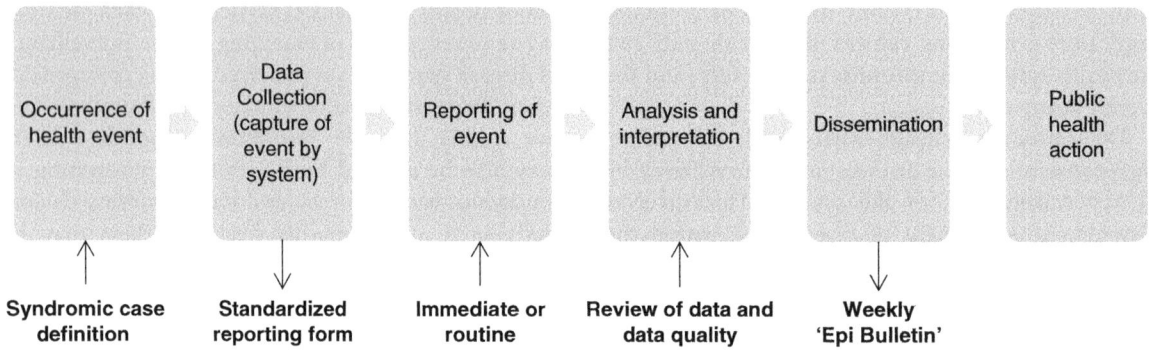

Figure 9.1 Components of a surveillance system

scenarios that warrant different surveillance strategies in advance can help smooth the transition from emergency to routine surveillance once the humanitarian emergency is over or in protracted emergency settings.

Activities

Surveillance systems are made up of the following main components:

- Data collection
- Reporting and transmission
- Analysis
- Interpretation and dissemination

There are shown in Figure 9.1. These traditional activities must be adapted and enhanced for emergency settings and for use among the affected population.

Data Collection

All data collection tools, including case definitions, patient registers, case verification and investigation forms, outbreak logs and databases, must be standardized to allow for proper data aggregation and data management. This is even more critical during emergencies when new health partners are involved and staff turnover is high. Standardized data collection procedures will allow different agencies to aggregate data the same way and provide the ability to compare data across different areas (urban versus rural), populations (host versus displaced) and time periods (dry versus rainy seasons). All new or revised data collection tools must be pretested among end-users and all personnel involved in data collection and reporting must be trained on the tools to ensure data quality

Case Definition

A case definition provides a standard criterion for identifying, diagnosing, and reporting health conditions. As previously stated, case definitions used in surveillance during emergencies should be based on clinical symptoms or syndromic surveillance rather than laboratory confirmation and may differ from case definitions used during routine surveillance. Standard case definitions are available but may need to be adapted based on the setting and the available resources. In some cases, rapid diagnostic tests (RDTs) may be used to diagnose a condition such as malaria, but availability of these tests must be universal. Case definitions must be simple, clear, and easy to apply so clinicians of varying qualifications may consistently use them. They should be broad enough to generate signals but easily distinguishable from other nonpriority conditions (WHO 2012). It is important to note these case definitions are for surveillance purposes only and not for case management.

Data sources

Ideally, surveillance should be from all possible sources. This may not, however, be possible during an emergency and in poor resource settings. To ensure data quality, it is recommended that surveillance of weekly trend data be collected from selected health facilities (sentinel surveillance). Sentinel surveillance captures a portion of all occurring cases or health events. Data collected from selected health facilities may not be representative of the affected population, but will allow efforts to focus on complete reporting and better data to follow trends from fewer sources. This may be necessary at the beginning of an emergency when resources are limited, additional facilities may be added as the situation stabilizes. Immediately notifiable conditions should be reported from all informal and formal sources such as fixed and mobile health facilities, the community, traditional healers, the media, etc. (exhaustive or universal surveillance). Exhaustive or universal surveillance tries to capture all occurring cases or health events from all sources. This is inherently representative, but it may lack reliability depending on the source. A combination of sentinel and exhaustive surveillance will allow for more complete reporting from fewer sources to track trends while still using all sources to detect alerts.

Passive versus Active Surveillance

- **Passive surveillance** is when the coordinating health agency receives reports from health facilities or other reporting units without solicitation; i.e. facilities submit reports on their own. Passive surveillance is inexpensive, easy to implement, and can cover large geographic areas; however, it is often dependent on the reporting unit and can result in incomplete or untimely reporting especially from geographically remote or inaccessible areas.
- **Active surveillance** is when data are actively solicited; that is, staff seeks information from targeted sources such as health facilities, community health workers, etc., by visits or reminders. This is often conducted during an outbreak. Active surveillance provides the most complete information, but it is also expensive and may not be practical during an emergency (Nsubuga et al. 2006).
- We often rely on a combination of passive and active surveillance during humanitarian emergencies depending on existing capacity, communication infrastructure, human and financial resources and access.

Data Reporting and Transmission

Frequency of reporting will depend on the alert threshold for a particular priority condition. A hreshold is defined by the minimum number of cases needed to signal or "alert" the occurrence of an unusual health event (more than normal) and may trigger the early stages of an outbreak. The alert threshold for some conditions, including acute flaccid paralysis, measles, and cholera, may be one or two cases, while endemic conditions may require trend analysis and review of baseline estimates such as malaria in a malaria endemic country.

With the exception of immediately notifiable conditions, daily reporting is not recommended for communicable disease surveillance in emergencies. Daily collation and aggregation of data not only add to the workload of health staff but are often not meaningful on their own and are rarely reviewed on a daily basis. Daily reporting is only recommended during an ongoing outbreak when information is needed to describe the etiology of the outbreak and to implement and assess impact of control measures.

A clear and realistic reporting schedule, reporting procedures, and dedicated surveillance staff should be assigned for reporting of surveillance data at every reporting level. Weekly reports should be submitted via the predetermined reporting chain for timely analysis and dissemination. Weekly data aggregation should not place a large burden on health staff since the number of cases of priority diseases should be very few. Zero reporting must be included in weekly reports to indicate no cases for a specific disease for the reporting period, as blank fields can be misinterpreted for missing data. Internal data quality review must also be incorporated as part of the reporting process. Routine monitoring is critical to ensure data integrity and follow-up of alerts that were not immediately reported (i.e., unreported alerts).

Alerts should be reported using the fastest means possible and to the most reachable public health personnel, often the surveillance staff, local health authority, and/or health officer. Alert notification should not wait until the end of the reporting week for investigation. Figure 9.2 shows data flow for weekly data and immediately notifiable alerts.

Data Analysis

Data must be analyzed quickly and at the field level where action can take place immediately. Essentially this means sorting and analyzing the data gathered in terms of person, place, and time. The comparison of epidemiological indicators, calculated over a given period of time, often a week or a month, with baseline, non-emergency values, is also part of data analysis. Surveillance analysis begins once the trends of these indicators can be followed over time.

Basic indicators to characterize the emergency and health status of the affected population include:

Section 2: Public Health Principles

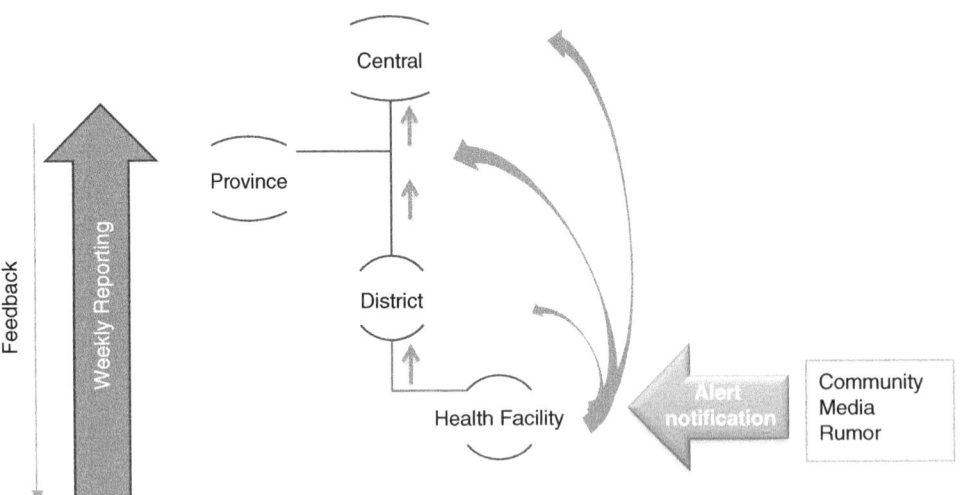

Figure 9.2 Data flow for weekly data and immediately notifiable alerts

- Who, when, where
- Trends on the most frequent pathologies via incidence rates, if accurate population estimates are available, otherwise proportional morbidity to determine trends or absolute number of cases for rare conditions
- Crude mortality rate, under-5 mortality rate, case fatality proportion, and attack rate during an outbreak

Data Interpretation and Dissemination

The analytical essence of surveillance data is based on their interpretation and the easiest way to interpret data is by producing graphs and charts on a regular basis. When interpreting data, especially emergency data, it is important to be cognizant of sudden fluctuations, not only because they may trigger the start or end of an outbreak, but because they may be due to reasons related to the emergency. For example, increases in cases may reflect an increase in population size, improved access, changes in the application of the case definition or enhanced reporting. Similarly, a decrease may be due to incomplete reporting because of conflict, security, access issues, etc. Furthermore, surveillance tools in emergency settings are often paper-based and can easily result in mistakes during data transfer. Thus, data during emergencies must be interpreted regularly, but with caution and attention to detail.

Dissemination is an essential part of surveillance. It is important to provide the findings to health professional/providers, policy makers, and donors. This is a critical step in linking data to public health action. It is equally important to share findings with those involved in collecting the information. Providing regular feedback will not only inform, but also motivate end users. Reports should be simple, composed of basic indicators, and interpreted within the context of the particular situation.

Challenges and Potential Pitfalls

An early warning surveillance system for populations affected by emergencies requires technical expertise, dedicated staff, and adequate funding to establish and operate optimally. However, one or more of these factors are often in short supply when an emergency occurs. These setbacks may be further compounded by insecurity, lack of access, weak health systems, poor infrastructure, and conflicting interests of health agencies involved in the emergency. This may adversely affect data quality and the system's ability to detect and respond to immediate health threats. Based on lessons learned from multiple evaluations of early warning systems implemented following acute and protracted emergencies, the main challenges can be grouped into three broad categories. These are not exhaustive, but rather meant to provide an overview of potential pitfalls and possible solutions for future emergencies.

Implementation Delays

Delays in implementation of early warning surveillance systems from a few weeks to several months are often too common in humanitarian crises. Delays tend to be more pronounced in slow-onset emergencies that steadily escalate into full-fledged humanitarian crisis such as simmering conflicts. These kinds of emergencies present with the dilemma of when to establish an early warning system as degradation of routine systems and impact on the population progressively worsens.

Once a decision has been made to establish an early warning disease surveillance system, other factors likely to delay implementation include:

- Lack of or slow funding mechanisms as disease surveillance is oftentimes not considered a top lifesaving priority intervention such as shelter, food and water in the early phase of a humanitarian crisis.
- Slow administrative processes because responsible international agencies and partner institutions do not adapt their administrative processes quickly enough to effectively address urgent needs of public health emergencies associated with humanitarian crisis. As a result, recruitment and deployment of staff and procurement of equipment and materials required for surveillance implementation is not timely. According to the UN grading system, for example, UN agencies can only mobilize skilled staff to support a member state when emergency reaches Grade 3 severity level by UN classification (www.who.int/hac/about/erf_.pdf), and this is often too late, especially for timely implementation of interventions that rely on additional human resources and capacity such as disease surveillance.
- Lack of agreement among stakeholders on system design, resistance from local authorities or discordance among health partners can delay system implementation. Local health authorities with little or no emergency experience may be unwilling to adapt or modify their existing surveillance system for the emergency. Alternatively, health partners responding to the emergency may have competing reporting priorities or alternative methods for surveillance making it difficult to reach consensus on reporting needs and methodology.
- Lack of a coordinating body due to the absence of a functioning ministry of health and/or lack of UN support due to civil conflict can not only delay implementation in non-government supported areas, but also complicate response efforts due to political sensitivities.

Poor Performance

Once implemented, effective operation of the surveillance system can be hampered by poor data quality, which can result in false alerts (thus reducing the positive predictive value), missed alerts (resulting in reduced sensitivity), and problems monitoring health trends (affecting the system's utility). Common reasons for poor performance of a surveillance system are in the following subsections.

Nonstandardized Reporting Forms

A nonstandardized reporting form complicates data aggregation and makes data incomparable across reporting facilities. Changes are often made to the surveillance reporting form at the central level without consultation, notification, training, or dissemination of revisions to field staff. Decisions made centrally may not be applicable or agreeable to provincial, district, or field level authorities. Additionally, health partners may have different reporting requirements and use their own reporting forms instead of the standardized emergency surveillance forms. This can result in multiple versions of the reporting forms and reporting mechanisms. Possible solutions for ensuring that a single standard surveillance reporting form is used by all reporting sites and stakeholders include involving users and implementers in the decision-making process and achieving buy-in from all administrative levels, effective communication of any revisions or modifications to reporting tools, and ensuring the form contributes to partner's minimum reporting requirements in order to minimize duplication and workload. Finally, indicating the version number on the most current form in circulation will facilitate easy reference.

Untimely Reporting

Insecurity, destruction of normal communication channels, political unrest, or geography can make access to target areas and the affected population challenging, thereby compromising timely reporting of surveillance data. Consider using only sentinel sites for data analysis in settings where infrastructure and communication is limited and obtaining reliable data from all health facilities is not possible. Furthermore, early warning systems cannot rely only on one type of reporting format, for example, electronic or paper-based. Web-based electronic systems or SMS-based systems have demonstrated capacity to address some challenges of reporting delays, poor data management, and analysis. However, it is also important to bear in mind that even technology can have its limitations such as IT support, training requirements and cost. A paper-based reporting system should always be maintained as a contingency when electricity, mobile services, and other communications mechanisms are down. Often, a combination of reporting mechanisms is necessary to compensate for the challenges encountered during an emergency. Most importantly, a high-tech data collection or reporting system is not a remedy for poor data quality. Without accurate and reliable data, "garbage-in" is "garbage-out" no matter what reporting format is used.

Inconsistent Application of Case Definitions

Inconsistent application of case definitions along with poor staff knowledge of priority conditions leads to subjective classification of diseases and missed outbreaks. Health care workers with different backgrounds training and skills may diagnose conditions based on their clinical training rather than the standard surveillance case definition. High staff turnover and limited or no training of new staff, lack of supervision and feedback, and dedicated funding for the surveillance activities exacerbates this problem. Health conditions/case definitions that are too broad or sensitive, such as acute respiratory illness (ARI) will generate numerous cases, reduce the ability to detect severe illnesses, and render the data unusable. Surveillance should include epidemic-prone diseases, that is, those that spread rapidly and have potentially high morbidity/mortality, in contrast to diseases of general public health importance, such as those with a high disease burden. In an emergency setting, case definitions should distinguish between these two, for example, suspected typhoid versus fever of unknown origin.

Inconsistent Reporting

Inconsistent, irregular, and duplicative reporting of cases may result in under or over reporting of cases, wide fluctuations in case counts, false alerts, or missed alerts. This may occur as a result of new health facilities emerging or old ones closing due to changes in partner activity, funding, or security. This tends to be more common during the early phases of an emergency when new partners arrive and attention on the emergency is high. This may be addressed by ensuring a mandatory and updated registration process of all health partners and health facilities and by including the numbers of reporting sites during analysis and interpretation of data. Duplicate reporting may result if patients seek care at multiple places for the same condition. A "patient card" can help track visits and minimize duplicate reporting for the same condition, especially in areas where health-seeking behavior is high.

Limited Public Health Action

Finally, a well-implemented and highly functioning system is only as good as the outcome it produces, that is, if it leads to public health action that helps reduce morbidity and mortality among emergency-affected populations.

Inadequate Data Analysis and Interpretation

Data analysis often only occurs at the central level resulting in missed alerts or late notification of alerts, and aggregated information is not granular enough to take action or identify field level trends. Limited capacity to analyze data at the field level or automated data analysis software transmits information up the reporting chain without adequate review and is often hampered by poor data quality. Management of surveillance at all levels should include well trained public health officers who can ensure optimal data quality and appropriate data analysis to guide public health response. Even if capacity does not exist at the health facility level, intermediate level staff should be encouraged to conduct their own basic analysis in order to initiate early action.

Limited Laboratory Support

Specimen testing requires specialized skills and equipment that are often unavailable or nonfunctional in emergency settings. Until adequate laboratory support can be obtained, it is necessary to ensure universal availability of rapid diagnostic tests (RDTs) for common epidemic-prone diseases (malaria, cholera).

Limited Supplies and Logistical Support

Lack of access and insufficient funding can severely hinder the ability to detect and respond to potential outbreaks. These challenges can be addressed by developing outbreak response plans beforehand, prepositioning emergency stockpiles for response activities such as specimen collection supplies, and securing adequate means for transportation and communication.

Poor Coordination among Partners

Poor coordination can result in unclear designation of roles and responsibilities among partners for outbreak investigation and response activities, uneven distribution of programs and provision of services in certain areas over other affected areas, and insufficient guidance to implement control measures. Coordination among partners for effective interventions can be improved through consensus on roles and responsibilities for outbreak investigation and response activities, assigning focal points for hard-to-reach/underserved areas, access to relevant guidance documents, and periodic meetings to discuss successes and failures for past outbreaks and responses.

Global Health Security

Vigilant surveillance during emergencies is also necessary to ensure adherence to key principles of global health security agenda. Spread of disease is not only a concern in crowded camp settings but is also a global concern. With the rising number of urban refugees, frequent cross-border movement of displaced populations, and increasing international trade and travel, the introduction and spread of new epidemics to other countries can occur very quickly and impact many parts of the world. Some of the recent examples include cholera in Haiti, polio in Syria, MERS-CoV in the Middle East, and Ebola in West Africa.

There is an increasing international effort to prevent, detect, and respond to outbreaks of infectious disease threat (Global Health Security Agenda, n.d.). The World Health Organization has termed such health events as *public health event of international concern* (PHEIC) (WHO n.d.). Member countries are mandated to report such events by the International Health Regulations to ensure adequate preparedness and timely response among countries at risk of cross border spread.

Conclusion

Populations affected by disasters are at an increased risk of disease outbreaks, especially in resource poor countries. The role of early warning disease surveillance systems to ensure early detection of and timely response to disease outbreaks in such settings cannot be overstated. However, implementing and ensuring optimal functionality of these systems in a disaster is always a new challenge.

The traditional approach of implementing early warning surveillance systems following a crisis in settings that experience rare or occasional humanitarian crises will continue to have a central role in humanitarian crisis. However, this model has been challenged recently both in countries that experience slow-onset emergences, such as the conflict in Syria or famine in the Horn of Africa, as well as in countries experiencing recurrent disasters such as floods in Pakistan and typhoons in the Philippines. Timely implementation may be difficult to achieve when the onset of an emergency is unclear, and donor fatigue may make it increasingly difficult to acquire funds for countries that experience recurrent disasters. In spite of these challenges in different emergencies, experience has shown that immediate deployment of skilled staff, appropriate system design, dissemination of standardized tools and training materials, timely procurement of emergency funds, effective monitoring and supervision, political support from local authorities, and collaboration among stakeholders are some of the critical success factors that should be considered when implementing such systems.

Planning for early warning disease surveillance as part of emergency preparedness can facilitate some of these factors and ensure that needed contingencies and resilience are built into the system. Disease surveillance in emergencies will always remain a challenge, as no two humanitarian emergencies are the same. Early warning disease surveillance principles, practices, and requirements specific for emergencies should be integrated into routine surveillance guidance documents and tools. MoHs, UN, and partner agencies responsible for implementing emergency disease surveillance systems should be better informed of implementation guidelines, especially at the country level. Investments in advocacy, partnerships, and coordination mechanisms plus development and dissemination of relevant guidance documents and tools would go a long way toward sensitizing local authorities and ensuring adequate local capacity for implementation and operation of surveillance in emergencies especially in countries that experience frequent crises.

Notes from the Field

Pakistan (2010)

The Disease Early Warning System (DEWS) in Pakistan was expanded nationally in response to the 2010 floods which displaced an estimated 20 million people, damaged 1.89 million homes and destroyed 82 districts. During the initial stages, central level stakeholders reached consensus on the priority conditions under surveillance. However, provincial health authorities, not part of the decision-making process, did not agree with the finalized list and were unwilling to use the revised reporting form. This resulted in problems with data aggregation. Cases of gastroenteritis, acute diarrhea and acute watery diarrhea from the district/province levels were aggregated as suspected cholera at the central level since each administrative level had a different category on their reporting form. Eventually, the list of conditions went through several iterations before all partners agreed and a new form was released – a process which took approximately three months and could have been prevented if all relevant stakeholders had been engaged from the onset.

Somalia (2011)

In response to the 2011 complex humanitarian emergency in Somalia, disease surveillance for the country was reorganized and revised into the early warning Communicable Disease Surveillance and Response (CSR) system. The revised system was implemented in January 2012. By 2013, CSR was collecting data from 195 sentinel health facilities. Due to mounting instability and insecurity in Central and South Zones, a simple monitoring plan was implemented to ensure minimum data quality assurances, particularly in hard to reach areas. However, funds dedicated for supervisory visits were redirected towards other health activities preventing routine checks and reviews. A 2014 evaluation of CSR revealed less than 75 percent agreement between data captured in health facility registers and data reported to the central level and 14 unreported alerts within the same reporting period, including a unreported case of "smallpox." Furthermore, insufficient funding compromised response capacity in Somalia. Regional surveillance officers and NGO staff reported the response component of the early warning system was lacking making the system ineffective. One regional officer in Somalia stated, "We are missing the 'R' in CSR! We cannot respond to alerts!" Budget procured for an emergency surveillance system must not only support weekly reports for disease monitoring, but must also account for alert verification, investigation, and the ability to implement control measures particularly in geographically remote and hard-to reach areas.

Nigeria (2012)

Unusually heavy rainfall that began in July 2012 led to severe flooding and waterlogging in 33 of the 36 States and the Federal Capital Territory in Nigeria. By October 2012, a national emergency was declared and the government of Nigeria made a request for international support. The floods displaced over two million persons, injured 18,200 people and led to 363 deaths across the affected states (OCHA 2012). Implementation of an early warning surveillance system was initiated immediately, but stalled due to lack of funds. Emergency funds were approved nearly two months later in December. By then, the recovery phase was already in progress and the number of internally displaced persons (IDPs) in evacuation centers had dropped by over 50 percent (OCHA 2012). A suspected cholera outbreak and increase of acute jaundice syndrome cases were detected by the early warning system once established, although the true magnitude of morbidity and mortality among the affected population prior to system implementation is unknown.

Philippines (2013)

The Philippines is in a region prone to hurricanes, typhoons, floods, earthquakes, and tsunamis. To prepare for such emergencies, the Department of Health developed Surveillance in Post Extreme Emergencies and Disasters (SPEED), a simplified system to monitor 21 health conditions in humanitarian crisis when the regular surveillance system is disrupted or stops working. It relies on daily reports via SMS, but also has online and manual reporting components in case of technology failures. In the case of typhoon Yolanda, the storm cut off power and decimated phone lines, so SMS and online reporting was not feasible in some parts of the affected area, particularly in the early phase of the crisis. In such areas, the manual paper-reporting component of SPEED was implemented, and "SPEED runners" were deployed to facilitate reporting. This consisted of men with motorcycles who would drive to the health facilities daily and pick up the forms. A survey of SPEED implementation in areas that experienced extensive destruction of the phone network in East Samar found that 2 weeks post-typhoon, 61 percent of facilities reported to SPEED using paper reporting forms and none were able to report via text; 4 weeks post-typhoon, 65 percent reported using paper forms and none reported via text; and 3 months post-typhoon, 50 percent of the facilities reported using paper forms and the other half used both paper forms and SMS, when cell network coverage became operational.

While problems with SPEED included too many health conditions to monitor effectively, relying on daily reporting instead of weekly and requiring mobilization of additional funds to maintain the SPEED runners, it does highlight the importance of an alternative or a combination of data transmission mechanisms in implementing an emergency disease surveillance system.

In addition, it was possible to deploy the system within two to three weeks in most of the areas affected by the typhoon, demonstrating the value of having a well-established humanitarian emergency surveillance system as a preparedness measure. Implement an early warning surveillance system from scratch post-Yolanda would have been an unimaginable challenge given the level of the devastation over many provinces.

Syria (2012)

Implementation of early warning surveillance in Syria and surrounding countries affected by the Syrian conflict offer lessons on both timely implementation and implementation delays. The Syrian civil conflict began in March 2011. The early warning emergency system was not implemented in government-controlled areas of Syria until September 2012 due to the slow escalation of violence and delayed realization of a humanitarian crisis underway. Despite the delay, emergency surveillance was quickly implemented once the decision was made due to good working relationship between the Syrian government and dedicated WHO country office staff with long experience in disease surveillance in emergencies. The situation was different in the northern part of the country that was under the control of opposition forces. Lack of government and UN presence in northern Syria not only delayed implementation of disease surveillance in these areas until 2013, but also prevented timely reporting and response activities due to ongoing insecurity and limited support from international community. Once established, it was this system that identified the initial cases of polio in northern Syria and eventually brought much-needed global attention to the area.

As the Syrian crisis worsened and refugees fled to neighboring countries, efforts to implement a similar early warning surveillance system were initiated in Iraq and Lebanon, and Jordan in June 2013. The system didn't become operational in Lebanon until January 2014, in Iraq until October 2014, and it was never fully adopted in Jordan. Human resource gaps and lack of consensus on system design affected optimal operation in Iraq. Local authorities' initial attempt to integrate early warning into a weak and dysfunctional preexisting routine system compromised capacity of both systems. This resulted in reporting delays, no alerts verifications, and poor data quality. For example, reported cases of suspected measles were arbitrarily classified as chickenpox without due process of appropriate verification and investigation. Eventually, a redesigned system with focus on the emergency-affected population and a dedicated focal point improved performance greatly. Delays in Lebanon were due to the government's reluctance to expand disease surveillance to affected refugee populations in efforts to discourage further influx. Refugees who made up an estimated 25 percent of the population of Lebanon and were housed in 1000 camps and informal settlements placed an enormous strain on public services and the social fabric of Lebanese society. Ultimately, some efforts to enhance the existing routine surveillance system to address the needs of the affected population were made; however, this does not substitute for an early warning disease surveillance system among the affected population.

Another example of delayed implementation was in a Syrian refugee camp in Jordan. A camp-based disease surveillance system was implemented in response to the increasing number of Syrian refugees. There were eight health partners from seven different countries, with varying areas of focus including injuries, primary care, reproductive health surgical trauma, etc., and distinctly separate reporting requirements. The main coordinating UN agency within the camp disseminated a standardized reporting form to facilitate data aggregation among the various partners; however, there was little initial investment in introducing the form and training. Health partners did not adopt the UN reporting form and continued to use their own data collection tools, making it difficult to understand disease trends among the affected population. Eventually, UN staff spent significant time with each health partner addressing questions and concerns on the standard form, adapting it to fit their needs, disseminating standardized case definitions, and conducting a two-day training and a mini-pilot in order to achieve buy-in.

The Syrian crisis offers a good illustration of how slow onset emergencies and civil conflict can mask the need for emergency interventions, confuse roles and responsibilities, and further exacerbate the deteriorating health status of the affected population. These experiences also show that time invested up-front in advocacy, partnerships, and coordination among all stakeholders can ease implementation efforts and minimize hurdles encountered later on.

References

Centers for Disease Control and Prevention (CDC). (2001). Considerations for distinguishing influenza-like illness from inhalational anthrax. *Morbidity and Mortality Weekly Report*, 50(44), 984–986.

Gayer, M., Legros, D., Formenty, P., and Connolly, M. A. (2007). Conflict and emerging infectious diseases. *Emerg Infect Dis*, 13(11).

Global Health Security Agenda (online). Available at: www.globalhealth.gov/global-health-topics/global-health-security/GHS%20Agenda.pdf (Accessed September 5, 2014).

Kamugisha, C., Cairns, K. L., and Akim, C. (2003). An outbreak of measles in Tanzanian refugee camps. *J Infect Dis*, **187**(Suppl 1), S58–S62.

Nsubuga, P., White, M. E., Thacker, S. B., et al. (2006). Public health surveillance: A tool for targeting and monitoring interventions, in D. T. Jamison, J. G. Breman, A. R. Measham, et al., eds., *Disease control priorities in developing countries*, 2nd edition. Washington, DC: World Bank, pp. 997–1015.

Office for the Coordination of Humanitarian Affairs (OCHA). (2012a). Nigeria: Floods, Situation Report No. 1 (online). Available at: http://foodsecuritycluster.net/sites/default/files/SITREP%20NIGERIA%20Floods%2001%20-%202012-11-06.pdf (Accessed September 21, 2015).

Office for the Coordination of Humanitarian Affairs (OCHA). (2012b). Nigeria: Floods, Situation Report No. 3 (online). Available at: http://reliefweb.int/sites/reliefweb.int/files/resources/Full%20Report_1165.pdf (Accessed September 21, 2015).

Refugee health: An approach to emergency situations. (1997). London: Macmillan Education.

Siddique, A. K., Akram, K., Zaman, K., et al. (1995). Why treatment centres failed to prevent cholera deaths among Rwandan refugees in Goma, Zaire. *The Lancet*, 345(8946), 359–61.

Teutsch, S. and Churchill, R. E. (2000). *Principles and practice of public health surveillance.* New York: Oxford University Press, p. 292.

Thacker, S. B., and Berkelman, R. L. (1988). Public health surveillance in the United States. *Epidemiol Rev*, 10, 164–90.

Toole, M. and Waldmann, R. (1990). Prevention of excess mortality in refugee and displaced populations in developing countries. *JAMA*, **263**(24), 3296–3302.

World Health Organization (WHO). IHR procedures concerning public health emergencies of international concern (PHEIC) (online). Available at: www.who.int/ihr/procedures/pheic/en/ (Accessed January 21, 2015).

World Health Organization (WHO). (2012). *Outbreak surveillance and response in humanitarian emergencies: WHO guidelines for EWARN implementation.* Geneva, Switzerland: World Health Organization, 6.

Chapter 10: Monitoring and Evaluation

Goldie MacDonald, Lori A. Wingate, and Susan Temporado Cookson

Introduction

In the wake of the 1994 genocide and civil war in Rwanda, a system-wide, multinational and multiagency evaluation identified significant shortcomings in the humanitarian response (Relief and Rehabilitation Network 1996). These included major deficiencies in coordination across United Nations (UN) agencies, inadequate preparation for the massive influx of refugees into Goma, Democratic Republic of the Congo (formerly Zaire), and underperformance of some international nongovernmental organizations (NGOs). A particularly concerning example was the finding that unprofessional and irresponsible behavior by some international NGOs most likely resulted in unnecessary loss of life (Relief and Rehabilitation Network 1996).

Evaluations of the response to events in Rwanda spurred discussions of the need for increased accountability and heightened attention to evaluation among humanitarian organizations. Several key initiatives followed:

- The Steering Committee for Humanitarian Response (SCHR), an alliance of international NGOs, the International Committee of the Red Cross, and the International Federation of Red Cross and Red Crescent Societies created in 1972, discussed self regulatory approaches for participating organizations.
- SCHR developed the first Humanitarian Charter and Minimum Standards, later known as The Sphere Project, and the Humanitarian Ombudsman Project evolved into the Humanitarian Accountability Partnership (HAP) to establish a voluntary certification process for NGOs.
- The Active Learning Network for Accountability and Performance in Humanitarian Action (ALNAP) was created in 1997 (Borton 2014).
- Seven international NGOs formed the Emergency Capacity Building Project "to improve the speed, quality, and effectiveness of the humanitarian community to save lives, improve welfare, and protect the rights of people in emergency situations" in 2004 (Emergency Capacity Building [ECB] 2011). One of the major aims of this initiative was to improve accountability and impact measurement (ECB 2011), resulting in *The Good Enough Guide* (ECB 2007).
- The Quality and Accountability Initiatives Complementarities Group formed, consisting of HAP, People in Aid, The Sphere Project, ALNAP, and others, in 2006 (Humanitarian Accountability Partnership 2014). As a result, People in Aid and HAP worked together to develop staff competencies, and HAP and The Sphere Project worked to align their respective standards.

Despite these and other multiorganizational and multinational initiatives, the need to improve capabilities and methods to evaluate responses to humanitarian emergencies remains. Hallam observed that the "full potential benefit of humanitarian evaluations is not being realized" and that far too many of these evaluations "exist as a disconnected process, rather than becoming embedded as part of the culture and mindset of humanitarian organizations" (Hallam 2011). Smith and Cosgrave echoed this sentiment and concluded that there is "little evidence that evaluation results lead to change of, or reflection on, policy and practice" (Smith and Cosgrave 2013). Still, many consider evaluation an essential activity for the continued improvement of organizations, humanitarian assistance, and ultimately the human condition. In 2013, United Nations Secretary-General Ban Ki-moon stated, "All of us share a responsibility to strengthen the evaluation function." He went on to say, "self-evaluation has to be part and parcel of our routine management work" (EvalPartners 2014).

Given the fundamental importance of program evaluation in public health, practitioners working in humanitarian emergencies need at least basic knowledge of the topic and how it is distinguished from other public health functions. This includes defining program evaluation and understanding its relationship to other public health functions, articulating the purposes and uses of program evaluation, describing key practices and methods common to program evaluation, and highlighting some of the challenges for program evaluation in the context of humanitarian emergencies.

Definitions

Program evaluation is related to, but distinct from, other data collection activities conducted to understand or track conditions in humanitarian emergencies, such as needs assessments, surveillance, and monitoring. There may be overlap in the information needed for these activities, and program evaluation, but they serve distinct purposes in the context of humanitarian emergencies. Needs assessments and surveillance are discussed in Chapters 7 and 9 respectively.

Program evaluation bears the specific connotation of a systematic approach to assessing or documenting an activity, set of activities, or intervention, whether simple or multifaceted, and reaching conclusions about its merit, worth, or significance. It is commonly used as an umbrella term to include evaluations of programs, policies, projects, activities or sets of activities, all of which are means to address a problem or improve a condition or situation. In the context of humanitarian emergencies, the program being evaluated is the response, or an aspect of the response, intended to reduce morbidity and mortality and promote return to normalcy following the emergency (The Sphere Project 2004). The Development Assistance Committee of the Organization for Economic Co-operation and Development (OECD–DAC) offers this comprehensive definition of evaluation:

- An evaluation is an assessment, as systematic and objective as possible, of an ongoing or completed project, program, or policy and its design, implementation, and results. The aim is to determine the relevance and fulfillment of objectives, developmental efficiency, effectiveness, impact, and sustainability. An evaluation should provide information that is credible and useful, enabling the incorporation of lessons learned into the decision-making process of both recipients and donors (OECD–DAC 1991).

Unlike the other activities, program evaluation focuses on documenting implementation and determining the effectiveness, impact, outcomes, or other aspects of a program intended to stabilize or improve conditions resulting from the emergency. This distinction is often overlooked or misunderstood amidst rapidly changing conditions and needs in these settings. The distinction cannot be overemphasized:

- Program evaluation is used to document, understand, and appraise the response to the emergency, not to document or understand the emergency itself.

The Development Assistance Committee (DAC) defined criteria for evaluating development assistance. While directed at development rather than emergency response, the criteria can be used in reference to humanitarian emergencies. They are shown in Table 10.1.

Evaluation vs. Monitoring

Program monitoring is often discussed in conjunction with program evaluation. Similar to other terms in public health, the operationalization and interpretation of these terms are likely to vary. The OECD–DAC offers this definition of monitoring:

- Program monitoring is the routine collection and analysis of information to detect changes in the health of the beneficiaries and inform managers, or other stakeholders, about the progress of an ongoing intervention intended to improve the health of beneficiaries (OECD–DAC 2002).

In some contexts, the terms monitoring and evaluation, or M&E, are used together to refer to a continuum of activities to determine how a program is implemented or performs and what a program achieves. In the literature on program evaluation, however, monitoring and evaluation are regarded as distinct activities. Davidson contrasts evaluation and monitoring by giving examples of the types of questions each might address, noting that a monitoring question regarding a program's outcomes might be: "What has changed since, and as a result of, program implementation?" while an evaluation's questions would be: "How substantial and valuable were the outcomes? Did they make a real difference in people's

Table 10.1 Development Assistance Committee (DAC) criteria for evaluating development assistance: Definitions and examples of related evaluation questions

Criterion	Definition	Examples of Evaluation Questions
Relevance	The extent to which the aid activity is suited to the priorities and policies of the target group, recipient, and donor	• To what extent are the objectives of the program still valid? • Are the activities and outputs of the program consistent with the overall goals and attainment of objectives? • Are the activities and outputs of the program consistent with the intended effects, outcomes, or impacts?
Effectiveness	The extent to which an aid activity attains its objectives.	• To what extent were the objectives achieved or are likely to be achieved? • What were the major factors influencing the achievement or nonachievement of the objectives?
Efficiency	Efficiency refers to the outputs, qualitative and quantitative, in relation to the inputs. It is an economic term to signify that the program or project uses the least costly resources possible in order to achieve the desired results. This generally requires comparing alternative approaches to achieving the same outputs to see whether the most efficient process has been adopted.	• Were activities cost-efficient? • Were objectives achieved on time? • Was the program or project implemented in the most efficient way compared to alternatives?
Impact	The positive and negative changes produced by an intervention, directly or indirectly, intended or unintended. This involves the main impacts and effects resulting from the activity on the local, social, economic, environmental and other development indicators. The evaluation should be concerned with both intended and unintended results and must also include the positive and negative impact of external factors, such as changes in terms of trade and financial conditions.	• What has happened as a result of the program or project? • What real difference has the activity made to the beneficiaries? • How many people has the program or project affected?
Sustainability	Sustainability refers to whether the benefits of an activity are likely to continue after donor funding has been withdrawn. Projects need to be environmentally as well as financially sustainable.	• To what extent did the benefits of a program or project continue after donor funding or the emergency ceased? • What were the major factors that influenced the achievement or nonachievement of sustainability of the program or project?

Source: OECD, 2014

lives?" and "Were the outcomes worth achieving given the effort and investment put into obtaining them?" (Davidson 2013) Program monitoring can be understood as a component of, or complement to, program evaluation.

A critical difference between these activities is that monitoring typically yields mostly descriptive information about a program while evaluation yields conclusions and judgments about the quality, value, or importance of a program.

Evaluation vs. Assessment

Assessment is often used synonymously with evaluation, but has different connotations in emergency settings. The Sphere Project describes assessment: "the priority needs of the disaster-affected population are identified through a systematic assessment of the context, risks to life with dignity and the capacity of the affected people and relevant authorities to respond" (The Sphere Project 2011).

Response personnel conduct Assessments to identify factors leading to or increasing vulnerabilities or needs among affected populations shortly after an emergency occurs. Depending on the purpose or timing of the assessment, it may be a needs assessment, initial assessment, or rapid assessment. In many cases, organizations and personnel use the results to make decisions about activities or programs needed in the initial phase of the emergency. Some assessments yield data that can be used for program evaluation purposes such as establishing a baseline for determining progress toward desired outcomes over time, for example. Assessments are discussed in detail in Chapter 7.

The Framework for Program Evaluation in Public Health

The CDC published the Framework for Program Evaluation in Public Health in 1999. The Framework delineates necessary steps and standards for program evaluation (CDC 1999). The steps are helpful for conceptualizing the elements and processes of program evaluation and aid in anticipating key decisions and necessary actions. The Joint Committee on Standards for Educational Evaluation developed the Program Evaluation Standards adopted by numerous evaluation organizations across the globe. In essence, the Program Evaluation Standards call for evaluations to be useful, practical, ethical, accurate, transparent, and fiscally prudent–qualities sought by many initiatives to improve program evaluation and accountability in humanitarian assistance worldwide. The Framework is not prescriptive with regard to focus, design, or methods used to evaluate a program. Moreover, application of this Framework is compatible with approaches and procedures recommended by various international organizations engaged in humanitarian action. The Framework posits that any program evaluation should include:

- Engaging stakeholders involved in or affected by the program and those who will use the evaluation results

- Describing the program to be evaluated, including the need, expected effects, activities, resources, stage of development, context, and logic model
- Focusing the evaluation design by defining its purpose, users, uses, questions, methods, and agreements related to administrative or procedural matters
- Gathering credible evidence with careful consideration of the data to be collected, the actions taken to assure data will be of adequate quality, and logistical considerations or issues related to the collection and handling of data
- Justifying conclusions by analyzing and synthesizing data, interpreting those data to reach judgments about the program based on established criteria or other points of reference including stakeholders' perspectives or values, and making recommendations for action or improvements relevant to the program and sensitive to its setting
- Ensuring use and share lessons learned by designing the evaluation with intended use and users in mind from the outset, preparing stakeholders to use information from the evaluation, encouraging input from stakeholders throughout the evaluation process, communicating and disseminating the evaluation results and lessons learned to relevant audiences, and supporting other uses of the evaluation process and results, as appropriate and necessary (CDC 1999; MacDonald 2014).

Recommended actions organized by steps in the Framework are shown in Table 10.6.

Purposes

Typically, program evaluation serves one or more of three broad and sometimes overlapping purposes:

- Formative evaluation to identify opportunities or ways to improve a program while it is underway
- Summative evaluation to determine the merit, worth, or significance of a more mature or completed program
- Accountability to document what was done and how resources were used

The US Centers for Disease Control and Prevention (CDC 1999, CDC 2013) emphasized two additional purposes of program evaluation in the work of public health:

- Determining whether a new activity, intervention, or strategy is viable for implementation more widely
- Using the evaluation process to bring about change in participants or other stakeholders including donor and partner organizations

In practice, organizations initiate program evaluations to serve a variety of purposes. Commonly identified purposes of program evaluation relevant to any type of program include the following (Weiss 1998):

- Providing data to support midcourse adjustments or corrections to the program
- Informing decisions about continuing or discontinuing, expanding, or reducing the program including the composition or reach of activities or services
- Recording the history of a program as a form of knowledge management
- Providing feedback for improvement to personnel
- Improving understanding of interventions

According to ALNAP, the principal purposes for evaluation of humanitarian action, specifically, include (Smith and Cosgrave 2013):

- Accountability for resources
- Drawing lessons from the inquiry to inform policy and practice in meaningful ways

Evaluation Design

In alignment with the stated purpose, it is important to identify key evaluation questions to focus the evaluation on the specific aspects of the program to be evaluated. Table 10.1 includes examples of evaluation questions matched to different criteria or types of evaluation. The questions addressed may be constrained by the evaluation's timing. An evaluation may be initiated early, as the response begins to unfold; ongoing as the intervention is occurring; midterm (or as nearly midterm as can be estimated); or at the conclusion of the response or post-intervention (Smith and Cosgrave 2013). Questions that speak to the characteristics or relevance of the response may be explored early on; in contrast, questions that explore the outcomes, impact, or sustainability of programing require investigation later in the response. Who performs the evaluation also varies; it could be done internally or, by an outside consultant or organization, or some combination of contributors that can include local personnel or other stakeholders. The planning and conduct of program evaluation, regardless of the conditions or speed of work required, must be a progression of informed, context sensitive technical decisions and related actions. At the outset of an evaluation, it is critical to clearly describe the program to be evaluated. This component of evaluation planning may be perceived as obvious or dismissed because those involved believe the program is already well known and understood. However, unchecked assumptions regarding the program are common and threaten the quality of the evaluation. This is especially true in humanitarian emergencies, as conditions beyond the control of program personnel can affect their ability to implement the program as intended. Thus, it is important to take time during evaluation planning to develop an accurate description of the program as a much-needed platform for subsequent decisions regarding its evaluation.

In the context of humanitarian emergencies, this step of describing the program to be evaluated is especially important. The typical boundaries of what constitutes a program and expectations about what should be evaluated may not be as clear in emergency situations as in nonemergency programming. As pointed out in OECD–DAC's *Guidance for Evaluating Humanitarian Assistance in Complex Emergencies*, evaluations of humanitarian assistance typically occur at one of four levels (OECD 1999):

- System-wide evaluation of the response by the whole system to a particular disaster event or complex emergency
- Partial system evaluation of a part of the system such as a thematic or sectorial study
- Single-agency response evaluation of the overall response to a particular disaster event or complex emergency by a particular agency
- Single-agency, single-project evaluation of a single project undertaken by a single agency

Therefore, a crucial step in defining the program to be evaluated is to determine at which of these levels the program operates and delineate the boundaries and components of the program clearly. Logic models are one of several tools that can be used to describe a program in advance of program evaluation (CDC 1999). Logic models depict the main elements of a program visually (inputs, activities, outputs, outcomes, and context) to illustrate how stakeholders and others expect resources dedicated to the program to contribute to desired changes (Taylor-Powell,

Table 10.2 Examples of program evaluations in humanitarian emergencies

Evaluation	Purposes or Objectives of the Evaluation
External Evaluation of the Haiti Emergency Relief and Response Fund (ERRF), 2008–2011	• Determine the extent to which the organization met objectives of the response • Identify strengths and weaknesses in operations relevant to the response (e.g., decision process for allocations of funds) • Assess adherence to criteria established by the OECD–DAC (e.g., effectiveness, efficiency) • Identify opportunities to improve or strengthen ERRF functioning, as well as ERRF strengths that might be systematized or applied in other settings
Inter-Agency Standing Committee (IASC) Real-Time Evaluation (RTE) of the Humanitarian Response to the Horn of Africa Drought Crisis – Ethiopia	• Provide real-time feedback to the Humanitarian Country Teams • Look at the lessons learned for the future and • Get the views of affected people on the quality of the response

Source: Morinière 2011, Sida et al. 2012

Jones, & Henert, 2002; Ladd et al., 2005). With this description in place and well understood among key stakeholders, the next task is to identify the purpose of the evaluation explicitly. Given the range of purposes that evaluation can serve and the fact that evaluation work is highly contextual, it is important for stakeholders to carefully consider and clearly define the purposes of an evaluation from the outset of planning. For example, The United Nations Office for the Coordination of Humanitarian Affairs (OCHA) conducts evaluations of humanitarian response "to promote transparency, accountability and learning through systematic and objective judgments about the relevance, efficiency, effectiveness and impact of humanitarian interventions" (OCHA 2014). The purposes of a particular evaluation may be stated generally or much more specifically to reflect the preferences of stakeholders, scope of the evaluation or intervention, or meet the precise information needs of specific users. Additional examples of program evaluations are shown in Table 10.2.

Whether expressed as evaluation objectives or purposes, it is necessary to articulate, at the earliest stages of planning, the aims, impetus, rational, or reasons why an organization resources and conducts an evaluation.

Data Collection

Common methods for collecting data in humanitarian emergencies for the purposes of program evaluation include, but are not limited to, surveys, interviews, focus group discussions, direct observation, and document review and analysis. These methods are defined in Table 10.3.

Common sources of data include program personnel, program beneficiaries or participants, nonparticipants, and program documents or records. These are shown in Table 10.4. In many cases, multiple entities or organizations operate programs in response to a single emergency. Efforts should be made to coordinate data collection to minimize the burden on those from whom information is requested, as well as to maximize use of often-limited resources dedicated to the evaluation. For evaluations that call for data on the health of populations impacted by a humanitarian emergency, utilizing a shared, easily accessible database can enhance efficiency. For example, the United Nations High Commissioner for Refugees established an online platform, called Twine, for managing and analyzing public health data collected in refugee operations (UNHCR, 2014b).

It is critical to understand that data collected or accessed from an existing source of information do

Table 10.3 Common methods of data collection in program evaluation in humanitarian emergencies

Method of Data Collection	Description
Survey	• The collection of standardized information from a population using a questionnaire at a single point in time (cross-sectional) or over time (longitudinal)
Interviews	• The collection of information by talking with and listening to participants, from highly-structured to more free-flowing formats
Document analysis	• Systematic review of written materials, such as reports, program materials, or websites, to extract key pieces of information
Observation	• First-hand experience or watching activities, behavior, characteristics, or events in a specific setting
Focus group	• An interview with a small group of people with shared characteristics or interests, designed to uncover information or insights regarding the program being evaluated

Source: Mathison 2005, Taylor-Powell and Steele 1996, CDC 2008a, CDC 2008b, Frechtling 2002

Table 10.4 Common sources of data for program evaluation

Source	Description
Staff	• Individuals involved in implementing the program
Participants or Beneficiaries	• Individuals participating in the program
Nonparticipants	• Individuals close to program participants or operations who do not participate in the program, whether due to ineligibility or choice
Documents or Materials	• Program records • Progress or status reports (e.g., implementation of the program, conditions within the emergency) • Budget or funding documents • Terms of Reference or Statements of Work used to describe the activity or program • Intake or processing forms (e.g., from a healthcare facility)

not automatically translate to findings and recommendations that are timely and usable by stakeholders. A process for analysis and interpretation of evaluation data and dissemination of results is necessary to ensure effective and efficient use of the data. Deriving meaning from data requires going beyond the information itself. Interpretation requires a comparison against something, which may be as informal as stakeholders' expectations for a program's performance or as formal as an agreed-upon, predetermined standard or value threshold for a certain program outcome often determined by looking at one or more indicators.

Indicators

Well-defined purposes of the evaluation and overarching evaluation questions are required to identify the specific data to be accessed or collected. Many organizations define and use indicators to answer evaluation questions. An indicator is a "documentable or measureable piece of information regarding some aspect of the program in question (e.g., characteristics of the program, facets of implementation or service delivery, outcomes)" (MacDonald 2013). An indicator identifies the specific data points needed to address evaluation questions and requires

Table 10.5 Criteria for selection of indicators for program evaluation

Criterion	Description
Accepted practice and history of use	• The degree to which use of an indicator is consistent with current and previous practices
Applicability in different settings	• The degree to which an indicator is relevant in diverse settings
Availability of data	• The degree to which data are accessible for use as part of the study
Burden of data collection on participants	• The degree to which data collection imposes burden on participants
Clarity of focus and meaning	• The degree to which a single indicator is unambiguous and reflects or represents the program accurately
Cultural appropriateness and Relevance	• The degree to which an indicator is culturally appropriate in terms of content or focus and related data collection activities
Data quality	• The degree to which information collected will be complete, reliable, and valid
Investment of resources	• The amount of resources (e.g., funds, personnel, time) needed for data collection, analysis, and use of data or findings
Non-directional language	• The indicator is written as neutral, not defined as positive or negative in advance of data collection
Opportunity to detect unexpected or unintended findings	• The degree to which an indicator (or set of indicators) allows for documentation of unexpected or unintended aspects of the program
Pathway for use of data	• The degree to which data use and users are known and agreed to
Relevance to evaluation questions	• The degree to which an indicator helps to address predefined evaluation questions
Strength of evidence or substantive merit	• The scope and quality of information supporting the indicator as an appropriate descriptor or measure of some aspect of the program
Value within a set of indicators	• The degree to which a single indicator adds meaning to a set of indicators

Source: MacDonald, 2013.

specification of how those data are to be collected. Table 10.5 provides example criteria for selection of indicators for program evaluation.

The Sphere Handbook includes key indicators to signal whether a minimum standard is achieved (The Sphere Project 2011).

The Sphere Project represents a major development in the use of a common set of standards as a benchmark or reference point for documenting humanitarian action. However, the Sphere standards and related indicators do not allow for examination of the characteristics or quality of implementation of the actions needed to achieve the minimum standards. The Sphere standards are *minimum* standards and the goal of programs should be to exceed them. To this end, while it is important to determine whether a minimum standard is met, there is still a need for additional information regarding the activities or interventions that should be collected via resource-efficient, rigorous program evaluation.

This and other information should be used to determine and ensure that programming meets the conditions and needs of the affected population. Given the multitude of sources and types of data common in humanitarian emergencies, the distinct value of program evaluation should be emphasized. Despite the regular use and exchange of various data in humanitarian emergencies, some organizations do not fully appreciate the need for program evaluation during or after the emergency.

Additional guidance for selection of indicators includes the Emergency Capacity Building (ECB) Project (2007):

- Use as few new indicators as possible
- Balance quantitative and qualitative information
- Collect only the information most needed
- Ensure that the indicators measure the aspect of the program or change of interest

As personnel explore options for indicators, including the logistics of data collection and analysis, it is especially important to consider use of existing sources of data and avoid duplication of effort with other organizations or partners. To do this, those tasked with evaluation planning must carefully consider the sources of information and means for gathering it prior to initiating data collection.

Interpretation of Results, Dissemination, and Recommendations

Typically, the process of interpretation of the evaluation data and deriving conclusions about the program requires consideration of several factors including:

- Comparison of current, observed conditions against preemergency levels
- Comparison of conditions with preestablished criteria or standards relevant to the program, populations served by the program, or its setting such as the minimum standards established by The Sphere Project
- Comparison of evaluation results with findings from other evaluations of similar programs in similar contexts
- Perceptions or opinions of people affected by the program, including those delivering the program and those served by the program

Because the factors considered when interpreting data will vary depending on the setting, type of emergency, and nature of the data used for the evaluation, it is especially important to be transparent about the analysis and interpretation process and to justify conclusions and recommendations including clearly explaining how and why conclusions about the program were reached. Stakeholder involvement in the interpretation process and consideration of their perspectives or understandings in relation to other comparison points helps ensure that conclusions are

Table 10.6 Recommended actions for program evaluation in humanitarian emergencies organized by steps in the Framework for Program Evaluation in Public Health

Framework For Program Evaluation In Public Health	Recommended Action
Step 1: Engage Stakeholders	• Identify existing agreements or requirements relevant to program evaluation in your setting • Identify intended users and uses of the evaluation
Step 2: Describe the Program	• Assure there is a sound description of the program to be evaluated • Use a logic model to link resources to results based on evidence or practice wisdom
Step 3: Focus the Evaluation	• Identify the purpose of the evaluation • Identify key evaluation questions, attending to process and outcome evaluation, as appropriate and resources permit
Step 4: Gather Credible Evidence	• Identify indicators (i.e., data or information) to be used to answer the evaluation questions • Use explicit criteria to select these indicators • Maximize use of existing sources of data and avoid duplication of efforts
Step 5: Justify Conclusions	• Collaborate with stakeholders to interpret the data • Convert findings to actionable, plain-language recommendations
Step 6: Ensure Use and Share Lessons Learned	• Assign responsibility for dissemination and follow-up • Disseminate the findings and recommendations to stakeholders not just donors

Source: Modified from CDC 1999.

accurate, appropriate, and relevant. The evaluation plan can include an opportunity for stakeholders to understand and interpret the data to ensure the accuracy, utility, and acceptability of the findings. This could take the form of a lessons-learned meeting to build agreement on key findings and identify changes needed (ECB 2007).

Finally, the findings and conclusions should be converted to actionable, plain-language recommendations specific to the purpose and objectives from the outset of the evaluation. For example, the United Nations Evaluation Group provided several checkpoints to ensure the quality of recommendations to be included in an evaluation report (United Nations Evaluation Group 2010):

- Recommendations are relevant to the object and purposes of the evaluation
- Recommendations are developed with the involvement of stakeholders
- The process to develop recommendations, including consultation with stakeholders, is well described
- Recommendations are firmly based upon evidence and conclusions drawn from the evaluation
- Recommendations are actionable, stated clearly, and include clear priorities for action
- Recommendations identify a target group for action
- Recommendations reflect an understanding of the commissioning organization and possible constraints to follow-up action

The evaluation should be designed in accordance with its purposes and intended uses. Release of information from the evaluation should be timely and directed at stakeholders to support those uses. If an evaluation is conducted concurrently with the response to a humanitarian emergency and is intended to inform decisions about the response, findings and conclusions from the evaluation should be shared with intended users as they become available. Ideally, the information can be used to improve the response and its outcomes. This information can be presented to stakeholders in various formats such as a traditional technical report, an executive report, a brief decision memo, or an oral presentation (CDC 2013). The format for conveying this information should be selected with the intended users in mind. Facilitating the use of the information may require more direct action than simply providing a report, such as a special meeting to focus on results, make decisions, and prepare action plans based on conclusions or recommendations.

Regardless of the eventual format, the evaluation team should deliver a debriefing of preliminary findings before leaving the emergency-affected area. To ensure the information reaches intended users, responsibility for dissemination and follow-up should be assigned purposefully. The assigned person, or persons, should disseminate the findings and recommendations to the full range of stakeholders, not just donors.

If an evaluation was done retrospectively or was not completed until a program concluded, the results of the evaluation can still be used to improve future actions and inform the community of agencies and organizations that respond to humanitarian emergencies. In fact, many agencies and organizations make evaluation information publicly available to support learning and improvement. Repositories of reports on evaluation of humanitarian actions include:

- The Active Learning Network for Accountability and Performance in Humanitarian Action (ALNAP) provides access to a collection of more than 100 evaluation reports searchable by agency, region, date, and language (www.alnap.org) (ALNAP 2006).
- OCHA maintains a collection of reports dating back to 2001 and includes both OCHA-specific and interagency evaluations (www.unocha.org).
- CARE International maintains a library of more than six hundred evaluation reports, searchable by country, language, year, evaluation type, and sector (www.careevaluations.org).
- UNICEF provides a database of evaluation information searchable by theme (www.unicef.org/evaldatabase).

Challenges

There are distinct challenges in the evaluation of programs in the context of humanitarian emergencies. Typically, attention to immediate needs and tasks limits attention to broader and long-term perspectives (Dabelstein 1996). The context of humanitarian emergencies is often chaotic with instability, insecurity, and uncertainty, all of which have significant implications for evaluation planning, implementation, and use of findings. Given these challenges, program evaluations in humanitarian emergencies should be done in consideration of (OECD–DAC 1999):

- The humanitarian space available
- The security situation
- Human rights abuses and protections

Humanitarian space is the general environments in which humanitarian actors operate (ATHA 2014). In humanitarian emergencies, this is fraught with lack of infrastructure, restricted movement, and limited access to resources. For example, access to the physical location of an activity or program may be limited due to unsafe or insecure conditions (Bamrah, et al. 2009). In these situations, security is a concern for individuals directly affected by the emergency, those engaged in programming, and those evaluating the program. As such, security and other risks need to be identified and considered when planning and conducting evaluations in these settings.

Sensitivity to issues and events surrounding a humanitarian emergency also present challenges to conducting program evaluation. Political, interpersonal, or cultural or ethnic tensions may run high, and individuals collecting data from program personnel, participants, and others must be aware of and responsive to these issues (Bamrah et al. 2009).

Information provided by individuals or organizations as part of an evaluation must be viewed with consideration of the intense feelings and polarization of the affected population (OECD–DAC 1999). Collecting data from a variety of respondents such as beneficiaries or participants, nonparticipants, and program staff, with diverse perspectives and using culturally appropriate data collection strategies enhance the validity of data gathered about sensitive topics (Bamberger et al. 2012). Evaluations should include attention to the adequacy of efforts intended to protect the most vulnerable segments of the population from abuses OECD–DAC (1999).

Those responsible for planning and conducting a program evaluation should be aware of the need to document possible unexpected or unintended outcomes or results, positive or negative. This may be particularly relevant to humanitarian emergencies. For example, an evaluation may find that aid or assistance is diverted from what was intended by the donor, identifying the need for critically important changes in operations. Similarly, an evaluation may document that assistance to those affected by the emergency spurs frustration or resentment among members of a host community. This finding adds to the understanding of the context and setting, and influences and subsequent implementation of programming or progress toward intended outcomes. For example, following the large influx of Syrian refugees into Mafraq, Jordan, some Jordanians observed refugees selling food aid and expressed a belief that the refugees were doing quite well, much better in fact than the majority of local residents. These Jordanians may not have understood that the refugees resorted to selling food to obtain other basic commodities (MercyCorps 2012). This tension in Mafraq is an example of unexpected and unintended effects of programming. Information like this can be used to inform or refine activities in productive ways across phases of the emergency.

Common limitations to conducting a program evaluation include constraints on budget, time, and availability of data. These issues, particularly with regard to data, are exacerbated in the context of a humanitarian emergency. Information on health in humanitarian emergencies is often "fragmented, lacking in standardization, not sufficiently geographically representative, or inaccurate" (Mock and Garfield 1999). There is often a lack of baseline or other comparison data against which change, or lack of change, can be determined. In some cases, it is possible to compensate for limited comparison data by reconstructing a baseline using secondary data. Possible sources of this secondary data include data collected previously for routine monitoring or surveillance purposes, data extracted from documents or records, data collected retrospectively, or data from geographic information systems or other georeferenced data (Bamberger et al. 2012).

Furthermore, in the context of a humanitarian emergency, there may be multiple contributors to, or providers of, programming or services. The resulting overlap or duplications makes it difficult to attribute changes, outcomes, or results to any single organization or program. Similarly, work in one sector may influence related outcomes in another sector. For example, blanket supplemental feeding programs and water, sanitation, and hygiene programs are believed to contribute to changes in morbidity and mortality among children less than five years of age, making it challenging to attribute an observed change to an individual program.

Finally, the humanitarian space often includes high turnover of personnel that may result in loss of information or institutional memory (Hallam 1998). This and other challenges require the conduct of program evaluation in a timely manner to meet the pressing need for information and findings while the program operates.

Conclusion

As financial investments in response to humanitarian emergencies have increased in the past two decades, donors and the public have called for improved accountability for use of these resources and their results (Oliver 2008). For this and other reasons discussed in the chapter, UN agencies, governments, and NGOs aim to conduct more and better evaluations of their programs. Even though program evaluations can appear as afterthoughts in humanitarian emergencies, these activities are vital for accountability to the beneficiaries as well as donors and the public.

Moreover, the information collected and lessons learned through systematic evaluation can be used to enhance current and future programming to improve the response to humanitarian emergencies. This chapter presents some recommended actions needed in any program evaluation. It is time to advocate for and promote evaluation and evidence-based policy-making at all levels and in all contexts including peacetime and emergency (International Evaluation Partnership Initiative 2014).

Notes from the Field

Kenya (2012)

In response to drought and famine in the Horn of Africa, the United States Centers for Disease Control and Prevention (CDC) was asked to evaluate the impact of blanket supplementary feeding programs (BSFP) in northern Kenya. The program was to last five months and included six rations for each participant. However, due to limited access because of insecurity, logistical and transportation challenges, and interruptions in the food pipeline, the program continued for eight months, necessitating a 30-day ration to cover up to 120 days.

The same security, logistical, and transportation constraints required CDC to evaluate and monitor the program remotely for the last five months of implementation. The program evaluation found that while the nutritional status of the cohort of participants improved, the blanket supplementary feeding program was not the sole reason for the improvement. There were other substantial programs in these counties, and return of the rains brought additional food supplies before the extended implementation of the BSFP ended. In this case, the evaluation demonstrated that it was important to acknowledge that the improvements should not be attributed to the BSFP alone.

References

Active Learning Network for Accountability and Performance in Humanitarian Action (ALNAP). (2006). *Evaluating humanitarian action using the OECD-DAC criteria: an ALNAP guide for humanitarian agencies.* London: Overseas Development Institute. Available at: www.alnap.org/resource/5253 (Accessed April 21, 2014).

Advanced Training Program on Humanitarian Action (ATHA). Humanitarian Space. Available at: www.atha.se/content/humanitarian-space (Accessed October, 28 2014).

Bamberger, M., Rugh, J., and Mabry, L. (2012). *Real world evaluation: Working under budget, time, data, and political constraints,* 2nd edition, Thousand Oaks, CA: Sage Publications.

Bamrah, S., Mbithi, A., Muhenje, O., et al. (2009). *The impact of post-election violence on HIV and other healthcare services, Kenya, January-February 2008.* Nairobi, Kenya: Medical Outreach, Inc.

Borton, J. (2014). Twenty years on: The Rwandan genocide and the evaluation of the humanitarian response. Humanitarian Practice Network, Blogs and Articles, 6 April 2014. Available at: www.odihpn.org/the-humanitarian-space/news/announcements/blog-articles/twenty-years-on-the-rwandan-genocide-and-the-evaluation-of-the-humanitarian-response (Accessed May 13, 2014).

Centers for Disease Control and Prevention. (1999, September). Framework for program evaluation in public health. *Morbidity and Mortality Weekly Report,* 48(RR-11). Available at: ftp://ftp.cdc.gov/pub/Publications/mmwr/rr/rr4811.pdf (Accessed May 13, 2014).

Centers for Disease Control and Prevention. (2008a). Data collection methods for program evaluation: focus groups. *Eval Briefs,* 13, 1–2. Available at: www.cdc.gov/healthyyouth/evaluation/pdf/brief13.pdf (Accessed July 1, 2014).

Centers for Disease Control and Prevention. (2008b). Data collection methods for program evaluation: observation evaluation. *Eval Briefs,* 16, 1–2. Available at: www.cdc.gov/healthyyouth/evaluation/pdf/brief16.pdf (Accessed July 1, 2014).

Centers for Disease Control and Prevention. (2012). Evaluation of a Blanket Supplementary Feeding Program in Two Counties in Kenya, August 2011 – March 2012. Available at: www.alnap.org/resource/9410 (Accessed June 19, 2014).

Centers for Disease Control and Prevention. (2013). *Evaluation reporting: A guide to help ensure use of evaluation findings.* US Dept. of Health and Human Services; Atlanta, GA. Available at: www.cdc.gov/dhdsp/docs/Evaluation_Reporting_Guide.pdf (Accessed June 20, 2014).

Dabelstein, N. (1996). Evaluating the international humanitarian system: rationale, process and management of the joint evaluation of the international response to the Rwanda genocide. *Disasters*, **20**(4), 287–294.

Davidson, J. Monitoring and evaluation: let's get crystal clear on the difference, 14 Jan 2013. Available at: http://genuineevaluation.com/monitoring-and-evaluation-lets-get-crystal-clear-on-the-difference/ (Accessed July 30, 2014).

Emergency Capacity Building Project. (2007). *Impact measurement and accountability in emergencies: The good enough guide.* Oxfam; Oxford, UK. Available at www.ecbproject.org/resource/18044 (Accessed February 24, 2015).

Emergency Capacity Building Project. (2011). The Project. Available at: www.ecbproject.org/the-project/theproject (Accessed May 13, 2014).

EvalPartners: The International Evaluation Partnership Initiative. Ban Ki-moon: "All of us share a responsibility to strengthen the evaluation function", April 16, 2013. Available at: http://mymande.org/evalyear/UNSG_Speech_Evaluation_EP (Accessed July 1, 2014).

Frechtling, J, (2002). *The 2002 user friendly handbook for project evaluation.* The National Science Foundation: Arlington, VA. Available at: www.nsf.gov/pubs/2002/nsf02057/nsf02057_4.pdf (Accessed July 1, 2014).

Hallam, A. (1998). Evaluating humanitarian assistance programmes in complex emergencies. Relief Rehab Network. Available at: www.odihpn.org/hpn-resources/good-practice-reviews/evaluating-humanitarian-assistance-programmes-in-complex-emergencies (Accessed May 13, 2014).

Hallam, A. (2011). Harnessing the power of evaluation in humanitarian action: An initiative to improve understanding and use of evaluation. Available at www.alnap.org/resource/6123 (Accessed October 27, 2014).

Humanitarian Accountability Partnership. (2014). The Core Humanitarian Standard. Available at: www.hapinternational.org/what-we-do/the-core-humanitarian-standard.aspx (Accessed May 13, 2014).

International Evaluation Partnership Initiative. (2014). 2015 declared as the International Year of Evaluation. Available at: http://mymande.org/evalyear (Accessed July 22, 2014).

MacDonald, G. (2013). Criteria for selection of high-performing indicators: a checklist to inform monitoring and evaluation. Available at: www.wmich.edu/evalctr/checklists/evaluation-checklists (Accessed July 1, 2014).

MacDonald, G. (2014). Framework for program evaluation in public health: a checklist of steps and standards. Available at www.wmich.edu/evalctr/checklists/evaluation-checklists (Accessed May 20, 2014).

Mathison, S., ed. (2005). *Encyclopedia of evaluation.* Thousand Oaks, CA: Sage Publications, Inc.

MercyCorps. (October 2012). Analysis of host community-refugee tensions in Mafraq, Jordan. Available at http://data.unhcr.org/syrianrefugees/download.php?id=2958 (Accessed November 12, 2014).

Morinière, L. (2011). External evaluation of the Haiti emergency relief and response fund (ERRF), 2008–2011. Available at: https://docs.unocha.org/sites/dms/Documents/ERRF%20Haiti%20Evaluation%20Report.pdf (Accessed May 20, 2014).

Oliver, M. L. (2008). *Evaluation of Emergency Response: Humanitarian Aid Agencies and Evaluation Influence.* Public Management and Policy Dissertations, Department of Public Management and Policy, Georgia State University, Paper 23. Available at: http://digitalarchive.gsu.edu/pmap_diss/23 (Accessed May 2, 2014).

Organisation for Economic Co-operation and Development—Development Assistance Committee. (1991). Principles for evaluation of development assistance. DAC High-Level Meeting, 3 and 4 December 1991, Paris. Available at: www.oecd.org/development/evaluation/2755284.pdf (Accessed June 20, 2014).

Organisation for Economic Co-Operation and Development—Development Assistance Committee. (1999). Guidance for evaluation humanitarian assistance in complex emergencies. Available at: www.oecd.org/development/evaluation/2667294.pdf (Accessed May 13, 2014).

Organisation for Economic Co-Operation and Development—Development Assistance Committee. (2002). Glossary of Key Terms in Evaluation and Results Based Management. Available at: www.oecd.org/dataoecd/29/21/2754804.pdf (Accessed June 20, 2014).

Organisation for Economic Co-operation and Development—Development Assistance Committee. (2014). DAC criteria for evaluating development assistance. Available at: www.oecd.org/dac/evaluation/daccriteriaforevaluatingdevelopmentassistance.htm (Accessed June 20, 2014).

Relief and Rehabilitation Network. (1996). The Joint Evaluation of Emergency Assistance to Rwanda: Study III Principal Findings and Recommendations, Network Paper 16. London: Overseas Development Institute. Available at: www.odihpn.org/index.php?option=com_k2&view=item&layout=item&id=2132 (Accessed May 13, 2014).

Sida, L., Gray, B., and Asmare, E. (2012). IASC real-time evaluation of the humanitarian response to the Horn of Africa drought crisis in Somalia. Available at: https://docs.unocha.org/sites/dms/Documents/IASC%20RTE%20Ethiopia%202012.pdf (Accessed May 20, 2014).

Smith, M. B. and Cosgrave, J. (2013). Evaluation of humanitarian action: Pilot guide. London: ALNAP. Available at: www.alnap.org/eha# (Accessed April 21, 2014).

Taylor-Powell, E. and Steele, S. (1996). Collecting evaluation data: an overview of sources and methods. U Wisconsin-Extension. Available at: http://learningstore.uwex.edu/assets/pdfs/g3658-4.pdf (Accessed July 1, 2014).

The Sphere Project. (2004). *Humanitarian charter and minimum standards in humanitarian response*. Geneva, Switzerland: Author.

The Sphere Project. (2011). *Humanitarian charter and minimum standards in humanitarian response*. Rugby, UK: Practical Action Publishing.

United Nations Evaluation Group. (2010). UNEG quality checklist for evaluation reports. Available at: www.unevaluation.org/document/detail/607 (Accessed March 27, 2015).

United Nations High Commissioner for Refugees. (2014a). Public health data: Balanced scorecard. Available at: www.unhcr.org/pages/49c3646ce0.html. (Accessed June 20, 2014).

United Nations High Commissioner for Refugees. (2014b). http://twine.unhcr.org/app/ (Accessed June 20, 2014).

United Nations Office for the Coordination of Humanitarian Affairs (OCHA). (2014). Thematic areas: evaluations of humanitarian response [website]. Available at: www.unocha.org/what-we-do/policy/thematic-areas/evaluations-of-humanitarian-response/overview (Accessed June 20, 2014).

Weiss, C. H. (1998). *Evaluation*, 2nd edition. Upper Saddle River, NJ: Prentice Hall.

Yarbrough, D. B., Caruthers, F. A., Shulha, L. M., et al. (2011). *The program evaluation standards: A guide for evaluators and evaluation users*, 3rd edition. Thousand Oaks, CA: Sage Publications.

Chapter 11

Water, Sanitation, and Hygiene (WASH)

Nicole Weber, Anu Rajasingham, Molly Patrick, Andrea Martinsen, and Thomas Handzel

Introduction

Water, sanitation, and hygiene (WASH)-related diseases account for a significant proportion of the global burden of disease, and diarrhea remains one of the leading causes of childhood mortality (WHO, 2017). As the fecal-oral route is the predominant mode of transmission of diarrheal diseases, much of the childhood diarrheal disease burden could be alleviated through effective WASH programming, including proper treatment and storage of drinking water, safe disposal of human excreta, and improved personal hygiene practices. Populations affected or displaced by humanitarian emergencies may be even more susceptible to diarrheal and other infectious diseases due to overcrowding, lack of adequate shelter, poor hygiene, and interrupted services. In the acute phase of a humanitarian emergency in some camp settings, diarrheal diseases may account for more than 40 percent of deaths (Connolly et al., 2004). Thus, immediate actions should be undertaken to minimize the risk factors contributing to WASH-related diseases.

Populations affected by humanitarian emergencies are especially vulnerable to outbreaks of waterborne diseases, such as cholera and shigellosis. In the absence of adequate water, sanitation, and hygiene, outbreaks of cholera can spread rapidly through a population. In the extreme case of Goma, in the Democratic Republic of Congo (formerly Zaire), in 1994, a large displacement of approximately 500,000 – 800,000 refugees resulted in extremely poor sanitary conditions and lack of potable water supplies. A cholera outbreak spread through the population. This was followed by an outbreak of shigellosis which also spread to surrounding countries. The impact of these two outbreaks had an enormous toll on both the refugee and host communities with an estimated 50,000 deaths (Goma Epidemiology Group 1995). Outbreaks of hepatitis E have also affected displaced populations in Chad, Sudan, Uganda, Kenya, South Sudan, and Ethiopia in recent years. Additional information about the transmission, symptoms, and case management of these diseases is discussed in Chapter 22.

This chapter provides an overview of WASH in humanitarian emergencies and is divided into five main sections including water supply and quality, sanitation, hygiene, WASH in health care facilities, and WASH monitoring. All of these areas must be addressed to ensure protection from waterborne diseases. It is also important to note that simply providing hardware infrastructure alone will not ensure positive outcomes. People affected by humanitarian emergencies must also have the knowledge, skills, motivation, and enabling environment to prevent WASH-related diseases.

Water Supply

The provision of an adequate supply of potable water is an essential component of the public health response to humanitarian emergencies. Moreover, this provision is usually one of the first priorities of response agencies as the threat of waterborne disease outbreaks, including but not limited to cholera, typhoid fever, and hepatitis are greater in the absence of safe water supplies. In addition, although a minimum amount of water is required for human survival, increased quantities of water may be associated with better hygiene practices and a lower incidence of WASH-related diseases (Stelmach and Clasen, 2015). Thus, a primary objective of the WASH response in a humanitarian emergency is to quickly provide access to a minimum amount of potable water and subsequently increase the amount to improve personal hygiene.

The minimum volume of water required for survival is dependent on climate, cultural practices, and

Table 11.1 Minimum water quantities per person for basic survival water needs (adapted from Sphere Project 2011)

Need	Amount	Variables
Basic survival- drinking and food	2.5–3 liters/day	Depends on climate
Basic hygiene	2–6 liters/day	Depends on cultural practices
Basic cooking	3–6 liters/day	Depends on cultural practices and food type
Total basic water needs	7.5–15 liters/day	

Table 11.2 Minimum water quantities for institutions and other uses (adapted from Sphere Project 2011)

Use	Amount
Schools	3 liters/pupil/day for drinking and hand washing
Mosques	2–5 liters/person/day for drinking and washing
Livestock	20–30 liters/large or medium animal/day
	5 liters/small animal/day

sanitation needs but is generally estimated at 7.5–15 liters per person per day (Sphere Project, 2011). This includes water for drinking, cooking, and basic hygiene needs. For humanitarian settings, Sphere guidelines maintain a minimum standard of 15 liters per person per day (l/p/d), a maximum distance from any household to the nearest water point of 500 m, and a maximum queueing time of 30 minutes. Thus, for example, a household of 6 persons should, on average, be able to collect 90 liters of water per day. For a camp population of ten thousand persons, that would equate to 150 m³ of water per day before accounting for any losses in the distribution system, which may be up to 20 percent, due to leaks and spillage (MSF, 2010). The 15 l/p/d indicator must be contextualized based on pre-crisis norms, climate and post-crisis conditions. Additional water is needed for institutions, including healthcare facilities, schools, and places of worship, which need to be incorporated into the total requirements for water quantity. Some of the minimum water quantity guidelines from Sphere are shown in Tables 11.1 and 11.2.

Water requirements may also depend on the type of sanitation system used. If flush toilets or pour flush latrines are used, additional water will be needed. In addition, in some cultures, water is used for cleansing in sanitation facilities, which may add to water needs. In some emergencies, the livestock of the affected population may be an important food security consideration and increased water may be warranted (LEGS, 2014).

An initial assessment should be performed to collect data on the population's practices involving water. This will help guide the planning of the emergency water supply interventions. Particular attention should be paid to vulnerable populations who may need additional water, such as people with disabilities or people living with HIV/AIDS (PLHIV). Some important components of the population assessment include:

- Where do they collect water?
- How do they collect water?
- How much water is normally collected precrisis?
- How they treat and store water?
- What gender roles are related to water?
- What is the physical environment of the site and the water sources available?

Water Access

In addition to an adequate quantity of water, equitable access to water points is also extremely important. Collection of water is a daily burden and is often performed by women and children. If water collection points are too distant, people may either collect less water than needed or turn to alternative sources that are closer, but unpotable. Long queuing times at the water point may also lead to use of alternative sources. Thus, standards on the maximum distance to the source, maximum queueing time, and minimal flow rate also exist (Sphere Project, 2011). Table 11.3 provides guidance on the recommended maximum number of people per water point according to water flow. Facility managers may also need to ensure that access to water points is not controlled by individuals or groups and that everyone has access.

Water Storage

Populations displaced from their homes during a humanitarian emergency will also need to have a

Table 11.3 Maximum number of people per water point according to water flow (adapted from Sphere Project 2011)

Maximum Number of People/Water Point	Water Flow (guidelines assume availability eight hours/day and constant during that time)
500 people/hand pump	17 liters/minute
250 people/tap	7.5 liters/minute
400 people/single-user open well	12.5 liters/minute

sufficient number of clean water containers for collecting and storing water. The minimum requirement per household is two containers each of 10–20 liters. This will likely need to be increased if the family size is large or if there are frequent interruptions in the water supply necessitating longer storage times. Containers should be easy to carry to and from a water source. Any distribution of water storage containers is usually accompanied with hygiene promotion on safe water storage.

The most common containers used in emergencies are jerry cans and buckets with lids; however, traditional clay pots are also suitable as long as they remain covered. Containers with a narrow opening or tap, to prevent dipping hands or cups into water of wide-mouth containers, can help prevent further contamination. A cap or lid should always be replaced when opening the container to prevent contamination from hands, dirt, and animals. Regular cleaning of water transport and storage containers with detergent or chlorine may be necessary to reduce contamination.

Water Sources

The water sources available during a humanitarian emergency will depend on location and environmental conditions. In some emergencies, such as in urban settings, there may be existing water supplies for which minor repairs and treatment may be needed to ensure an adequate supply of potable water to the affected population. Surface water (lakes, ponds, rivers, etc.) may be the only or most available source of water during the acute phase of an emergency in many settings. Although it is easily extractable and often available in large quantities, surface water is not an ideal water source as it is highly vulnerable to microbiological, chemical, and physical contamination and generally requires multiple treatment steps to ensure potability.

Other options may include the use of groundwater including drilled wells, hand-dug wells, and springs. The quality of groundwater is variable but the amount of treatment that is required is usually less than surface water as it is generally low in turbidity and often requires only disinfection for treatment. Rainwater in nonindustrial and nonurban areas is often of high water quality and could be a viable source of water under some circumstances. However, rainfall is unpredictable and requires both catchment systems and storage capacity. Rainwater may also require rationing to provide ongoing access to water through the dry season. Table 11.4 provides a comparison of the advantages and disadvantages of the major water source types in emergencies (Davis and Lambert, 2002).

Water Trucking

Water trucking may play an important role in water provision in the early days of a humanitarian emergency when on-site water supplies are insufficient and other options do not exist. Water trucking can be an expensive option as it may require a large number of vehicles and transport over long distances. In addition, transporting water requires adequate roads and other infrastructure. For example, adequate storage tanks need to be in place to receive and distribute the water. However, in many emergency settings water trucking continues to play a key role. In 2010 post-earthquake Haiti, for example, water tankers were extremely useful in providing potable water to hundreds of internally displaced person (IDP) camps in Port-au-Prince. Water trucking should only be considered as a short-term response while longer-term water supply solutions are developed.

Water Treatment

In most emergency contexts, treatment of water supplies is required to ensure that the water is potable. This is often performed at centralized points for bulk water treatment but it can also be done at the point-of-collection or at the point-of-use (PoU) (household water treatment). Centralized bulk treatment is often preferred during an emergency response as it provides broad protection to affected populations without placing the responsibility of daily water treatment on the

Table 11.4 Comparison of water sources (Davis and Lambert 2002)

Water Source	Advantages	Disadvantages
Surface	• Quick access • Easily extractable in large quantity	• Exposed to potential microbiological and chemical contamination • Multiple treatment steps may be required
Hand-Dug Well	• Groundwater may be higher quality than surface water • Can be dug using locally available tools, materials, and labor • Low cost	• Water table subject to seasonal variability • May be subject to surface contamination if not well protected
Borehole	• High water quality and less susceptible to contamination than shallow wells • More consistent supply of water if aquifer is penetrated	• Requires drilling equipment and skilled staff to identify sites • May be high in minerals, affecting taste or water quality • Pumps for extraction require operation and maintenance
Spring or Seep	• High water quality • Lower operational costs if gravity-fed system is used	• Risk of contamination if spring is not adequately protected • Flow may vary depending on season • Location may be far away from population
Rain	• Lower risk of pollutants in rural and nonindustrial areas • Low cost and easy to maintain	• Difficult where rainfall is limited or unpredictable • Limited to available storage capacity

household themselves. The primary goal of water treatment interventions in emergencies is to remove or inactivate disease-causing organisms.

Disinfection of water supplies with chlorine is the most common water treatment process in emergency settings. Chlorination is most effective when the water is relatively clear or has turbidity generally less than 5 nephelometric turbidity units (NTU) (WHO, 2011). If water is turbid, additional treatment steps may be required prior to chlorination, both to ensure adequate disinfection and avoid potentially harmful disinfection by-products. These additional steps may include flocculation, sedimentation, or filtration. Additional references for water treatment in humanitarian emergencies are available (MSF, 2010).

Chlorine Disinfection

Chlorine is a powerful oxidant that will inactivate most microorganisms and, when dosed accordingly, will leave a residual that protects the treated water from recontamination during collection and storage. Chlorine is available in multiple forms and concentrations. High test hypochlorite powder, or HTH (65%–70% available chlorine), is often used in emergencies to treat bulk water supplies while liquid bleach (commonly 5.25% available chlorine) can also be used for small volumes of water. Chlorine gas may be used in larger water treatment facilities in urban settings, but must be handled with extreme care, as chlorine is very dangerous in gaseous form.

The amount of chlorine needed to treat a particular volume of water depends on the chlorine demand of the water and the desired residual chlorine after treatment. In practice, the appropriate chlorine dosage is determined by testing a small amount of water and then calculating the appropriate dose needed for bulk treatment. This process is commonly called a Jar Test. In most emergency settings, the free chlorine residual (FCR) should be 0.5 mg/L after a minimum of 30 minutes of contact time at water collection points. Both organic and inorganic materials, as well as microorganisms in the water, will consume chlorine, so the required chlorine dosage may be higher to leave a minimum FCR of 0.5 mg/L. Testing the chlorine demand is recommended – for example, dosing at 1.5 mg/L, testing the resulting residual after 30 minutes, and adjusting the dose accordingly. It is important to note that chlorine is less effective as a disinfectant at higher pH values. If treating water with a pH of 8.0 or greater, the contact time may need to be extended beyond 30 minutes to ensure the same chlorine effectiveness (WHO, 2011).

A higher FCR is recommended during a waterborne disease outbreak. For example, during cholera outbreaks WHO recommends a FCR of 1.0 mg/L at water collection points and 2.0 mg/L for water trucks (WHO, 1993). At higher chlorine concentrations, users may find the taste and smell unacceptable and refuse to drink it. However, the taste threshold is lower than the WHO health-based threshold, which specifies a maximum of 5 mg/L. Therefore, it is important that the FCR concentrations are monitored closely to ensure that it is neither too high nor too low.

Shock Chlorination

Shock chlorination of drinking water wells is sometimes used during waterborne disease outbreaks where wells are suspected to be contaminated. In this procedure, the well is treated with a high concentration of chlorine (for example, 50 mg/L), based on the volume of water in the well. The well is then closed for 1–2 days and pumped until chlorine levels are within an acceptable range for drinking. This method provides only limited protection as chlorine concentration will dissipate, particularly in the case of unlined, hand-dug wells. In addition, shock chlorination only disinfects the well and water in the well itself, not the surrounding groundwater supplying the well. Further, if the well is prone to recontamination, repeated treatments will be needed.

If the groundwater supply itself is contaminated, further remediation efforts may need to be taken in addition to regular treatment of the water prior to consumption. An additional disadvantage of shock chlorination of wells is that it may give a false perception or sense of security to the population that the water is potable and that additional treatment (e.g., at the household level) is not necessary.

Point-of-Collection Disinfection

Drinking water may also be disinfected at the point-of-collection. Two examples of this are bucket chlorination and chlorine dispensers. In bucket chlorination, trained individuals dose water containers once they are filled at the water point. The attendant is usually situated at a water source with water purification tablets or a stock solution of chlorine and a measuring device (syringe or similar device). As people collect water from the water source they pass by the attendant who dispenses the correct amount of chlorine into the vessel. Bucket chlorination permits an implementing agency to have more control over free chlorine residual at the individual level, as opposed to PoU chlorination whereby each person treats their own water at the household level. However, bucket chlorination can be labor intensive and expensive as there may be multiple water points, and water may be collected throughout the day. In addition, attendants must be trained on how to correctly dose various sized containers. Finally, there is substantial evidence that treated water may be recontaminated during transport between source and the PoU (Wright et al., 2004). While bucket chlorination has been used in numerous emergencies and disease outbreaks, there is only limited evidence on the effectiveness of this intervention (Ali and Kadir, 2016). Bucket chlorination is also discussed in Chapter 22.

Chlorine dispensers are an alternative method of chlorinating water at the point-of-collection and have been used in several recent humanitarian emergencies. A dispenser is set up next to the water source. The user turns a lever to automatically add a predetermined amount of chlorine to the water in the water collection vessel. The consistent use of chlorine dispensers in an emergency remains a challenge, as users may not use them. Across seven evaluations in four emergencies (including three cholera emergencies), the reported effective use of the dispensers ranged widely (Yates et al., 2015).

Point-of-Use/Household Water Treatment

Point-of-use or household water treatment methods are commonly used in emergencies, especially in the acute phase, in both urban and rural settings where centrally treated bulk water supplies are not available. Options include boiling, chlorination, flocculation with chlorination, filtering, and solar disinfection. Contrary to centralized or point-of-collection treatments, PoU treatment transfers the responsibility of water treatment from the water provider to the consumer and requires the consumer to consistently treat their own water. In all cases, however, the user is solely responsible for ensuring safe water storage to prevent recontamination at the household. The effectiveness of PoU treatment depends on the correct, consistent, and sustained use of the product (Ali and Kadir, 2016). PoU treatment interventions have the greatest potential for success when used in households that are familiar with the intervention prior to the emergency and have the training and supplies necessary to use the intervention during and after the emergency (Lantagne and Clasen, 2012).

PoU treatment options are generally less effective under field conditions than in laboratory settings. The available literature from nonemergency settings suggests that household water treatment reduces diarrheal disease but with wide ranges. Observed diarrheal disease reduction was 9%–35% (before controlling for blinding) for disinfection products, 41%–62% reduction for PoU filtration systems, and 6%–58% for solar water disinfection (Clasen et al., 2015).

Boiling

Boiling is a common household water treatment practice and is effective against waterborne pathogens, including cryptosporidium. Acceptability may be high as there is minimal change in the taste of the water, and the affected population may already have practiced boiling (Lantagne and Clasen, 2009). However, boiling requires fuel, which can contribute to deforestation if using charcoal or wood. Boiled water is also susceptible to recontamination if not safely stored, as there is no residual protection. Microbiological field testing has shown that water postboiling may still have pathogens due to inconsistent boiling, not bringing the water to a high enough temperature, or recontamination postboiling (Lantagne and Clasen, 2009).

Chlorination

Chlorine is one of the most commonly deployed PoU treatment in emergencies. It can be found in tablet form, also known as NaDCC (Aquatab™, Medentech, Wexford, Ireland), liquid, and powder form and is effective against bacteria and viruses. The chlorine residual provides additional protection against recontamination. Chlorine options are relatively low cost depending on the product used. However, the large variety of products and sizes with varied dosages, challenges with ensuring a consistent supply chain, inconsistent or incorrect use at the household level, and inadequate training of beneficiaries are barriers to its effectiveness (Ali and Kadir 2016). Additionally, the chlorine taste may prevent some users from consistently using chlorine.

Flocculant Disinfectants

Flocculant/disinfectant sachets, such as P&G Purifier of Water™ (Procter & Gamble Company, Cincinnati, US) or Watermaker™ (Control Chemicals, Johannesburg, South Africa), permit the treatment of turbid water and remove most bacteria, viruses, and protozoa. The contents of the sachet are poured into the water and then slowly stirred, allowing floc formation. The floc is then allowed to settle to the bottom of the bucket and the supernatant (liquid that has been separated) is poured off through a cloth or mesh fabric into a second container. The second component of the sachets is a chlorine-based compound that releases chlorine into the treated water. Thus, the sachets both reduce turbidity and disinfect the water. Flocculant disinfectants have been distributed in many emergency settings. They require a higher involvement by the user than other chlorine-based PoU, as multiple steps are required, as well as more time and containers, as the water must be stirred and poured into separate containers. They are also usually more expensive than tablet or liquid chlorine products. Taste and odor may be issues, similar to chlorine products (Lantagne and Clasen, 2009).

Filtration

Filters mechanically remove materials and pathogens, including bacteria, protozoa, helminths, and turbidity, and are effective against some viruses. Examples include ceramic, biosand, membrane, and fiber membrane filters. They improve the taste, color, and smell of water and may be produced locally. Many filter systems also provide safe storage for treated water, although they do not provide residual protection. Some disadvantages include the relatively high cost and difficulty in transport and storage. Furthermore, the breakage of filters, as well as the slow flow rate, especially with turbid water, are barriers to consistent use at the household level. Filters often require replacement parts, which must be accessible to affected populations and integrated into the deployment plan. Filter performance decreases if not properly cleaned and maintained, and high turbidity and high levels of iron may require frequent cleaning as fouling of the filters may occur. The effectiveness of ceramic filters also depends on the production quality, which can vary from factory to factory (Lantagne and Clasen, 2009). Filters may be well suited to protracted emergencies where treatment is focused on the household level, households receive ongoing support in appropriate use, and chlorine-based products are less accepted by the population or not as effective due to high turbidity.

Solar Disinfection

Solar disinfection, also referred to as SODIS, may be effective against viruses, bacteria, and protozoa and is a low-cost, easy to use method of PoU treatment. Users fill clean, clear polyethylene terephthalate (PET) plastic or glass bottles with low-turbidity water, shake to oxygenate, and place outdoors for six hours (if sunny) or two days (if cloudy). The user must plan ahead to prepare and fill bottles to place in the sun hours or days before consumption. If households do not clean their bottles, there can be microbial growth (Islam et al., 2015). Plastic bottles can also become less transparent over time, reducing effectiveness. Additional barriers to use include time to treat water if sunlight is limited, decreased efficiency for turbid water, and the volume limited to the size and number of bottles available. SODIS is not commonly promoted during the acute phase of emergencies due to these complexities.

Water Quality

Monitoring the microbiological water quality is of utmost importance in emergency settings in order to prevent the transmission of waterborne diseases, including those of outbreak potential. Water provided in humanitarian emergencies should be free from disease-causing organisms and meet WHO drinking water standards (WHO, 2011). Sanitary surveys, which should be conducted for all water sources, are used to identify likely sources of contamination and provide recommendations on how to remove these potential contaminants. It is usually not possible to routinely test water directly for pathogenic organisms. Therefore, indicators are used, such as fecal coliforms (thermotolerant coliforms) or *E. coli*. These organisms are found in the gut of warm-blooded animals and their presence in water samples indicates potential fecal contamination. Portable water testing kits are available to analyze water samples for these indicators. Typically, a 100 mL sample of water is tested. According to WHO and Sphere standards, no fecal coliforms or *E. coli* should be detected in a 100 mL sample of drinking water (WHO 2011, Sphere Project, 2011).

If the water is chlorinated, it is often not necessary to conduct microbiological tests if the presence of residual chlorine is confirmed. As most drinking water supplied to emergency affected population is chlorinated, tests for free chlorine residual are commonly used to monitor the quality of water. As the effectiveness of chlorine is affected both by the pH and turbidity of the water, these two parameters are also included. Each of these tests can be conducted in the field with portable field kits. If chlorinated, water supplies should have a free chlorine residual of at least 0.5 mg/L at the point of collection. Table 11.5 summarizes the standard water quality levels and rationale for the basic parameters.

Total dissolved solids (TDS) may also be tested early in an emergency, as high salinity levels may discourage use of particular water sources.

Chemical parameters, such as arsenic, fluoride, iron, manganese, nitrate, nitrite, aluminum, or zinc, are usually only tested after the initial phase of an emergency or when new water sources such as drilled wells are brought online. Water in urban settings may have specific chemical contaminants that require additional treatment. However, these chemical properties may be of lower concern for short-term exposure than microbiological indicators of fecal contamination that pose acute health risks.

Filtration with different media types, activated carbon, and different coagulants may remove certain chemical contaminants (Ali and Kadir, 2016). Advanced technologies such as reverse osmosis or nanomembrane filtration may be required to address certain chemical parameters.

Sanitation

Providing adequate sanitation infrastructure and accompanying behavior change interventions during a humanitarian emergency are paramount to reducing the incidence of fecal-oral disease and transmission and to ensuring a safe environment. Particular attention should be paid to the containment of human excreta; though, the management of wastewater and solid waste pose challenges as well.

Table 11.5 Basic water quality standards in emergencies

Test	Standard	Justification
Free chlorine residual (FCR)	0.5 mg/L in general; >1.0 mg/L during outbreaks at the point of collection (Sphere, 2011)	Chlorine is the most commonly used disinfectant in emergencies. FCR should be tested at the point of collection and at the household level. UNHCR recommends that WASH actors monitor free chlorine residuals on a daily basis for the first eight weeks before moving to the monthly monitoring schedule suggested by WHO (1997).
Fecal coliform or E. coli	0 per 100 ml (Sphere, 2011)	Fecal coliforms and *E. coli* are an indicator of the level of human and/or animal waste contamination in water and the potential presence of harmful pathogens.
Turbidity	<5 NTU	Ideally, the turbidity should be <5 NTUs. If turbidity >20 NTUs, then some form of pretreatment should be carried out. WHO recommends dosing clear water (<10 NTU) with chlorine at about 2 mg/L and dosing turbid water (>10 NTU) at 4 mg/L due to higher chlorine demand (WHO, 2011).
pH	Between pH 6.5 to 8.5	Chlorination is less effective when the pH is >8. Contact time or initial dose may need to be increased based on pH level (WHO, 2011).

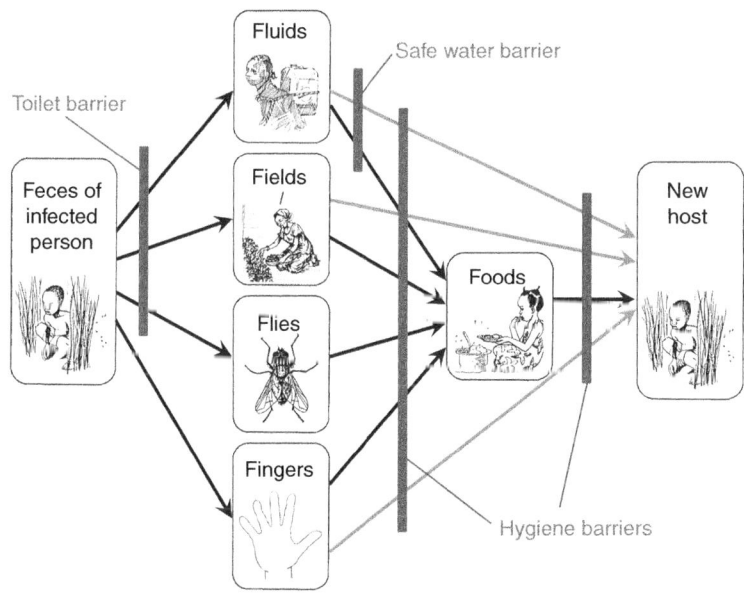

Figure 11.1 F-diagram of key fecal-oral transmission routes and protective barriers

Human excreta, which includes both urine and feces, can transmit many infectious diseases; however, in general, feces are more dangerous than urine and thus a higher priority for containment. Inadequate access to sanitation may lead directly to contamination of drinking water supplies and food as well as increased person-to-person transmission. Figure 11.1 illustrates the key fecal-oral transmission routes, often referred to as an *F-diagram*. The F-diagram is also shown in Chapter 22.

A simple sanitation program can be built upon as the emergency develops, but it is important that the population is involved so that culturally appropriate measures can be properly implemented. Shared or household latrines may take more time than communal latrines to install because the construction of latrines requires substantial materials and tools. These materials may need to be supplied from outside the affected area and require time and resources to transport on-site. Once on-site, latrine pits will need to be dug, covered with slabs and superstructures assembled.

The Sphere standards specify 50 persons per latrine during the acute phase and 20 persons per latrine, once the situation has stabilized. To put this into perspective, a camp of ten thousand persons would require two hundred latrines to meet the emergency standard and five hundred latrines to reach the standard for the postemergency phase (Sphere Project, 2011). Latrines should be a minimum of 30 meters from any water source to reduce the potential for contamination. In addition, to prevent contamination of groundwater, the bottom of the latrine pit should be at least 1.5 meters above the water table (Sphere Project, 2011). Latrines are also discussed in Chapter 22.

The acceptability of sanitation facilities is a major consideration in any emergency. Excreta disposal facilities must be culturally appropriate and acceptable to the affected population, otherwise use may be low and facilities may become grossly contaminated. This includes the design of the latrines or toilets themselves, as well as other considerations such as location and distance from users, lighting, and separation of male and female facilities. During the initial assessment, data should be collected to inform sanitation decisions, such as population demographics, the environment of the site, and cultural practices, including anal cleansing and menstrual hygiene management habits. Factors and key issues that should inform these decisions are shown in Table 11.6.

Sanitation During the Acute Phase

In the acute phase of an emergency, one of the first priorities is to reduce open defecation. If that is not possible, care should be taken to prevent fecal contamination of drinking water sources and food supplies. Interventions can include creating barriers around water storage and treatment facilities, crop fields, and food storage areas and directing people to defecate in well-defined spaces, such as in defecation fields.

Defecation Fields

At the onset of an acute emergency, demarcated open areas or fields surrounded by screening may be set up for open defecation. The purpose of a defecation field is to contain feces to a particular area, to reduce the risk of exposure to the general population, and to reduce the risk of contaminating water supplies.

Full-time supervision of the fields by paid attendants should be organized. Attendants guide individuals to the correct areas and to handwashing facilities. Internal partitions can be made to segregate areas for men and women and to provide privacy (MSF, 2010). Water and buckets/pots for anal cleansing and receptacles for any materials used may be needed. Defecation fields are rapid to implement and can minimize indiscriminate open defecation; however, there is lack of privacy for users, a large space requirement, and a potential for cross-contamination of users (Harvey, 2007). This is a temporary solution until safer sanitation options can be installed (MSF, 2010).

Communal Latrines

Communal latrines are often a temporary solution to allow time for either shared or household facilities to be built. They typically consist of blocks of latrines placed over larger pits and are shared by a large number of households. Sanitation committees or paid attendants may be required and provided supplies to organize regular cleaning of latrines. If latrines are not well maintained and clean, people may seek alternatives or chose open defecation over using the latrines.

Shared or Household Latrines

As soon as feasible, shared or household latrines should be built. Shared latrines are usually for a maximum of four households, or 20 persons, per latrine. A smaller number of users and increased ownership may present fewer problems in terms of maintenance and hygiene. The proximity to the household also promotes use.

Evidence from a systematic review suggests that households with shared sanitation facilities (used by two or more families) compared with individual household latrines are at increased risk of adverse health outcomes, including diarrheal diseases. There are methodological limitations to the evidence base and these results are likely to vary depending on number of users, quality of the latrine construction, and maintenance and management of the latrines (Heijnen et al. 2014).

In another study, Demographics and Health survey data from 51 countries was used to compare children from households with individual latrines and those with shared latrine facilities. In most countries, the prevalence of diarrhea was higher among households sharing a toilet facility. However, the effect varied across countries, suggesting that cultural, economic and social context are important factors (Fuller et al., 2014).

For health, operations and maintenance reasons, the ideal is to have household latrines. However, it may not always be possible because of population density, lack of space, or resources. In that case, shared or communal latrines may be implemented accompanied with adequate hygiene promotion.

Sanitation During Protracted Emergencies

In chronic emergencies or stabilized situations, community participation is imperative for culturally appropriate and effective management of excreta disposal. An in-depth consultation with intended users is critical. Table 11.6 includes factors and issues that should inform decisions before implementing a safe excreta disposal strategy in middle and long-term emergencies (Adapted from MSF 2010). Users should be included as much as possible in the choice, maintenance, and implementation of the excreta disposal facilities. Information on whether or not users can provide their own anal cleansing material should be gathered, and if not, agencies may need to supply these materials.

Pit Latrine

Pit latrines are commonly used in emergencies. They have a dug or raised pit, slab to cover the top of the pit, and a latrine superstructure for privacy. There are several types of pit latrines including simple pit latrines, ventilated-improved pit (VIP) latrines, and raised-pit latrines.

Pour-Flush latrines

Pour-flush latrines may be used in settings where pour-flush latrines are the norm and the quantity of

Table 11.6 Factors and issues to inform sanitation decisions (Adapted from MSF 2010)

Factor	Key Issue(s)

Demographics and specific needs	• Number of users by gender and age
	• Number of users with specific needs
	  • Disabled and physically impaired people and PLHIV, and the elderly may need specifically adapted excreta disposal sites in terms of distance, space, equipment (handrails)
	  • Children should have latrines suited to their size
	  • Women require accommodations during pregnancy, for menstruation, and personal safety

Social, cultural, and religious	• Separation of facilities by gender • Need for privacy • Preferred position for toilet (sitting or squatting) • Method of anal cleansing (wipers or washers), material used and disposal method • Menstruation (material used, its disposal, single-use or reusable) • Orientation of latrine • Taboo practices or locations (i.e., defecating on top of others' excreta) • Acceptability of emptying latrine
Physical environment/ site	• Available space for latrine – communal, shared, or family type • Soil type, available depth and ease to excavate, infiltration rate, stability, soil bearing capacity (i.e., able to support heavy superstructure) • Water resources, including proximity to groundwater and other resources • Sufficient quantity of water for anal cleansing and pour-flush latrines • Risk of flooding • Preexisting sanitation infrastructure (e.g., sewage conveyance and treatment)
Climate	• Precipitation patterns (i.e., rainy season) • Temperature (for vector control) • Main wind direction (odor)
Available resources	• Financial (material and labor costs) • Materials and tools (what is locally available) • Human capital (skills and experience to construct facilities)

water available is adequate. Following defecation, the user pours a small amount of water to flush excreta into the tank. They often require a septic tank, drainage pit, or sewage collection system (MSF, 2010). They work well for communities that use water for anal cleansing.

Septic Tanks

Where pour-flush latrines or flush toilets are used, below-ground septic systems or holding tanks may be constructed to collect and/or treat wastewater. In the case of septic systems, feces will decompose anaerobically within the septic tank and the liquids are directed from the tank for infiltration into the ground via a septic drain field or leach field. Where space is constrained or the water table is high, tanks may be enclosed and function simply as holding tanks which require periodic emptying and a safe disposal site for the sludge that is removed.

Additional Considerations

Children's Excreta

A common belief in some settings is that children's feces are not harmful and thus less attention will be paid to its safe disposal. This can contribute to environmental contamination and spread of disease. Therefore, hygiene and sanitation campaigns should include safe disposal of children's feces, handwashing after changing a child's diaper or emptying a child's potty, and safe laundering practices. Distributions to households with children should include culturally appropriate child feces management supplies, such as potties, diapers, or small shovels to scoop up feces.

Women and Sanitation

Special considerations should be made for women around menstrual hygiene, sanitation, privacy, and safety. It may be important to include washing basins and drying lines within female sanitary areas to wash reusable sanitary towels. A waste receptacle in or near the sanitary facilities may be included for the disposal of single-use sanitary towels. Disposing of menstrual hygiene materials into the latrine should be actively discouraged as this will compromise latrine effectiveness and poses significant challenges if desludging is required. See "A toolkit for integrating menstrual hygiene management (MHM) into humanitarian responses" for more details Sommer et al., 2017).

Providing locks on the inside of the latrines, adequate lighting in and around latrines, and reducing the distance to latrines may improve privacy and reduce the risk of sexual violence (House et al., 2012).

Sanitation and Disabilities

People living with disabilities can face social and physical barriers to sanitation. Barriers depend on the cultural and geographical context, as well as on the disability (Groce et al., 2011). Latrines are often too small to enter with wheelchairs or crutches. Steps or steep ramps up to latrines and slippery floors are also barriers. Low-cost modifications to latrine design are possible, such as constructing latrines with handrests and seats, using less slippery surfaces for floors and building ramps up to the latrines (MSF, 2010). At least 10 percent of sanitation facilities in emergencies should be accessible to people with disabilities (Handicap International, 2009).

Challenging Environments

In some emergency settings, installation of traditional below-ground sanitation options may be difficult. This may include difficult environments with flooding, high water table, sandy soils or rocky areas. In these areas, digging pit latrines may be expensive, time- and labor consuming, or impossible in some cases. Dense urban environments also present sanitation challenges in terms of insufficient space, land ownership issues, or environmental restrictions. Sanitation systems in the urban context often need frequent emptying and cleaning (desludging), which requires considerable resources (e.g., logistical, financial) and safe disposal sites.

In these settings, the use of alternative sanitation options may be preferred. Some of these technologies include chemical toilets or disposable biodegradable bags (i.e., Peepoo™ bags (Peepoople, Stockholm, Sweden)) in the acute phase, as well as ecological sanitation options such as above-ground dry or composting toilets in the stabilized phase of the emergency. User education and a well-managed sanitation chain for waste disposal and treatment is needed for these technologies. Collection of waste may require desludging equipment as well as a final disposal site.

Chemical Toilets

Chemical toilets are portable, premade, above-ground sanitation units that consist of a sit-down toilet or a squatting pan, depending on local cultural practices. Chemical toilets have been used as temporary solutions where pit latrines or septic tanks are unsuitable or unacceptable, for example in areas with heavy flooding or in densely populated urban areas. These units are placed above a water-tight excreta-holding tank, which contains a chemical solution to aid in digestion of excreta and to reduce odor. Desludging equipment and personnel are needed to empty and take away for disposal. Additionally, a safe disposal site for waste is required. As an example, chemical toilets were utilized in Haiti after the 2010 earthquake. However, their use was limited in time due to high maintenance costs and limited storage capacity (Oxfam, 2011).

Disposable Biodegradable Bags

Biodegradable bags can be used at the household level for defecation. Peepoo™ (Peepoople, Stockholm, Sweden) bags are one type which have been piloted in emergency settings. They contain urea, which inactivates fecal pathogens. Safe collection methods and disposal or composting sites for used bags should be identified in advance. The use of Peepoo™ bags has been piloted in sudden onset emergencies in Haiti (Patel et al., 2011), Pakistan, Philippines, as well as in refugee camp settings in Kenya, Syria, and South Sudan (Peepoople, 2016).

Urine Diversion Dry (or Dehydration) Toilets

Urine-diversion dry toilets (UDDTs) are a type of ecological sanitation designed for dry excreta management. The technology is comprised of two primary design components: source separation of urine and feces via the user interface (squatting slab or seat) and ventilated, above-ground vault(s) or containers for feces storage. One advantage of separating urine from feces is to reduce potential odors as well as reducing volume. During a prolonged storage period, the solid fecal waste becomes inert, primarily via desiccation. Additives, such as ash, are often added to the vault on an ongoing basis during use to enhance the physical-chemical inactivation process as well as reduce odors. Urine can either be collected for fertilizer or drained into a soak pit. Treated solid waste can be landfilled or potentially reused for agriculture, depending on levels of pathogen inactivation per WHO reuse guidelines (WHO, 2006). The treated waste may also be used as a fuel source. During a recent project in Kakuma Refugee Camp, fecal waste was collected in UDDTs and then sanitized in solar concentrators. Waste was then compressed into briquettes to use for cooking. Briquettes were reported to burn longer than wood and charcoal and had high user satisfaction (Foote et al., 2016).

Composting Toilets

An alternative type of Eco-San is the composting toilet, which is designed to turn excreta into compost. These toilets can be urine diverting or not. Similar to UDDTs, there are single- and double-vault composting toilets. Pathogens are subject to biological decomposition under aerobic conditions, either by naturally-occurring microorganisms or introduced earthworms (referred to as vermi-composting) The addition of soil, leaves, or other organic matter can help the composting process by ensuring appropriate nutrient ratios for the biological activity (Harvey 2007). It is also important to ensure appropriate temperature, moisture, and aeration levels. Waste can either be composted in the vault or pit directly, or be moved off-site to compost in piles. An example of an in-pit composting toilet is the fossa alterna, which has two alternating permanent pits. When the first pit is full, the toilet superstructure and slab is moved on to the second pit. Top soil is placed over the contents of the first pit which is then left to compost. The second pit is used while the contents of the first pit are composting. The use of urine-diversion composting toilets with a centralized (i.e., off-site facility requiring transport of waste) composting process has been piloted recently in an urban emergency setting in Haiti. An evaluation conducted in Port-au-Prince showed an inactivation of *E. coli* and *Ascaris* within 16 weeks. Warm temperatures throughout the composting beds led to faster inactivation than in previous studies (Berendes et al., 2015).

Disposal

Many of the sanitation options described above require emptying, and therefore an additional final disposal site. Options for transport and disposal of waste should be investigated at the onset of an emergency before a large amount of material needs to be disposed. If existing disposal facilities are available, the feasibility of adding additional material should be assessed. If there are no disposal sites available within feasible transport distances, one may need to be developed. This should be done in conjunction with a hydrogeologist and/or soils expert to ensure that contamination of groundwater or the environment do not occur. Proper operating practices, such as covering material with soil, will also need to be implemented.

Solid Waste Control

Solid waste during an emergency includes organic waste such as food scraps, market and household refuse, and sweepings, and may also include packing material and plastic bags and bottles. Solid waste can attract disease vectors if not properly managed. Urban areas with high population density have particular issues with solid waste accumulation. Efforts should include organizing waste collection by teams, equipping teams with trucks for removal, and creating a landfill system with pits or trenches where waste is safely disposed of and covered daily with soil. Refer to the WASH in healthcare facilities section for more information on medical waste management. Solid waste indicators from Sphere include (Sphere Project 2011):

- All households have access to garbage receptacles that are emptied twice per week at minimum. These receptacles should be no more than 100 meters from a communal refuse pit.
- All waste of those living in settlements is removed from the living environments at least twice a week.
- At least one 100-liter refuse receptacle is available per ten households, where domestic refuse is not burned.
- There is timely and controlled safe disposal of solid waste from the environment.

Hygiene

Social and behavior change interventions that target key hygiene practices are crucial in humanitarian emergencies to reduce disease transmission. They complement water and sanitation interventions and are essential to ensure that the benefits of improved facilities are realized by the population. For example, if household latrines are constructed, but not hygienically maintained or systematically used, their benefits for diarrheal reduction will be limited, and they may become sources of contamination close to households. If water is treated at the source but then not safely transported or stored at the household level, the impact of centralized water treatment on diarrheal disease reduction will also be limited.

Hygiene promotion includes providing households with the means to wash their hands, bathe, store water safely in the home, dispose of child and adult feces hygienically, and protect food from contamination. Furthermore, it includes providing the knowledge, skills, and motivation to take appropriate steps to reduce the risk of becoming infected. For example, the provision of chlorinated water at tap stands might seem sufficient to elicit behavior change among displaced populations; however, there may be other factors that affect users' decisions to use treated water, including the lack of understanding of the role of treated water in disease prevention, distance to water source, or the taste of chlorinated water.

The Sphere Project defines hygiene promotion as a "planned, systematic approach to enable people to take action to prevent and/or mitigate water, sanitation, and hygiene-related diseases" (Sphere Project, 2011). Traditional hygiene approaches have included health messaging and knowledge-based approaches. However, studies show that health knowledge does not necessarily result in improved hygiene practices; there is a shift toward including psychosocial factors in hygiene interventions. This is because health-related motivations may not be the key reason that explains why people practice good hygiene. Emotional drivers, such as feelings of disgust towards feces, and comfort, nurturing, and social/cultural norms may have a greater influence on hygiene practices (Curtis et al., 2009). Factors important to successful hygiene promotion are shown in Figure 11.2.

Behavior change may occur more rapidly in emergency settings, due to an increased perception of susceptibility or risk, severity of the situation, or because of environmental changes that present opportunities for new behaviors. Thus, emergencies may also offer a public health opportunity to encourage improved hygiene practices that could continue after the emergency. There is considerable evidence in nonemergency settings that health behaviors can be effectively modified through behavior change interventions. Behavior change programming that accompanies hardware interventions can inform, motivate, and equip affected communities with skills to reduce the risk of disease transmission.

However, evidence from nonemergency settings suggests that the sustainability of behavior change in

- Ensure a bottom-up, participatory approach
- Provide hygiene and behavior change technical support
- Focus the intervention to target the behavioral determinants (motivators and barriers) rather than on the health benefits of the behavior
- Continue regular monitoring and long term follow-up
- Ensure regular and frequent contact with a health promoter
- Mix interpersonal and mass media communication channels
- Monitor and measure actual behavior change
- Accompany all hardware interventions or distributions with hygiene information and communications on how to use the hardware and to motivate use

Figure 11.2 Factors important to successful hygiene promotion

Adapted from Hulland et al. 2015 and UNICEF 2009

response to interventions is limited, with effects diminishing over time (Kwasnicka et al., 2016).

Hygiene promotion activities will likely not be effective if implemented without repetitive understanding the cultural background of the beneficiaries. The location (urban, peri-urban, and rural), the type (political, economic, or environmental), and duration of the emergency, and the demographics of the affected population may influence the hygiene priorities. Formative research can help shape programming.

Pretesting hygiene messages, visual aids, and checking for translation accuracy before mass diffusion may help ensure that messages serve their intended purpose. Once pretested and refined, diffusing messages through trusted channels identified during the assessment may improve their credibility and impact on the population (see Social and Behavior Change Communication for Emergency Preparedness Implementation Kit, http://sbccimplementationkits.org/sbcc-in-emergencies/).

Many settings experience recurring emergencies. Development partners may be present and might have preemergency data on hygiene practices, knowledge, and attitudes. Some information could be transferable to the new emergency. This prevents the duplication and misdirection of efforts and resources and is likely to lead to more effective programming. Hygiene promotion is also discussed in Chapter 22.

Key Hygiene Items

An important part of hygiene intervention in the acute phase of an emergency is the availability of key hygiene items that may be included as part of a hygiene kit or provided separately as part of nonfood item (NFI) distributions. Soap for handwashing is essential and needs to be supplied at regular intervals if households are unable to access it themselves. Men, women, boys, girls, and individuals living with disabilities should be consulted regarding their needs for hygiene materials. Table 11.7 lists the basic minimum hygiene kit, usually containing water storage vessels, soap for handwashing and laundry, and menstrual hygiene materials (Sphere Project, 2011).

Additional hygiene kit items may be distributed depending on availability and circumstances. For example, this could include chlorine tablets or flocculant-disinfectant sachets where household water treatment is promoted. Hygiene kits are also discussed in Chapter 22.

Other items may include toothpaste, toothbrush, shampoo, lotion, disposable razor, underwear, hairbrush/comb, diapers/potties, nail clippers, and Oral Rehydration Solution (ORS) packets (Sphere Project 2011). Programming will need to anticipate when and how consumables in hygiene kits will be replaced. Postdistribution monitoring should also be conducted on use and satisfaction with the distributed kits.

Cash transfers or voucher programs may be alternatives to distributing hygiene kits. This is an option where products are available in suitable quality and quantity on the local market. This may include urban areas or where markets are functioning. This approach can have a multiplier effect on the local economy and may offer greater dignity and flexibility to the affected population, allowing them to select their preferred hygiene products based on their needs. Recent examples in cash/voucher programming for WASH in emergencies include Haiti, Palestine, Jordan, Ethiopia, Lebanon, the Philippines, Somalia, Iraq,

Table 11.7 Basic hygiene kit (Sphere Project 2011)

Item	Description
10–20 liters capacity water containers	Two per household (one for transport and one for water storage)
250 g bathing soap	Per person per month
200 g laundry soap	Per person per month
Acceptable material for menstrual hygiene	For all women of menstruating age; will depend on type of material used, disposable or reusable

Benin, Bangladesh, and Cambodia. In some contexts, cash or voucher programming covered either water, sanitation or hygiene, while in other contexts, programming provided one complete WASH package altogether (Juillard and Islam Opu, 2015).

Handwashing Hardware

Handwashing with soap and water is a key public health intervention and hygiene activity. Proper and consistent handwashing can have a large impact on reducing the risk of fecal-oral diseases. Systematic reviews have consistently reported the benefits of hygiene and handwashing. Studies from nonemergency settings in low- or middle-income countries reported that community handwashing promotion interventions were associated with a reduction in diarrheal episodes by 17%–38% (Ejemot-Nwadiaro, et al. 2015). Hand hygiene may also reduce respiratory infections by 5% to 32% (Aiello et al., 2008).

Handwashing promotion includes both the introduction of hardware and the use of soap, as well as behavior-change interventions, which may include instructions in proper handwashing techniques plus messaging to address psychosocial drivers and barriers to handwashing. The distribution of soap to affected households may be sufficient to elicit handwashing at key times. However, soap may be valued for other purposes such as doing laundry. Thus, any soap distribution will need to include soap for personal use and laundry use and will likely need to be accompanied with behavior change activities to target this core behavior.

In order to make handwashing easier and more attractive, a number of handwashing station models have been deployed to the field. These include handwashing bags, tippy taps, and buckets with lids and taps (e.g., the Oxfam bucket and Handy Wash). Ease of transport, durability, beneficiary acceptability, and minimum setup required are important considerations for handwashing stations in emergency situations. Handwashing stations are needed adjacent to latrines for handwashing after defecation; at the household level for handwashing before eating and preparing food; and during childcare (feeding children and managing child feces).

Handwashing Bags

Handwashing bags are lightweight, easily portable, and suitable for household use. A recent pilot of the handwashing bag among Sudanese refugees in Ethiopia reported high acceptability. However, a number of drawbacks were also noted as some participants complained that it was difficult to hang the bag, the bag was too small or defective, soap was not always available, and the bag was not adequately promoted (Husain et al., 2015).

Tippy Tap

Tippy taps can be made using old jerry cans or plastic bottles. A hole is made in the container near the cap to hang it. A foot pedal is installed to release water without touching the tap. Experience from the field has shown that the hands-free aspect of this technology is appealing to households (Ramos et al., 2016).

Buckets with Lid and Tap

Simple plastic buckets with lids and taps allow users to easily wash hands. The Oxfam buckets are a field ready example. These buckets are made of UV resistant plastic and have a built-in cap allowing water to be restocked without taking off the lid. The bucket is also designed to be easily cleaned and stackable for distributions. Another technology available is the handy wash device. This compact tap can be fastened to any locally available container. Because it automatically stops water from flowing once the push control is released, water loss is minimized. The Handy Wash has been piloted in Liberia, Kenya, and South Sudan.

Handwashing Products

In some cases, bar soap may not be available in sufficient quantity or quality needed for the emergency. Some alternatives to bar soap include alcohol-based hand rub, ash, chlorine solution, and soapy water.

Alcohol-based Hand Rub

Alcohol-based hand rub may be an option where access to water is very limited or for use in institutional settings, such as healthcare facilities. In Tanzania, testing among mothers showed that alcohol-based rub was as effective against microbes as handwashing with soap (Pickering et al., 2010). To date, the use of alcohol-based hand rub is not common in the emergency context, given the cost, as well as the potential logistical challenges of importation. Of note, the World Health Organization (WHO) has produced guidelines for local manufacturing of alcohol-based hand rubs, particularly for health care facilities, which may increase the feasibility of this soap alternative in some emergency contexts in the future.

Ash

In some settings, if soap is not available, ash can be promoted for handwashing as an alternative. Studies in Bangladesh and India have demonstrated that the abrasive properties of ash were effective in removing fecal coliforms from hands (Nizame et al., 2015). However, there is limited evidence of its effectiveness across pathogens. There may be some resistance among some populations to using ash for handwashing.

Chlorine Solution

In specific cases, for example during outbreaks of highly infectious disease (e.g., Ebola), a dilute chlorine solution (0.05%) may be used for hand hygiene in emergencies. This alternative to soap has been primarily used in healthcare facilities, but during the 2014–15 West Africa Ebola outbreak it was extended to the community level. There has been some concern that the use of a chlorine solution for hand hygiene may cause skin irritation over time. However, there is limited evidence of this to date. A recent study of participants that washed their hands ten times daily with chlorine solutions over a four-week period suggested that chlorine solutions did not compromise skin integrity (Wolfe et al., 2016).

Soapy Water

Soapy water may be a low-cost alternative to bar soap. Powdered soap, such as laundry soap, can be mixed with water to make a soapy water solution. Soapy water ensures that everyone who rinses hands with water is receiving the added benefit of contact with soap. Soapy water may also be less likely to be stolen than bar soap from handwashing stations, such as at communal latrines in camp settings. Qualitative research has shown soapy water to be acceptable in some contexts due to the ease of use and low cost (Amin et al., 2014). The ratio of powered soap to water may vary. In a field trial among mothers in urban Dhaka, Bangladesh, 30 g of powdered detergent was mixed with 1.5 liters of water. This trial found that soapy water removed fecal coliforms at rates similar to bar soap after washing for 15 seconds (Amin et al. 2014)

In addition to providing handwashing hardware and soap-like products, implementers can strengthen the enabling environment through behavioral interventions to elicit behavior change. One of these interventions is known as nudging. Nudges are simple clues in the environment to trigger behavior change (Dreibelbis et al., 2016). For example, latrines can be connected to handwashing stations via brightly colored pathways or by painting footsteps on the paths from the latrine to the handwashing station that "nudges" the latrine user to wash their hands. Brightly colored handwashing stations with soap strategically placed can also serve as nudges. Although nudges have been shown to be effective in other health domains, their use in handwashing is still being explored with early trials in schools in Bangladesh (Dreibelbis et al. 2016), camps in Democratic Republic of the Congo (DRC), and in interventions to target open defecation (Neal et al., 2016).

Hygiene During Acute Phase

During the acute phase of an emergency, hygiene promotion activities focus on targeting core WASH behaviors that are lifesaving and stop fecal-oral transmission. These will include handwashing with soap and water, safe disposal of adult and child feces, clean (treated) water use and storage, control of flies and vectors, and personal hygiene (including menstrual hygiene management and food hygiene). Behaviors and audiences need to be well defined. For example, handwashing campaigns must target all members of the community, but messaging for menstrual hygiene management will be geared towards women and girls while also sensitizing community management on the need to provide disposal options.

At the onset of an emergency, rapid multisectorial or WASH assessments may be conducted and may include questions to identify current hygiene practices, as well as beliefs, motivators, and barriers to these practices. These rapid assessments can be accompanied by more in-depth methods, such as interviews, discussion groups, community mapping, or environmental walks. There may not be enough time or resources when initially launching emergency operations to use full in-depth qualitative tools. However, over time, additional formative research can be conducted to identify the perceptions, beliefs, barriers, and motivators of the affected population towards these essential hygiene practices. Formative research may ask questions such as:

- What are trusted channels that the population uses to seek information?
- What are the perceived advantages and disadvantages of specific hygiene practices?
- What are the perceived causes of waterborne diseases?
- How do their peers feel about these behaviors and diseases?

This research can be used to develop hygiene materials such as community mobilization sessions, visual aids, theater performances, social media, and mass media messages. Research in humanitarian contexts, such as in refugee camps in South Sudan, has shown that even when knowledge and soap is present, there may be a need for further qualitative research to understand the drivers, motivators, and barriers of handwashing with soap (Phillips et al. 2015). During an emergency, key messages can be misunderstood or distorted. Pretesting hygiene messages, visual aids, and checking for translation accuracy before mass diffusion may help ensure that messages serve their intended purpose. Once pretested and refined, diffusing messages through trusted channels identified during the assessment may improve their credibility and impact on the population (see further reading: Social and Behavior Change Communication for Emergency Preparedness Implementation Kit, http://sbccimplementationkits.org/sbcc-in-emergencies/).

Selecting a limited number of behaviors to target concurrently has been shown to be the most effective in health and behavior change. Complex behaviors may be broken down into simpler and more accessible components targeted at the onset of an emergency, as people rarely go from current practices to ideal behaviors immediately. The ideal behavior can be broken down into components that are considered feasible by the member of the household from his or her perspective. Over time, additional components are targeted to eventually arrive at the ideal behavior. In the example of handwashing, the ideal behavior is washing hands with soap and running water at all critical times (after defecation, before cooking or eating, before feeding a child, and after changing a child's diaper). At the beginning of the hygiene campaign, messaging could target one component of this multifaceted behavior, such as washing hands with soap after defecation. Once the population practices this handwashing behavior, another component could be added, such as handwashing before eating. This continues until all components of the ideal behavior are included.

Hygiene promotion is usually interactive and includes dialogue oriented methods rather than focusing exclusively on the mass dissemination of messages (Sphere Project, 2011). During an acute phase, there will likely be a mix of behavior change approaches. They generally contain a component of community mobilization, mass media, and/or visual aids as described below. Selected approaches should be based on assessments.

Community Mobilization

Community mobilization or interpersonal communication is a major component of hygiene activities and may include multiple methods, such as door-to-door visits and community gatherings facilitated by hygiene promoters or community health workers (CHWs). Sphere standards recommend two hygiene promoters/community mobilizers for every one thousand persons in a camp or similar situation (Sphere Project, 2011). Trained hygiene promoters or mobilizers may already be present in the community and should be identified during the assessment phase. However, during some humanitarian emergencies, stakeholders may request their assistance with a wide range of response activities. Therefore, close consultation with the Ministry of Health as well as with other humanitarian and health actors is imperative to ensure that the community mobilizers or volunteers are not overburdened.

Visual Aids and Print Materials

At the beginning of a response, generic visual aids and simple print materials such as flyers, posters, or billboards may be used to promote key hygiene practices. However, as soon as possible, materials need to be adapted to the local context and to address the key motivators and barriers as identified by the affected population. Local artists can be recruited to tailor scientific material to the local context, beliefs, barriers, and motivators.

Mass Media and Social Media

Mass media channels and social media platforms can be effective tools to rapidly reach a large population. Channels can include radio, television, websites, applications, mobile phone, megaphones, or theater performances. Their utility will depend on the assessment findings, such as the population's trust of mass media communication channels and coverage of these channels. Trusted communications channels should be engaged to relay key behavior change messages whenever possible. Campaigns that involve frequent transmissions on popular channels can help ensure that messages are captured, recalled, and serve as cues to action (Naugle and Hornik, 2014).

Hygiene During Protracted Emergencies

As with the acute phase, hygiene activities will likely continue to target key behaviors during protracted emergencies. However, these behaviors may be targeted by additional approaches. Commonly used hygiene promotion approaches, in protracted emergencies, include Community Lead Total Sanitation (CLTS), Participatory Hygiene and Sanitation Transformation (PHAST), peer education groups such as child-based approaches, mother leader groups, community health clubs, and social marketing. There may also be a mass media component. With the exception of mass media, these approaches will likely be used after the acute phase as they usually require trained facilitators, time, resources and a stable population. However, if the affected population had been previously trained in one of these methods, they may be implemented sooner in the emergency. To date, there is limited rigorous evidence on the effectiveness of these approaches in emergencies and which factors contribute to their effectiveness (Taylor et al., 2015). Successful interventions may have some key factors in common, including community participation, formative research based on behavior change theories or models, and the integration of hardware and software components.

WASH in Healthcare Facilities

WASH in healthcare facilities is essential to providing quality healthcare and basic infection prevention and control (IPC). Nevertheless, in a 2015 review of 54 low- and middle-income countries, coverage of basic WASH services in healthcare facilities was found to be very low, which creates health risks to both patients and staff alike (WHO/UNICEF, 2015). Of the approximately 66 thousand facilities assessed in the review, 38 percent lacked access to basic WASH services. In humanitarian emergencies, adequate WASH services in healthcare facilities is even more imperative given the potential for sudden overcrowding by emergency-affected persons suffering from injury (e.g. conflict-related) and/or illness (e.g. infectious disease outbreak). In the absence of basic WASH services to enable IPC practices, healthcare facilities can become epicenters of disease transmission during public health emergencies. In the recent Ebola epidemic in West Africa, healthcare workers were considerably more likely to become infected than the general population (WHO, 2015).

The World Health Organization (WHO) has provided key domains and minimum standards for WASH services in healthcare facilities in low- and middle-income settings (WHO 2008). Guidance specific to emergency situations has been adapted from the 2008 Essential Environmental Health Standards in Health Care (WHO, 2008).

Water Quality, Quantity, and Access

Adequate quantities of water from improved sources should be available at health facilities, either on the facility grounds or within 500 m, for essential IPC activities, including handwashing, environmental cleaning, laundry and personal hygiene, in addition to water for drinking, cooking, and specific medical activities. If water has to be hauled to health facilities, extra attention is needed to ensure adequate quantities of water are available. Water for consumption

Table 11.8 Water requirements for health care facilities (WHO, 2008)

Staff	5 liters/person/day
Outpatients	5 liters/consultation
Inpatients	40 – 60 liters/patient/day
	15 liters/carer/day
Operating theater or maternity unit	100 liters/intervention
Dry or supplementary feeding center	0.5–5 liters/consultation (depending on waiting time)
Wet supplementary feeding center	15 liters/consultation
Inpatient therapeutic feeding center	30 liters/patient/day
	15 liters/carer/day
Cholera treatment center	60 liters/patient/day
	15 liters/carer/day
Severe acute respiratory diseases isolation ward	100 liters/patient/day
	15 liters/carer/day
Viral hemorrhagic fever isolation ward	300–400 liters/patient/day
	15 liters/carer/day

Carer refer to families, friends or volunteers who care for a patient at the health care facility. They provide basic non-professional care and they may cook, clean and care for patients in the health care setting.

should be treated to national microbiological standards by approved treatment processes, such as filtration and/or disinfection. In some cases, there may be specific water quality standards required for certain medical procedures such as hemodialysis. In emergencies, the most commonly used disinfectant is chlorine, which is highly effective at inactivating and destroying disease-causing microorganisms, if dosed appropriately. Monitoring free chlorine residual is an affordable test that can be used to ensure that water has been adequately disinfected with chlorine. In general, drinking water should have a free chlorine residual of at least 0.5 mg/L at the point of collection. During waterborne disease outbreaks, the minimum level is increased to 1.0 mg/L at the tap (WHO 1993). Minimum water quantities for specific services is summarized in Table 11.8. During emergencies and as a general preparedness measure, it is recommended to have on-site water storage capacity for two days of services. This allows a buffer in the event of damage to water supply infrastructure or power outages impacting the delivery of water to the facility.

Handwashing

In healthcare facilities in emergencies, there should be functional handwashing stations at all locations where healthcare is provided, such as delivery rooms and isolation wards, and in service areas, such as toilets and waste zones. Functional handwashing stations include water, soap, and safe wash water disposal to prevent environmental contamination. In an emergency setting, this may be as simple as a jug of water, soap, and a basin. When hands are not visibly soiled, the use of an alcohol-based hand rub solution for clinical handwashing is also recommended. In the case of infectious disease outbreaks, such as cholera or viral hemorrhagic fever, hand hygiene is extremely important. The use of 0.05 percent chlorine solutions for handwashing is also used as an alternative during infectious disease outbreaks because it is rapidly scalable and inexpensive (UNICEF, 2013).

Excreta and Wastewater Disposal

There should be functional, safe, accessible, and appropriate forms of improved sanitation facilities available for patients, staff, and caregivers. This can be as basic as improved pit latrines with adequate privacy. If possible, facilities should be separated by gender and by patient and staff. It is highly recommended to have separate toilets for patients during outbreaks of diarrheal disease, such as cholera, or highly infectious diseases such as viral hemorrhagic fever. Safe excreta disposal, which does not contaminate the healthcare setting or surrounding environment, is critical during emergencies, especially in the case of diarrheal disease outbreaks. Traditionally, super chlorination has been used for on-site treatment of wastewater generated during infectious disease outbreaks, but the effectiveness of this procedure for disinfecting wastewater is not proven. However, novel on-site treatment protocols for wastewater in infectious disease outbreaks are currently in development and may provide more effective options in the future (Sozzi et al., 2015).

Wastewater also includes that from handwashing, personal hygiene (bathing) facilities, cleaning, and laundry activities. It is important that this water is disposed of rapidly and safely on the healthcare facility grounds to prevent this contaminated water from impacting the surrounding community. This is especially important during outbreaks of highly infectious diseases. During an emergency, this can be as simple as installing soak-away pits with grease traps.

Healthcare Waste Management

It is important to ensure that solid waste from healthcare facilities is segregated at the point of generation to separate and isolate infectious materials (such as sharps and materials contaminated with bodily fluids). Infectious waste should be safely collected, transported, and ideally treated on-site before disposal. Disposal sites should be designed to adequately contain waste, whether they are on-site or off-site. Country-specific standards may provide guidance on appropriate treatment or disposal technologies; however, in their absence, WHO has developed guidance to assist with waste management and technology selection (WHO, 2014). Additional major considerations for WASH in healthcare facilities in emergencies include isolation wards, disposal of dead bodies, and vector control.

WASH Monitoring

The routine monitoring of WASH interventions is essential to ensuring that minimum standards are being met and health gains are realized. Monitoring is also useful in identifying gaps in coverage or areas that need strengthening and can document whether progress is being made in terms of access or coverage of WASH services. It can also contribute to accountability towards beneficiaries, improve coordination of the response, allow for readjustment of activities, and help to prioritize WASH resources. However, similar to the collection of surveillance data, monitoring of WASH activities should target essential data that will be used to strengthen WASH programming and not burden staff or the affected population with the collection of unnecessary data.

All monitoring data collected should be harmonized using common methodologies and tools to ensure that information can be compared and used to define priorities. Depending on the circumstances, the WASH Cluster or a WASH sector lead may play this coordination role.

Key WASH Indicators

Key WASH indicators likely to be included in routine monitoring include the quantity of water provided (l/p/d), distance to the water source, the quality of water provided (free chlorine residual testing or microbiological testing of source water), access to latrines (persons per latrine or toilet facility characteristics), availability of water storage vessels, and availability of handwashing stations and soap.

Data Sources and Methods

Monitoring data can come from a variety of sources including regular reporting from implementing agencies, separate monitoring activities, sanitary surveys, observations at key WASH infrastructure, and collection of household level data via surveys. Often several sources are combined or triangulated to provide a more complete picture of access to and use of essential WASH services. For example, reports of new latrines constructed within a camp can be combined with population updates to monitor the number of persons per latrine over time. Direct observations can verify their installation and use and household surveys or focus group discussions can provide evidence on whether they are used and by what members of the family.

Another key example of the variety of data sources required for effective monitoring is measuring access to sufficient quantities of water. The agency responsible for this activity can provide data on the total quantity of water available to the population. This information can then be combined with observations, as well as measurements at water collection points. Measurements may include observing the length of time spent queuing for water at peak collection times or the flow rate at tap stands. However, these figures do not provide any information on whether access to water is equitable, the availability of water throughout the day, or the use of unsafe sources. Household surveys can help to provide this information and to estimate the total water use per person.

In emergencies in which household water treatment products are distributed, household level monitoring is especially important as individual households are responsible for treating their drinking water. Both the availability of water treatment products and the knowledge of how to use them appropriately are essential. Household level monitoring can determine whether the products were actually received, whether they understand how to dose appropriately, whether they have the appropriate water storage vessels, and whether they understand the importance of drinking and cooking with the treated water. Testing for FCR can also be used to ensure that the correct dose has been used.

Other Considerations

Following any distribution of water treatment products, soap, cash transfers/vouchers, or hygiene kits, postdistribution monitoring can be useful to identify any gaps in coverage, establish usage patterns, collect beneficiary opinions, and identify unmet needs. It can also reinforce accountability by checking if the planned distributions have been received by the intended beneficiaries or not. Monitoring visits can also identify protection risk, if people felt safe during and after distributions.

It is important to understand how equitable the distribution of resources is and if particular groups of people or geographic areas are not being reached. Likewise, one may want to know what is happening at the household level – are items included in distributions actually being received? Are they being used? If not, why not? For this type of information, household surveys, such as knowledge, attitudes, and practices surveys (KAP) may be useful. At the time of writing of this chapter, a KAP training guide for WASH emergencies is under development by CDC in collaboration with partners.

Although the ultimate goal of WASH interventions is to reduce WASH-related diseases, it may be difficult to directly monitor the health impact during emergencies due to methodological challenges (UNICEF 2007). Evaluating the health impacts of WASH interventions in any setting is difficult due to potential recall bias of self-reporting of health events, but data collection during emergencies is often more difficult when the primary focus is lifesaving interventions.

Conclusion

Improving access to potable water, sanitation, and hygiene is an essential activity in humanitarian emergencies. The interventions described here are not novel and are based on effective WASH interventions in non-emergency settings. However, due to the risk of disease outbreaks, the implementation of these interventions must be rapid and efficient requiring strong logistic support and good coordination among implementing partners. Without adequate coordination, resources may not be efficiently targeted to those most in need. Additionally, more operational research is needed as the evidence base for the effectiveness of WASH in humanitarian emergencies on health outcomes, including the reduction of diarrheal diseases, is limited at this time (Ramesh, 2015).

Although much attention goes to the installation of hardware and distribution of commodities, the importance of hygiene promotion and social mobilization cannot be underestimated. These software interventions are essential to ensure that affected populations have the knowledge and understanding on how they can reduce their risk of contracting WASH-related diseases.

Notes from the Field

Tanzania (2015)

In August 2015, Tanzania detected a cholera outbreak that began in Dar es Salaam and spread into 22 of 25 mainland regions throughout Tanzania resulting in over twenty-two thousand cases and 350 deaths by the end of 2016 (MoHCDGEC, 2016). Dar es Salaam reported 5,106 cases alone or 22 percent of the mainland total. Morogoro, another heavily affected region, reported 3,385 cases or 14 percent of the mainland total.

At the start of the outbreak, it was estimated that only 10 percent of the residents in Dar es Salaam and 20 percent of residents in Morogoro had in-home running water from the municipal drinking water utility. The remainder of residents, especially those in cholera affected areas, obtained drinking water from a variety of sources, including private water vendors. These vendors stored water in large volume tanks that ranged in size from 1,000 to 15,000 liters and sold water to community members in 20 liter increments. Private water vendors used a variety of sources to fill their tanks, including piped water from the municipal utility, private boreholes, or trucks delivering municipal water.

During a cholera outbreak, access to safe drinking water is critical and chlorine is an effective chemical to disinfect and protect water supplies from recontamination (WHO, 1993). Many challenges were identified that compromised the chlorination levels of the drinking water supply in both Dar es Salaam and Morogoro. First, although water supplied by the utilities was chlorinated, free chlorine residual levels observed throughout the network were inconsistent. At the peak of the outbreak, spot checks from the water systems and vendors detected low or no chlorine residual. Second, vendor tanks that were filled from boreholes were not chlorinated.

In response to these challenges, the Ministry of Health, Community Development, Gender, Elderly and Children (MoHCDGEC) of Tanzania, UNICEF, and the Centers for Disease Control and Prevention (CDC) collaborated to use 8.68 gm sodium dichloroisocyanurate (NaDCC) tablets to treat large volumes of drinking water supplied by water vendors to improve chlorination during this outbreak. A three-month supply of chlorine tablets was distributed to more than 850 water vendors in cholera affected wards of Dar es Salaam and Morogoro. Routine monitoring of vendor tanks was conducted by ward health officers throughout the three-month period. An evaluation of the program conducted after the implementation period found evidence of high acceptability and use of the tablets. Overall, three months after free tablet distribution, the free chlorine residual ≥ 0.1 mg/L was detected in 68.8 percent of all vendor tanks and in 81.7 percent of tanks that were reported to be treated. These results indicate that chlorination targeting bulk water providers, such as water vendors, could be a feasible mechanism to address chlorination gaps at the community-level during emergencies, or as a prevention measure during cholera outbreaks.

Pakistan (2005)

Following the 2005 earthquake in Pakistan, Oxfam GB consulted internally displaced women in tented villages on their menstrual and sanitation needs. Based on these consultations, hygiene units were included in some of the toilet and bathing units for washing and drying menstrual cloths. Women recommended design changes to improve the security, privacy, and comfort of the facilities. For security, having an internal lock and wooden doors instead of plastic sheeting was important. In terms of comfort, some women requested a mirror, piped water into the unit, a seat, and rack to hang their bathing towel. Privacy was essential to ensure that people outside the units or on higher grounds couldn't see into the facility nor see the wastewater leaving from the unit (Nawaz et al. 2010).

Ethiopia (2012)

Oxfam installed double vault UDDTs at a pilot scale in a Somali refugee camp in Dollo Ado, Ethiopia in 2012 due to difficult soil conditions. After demand was generated by the pilot and an assessment of uptake and acceptability, the program has since scaled up considerably with installation of UDDTs designed for use by two families. To date, approximately one thousand UDDTs are in-use, serving roughly 20 percent of the camp population. UDDTs are also being introduced into other refugee camps in Ethiopia.

Haiti (2010)

Following the earthquake and cholera outbreak in Haiti, humanitarian actors used multiple communication channels to promote handwashing. One study examined the effectiveness of eleven of these communication channels. Six channels suggested a positive association with handwashing behavior: hygiene radio spots, radio programs with experts answering listener's questions, material distributions with instructions for use, information from friends or neighbors, theater, and community clubs. Five of the promotional channels suggested a negative association with handwashing. Respondents who experienced a focus group, stickers, posters and paintings, hygiene songs, special hygiene days, and home visits tended to wash their hands less often (Contzen and Mosler, 2013). The study results show that effectiveness of interventions may depend on the context. Real-time monitoring, which is available immediately, can provide decision makers with evidence to modify programming to use the most effective channels identified in specific contexts.

Acknowledgments

The authors would like to thank Melissa Opryszko and Rick Gelting for their review and comments on the chapter.

References

Aiello, A. M., Coulborn, R. M., Perez, V., and Larson, E. L. (2008). Effect of hand hygiene on infectious disease risk in the community setting: A meta-analysis. *American Journal of Public Health*, **98**(8), 1372–1381.

Ali, S. I. and Kadir, K. (2016). *Water treatment*. WASH in emergencies problem exploration report. Humanitarian Innovation Fund (online). Available at: www.elrha.org/wp-content/uploads/2016/01/Water-Treatment-WASH-Problem-Exploration-Report.pdf (Accessed on November 29, 2016).

Amin, N., Pickering, A. J., Ram, P. K., et al. (2014). Microbiological evaluation of the efficacy of soapy water to clean hands: A randomized, non-inferiority field trial. *American Journal of Tropical Medicine and Hygiene*, **91**(2), 415–423.

Berendes, D., Levy, K., Knee, J., Handzel, T., and Hill, V. R. (2015). Ascaris and Escherichia coli inactivation in an ecological sanitation system in Port-au-Prince, Haiti. *PLOS ONE*, 10(5).

Connolly, M. A., Gayer, M., Ryan, M. J., et al. (2004). Communicable diseases in complex emergencies: impact and challenges. *The Lancet*, **364**(9449), 1974–1983.

Contzen, N. and Mosler, H. J. (2013). Impact of different promotional channels on handwashing behaviour in an emergency context: Haiti post-earthquake public health promotions and cholera response. *Journal of Public Health*, **21**(6), 559–573.

Curtis, V. A., Danquah, L. O., and Aunger, R. V. (2009). Planned, motivated and habitual hygiene behaviour: An eleven country review. *Health Education Research*, **24**(4), 655–673.

Davis, J. and Lambert, R. (2002). *Engineering in emergencies*. 1st edition. London: ITDG.

Dreibelbis, R., Kroeger, A., Hossain, K., Venkatesh, M., and Ram, P. (2016). Behavior Change without Behavior Change Communication: Nudging Handwashing among Primary School Students in Bangladesh. *International Journal of Environmental Research and Public Health*, **13**(1), 129.

Ejemot-Nwadiaro R. I., Ehiri, J. E., Arikpo, D., Meremikwu, M. M., and Critchley J. A. (2015) Hand washing promotion for preventing diarrhoea. *Cochrane Database of Systematic Reviews*, 9.

Foote, A., Woods, E., Lokey, H., Hakspiel, D., and Earwaker P. (2016). Lessons learned: Designing and implementing a new approach to sanitation in Kakuma Refugee Camp (online). Available at: https://sanivation.app.box.com/v/LessonsLearnedKakuma (Accessed on November 29, 2016).

Fuller, J. A., Clasen, T., Heijnen, M., and Eisenberg, J. N. (2014). Shared sanitation and the prevalence of diarrhea in young children: Evidence from 51 countries, 2001–2011. *American Journal of Tropical Medicine and Hygiene*, **91**(1), 173–180.

Goma Epidemiology Group. (1995). Public health impact of Rwandan refugee crisis: what happened in Goma, Zaire, in July, 1994? *The Lancet*, **345** (8946), 339–344.

Groce, N., Bailey, N., Lang, R., Trani, J. F., and Kett, M. (2011). Water and sanitation issues for persons with disabilities in low- and middle-income countries: a literature review and discussion of implications for global health and international development. *Journal of Water and Health*, 09.4, 617–627.

Handicap International (2009). Accessibility for all in an emergency context (online). Available at: www2.wpro.who.int/internet/files/eha/toolkit/web/Technical%20References/Disabilities/Accessibility%20for%20All%20in%20Emergency%20Context%202009.pdf (Accessed on March 15, 2017).

Harvey, P. (2007). *Excreta disposal in emergencies*. Leicestershire: WEDC, Loughborough University.

Heijnen, M., Cumming, O., Peletz, R., et al. (2014). Shared sanitation versus individual household latrines: A systematic review of health outcomes. *PLoS ONE*, **9**(4).

House, S., Mahon, T., and Cavill, S. (2012). *Menstrual hygiene matters: A resource for improving menstrual hygiene around the world*. WaterAid (online). Available at: www.wateraid.org/mhm. (Accessed on November 29, 2016).

Hulland, K., Martin, N., Dreibelbis, R., et al. (2015) What factors affect sustained adoption of safe water, hygiene and sanitation technologies? *A systematic review of literature*. EPPI-Centre, Social Science Research Unit, UCL Institute of Education, University College London (online). Available at: http://eppi.ioe.ac.uk/cms/Portals/0/PDF%20reviews%20and%20summaries/WASH%20technologies%202015%20Hulland%20report.pdf?ver=2015-06-10-141853-910 (Accessed on July 7, 2017).

Husain, F., Hardy, C., Zekele, L., et al. (2015). A pilot study of a portable hand washing station for recently displaced refugees during an acute emergency in Benishangul-Gumuz regional state, Ethiopia. *Conflict and Health*, **9** (26).

Islam, M. A., Azad, A. K., Akber, M. A., Rahman, M., and Sadhu, I. (2015). Effectiveness of solar disinfection (SODIS) in rural coastal Bangladesh. *Journal of Water and Health*, 13(4), 1113–1122.

Juillard, H. and Opu, M. I. (2015). *Scoping study of emergency cash transfer programming in the WaSH and shelter sectors*. Cash Learning Partnership (online). Available at: www.cashlearning.org/downloads/scopingstudy-emergencyctpinwashandshelter.pdf (Accessed on November 29, 2016).

Kwasnicka, D., Dombrowski, S. U., White, M., and Sniehotta, F. (2016). Theoretical explanations for maintenance of behaviour change: a systematic review of behaviour theories. *Health Psychology Review*, **10**(3), 277–296.

Lantagne, D. S. and Clasen T. F. (2009). *Point of use water treatment in emergency response*. London School of Hygiene and Tropical Medicine (online). Available at: http://pdf.usaid.gov/pdf_docs/Pnads134.pdf (Accessed on July 7, 2017).

Lantagne, D. S. and Clasen, T. F. (2012). Use of household water treatment and safe storage methods in acute emergency response: Case study results from Nepal, Indonesia, Kenya, and Haiti. *Environmental Science & Technology*, **46**(20), 11352–11360.

Livestock Emergency Guidelines and Standards (LEGS), Second edition. (2014). Accessed December 1, 2017. Available at: http://www.livestock-emergency.net/download-legs//

MoHCDGEC. (2016). Cholera outbreak summary. United Republic of Tanzania Ministry of Health, Community development, gender, elderly, and children. December 11, 2016, update # 415.

MSF. (2010). *Public health engineering in precarious situations*. 2nd edition, Paris: Médecins Sans Frontières.

Naugle, D. A. and Hornik, R. C. (2014). Systematic review of the effectiveness of mass media interventions for child survival in low- and middle-income countries. *Journal of Health Communication*, **19**, 190–215.

Nawaz, J., Lal, S., Raza, S., and House, S. (2010). Oxfam experience of providing screened toilet, bathing and menstruation units in its earthquake response in Pakistan. *Gender & Development*, **18**(1), 81–86.

Neal, D., Vujcic, J., Burns, R., et al. (2016). *Nudging and habit change for open defecation: new tactics from behavioral science*. World Bank Group (online). Available at: http://documents.worldbank.org/curated/en/905011467990970572/Nudging-and-habit-change-for-open-defecation-new-tactics-from-behavioral-science (Accessed on January 18, 2017).

Nizame, F. A., Nasreen, S., Halder, A. K., et al. (2015). Observed Practices and Perceived Advantages of Different Hand Cleansing Agents in Rural Bangladesh: Ash, Soil, and Soap. *American Journal of Tropical Medicine and Hygiene*, **92**(6), 1111–1116.

Oxfam (2011). Urban WASH Lessons Learned from Post-Earthquake Response in Haiti (online). Available at: www.alnap.org/pool/files/tbn20-wash-urban-lessons-learnt-haiti-06052011-en.pdf (Accessed on January 18, 2017).

Patel D., Brooks, N., and Bastable, A. (2011). Excreta disposal in emergencies: Bag and Peepoo trials with internally displaced people in Port-au-Prince. *Waterlines*, **30**(1).

Peepoople (n.d.). Peepoople (online). Available at: www.peepoople.com/ (Accessed on December 20, 2017).

Phillips, R. M., Vujcic, J., Boscoe, A., et al. (2015). Soap is not enough: handwashing practices and knowledge in refugee camps, Maban County, South Sudan. *Conflict and Health*, **9**(1).

Pickering, A. J., Boehm, A. B., Mwanjali, M., and Davis, J. (2010). Efficacy of waterless hand hygiene compared with handwashing with soap: A field study in Dar es Salaam, Tanzania. *American Journal of Tropical Medicine and Hygiene*, **82**(2), 270–278.

Ramesh, A., Blanchet, K., and Ensink, J. H. J. (2015). Evidence on the Effectiveness of Water, Sanitation, and Hygiene (WASH) Interventions on Health Outcomes in Humanitarian Crises: A Systematic Review. *PLOS ONE*, **10**(9).

Ramos, M., Benelli, P., Irvine, E., and Watson, J. (2016). *WASH Problem exploration report: Handwashing*. Humanitarian Innovation Fund (online). Available at: www.elrha.org/wp-content/uploads/2016/01/Handwashing-WASH-Problem-Exploration-Report.pdf (Accessed on December 20, 2016).

Sommer, M., Schmitt, M., Clatworthy, D. (2017). A toolkit for integrating Menstrual Hygiene Management (MHM) into humanitarian response. (First edit). New York: Columbia University, Mailman School of Public Health and International Rescue Committee

Sozzi E., Fabre K., Fesselet J. F., Ebdon J. E., and Taylor, H. (2015). Minimizing the risk of disease transmission in emergency settings: Novel in situ physico-chemical disinfection of pathogen-laden hospital wastewaters. *PLOS Neglected Tropical Diseases* **9**(6).

Sphere Project. (2011). Sphere Handbook: Humanitarian Charter and Minimum Standards in Disaster Response (online). Available at: www.sphereproject.org/handbook/ (Accessed on October 12, 2016).

Stelmach, R. D. and Clasen, T. (2015). Household water quantity and health: A systematic review. *International Journal of Environmental Research and Public Health* **12**(6), 5954–5974.

Taylor, D. L., Kahawita, T. M., Cairncross, S., et al. (2015). The impact of water, sanitation and hygiene interventions to control cholera: A systematic review. *PLOS ONE*, **10**(8).

UNICEF. (2007). WASH cluster M&E toolkit for hygiene indicators (online). Available at: http://toolkit.ineesite.org/toolkit/INEEcms/uploads/1071/Indicators_for_monitoring_Hygiene_Promotion.pdf (Accessed on November 29, 2016).

UNICEF. (2009). Introduction to hygiene promotion: Tools and approaches (online). Available at: www.unicefinemergencies.com/downloads/eresource/docs/WASH/WASH%20Introduction%20to%20Hygiene%20Promotion.Tools%20and%20Approaches.pdf (Accessed on Nov. 29, 2016).

UNICEF. (2013). Cholera toolkit. Available at: www.unicef.org/cholera_toolkit/ (Accessed on November 29, 2016).

Wolfe M. K., Wells E., Mitro B., et al. (2016) Seeking Clearer Recommendations for Hand Hygiene in Communities Facing Ebola: A Randomized Trial Investigating the Impact of Six Handwashing Methods on Skin Irritation and Dermatitis. *PLoS ONE*, 11(12).

World Helath Organization. (1993). Guidelines for Cholera Control. Available at http://apps.who.int/iris/bitstream/10665/36837/1/924154449X.pdf (Accessed January 22, 2018).

World Health Organization. (1997). The guidelines for drinking-water quality Volume 3—Surveillance and control of community supplies (online). Available at: www.who.int/water_sanitation_health/dwq/gdwqvol32ed.pdf (Accessed on December 12, 2016).

World Health Organization. (2006). Guidelines for the Safe Use of Wastewater, Excreta, and Greywater: Volume 4 Excreta and greywater use in agriculture (online). Available at: www.who.int/water_sanitation_health/publications/gsuweg4/en/ (Accessed on December 12, 2016).

World Health Organization. (2008). Essential environmental health standards in health care (online). Available at: www.who.int/water_sanitation_health/hygiene/settings/ehs_health_care.pdf.pdf (Accessed on November 29, 2016).

World Health Organization. (2011) Guidelines for drinking water quality, 4th edition (online). Available at http://apps.who.int/iris/bitstream/10665/44584/1/9789241548151_eng.pdf (Accessed on November 29, 2016).

World Health Organization. (2014). Safe management of wastes from health-care activities (online). Available at: http://apps.who.int/iris/bitstream/10665/85349/1/9789241548564_eng.pdf?ua=1&ua=1 (Accessed on November 29, 2016).

World Health Organization. (2015). Health worker Ebola infections in Guinea, Liberia and Sierra Leone (online). Available at: www.who.int/hrh/documents/21may2015_web_final.pdf (Accessed on November 29, 2016).

World Health Organization and UNICEF (2015). Water, sanitation and hygiene in health care facilities Status in low- and middle-income countries and way forward (online). Available at: www.who.int/water_sanitation_health/publications/wash-health-care-facilities/en/ (Accessed on November 29, 2016).

WHO. (2017). Diarrhoeal disease. Available at: http://www.who.int/mediacentre/factsheets/fs330/en/ (Accessed on January 22, 2018)

Wright, J., Gundry, S., and Conroy, R. (2004). Household drinking water in developing countries: a systematic review of microbiological contamination between source and point-of-use. *Tropical Medicine and International Health*, 9(1), 106–117.

Yates, T. M., Armitage, E., Lehmann, L. V., Branz, A. J., and Lantagne, D. S. (2015). Effectiveness of chlorine dispensers in emergencies: Case study results from Haiti, Sierra Leone, Democratic Republic of Congo, and Senegal. *Environmental Science & Technology*, 49(8), 5115–5122.

Nutrition

Leisel E. Talley and Erin Boyd

Introduction

Malnutrition refers to a state of physiologic disruption caused by inadequate or deficient diet. Malnutrition includes both overconsumption and underconsumption of nutrients resulting in an imbalance between a person's nutritional intakes and his/her nutritional needs. *Undernutrition* includes acute malnutrition, chronic malnutrition or growth failure, micronutrient malnutrition and interuterine growth restriction (IUGR). During humanitarian emergencies, emergency nutrition response addresses undernutrition, which in these settings is energy intake below metabolic requirements and also expenditure.

An estimated 52 million children under five are wasted; 35.1 million affected by moderate acute malnutrition (MAM) and 16.9 million by severe acute malnutrition (SAM); and 155 million children under five are stunted (UNICEF/WHO/World Bank 2017). Children with acute malnutrition are between 4.5 for MAM and 9 for SAM times more likely to die, and therefore, levels of acute malnutrition in children under five are often used as proxy indicators for determining the severity of a crisis. Levels of undernutrition are indicative of food security, morbidity, care, and the environmental situation for people affected by the humanitarian emergency.

This chapter provides an overview of the key terms and concepts associated with nutrition in humanitarian emergencies. In order to understand the different types of undernutrition, a brief description of undernutrition is presented, followed by an examination of risk factors, vulnerabilities, and the measurement of acute malnutrition, as well as a description of how it is used to determine the scope of nutritional problems in crisis-affected populations.

Finally, an overview analysis of nutrition response and prevention options during humanitarian emergencies is presented. Nutrition programming is most closely linked to food security health programming and treatment of malnutrition; however, important interactions exist between nutrition and communicable diseases, water, sanitation and hygiene, as well as surveillance in humanitarian emergencies. Food security and malnutrition are discussed in Chapters 13 and 25 respectively.

Nutrients and Food Groups

There are two types of nutrients: macronutrients and micronutrients. Macronutrients include carbohydrates, fats, and protein and are the basis of energy required for a body to function.

Macronutrients

There are three main types of macronutrients:

- Carbohydrates make up the majority of diets in developing countries, and are an important source of energy (1 g carbohydrate provides approximately 4 kcal).
- Fats contribute to cell structure and provide main energy stores of the body (1 g fat provides 9 kcals).
- Proteins provide the building blocks of body tissues and a source of energy. Higher levels of protein are needed at different times in an individual's life, such as during growth in infancy and early childhood, adolescence, pregnancy and lactation, and in illness (1 g protein provides 4 kcals).

Micronutrients

Micronutrients include vitamins and minerals and are required in small amounts for a range of critical body functions. There are two main types of micronutrients:

- Vitamins are required for essential metabolic processes. The two types of vitamins include water-soluble such as Vitamin C and B vitamins, which are not stored in the body for long periods of time, and fat soluble vitamins, which include A, D, E, and K, and are stored in the body for longer

periods of time. Sources of A, D, E, and K include animal products.
- Minerals are essential constituents of some hormones, enzymes, and body tissues.

Food Groups

There are six main categories of food groups:

- Cereals consist mainly of carbohydrates and low quality protein. Examples include sorghum, rice, maize, barley, and wheat.
- Pulses have approximately twice as much protein as cereals and are rich in the B-complex vitamins and iron. Examples include lentils, beans, groundnuts, soya beans, sesame, and sunflower seeds.
- Tubers and roots provide mainly carbohydrates with low protein content. Examples include yams, taro, cassava, sweet potato, and potatoes.
- Fruits and vegetables are an excellent source of vitamin A, vitamins B and C, iron, and calcium.
- Animal products provide high quality protein, but are usually only eaten in small amounts in developing countries. Examples of animal products are meat, eggs, poultry, fish, and dairy products.
- Oils and fats improve the palatability of the diet and are a concentrated source of energy. Fat from milk is a rich source of vitamins A and D. Vegetable oils and fats do not contain vitamin A and D unless fortified. An exception is red palm oil that contains vitamin A naturally. Examples of oils and fats are groundnut oils such as peanut, soya, sunflower, rapeseed, and butter.

Both the understanding of causes of malnutrition and approaches to manage malnutrition have changed over the past decades. Previously, malnutrition was thought to be directly related directly to a lack of food intake, specifically protein. In the late 1980s evidence from different contexts began to refute these ideas (WHO et al. 2000). Nutritionists found that malnutrition occurred where food was available, and the link between disease and malnutrition was increasingly understood. In 1990, the UNICEF conceptual framework was developed and further revised in 2008 (Black et al. 2008b). This conceptual framework outlines three levels of causes of malnutrition:

- Direct/immediate causes of malnutrition include inadequate food intake and disease.
- Underlying causes of malnutrition include inadequate household food security, the social and care environment (which covers infant and young-child feeding practices, health-seeking behavior, and lack of access to healthcare), and a poor health environment (which includes quality and safety of water as well as sanitation and hygiene).
- Basic causes include formal and informal infrastructure, political ideology and resources.

This framework has provided a lens through which to analyze nutritional risks, as well as make response decisions. It is shown in Figure 12.1.

Agencies in Emergency Nutrition

The main body with the mandate to address the nutritional needs of a population in a specific country is usually the Ministry of Health (MoH). MoH-supported nutrition programs are normally integrated into the health system, focused on prevention of malnutrition, and may include growth monitoring and promotion at community level health clinics, training on optimal infant and young child feeding (IYCF) for healthcare professionals and vitamin A supplementation campaigns often linked to vaccination campaigns. In many countries affected by humanitarian emergencies, the MoH has neither the financial nor human resources to adequately meet the needs of the malnourished population. In these cases, the humanitarian community is involved in augmenting the services available for nutritionally vulnerable populations.

The humanitarian community includes several United Nations (UN) agencies and nongovernmental organizations (NGO) that are directly involved in the provision of emergency nutrition assistance during crises.

United Nations Agencies

- Food and Agriculture Organization (FAO) mainly addresses macrolevel and some household-level food security, and links initiatives for the prevention of malnutrition through these interventions.
- United Nations High Commissioner for Refugees (UNHCR) has the mandate to meet the emergency nutrition needs of refugee populations and often supports a range of nutrition interventions in refugee camp and noncamp settings.

Chapter 12: Nutrition

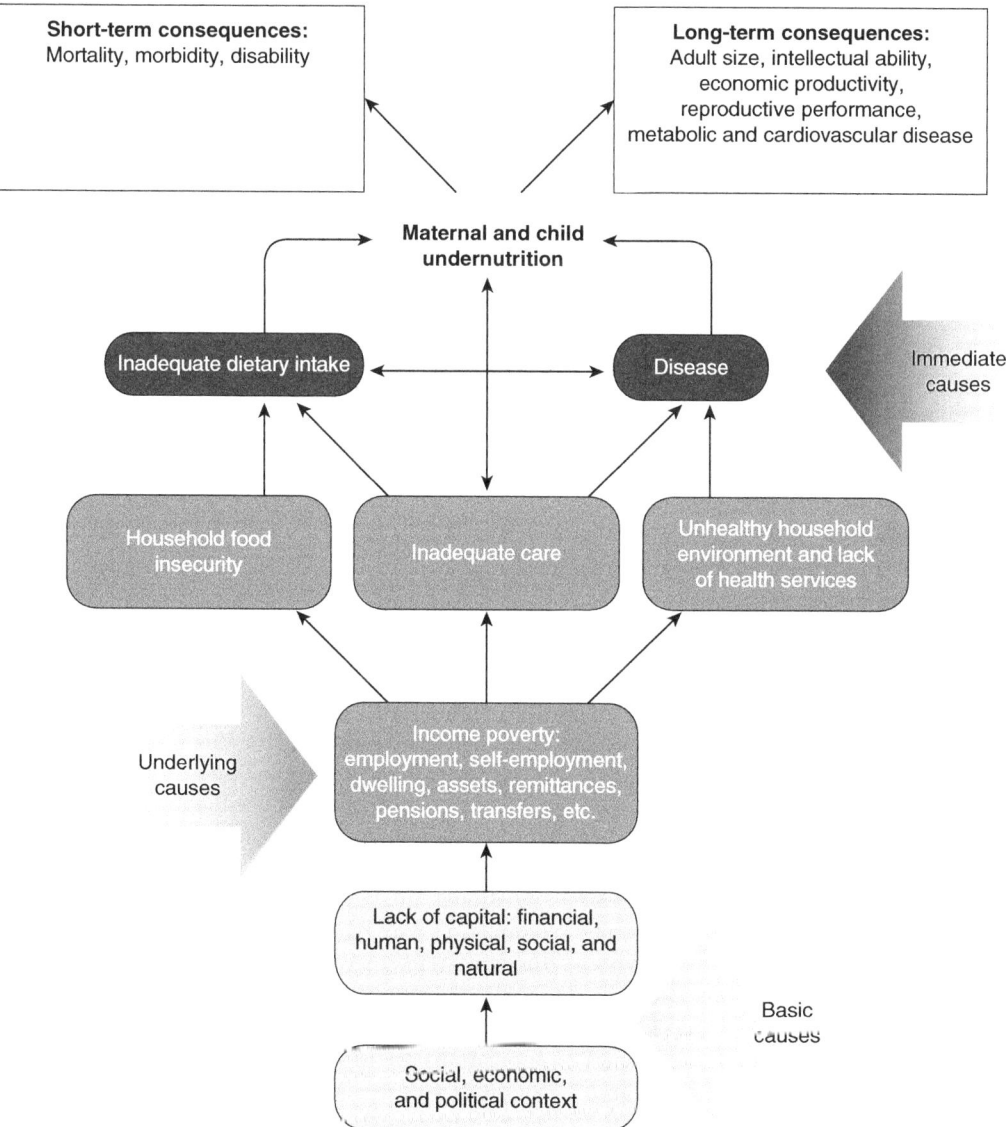

Figure 12.1 Conceptual framework of three levels of causes of malnutrition

- United Nations Children's Fund (UNICEF) has the mandate for supporting the MoH to implement nutrition interventions aimed at protecting children and addressing: optimal IYCF, micronutrient deficiencies, nutritional surveillance, and the management of severe acute malnutrition.
- World Food Programme (WFP) is the UN agency responsible for ensuring household level food security, which often entails supporting general food distributions (GFD) or providing cash assistance aimed at securing household level food security. WFP is also responsible for the management of moderate acute malnutrition (MAM) and preventive blanket supplementary feeding (BSFP).
- World Health Organization (WHO) provides technical support to build the capacity of MoH staff, particularly at a tertiary level, which includes supporting medical professionals to receive training on the management of acute malnutrition.

Nongovernmental Organizations

International nongovernmental organizations (INGO) are often the implementing partners in collaboration with the MoH and UN agencies. INGOs often directly implement nutrition interventions either through existing health structures or in parallel where the health structures are nonfunctioning. Major INGOs working in nutrition include Action Contre la Faim, Concern, GOAL, International Medical Corps, Alima and International Rescue Committee, Save the Children, and World Vision. There are also national NGO and civil society groups, specific to each country, that support nutrition interventions on their own and/or in direct collaboration with INGO, MOH, and UN agencies.

Depending on the country, national NGO and civil society groups may have significant nutrition experience and relationships with communities, which can be particularly useful in reaching more people and understanding underlying causes of malnutrition. Additionally, governments and donors also play an important role.

Risk Factors

Vulnerable Populations

Nutritional vulnerability can be divided into different categories when discussing humanitarian emergencies. The first category is physiologic vulnerability, defined as the section of the population with increased nutrient needs or reduced appetites. This includes infants between zero and 6 months of age, and children from 6 to 59 months of age, as both have high nutritional needs as result of their rapid growth and development. Exclusive breastfeeding of children 6 months and younger is the best protection against malnutrition. Older children are at greater risk of infection as they transition from exclusive breastfeeding to complimentary foods. In humanitarian emergency settings, high rates of acute malnutrition are seen in children 6–24 months. Pregnant and lactating women are also vulnerable to acute malnutrition as their nutritional needs increase during pregnancy and lactation. As a general rule, the additional caloric requirements are 300 calories per day for pregnant women and 500 calories per day for lactating women (WHO et al. 2000). Malnutrition in pregnancy can result in low-birth-weight babies, who are in turn vulnerable to acute malnutrition. Energy reserves and additional intake support the production of breast milk and optimal nutrition in infants.

Another physiologically vulnerable group is adolescents. Like infants and young children, adolescents are in a period of rapid growth and development. Menstruation further increases micronutrient demands in adolescent girls as a result of iron losses. Perhaps the greatest nutritional demand is in a pregnant adolescent girl. The additional nutritional demands from pregnancy in conjunction with the nutritional requirements for continued growth in adolescence increases the risk of malnutrition in the mother and delivering a low-birthweight baby at increased risk of malnutrition (United Nations System Standing Committee on Nutrition 2010).

Older people, as well as those living with a disability are also at increased risk, often from reduced appetites or difficulty with the mechanics of eating including chewing and swallowing. This can significantly reduce the nutrient intake in these populations. In previous humanitarian emergencies, such as during the war in Bosnia in the nineties, the elderly with limited social support were at greatest risk of acute malnutrition even when compared with children under five years of age. Finally, individuals with chronic diseases such as HIV/AIDS and tuberculosis have increased nutritional demands, but often reduced appetites or reduced ability to eat. Poor absorption of nutrients, metabolic disturbances and side effects of medications can all impact the overall nutritional intake of chronically ill patients. This population may quickly deteriorate in the setting of humanitarian emergency.

Other vulnerabilities that exist in relation to acute malnutrition include geographic vulnerability where populations are inaccessible or live in harsh climatic conditions (desert or extreme cold) altering the nutrient requirements. People with disabilities may also be at risk of malnutrition due to physical inability to access food or marginalization in a community due to stigma. Political or social vulnerability where a specific population may be underserved or excluded based on their political affiliations, ethnicity, religion or gender. And finally refugees and internally displaced persons who are unable to access preventive and curative services, as well as their regular livelihoods, increasing their vulnerability.

Nutritional vulnerability and risk can extend beyond a single generation and is known as the intergenerational cycle of growth failure, shown in Figure 12.2 (Action Contre la Faim International 2010). This concept is based upon stunted girls

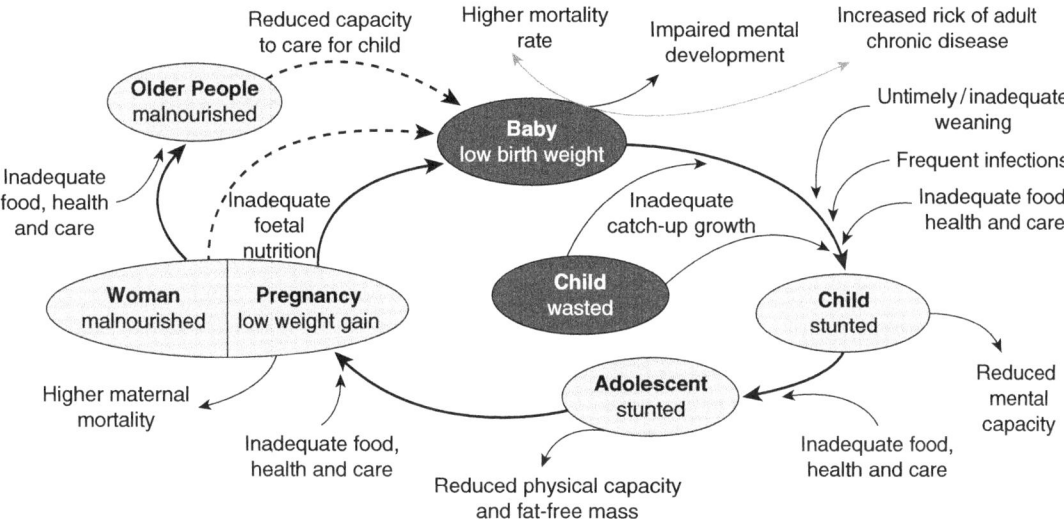

Figure 12.2 Intergenerational cycle of growth failure

becoming small women who are more likely to have low-birthweight babies at increased risk of both acute and chronic malnutrition. Pregnancy during adolescence can further contribute to the risk of low-birthweight as described above. This cycle continues across generations. To properly address and interrupt this cycle, the nutritional status of young girls, pregnant women and mothers needs to be improved, in addition to delaying the age of first pregnancy (United Nations System Standing Committee on Nutrition 2010).

Malnutrition-Infection Cycle

Malnutrition and infection interact in two important ways. First, when a person is malnourished, they are more susceptible to infection due to atrophy of the thymus, reduced cell numbers, and subsequently underdeveloped peripheral lymphoid organs that reduce immunity (Schaible 2007). Additionally, a person who is suffering from an infection often has increased energy requirements and decreased appetite, and is therefore more likely to become malnourished. Once a person is malnourished, it is more difficult to recover from infection as their immune system is weakened. During illness, immune cells are propagated, and additional protein synthesis is necessary increasing energy requirements (Schaible 2007). Undernutrition contributes to approximately half of under-five child deaths (UNICEF 2013).

This cycle is particularly relevant for children under five, whose immune systems are less developed. The most common infections in children under five include malaria, measles, acute respiratory infections, and diarrhea. These diseases all have malabsorption as one of the symptoms (Schaible 2007). Malnutrition is often an underlying cause or contributing factor of mortality associated with these diseases. Measles is of particular concern because of its contagiousness and high case fatality rate among malnourished children. In humanitarian emergencies, mass measles vaccination in nutritionally vulnerable populations should be a priority (Salama et al. 2001). Tuberculosis and HIV/AIDS may cause persistent malnutrition and often require modified prevention and treatment of acute malnutrition.

Water, Sanitation, and Hygiene Practices and Health Services

The conceptual framework of malnutrition shown in Figure 12.1 identifies the environment and lack of health services as underlying causes of malnutrition. Water, sanitation, and hygiene practices and health risk factors all contribute to risk of malnutrition. Poor quality and limited quantity of water, poor water storage practices, such as open defecation increase the risk of diarrheal disease and other fecal-transmitted infections, increasing the risk of malnutrition. Health services include both the availability and accessibility of healthcare, as well as the quality and reliability of services. If populations have limited access to preventative and curative health services, the delay in treatment for preventable and treatable diseases may also increase the risk of malnutrition. Access to vaccines and prompt treatment of diarrheal disease, acute respiratory infections, measles, and malaria can improve the overall health and nutritional status of a child.

Social and Care Environment

Also highlighted in the conceptual framework of malnutrition as one of three underlying causes in the social and care environment, which includes feeding practices and health seeking behavior of caretakers. IYCF practices refer to how children are fed from birth until at least two years of age, including exclusive breastfeeding and/or optimal use of breast milk substitutes (BMS), appropriate introduction of nutritionally adequate complementary foods, and minimum meal frequency and diversity. In many cultures, new mothers may rely on their mothers and/or mothers-in-law for guidance on how to breastfeed and feed young children. A common example of how social dynamics can influence IYCF practices is when grandmothers tell new mothers not to offer newborns colostrum following birth because it is "dirty" (Walia et al. 2009). If new mothers listen to this advice, they will deprive their infant of important first milk, which provides important immune and growth factors as well as essential nutrients. The social and care environment also includes health-seeking behavior, which relates to when a caregiver decides to consult a medical professional concerning their child's health. As a result, the status of women is a significant predictor of malnutrition. In societies where women are more empowered, they can make the decision to take their child to a healthcare provider; whereas in societies where women have less autonomy, they may have to convince a father or grandmother before visiting a healthcare professional. This can result in delayed access to lifesaving medicine for young children. Additionally, maternal literacy is directly correlated with the risk of a child being malnourished (Makoka 2015).

Seasonality

Seasonality refers to predictable climatic changes that are linked to increases in levels of acute malnutrition at specific times of the year. Most often, malnutrition rises during the rainy season, when the risk of communicable disease increases with worsening sanitation conditions, including diarrheal disease. Many countries have rainy seasons which last for 1–3 months, either once or twice a year. The lean season refers to the agricultural cultivation period, which overlaps with the rainy season when food is less available. Mothers and other caregivers are engaged in planting activities and sometimes absent from the home. This can leave young children in the care of older siblings, increasing their exposure to inadequate feeding practices. While the harvest period yields increased food availability, the impact on levels of malnutrition will not be immediate.

In the Darfur region of Sudan, during the rainy season the levels of acute malnutrition increase by as much as ten percentage points. The people of Darfur have developed several coping mechanisms: reducing meal frequency, eating wild foods that may stave off hunger, and migration to areas where food may be more available.

Types of Malnutrition

Acute Malnutrition

Acute malnutrition is an acute event that results in rapid weight loss. This may be a result of decreased dietary intake or reduced appetite and increased metabolism in relation to infectious disease. A young child can lose a significant amount of their body weight in a short period of time. Acute malnutrition is the type of undernutrition of most concern in emergencies as it carries an immediate risk of mortality, which can be prevented with appropriate and timely treatment.

On a population level, acute malnutrition is divided into two categories. The first is global acute malnutrition (GAM) that includes all cases of malnutrition: moderate, severe, and bilateral pitting edema. GAM is a main indicator of the scale of the emergency or crisis and is reported in almost all emergencies. The second category is severe acute malnutrition or SAM that includes all cases of severe acute malnutrition and bilateral pitting edema. Both GAM and SAM have thresholds associated with them to indicate critical and emergency levels of acute malnutrition.

On an individual level, acute malnutrition may present in three different forms. Marasmus or wasting is perhaps the most well-known because of the easy visual identification of the most severe cases.

In marasmus, the body consumes muscle and fat to provide energy and results in the very thin appearance of the child. This is the most common form of acute malnutrition in emergency contexts. A child may either be moderately or severely malnourished defined as a weight-for-height Z-score of <−2 and ≥−3 or <−3, respectively. Additionally, the mid upper arm circumference (MUAC) of a child can be used as a criteria of moderate and severe wasting: <125 to ≥115 mm or <115 mm, respectively. The definitions of malnutrition are shown in Table 12.1.

Kwashiorkor or nutritional edema, defined as bilateral pitting edema, is the second form of acute malnutrition. Kwashiorkor's main characteristic is edema, where the body of the child swells with fluid. Initially, edema is limited to the feet, but may progress up the body to the hands and face in more severe cases. At first glance the child may not appear acutely malnourished due to their plump and bloated appearance, but kwashiorkor has a high mortality rate. A child with this form of malnutrition is often described as having a "full moon face." In some cases severe skin lesions prone to secondary infection may develop, and a child's hair may be discolored lighter than normal and brittle. Marasmic kwashiorkor is the third presentation of acute malnutrition. In this form, a child is both wasted and has edema.

Chronic Malnutrition

Chronic malnutrition, also known as growth failure or stunting, is the most pervasive form of undernutrition, with a global estimate of 170 million moderately or severely stunted children (Olofin et al. 2013). Chronic malnutrition results in a child that is too short for his/her age. Additionally, chronic malnutrition can affect the cognitive development of a child. The process of growth failure leading to stunting is complex and occurs over time. A child may have both acute and chronic malnutrition. The growth period between birth and two years of age is the most critical time in preventing or minimizing the effect of chronic malnutrition (Bhutta et al. 2008, Black et al. 2008a, Black et al. 2008b, Bryce et al. 2008, Morris et al. 2008, Victora et al. 2008). After two years of age, it is believed that most stunting is irreversible. In the acute phase of an emergency, chronic malnutrition is not the highest priority as the immediate risk of death is lower than that of acute malnutrition. However, in protracted situations chronic malnutrition is important and should be addressed. UNHCR has developed guidance on programming to addressing stunting in refugee contexts (UNHCR 2011). On a global level, programming has begun to focus on the first 1,000 days of life, the period from conception to two years of age, as a way to reduce the impact

Table 12.1 Definitions of malnutrition

Type of Malnutrition	Indices	Definition
Underweight	Weight-for-age	Moderate: <−2 to ≥−3 Z-score
		Severe: <−3 z score
Chronic (stunting)	Height-for-age	Moderate: <−2 to ≥−3 Z-score
		Severe: <−3 z score
Acute (wasting)	Weight-for-length/height	Moderate: <−2 to ≥−3 Z-score
		Severe: <−3 z score
	MUAC	Moderate: <125 to ≥ 115 mm
		Severe: <115 mm
	MUAC for pregnant/lactating Women[+]	Range: <18.5 cm to <23 cm
	Body Mass Index (BMI) for child age 5–19 years	Thinness: <−2 to ≥−3 Z-score
		Severe Thinness: <−3 Z-score
	Body Mass Index (BMI) for adult	Moderate: <17 to ≥ 16 kg/m^2
		Severe: >16 kg/m^2
Acute (Kwashiorkor)	Bilateral pitting edema	Severe

Note: "Children" defined as age 6–59 months unless otherwise noted. [+]There is no internationally agreed upon cutoff for acute malnutrition in pregnant or lactating women based upon MUAC.

of overall undernutrition levels, including growth failure (Bhutta et al. 2008, Black et al. 2008a, Black et al. 2008b, Bryce et al. 2008, Morris et al. 2008, Victora et al. 2008).

Stunting-Wasting Linkages

Both stunting and wasting carry increased risk of mortality. Children are 2.3 and 5.5 times more likely to die if they are moderately or severely stunted, respectively (Olofin et al. 2013). The risk is even greater for wasted children – 4.5 for moderately wasted and 9 for severely wasted children (Black et al. 2008b, United Nations Children's Fund, 2012). The child that is both wasted and stunted is in a most precarious state with an increased risk of mortality of 12.3 (Khara and Dolan 2014, Olofin et al. 2013). While wasting has been the primary focus of emergency nutrition programming with the objective to minimize acute morbidity and mortality, addressing stunting in the acute phase of a humanitarian emergency is not a priority. However, there is a movement to assess stunting and implement more preventive programming in emergency settings.

Underweight

Underweight, another form of undernutrition, is assessed by the wight-for-age. It is a composite measure of acute and chronic malnutrition and was widely used in many community programs until recently. Based on this anthropometric indicator, one cannot determine if a child is too thin for his height or too short for his age. Underweight is most often used in growth monitoring of infants and young children where repeated measures are taken to track the growth of a child. In some situations, the prevalence of underweight may be the only available nutritional data on the affected population.

Micronutrient Malnutrition

Micronutrients are vitamins and minerals required by the body to carry out all biochemical and metabolic processes. Unlike energy, they are required in very small amounts. Micronutrients can be divided into 2 categories: Type 1 and Type 2. The simplest explanation of the difference is that Type 1 nutrients affect metabolism and immune response and have nutrient-specific clinical manifestations; whereas Type 2 nutrients affect metabolism and have the same non-specific manifestation – growth failure (Golden 1995). Requirements of micronutrients vary by age and sex, as well as stage of life. Periods of rapid growth (infancy, early childhood, adolescence, pregnancy and lactation) or illness (caused by diarrhea, malaria, helminth infections, and tuberculosis) can increase the demand for micronutrients. Micronutrient malnutrition is a type of undernutrition which is a result of inadequate intake, absorption, or utilization of specific micronutrients. Micronutrient deficiency disease (MDD) is when a clinical disease occurs because of the lack of a specific micronutrient (NutritionWorks; et al. 2011). MDD treatment will be discussed in Chapter 25.

Micronutrient malnutrition persists in both emergency and nonemergency contexts and is often referred to as silent malnutrition. This form of malnutrition and deficiencies contribute to acute morbidity and mortality in this context and produce long-term health effects, such as reduced cognitive capacity and work capacity. A key concept in micronutrient malnutrition is that an individual may meet their energy requirements, but be unable to meet their micronutrient needs (NutritionWorks; et al. 2011). Emergency affected populations are often at greater risk because of factors such as diarrheal disease, (where repeated episodes affect gut function and absorption micronutrients), other infectious diseases (such as malaria or helminth infections that cause iron deficiency), unvaried diets (due to limited access or inadequate food rations which do not contain fortified foods), low micronutrient bioavailability or inhibitors to absorption, and poor compliance with supplementation (NutritionWorks et al. 2011).

Epidemiology

Malnutrition

Globally, the most prevalent form of micronutrient malnutrition is iron deficiency anemia. The WHO estimates that two billion people are anemic, mostly due to iron deficiency (WHO 2017a). Vitamin A deficiency also affects up to 250 million preschool age children, increasing their risk of mortality from severe infections and is the leading cause of preventable blindness in this population (WHO 2017b). While iron and vitamin A deficiency affect populations globally, there are some deficiencies rarely seen outside of emergencies. These include deficiencies of vitamin C (scurvy), niacin (pellagra), riboflavin (angular stomatisis) and thiamin (beri-beri). Additionally, zinc is a particularly important micronutrient for all populations. Evidence has shown that zinc supplementation results in a reduction of all-cause mortality in children with the greatest impact on diarrheal- and pneumonia-related mortality, as well as a reduction in diarrheal and pneumonia incidence (Black et al. 2013). Additionally, zinc may play a role in preventing stunting. As diarrheal disease is a prominent cause of morbidity in young children and emergency populations and can lead to weight loss (see malnutrition infection cycle), zinc supplementation is a key nutritional intervention. It is important to note that outbreaks continue in emergency populations, for example, the large scale outbreak of angular stomatitis in the Karamoja Region of Uganda in 2009/2010 (Nichols et al. 2013).

Overnutrition

Overweight and obesity is a growing global epidemic with more than one billion overweight adults and six hundred million adults classified as obese and 41 million overweight children under five years of age (Black et al. 2013, WHO 2017c). This type of malnutrition has not typically been a focus of nutrition programming in emergencies; however, the international community must begin to consider its impact in future emergencies. More countries, including those in South East Asia, Africa, and the Middle East and emergency affected populations are experiencing the phenomenon known as the *double burden of malnutrition* where overnutrition and undernutrition coexist, even within the same household. Grijalva-Eternod et al. documented this occurrence in the long-standing Sahwari refugee population in Algeria where there were high rates of obesity in women while young children were acutely and/or chronically malnourished (Grijalva-Eternod et al. 2012). As more emergencies occur in middle income countries and urban populations, for example, Syria, and refugee situations are protracted, programs need to begin to address overnutrition and the associated morbidities like hypertension, cardiovascular disease and type 2 diabetes.

Measuring Nutritional Status

Anthropometry

Anthropometry is the measurement of body parameters – height or length, weight, mid upper arm circumference (MUAC), age and sex. When two measurements are combined, they produce an anthropometric index such as weight-for-height, height-for-age and weight-for-age. These indices form the basis for the nutritional assessment of both individuals and populations. These indices are used to classify the nutritional status of individuals, albeit they do not account for edema or micronutrient deficiencies. What is measured is dependent upon the type of undernutrition being assessed.

Children 6–59 months of age are the subset of the population most commonly measured. Infants less than 6 months are not routinely included in population assessments in emergencies, but may be assessed on an individual basis for enrollment into therapeutic feeding programs for the management of acute malnutrition. Clinical signs of acute malnutrition including visible wasting, edema, and lack of weight gain are primarily used in place of anthropometric measurements in infants under 6 months of age. The Management of Acute Malnutrition in Infants project is leading research into assessment guidance for this age group (Kerac et al. 2010).

Standard procedures and equipment have been developed for anthropometric assessment as well as age estimation and determining the presence of bilateral pitting edema (WHO Multicentre Growth Reference Study Group 2006). Height boards are used to assess both length and height of children. If a child is less than two years of age or 87 cm, or if the age is unknown, his/her length will be measured lying down; otherwise standing height is measured. There are two main types of scales used for assessing weight. A spring scale can be used but can be difficult to use and record accurate weights. High quality electronic scales have replaced spring scales in many surveys and programs. These scales come equipped with tare functions and can be used to measure adults and children, as well as infants in the arms of a caregiver. In some clinics or inpatient programs, balance or beam scales for infants may be available.

MUAC is the measurement of the circumference of the mid upper left arm. It is an indicator of wasting and assesses lean body mass. MUAC has also been shown to be correlated with the risk of mortality, particularly in young children. MUAC is biased toward the identification of younger children as acutely malnourished because they biologically have smaller arms; however, these children are often at the greatest risk of mortality. This bias is accepted as MUAC is most often used to identify those at greatest risk of death and in need of treatment (Goossens et al. 2012). MUAC-for-age tables are available for use, but rarely used in emergency contexts (WHO Multicentre Growth Reference Study Group 2006). The primary use of MUAC is among children 6–59 months and pregnant and lactating women. Unfortunately, there are no cutoffs for children 5–19 years of age. Among pregnant and lactating women, MUAC is used to identify malnutrition since body mass index is not a true reflection of the nutritional status in this population. Cutoffs defining malnutrition in this population vary by agency and country and is not standardized (Ververs et al. 2013).

MUAC assessment requires little equipment, only MUAC tapes. However, the minimal equipment should not oversimplify the process and required training. MUAC measurements are prone to significant inter- and intrameasurement error. Very small changes in the measurement can result in misclassification of the nutritional status of the child and potentially his/her access to appropriate treatment. MUAC tapes are widely available from different manufacturers.

At present, MUAC is used to identify wasted individuals. It is often used to quickly and efficiently screen large groups of children for admission into therapeutic feeding programs. Collection of MUAC data is encouraged in population-based surveys to inform programs, but it is not recommended that this data be used as the estimated population prevalence of acute malnutrition.

Once anthropometric indices are calculated, they need to be compared to a standard or reference for interpretation. For example, the weight-for-height index of the assessed child is compared to median weight of children with the same sex and height/length in the reference or standard population. Currently there is the National Center for Health Statistics (NCHS) growth reference and the WHO growth standards. The WHO growth standards and the use of Z-scores are recommended, and many national MOHs have adopted the use of these standards. A weight-for-height Z-score in conjunction with standard deviation information for the reference population indicates how far away positively or negatively a child is from the median. Within the WHO growth standards, 95% of the population lies between −2 and +2 Z scores, indicating normal nutritional status for weight-for-height, height-for-age, and weight-for-age. Once an individual has an index below −2 Z-scores, they are considered undernourished, acutely malnourished, stunted, or underweight.

Community Mobilization and Screening

Research has shown that the earlier children are identified as malnourished, the better their response to treatment (Collins et al. 2006). On a programmatic level, it is more cost-effective to treat a child with MAM than a child with SAM, and even more than with complicated SAM. Two program components are critical to early detection of cases: community mobilization and screening. Community mobilization is a critical component of nutritional programming in all contexts, but especially when programs are rapidly implemented or scaled-up during emergencies. Community mobilization is meant to sensitize the community to the management of malnutrition as well as nutrition in general. In acute emergencies where malnutrition rates are high, there is often a large caseload for treatment programs. Active case finding in the community or camp can be implemented to identify malnourished children. Depending on the context, these screenings may be carried out biweekly or monthly by community health workers. They can also be conducted at various population gatherings such as general or blanket food distributions or during immunization campaigns. Community screenings offer a quick and efficient method of screening large numbers of children across geographic areas in a relatively short amount of time. MUAC is the most common indicator used in screenings to refer children to treatment. Screenings may identify children with severe or moderate wasting as well as kwashiorkor. Children meeting referral or admission criteria are referred to treatment programs for further evaluation. Malnutrition is discussed in Chapter 25.

Assessing the Nutritional Status of the Population

Just as individuals are assessed for the presence of acute malnutrition, populations are also assessed as well to determine the prevalence of acute malnutrition and the severity of the situation. The three main methods that can be used to assess the nutritional status of a population are covered in the next three sections.

Rapid Assessment

Rapid assessment (RA), as the terminology implies, is a very quick look at the population. This type of assessment may be carried out at the very beginning of an emergency, when new areas of vulnerability and perceived risk or need are identified, or as security improves and access is gained. In many contexts, time on the ground is limited and data must be collected rapidly to determine the presence of a crisis. Key informants provide crucial information during the RA. Qualitative data on the status of the population are gathered – population size, displacement, access to food, water, shelter, healthcare and available resources, as well as more detailed information on nutrition and food security, such as signs of malnutrition, cases of malnutrition, food stocks, use of wild foods, and other coping mechanisms. A quick MUAC assessment of children age 6–59 months may be carried at the household level. Data should be cautiously used from these assessments as they are not a representative sample. However, this data can be used to determine the need for further assessment of the population. While there is no globally agreed upon standard for RA, there are some new methodologies (SMART Methodology 2014) and the Multi Cluster/Sector Initial Rapid Assessment (MIRA) tool developed in an effort to streamline data collection, reduce redundancy, and improve effectiveness in the initial days of a humanitarian response (Inter-Agency Standing Committee 2012, SMART Technical Advisory Group 2006). Rapid assessments are discussed more generally and in greater detail in Chapter 7.

Surveys

Surveys are the most frequently used form of data collection for assessing the nutritional status of a population. Cross sectional surveys offer a one-time "snapshot" of the current situation. In recent years, standardized data collection methodology for anthropometric and mortality surveys have been developed and are now in widespread use (SMART Technical Advisory Group 2006). Nutritional surveys should be representative of the population of interest, which might include refugees, internally displaced persons, or other identified vulnerable groups, and collect data in a timely fashion. In highly dynamic settings, like the initial phase of an emergency, nutrition data can become quickly outdated as the nutritional status of the population can change significantly over a relatively short period of time. Nutritional surveys range from extremely simple surveys that assess anthropometry and mortality with a few key questions related to immunization, morbidity and access to food, to very complex multisector surveys such as the WFP Emergency Food and Nutrition Assessments (WFP 2009).

When widespread micronutrient deficiencies or an outbreak of micronutrient deficiency disease are suspected, a micronutrient survey may be conducted. Unless there is an acute outbreak such as pellagra or scurvy, for example, micronutrient assessments are more frequently implemented after the acute phase of the emergency. These surveys require biochemical data collection, including venipuncture, lab supplies, and often access to a cold chain in country. While there has been progress in the development of more field friendly tests, such as Hemocue®, the cost of a micronutrient survey can be prohibitive, doubling or tripling the cost of an anthropometric survey. The simplest micronutrient surveys assess the prevalence of anemia in young children and women of reproductive age by measuring hemoglobin concentration using HemoCue® that requires collecting a few drops of blood from the finger. Some surveys will include clinical signs of micronutrient deficiencies; however, only a small percentage of the deficient population will show clinical signs (UNHCR 2011, Gorstein et al. 2007). Surveys are discussed more generally and in greater detail in Chapter 8.

Surveillance

Surveillance by definition is the routine systematic collection of data that is analyzed, interpreted, reported, and disseminated in a timely manner and used to inform programs. Nutritional surveillance can take many forms including repeated large scale nutrition surveys, repeated small scale surveys, clinic-based data, data from therapeutic feeding programs for acute malnutrition, sentinel sites, or a combination of these. Each of these forms of data has their own limitations (Bilukha et al. 2012). Trend analysis is a key component of nutritional surveillance and critical in the interpretation of the data. Seasonality significantly influences nutritional status, and it is essential to take this into account during the interpretation of the data. Nutritional data is often incorporated into early warning systems, such as the Famine Early Warning Network. One of the greatest challenges of nutritional surveillance is the ability to predict crises. By the time the nutritional status of a population has deteriorated to meet the definition of a nutritional crisis, there has been a significant series of events and missed opportunities for mitigation. Surveillance is discussed more generally and in greater detail in Chapter 9.

Nutritional Crisis

Humanitarian emergencies arise from many different causes from acute natural and manmade disasters, to slow onset emergencies, including famine. Nutritional crises occur when there is an underlying vulnerability in the population. Often, these crises are a combination of acute food shortages and large-scale outbreaks of epidemic diseases, such as measles. It is important to remember that nutritional status is not solely linked to the availability of food, but rather is a complex interaction of food security, morbidity, caring practices, water and sanitation, preventive and curative services, and physical security.

A nutritional crisis may occur when a population experiences an acute onset natural disaster such as the widespread flooding that destroyed crops, grain reserves, and homes, with displacement of the population in Pakistan in 2010. Other natural disasters (volcanoes, hurricanes, typhoons, and earthquakes) may also have an impact through disruption of agricultural activities from planting to harvest, destruction of crops and food stores, and disruption of markets. Some of these impacts may be long-lasting in terms of livelihoods and food security. Food Security is discussed in Chapter 13.

Drought is a cyclic event in many regions of the world including the Sahel and Horn of Africa. This form of natural disaster can be thought of as a slow onset emergency as failures in rains and crop production occur over a period of time. In many places, the interval between droughts has been decreasing, diminishing the population's ability to recover on a physiological, household, and economic level.

Political and economic events may also result in increased vulnerability and rates of acute malnutrition. For example, the combination of global high food prices and increasing fuel prices in 2008 resulted in an increase in the number of vulnerable and food insecure households. As prices rose, the purchasing power of households declined. For the poorest households already spending 60% of their income on food purchases, the crisis placed them at increased risk. Countries that heavily relied on food imports were also greatly affected. Studies postcrisis indicated that in some of the most affected countries, child acute malnutrition rose by 50% in the most vulnerable households (Compton et al. 2010).

Political failures are often intertwined with conflict and displacement. This combination may result in a nutritional crisis. The impact of conflict on the nutritional and health status and food security of a population is multifaceted. For example, conflict may disrupt livelihoods and agricultural production. Crops may not be planted because of insecurity or population displacement, increasing food insecurity. Food security is discussed in detail in Chapter 13. Populations may not be able to access preventive or curative health services because of the targeting of health facilities, lack of personnel or medications, and physical barriers to accessing facilities. In some circumstances, populations maybe under siege for extended periods of time without access to regular access to food. Such a situation occurred in Sarajevo from 1992–96 and more recently in Yarmouk refugee camp in Syria in 2013–14 (United Nations Office of the High Commissioner for Human Rights 2014).

There are areas of the world that face chronic emergencies continuing for years or decades. In these complex situations, the cyclic impact of drought with a lack of development, lack of national resources, and high levels of poverty exacerbate the status of already vulnerable populations. In many of these situations, levels of acute malnutrition remain elevated throughout the year and may increase two- or threefold during a humanitarian emergency. The Sahel region of Africa is an example of this type of chronic emergency.

While nutritional crisis is a consequence of many humanitarian emergencies, this is not always the case. For example, following the 2011 Japanese tsunami there was no large-scale nutritional emergency. Similarly, following the earthquake in Haiti in 2010 that devastated Port-au-Prince and the surrounding area, there was no increase in the level of acute malnutrition postearthquake. While preexisting undernutrition (specifically micronutrient malnutrition and chronic malnutrition) persisted, there was no widespread nutritional crisis after the earthquake.

The most commonly used thresholds for defining the severity of a nutritional crisis are a wasting (weight-for-height <−2 z scores) prevalence of 10%–14% for a serious situation and a prevalence of 15% or greater for a critical situation (WHO et al. 2000). These thresholds are based purely on prevalence and do not take into account the context of the situation. There are classification systems that include more than the prevalence of wasting and incorporate crude mortality. Two examples, the Integrated Food Security Phase Classification (IPC) and the IPC for acute malnutrition are increasingly used to define the context in which malnutrition prevalence estimates are occurring (IPC Global Partners 2012). Several of the classification systems used to define the severity of a nutritional crisis are shown in Table 12.2 (Howe and Devereux 2004, IPC Global Partners 2012, WHO et al. 2000).

Two critical indicators that assess the severity and magnitude of a humanitarian crisis at the population level are the crude mortality rate and the prevalence of acute malnutrition among children under five years of age. These two pieces of data are used universally across donor agencies, governments, UN agencies, and NGOs.

Response and Control

Preventing acute malnutrition and mitigating its impact in a population has become a priority during the response to a humanitarian emergency, particularly in the last decade. In many countries there are ongoing public nutrition interventions that have the benefit of preventing acute malnutrition. Often these interventions are supported and implemented by the MoH, in some cases with financial support from UN agencies, donors such as foreign governments, or the World Bank. A country may implement a variety of nutrition programs integrated into the health system. Some examples include infant and young child feeding (IYCF) awareness, nutrition counseling and support, growth monitoring and promotion, micronutrient campaigns, sanitation and hygiene interventions, and deworming. Additional programming may include general food distribution, community and household food security interventions, and livelihoods programs, supported by different entities such as the Ministry of Agriculture, UN agencies, and NGOs.

A number of programs implemented in emergencies to address acute and micronutrient malnutrition, both preventive and curative, are shown in Figure 12.3. The management of acute malnutrition and treatment of specific micronutrient deficiencies are discussed in Chapter 25.

Blanket Supplementary Feeding Programs (BSFP)

One of the most common interventions in emergencies is a Blanket Supplementary Feeding Program (BSFP). This option has become increasingly implemented in the last decade (MAM Taskforce of the Global Nutrition Cluster 2012). Although BSFP should be conducted to prevent malnutrition, BSFP is generally a late intervention like most nutritional interventions in emergency nutrition. The concept of BSFP is to provide extra calories and micronutrients to protect the nutritional status of a vulnerable population. Individuals targeted in this intervention are most often children 6–59 months and pregnant/lactating women. When resources are limited, children 6–23 or 6–36 months of age may be targeted, as they are the most vulnerable to acute malnutrition. When possible, all children 6–59 months should be included (MAM Taskforce of the Global Nutrition Cluster 2012). The ration is distributed on a biweekly or monthly basis. The two types of BSFP are wet and dry. Wet BSFP are implemented only in extreme circumstances, including insecurity where a population would be at risk of attack while transporting dry rations, or in situations where cooking is not an option for the affected population. The development and use of ready-to-use foods has greatly reduced the need of wet BSFP. Where feasible, dry rations are the program option of choice. Dry rations consist of a fortified blended food (FBF) with oil and sugar or in some circumstances an improved FBF for children 6–23 months of age. FBFs are partially precooked milled cereals and pulses such as soya or beans that are fortified with micronutrients (MAM Taskforce of the Global Nutrition Cluster 2012). Improved FBF consists of maize, de-hulled soya beans, dried skimmed milk powder, sugar, vegetable oil, and micronutrients and is formulated to meet the nutritional needs of children 6–23 months of age (MAM Taskforce of the Global Nutrition Cluster 2012). When FBF is distributed, the energy content is typically one thousand calories per person per day. This is higher than the required individual needs, but accounts for sharing at the household level. Medium quantity lipid-based nutrient supplement (LNS) may also be distributed as a dry ration. Medium quantity

Table 12.2 Classification of nutritional and food security emergencies

Source	Classification	Indicator and Threshold
United Nations (UN)	Serious	Wasting 10–14% (<−2 WHZ)
	Critical	Wasting >15% (<−2 WHZ)
Howe Devereux Famine Magnitude Scale	Food security conditions	CMR < 0.2/10,000/day and Wasting <2.3% (<−2 WHZ)
	Food insecurity conditions	CMR >0.2 but <0.5 /10,000/day and/or Wasting >2.3 but <10% (<−2 WHZ)
	Food crisis conditions	CMR >0.5 but <1 /10,000/day and/or Wasting >10 but <20% (<−2 WHZ) and/or edema
	Famine conditions	CMR >1 but <5 /10,000/day and/or Wasting >20 but <40% (<−2 WHZ) and/or edema
	Severe famine conditions	CMR >5 but < 15 /10,000/day and/or Wasting >40 but <40% (<−2 WHZ) and/or edema
	Extreme famine conditions	CMR >15/10,000/day
Integrated Phase Classification 2012	Minimal	CDR <0.5/10,000/day U5DR <1/10,000/day Acute malnutrition <5% (<−2 WHZ and edema)
	Stressed	CDR <0.5/10,000/day U5DR <1/10,000/day Acute Malnutrition 5–10% (<−2 WHZ and edema)
	Crisis	CDR 0.5–1/10,000/day U5DR 1–2 /10,000/day Acute Malnutrition 10–15% or >usual and increasing (<−2 WHZ and edema)
	Emergency	CDR 1–2/10,000/day or >2x reference U5DR 2–4 /10,000/day Acute Malnutrition 15–30% or usual and increasing (<−2 WHZ and edema)
	Famine	CDR >2/10,000/day or >2x reference U5DR >4 /10,000/day Acute Malnutrition >30% (<−2 WHZ and edema)

From: Howe and Devereux 2004, IPC Global Partners 2012, World Health Organization et al. 2000.

LNS is a supplement that comes in a paste form made from peanuts/soy/chick pea, vegetable fat, skimmed milk powder, whey, maltodextrines, and sugar (MAM Taskforce of the Global Nutrition Cluster 2012). Medium quantity LNS is packaged in a pot that contains a one-week ration with energy content of 247 calories per child per day. This is significantly less than a FBF ration, but sharing, in theory, should be reduced as the LNS is prepackaged is ready to consume and does not have to be cooked.

BSFP is implemented when levels of GAM are significantly increased by 20 percent or greater (MAM Taskforce of the Global Nutrition Cluster 2012). They can also be implemented when a general food ration has not yet been implemented. Another scenario for BSFP is during seasonal malnutrition.

Chapter 12: Nutrition

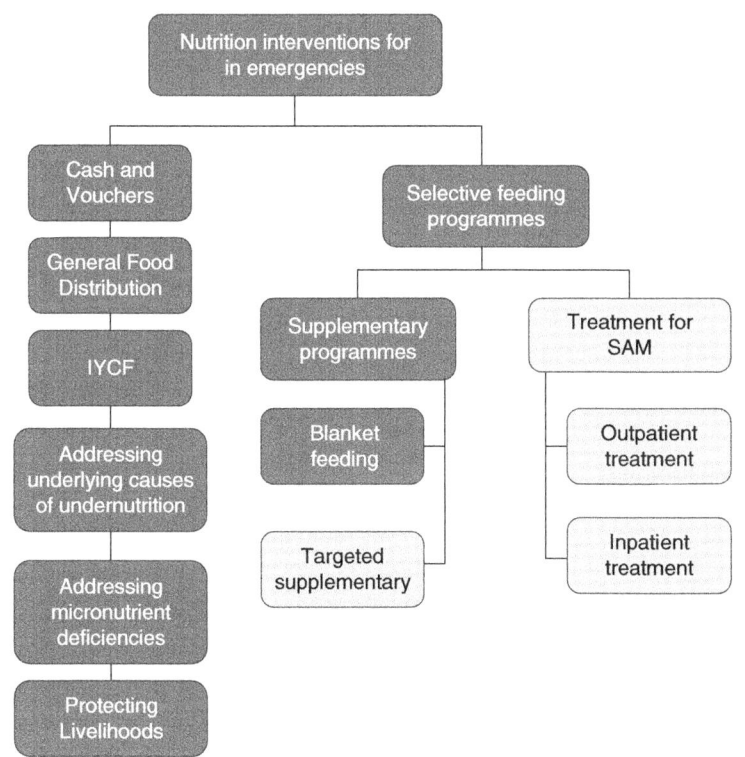

Figure 12.3 Programs implemented in emergencies to address acute and micronutrient malnutrition

As described above, many populations experience cyclic increases in acute malnutrition preceding harvest time. In this context, BSFP is designed to start a month or two before the peak of malnutrition and continue through the lean season. In general, BSFP should be implemented for three to six months with a clear exit strategy designed from the start of the program; however, the context of the situation should dictate the length of the program.

In certain circumstances, non-food aid assistance will have a greater impact on the health and nutritional status of the affected population than the provision of food commodities. Cash and vouchers are now standard practice in emergency response (MAM Taskforce of the Global Nutrition Cluster 2012). Cash and vouchers come in two forms, restricted and unrestricted. Restricted cash and vouchers are designed to be spent on specific commodities, for example, fresh fruits and vegetables, bread, or milling. Additionally, conditionality may require beneficiaries to participate in some type of specified activity, such as an IYCF training session, in order to qualify for the cash. In contrast, unrestricted vouchers have no commodity assigned to them and may be spent on what the household deems the greatest need. The World Food Program is increasingly moving towards vouchers and cash in their general ration distribution programs in place of actual foodstuffs. For this approach to be successful there must be functioning market systems, and the purchasing power of the targeted population must be secure. Food for work is another form of assistance where food is provided in exchange for participation in public work activities such as road construction or digging of canals. These programs are discussed in greater detail in Chapter 13, Food Security.

Infant and Young Child Feeding (IYCF)

IYCF is another type of program that might be implemented during a humanitarian emergency. It is well established that breast milk is the best option for feeding infants as it contains complete nutritional requirements and also is protective against infection (WHO 2004). Therefore, optimal IYCF practices include exclusive breastfeeding, with no provision of water, for six months followed by continued breastfeeding for two years and beyond with timely introduction of appropriate complementary foods, feeding a child three to four small meals a day, and responsive feeding of a child when sick. These IYCF practices may be difficult for the mother to follow for a variety of reasons, including a woman's social status, lack of knowledge and appropriate healthcare, competing priorities of other children, work, and lack of availability of quality and adequate complementary foods.

IYFC has been directly linked to the nutritional status of children less than two years of age (Bhutta et al. 2008, Victora et al. 2008, Golden 1991). Children between 6 and 23 months are most likely to be acutely malnourished after the introduction of complementary foods at six months because the introduction of complementary foods exposes infants to bacteria and other pathogens for the first time, often resulting in diarrhea or other fecal transmitted infections. Malnutrition often occurs in this age group even in populations where food security is not a problem (FAO 2011). Therefore, one way to prevent malnutrition in children under two includes improving the IYCF practices of mothers in order to protect the nutritional status of their children.

IYCF counselling and support includes health workers providing one-on-one consultation with mothers to support them in optimal feeding of infants up to the age of two. IYCF counseling refers to healthcare workers explaining what mothers should do to optimally feed their child and how to do it. IYCF support refers to what healthcare workers do when a problem linked to IYCF arises. This may include lactation support, which can involve physical manipulation to support newborns to latch on to the breast. Lactation support is often needed on a continual basis. IYCF support can also include clinical support for a child under two who is having difficulties with complementary feeding.

IYCF also includes awareness raising activities that are community-level advocacy campaigns to inform households of ideal IYCF practices. Awareness raising activities may include radio messages, billboards, pamphlets, and other informational materials that are distributed. It is important to include grandmothers and fathers who may be critical in household decision-making and can greatly influence how a mother feeds her children. It is important to note that IYCF awareness-raising activities alone have not been proven to have sustainable impact on improving IYCF practices.

During humanitarian emergencies, IYCF counseling, support, and awareness are often conducted. Additionally, special Infant and Young Child Feeding in Emergencies (IYCF-E) interventions should be considered. In humanitarian emergencies, there are often large donations of powdered infant formula (PIF) that are dangerous in settings where sanitation and hygiene conditions do not allow for safe preparation of infant formula. Additionally, the availability of PIF and other breast milk substitutes (BMS) often deter women from breastfeeding, which puts infants at risk since they do not benefit from increased protection from breast milk. In some humanitarian emergencies, there are a large number of orphaned or separated infants due to massive displacement or death. In this case, alternatives to mothers' breast milk needs to be secured. In these rare circumstances, the emergency nutrition response may include provision of BMS for a limited duration to infants who meet strict criteria. Recently, there have been emergencies where large numbers of infants were not breastfed prior to the shock, for example in the Syrian Crisis and its spillover into surrounding countries and Europe. Special programs to address the needs of extremely vulnerable nonbreastfed infants should be developed along with appropriate guidance to provide safer artificial feeding (UNICEF, UNHCR 2015).

Complementary Feeding

With the recognition of the importance of the first one thousand days of life and the lasting nutritional impact of gains and losses during this time period, more attention has been focused on complementary feeding. The time when complementary feeding begins, when a child moves from exclusive breastfeeding to the introduction of foods at 6–9 months of age, corresponds with the peak of acute malnutrition. With the introduction of complementary foods, young children are exposed to pathogens in food and water as well as through the regular development processes of becoming more mobile and mouthing objects. Not specific to emergencies alone, complementary foods are typically void of the very micronutrients and growth promoting essential fatty acids needed for robust linear growth. Many complementary foods are porridges made from staple grains with limited micronutrients and contain inhibitors to absorption of micronutrients. This can be compounded when a population is dependent upon a sole general food ration containing little variety and limited fortified foods. In addition, in this context, the energy density versus stomach capacity of young children may be a contributing factor to malnutrition. Ideally foods would be energy dense in a small quantity. However, in the case of porridges and similar foods, the necessary volume required to meet energy and micronutrient requirements are not achievable in young children.

In response to these challenges, new specialized nutritious foods (SNF) have been developed for children 6–23 months of age. It is important to note, that these SNF are not meant to replace the calories and nutrients received from breastfeeding, but to supplement the overall nutritional intake. SNF includes the improved fortified blended food used in BSFP. It is specifically formulated to meet the needs of children 6–23 months of age. In emergency contexts, this product may be used in either the treatment of moderate acute malnutrition in children 6–59 months or for prevention of acute malnutrition in children 6–23 months.

In addition, there is a second SNF called low-quantity lipid-based nutrient supplements (LNS) that may be used to prevent micronutrient malnutrition and stunting in children 6–23 months of age (UNHCR 2011). These products contain the essential fatty acids and micronutrients necessary for growth in young children that are often missing or insufficient in their diet. The supplement is in the form of a paste and is typically made of peanuts, sugar, vegetable fat, skimmed milk powder, maltodextrin and whey, enriched with various micronutrients. LNS can be mixed into precooked food or consumed directly from the package. In protracted emergency settings, LNS distributions are commonly implemented to attempt to prevent or minimize stunting (UNHCR 2011).

Micronutrient Supplementation

As previously described, micronutrient malnutrition is a significant public health issue in populations affected by humanitarian emergencies. Treatment of clinical micronutrient deficiency diseases is discussed in greater detail in Chapter 25. On a population level, micronutrient supplementation is often put in place when levels of specific deficiencies are reached. Micronutrient supplementation can be carried out with two different SNF, but only one SNF should be used in a population at a time. The first SNF, described above in complimentary feeding, has the dual benefit of providing both micronutrients and essential fatty acids needed for growth. The second option is multiple micronutrient powders (MNP), which is a powdered formulation of 15 vitamins and minerals agreed upon by UNICEF, WHO and WFP. The exact formulation can be adjusted based on the context. For example, the vitamin A content may be reduced if vitamin A fortified oil is distributed to the population. MNP may be distributed at health centers by healthcare providers, purchased in the private market, or distributed through community-level campaigns.

In addition to MNP, single micronutrient supplements are even more widely used for prevention of malnutrition. The most common supplements include: iron and folic acid (IFA), vitamin A, iodine supplements, B vitamins, and vitamin C. Iron deficiency and anemia are extremely common worldwide due to inadequate intake of iron-rich foods, including animal sourced protein, as well as from common infections. Iron tablets or iron and folic acid supplements are commonly given to pregnant and lactating women through health centers. Vitamin A deficiency is common due to a lack of intake of vitamin A rich foods such as green leafy vegetables and noncitrus orange fruits and vegetables. Vitamin A supplementation is also known to reduce mortality associated with specific diseases, particularly measles (Bhutta et al. 2008). Vitamin A supplements are widely used in prevention activities and are often distributed household to household during polio or measles vaccination campaigns, ideally twice per year. Iodine supplements, in the form of oil capsules, are distributed in areas where iodine deficiency or goiter is common. More commonly, iodized salt is provided as part of a general food ration. In these settings, salt should always be iodized. Fortification of general food rations with B vitamins is considered best practice to prevent the development of pellagra and beriberi that results from deficiencies of niacin (B3) and thiamine (B1), respectively. Finally, vitamin C deficiency, which manifests as scurvy in its extreme form, can be prevented through vitamin C supplement distribution, but these are expensive and not common. More common is encouraging or facilitating access to vitamin C rich foods such as citrus fruits.

Notes from the Field

Africa (2016)

In 2016, the effects of El Niño in Southern Africa resulted in severe drought conditions in eleven countries, negatively impacting the communities dependent on rain-fed agriculture. Nearly 21 million people were estimated to be in need of emergency food assistance due to El Niño and a poor harvest in 2014/15 and half-million children were suffering from severe acute malnutrition. Chronic vulnerability due to poverty, ongoing effects of climate change, and high levels of HIV/AIDS have historically contributed to high levels of stunting in many parts of these countries, but acute malnutrition was limited to small pockets in southern Madagascar and Angola. Due to the anticipated increase in acute malnutrition, Angola, Lesotho, Madagascar, Malawi, Mozambique, Swaziland, and Zimbabwe started to support increased nutritional surveillance, worked with Ministries of Health in order to support capacity around preventing undernutrition, supported the scale-up of the Community Management of Acute Malnutrition (CMAM), and worked to ensure that food security and nutrition indicators were linked to programming. As of August 2016, 52,000 children in the seven countries had been treated for acute malnutrition.

Conclusion

?A3B2 tlsb -0.01w?>Despite the evidence linking malnutrition to infection, and implementation of programs to address both of the immediate causes of malnutrition (disease and inadequate diet), malnutrition often remains incorrectly associated solely with food availability at a macro level. As a result, food continues to be the main form of humanitarian assistance in humanitarian emergencies. In the past, the US and other governments supported grain surpluses through the provision of subsidies, and excess food was shipped to developing countries. More recently the Office of Food for Peace (FFP), within USAID, provides this food to different agencies in receiving countries for distribution. WFP remains the main UN body responsible for receiving food aid from FFP and distribution through NGOs. Recently, there has been a shift towards local purchasing and cash and voucher programs for beneficiaries in place of general food distributions. This is discussed in greater detail in Chapter 13. Additionally, there is emphasis on integrating health and nutrition programming to achieve maximum effectiveness.

References

Action Contre La Faim International. 2010. Taking action. Nutrition for survival, growth and development, white paper.

Bhutta, Z. A., Ahmed, T., Black, R. E., Cousens, S., Dewey, K., Giugliani, E., Haider, B. A., Kirkwood, B., Morris, S. S., Sachdev, H. P., and Shekar, M. Maternal & Child Undernutrition Study Group. (2008). What works? Interventions for maternal and child undernutrition and survival. *Lancet*, **371**, 417–440.

Bilukha, O., Prudhon, C., Moloney, G., Hailey, P., and Doledec, D. (2012). Measuring anthropometric indicators through nutrition surveillance in humanitarian settings: Options, issues, and ways forward. *Food Nutr Bull*, **33**, 169–176.

Black, M. M., Walker, S. P., Wachs, T. D., Ulkuer, N., Gardner, J. M., Grantham-McGregor, S., Lozoff, B., Engle, P. L., and De Mello, M. C. 2008a. Policies to reduce undernutrition include child development. *Lancet*, **371**, 454–455.

Black, R. E., Allen, L. H., Bhutta, Z. A., Caulfield, L. E., De Onis, M., Ezzati, M., and Mathers, C., Rivera, J., Maternal & Child Undernutrition Study Group. (2008b). Maternal and child undernutrition: Global and regional exposures and health consequences. *Lancet*, **371**, 243–260.

Black, R. E., Victora, C. G., Walker, S. P., Bhutta, Z. A., Christian, P., De Onis, M., Ezzati, M., Grantham-McGregor, S., Katz, J., Martorell, R., and Uauy, R. Maternal & Child Nutrition Study Group. (2013). Maternal and child undernutrition and overweight in low-income and middle-income countries. *Lancet*, **382**, 427–451.

Bryce, J., Coitinho, D., Darnton-Hill, I., Pelletier, D., and Pinstrup-Andersen, P., Maternal & Child Undernutrition Study Group. (2008). Maternal and child undernutrition: effective action at national level. *Lancet*, **371**, 510–526.

Collins, S., Dent, N., Binns, P., Bahwere, P., Sadler, K., and Hallam, A. (2006). Management of severe acute malnutrition in children. *Lancet*, **368**, 1992–2000.

Compton J, Wiggins S., and Keats S. (2010). *Impact of the global food crisis on the Poor: What is the evidence?* London, UK: Overseas Development Institute. Available at: www.odi.org/publications/5187-impact-global-food-crisis-poor-evidence. (Accessed on July 17, 2017).

Food and Agricultural Organization (2011). *Complementary feeding for children 6–23 months*. Food and Agricultural Organization; Rome, Italy.

Golden, M. H. (1991). The nature of nutritional deficiency in relation to growth failure and poverty. *Acta Paediatr Scand Supplement*, **374**, 95–110.

Golden, M. H. (1995). Specific deficiencies versus growth failure: Type I and Type II nutrients. *Scn News*, **12** 10–14.

Goossens S. B. Y., Yun, O., Harczi, G., Ouannes, M. et al. (2012). Mid-upper arm circumference based nutrition programming: evidence for a new approach in regions with high burden of acute malnutrition. *Plos One*. Available at: https://doi.org/10.1371/journal.pone.0049320. (Accessed on July 17, 2017).

Gorstein, J., Sullivan, K. M., Parvanta, I., and Begin, F. (2007). *Indicators and methods for cross-sectional surveys of vitamin and mineral status of populations.* The micronutrient initiative (Ottawa) and the Centers for Disease Control and Prevention (Atlanta).

Grijalva-Eternod, C. S., Wells, J. C., Cortina-Borja, M., Salse-Ubach, N., Tondeur, M. C., Dolan, C., Meziani, C., Wilkinson, C., Spiegel, P., and Seal, A. J.. (2012). The double burden of obesity and malnutrition in a protracted emergency setting: a cross-sectional study of Western Sahara refugees. *Plos Med*, **9**, E1001320. Available at: https://doi.org/10.1371/journal.pmed.1001320. (Accessed on July 17, 2017).

Howe, P. and Devereux, S. (2004). Famine intensity and magnitude scales: A proposal for an instrumental definition of famine. *Disasters*, **28**, 353–372.

Inter-Agency Standing Committee. (2012). Multi-cluster/sector initial rapid assessment (MIRA). *Provisional Version March 2012.* Inter-Agency Standing Committee; Geneva, Switzerland.

IPC Global Partners. 2012. *Integrated food security phase classification technical manual. Version 2.0. Evidence and standards for better food security decisions.* FAO; Rome, Italy. Available at: www.ipcinfo.org/fileadmin/user_upload/ipcinfo/docs/ipc-manual-2-interactive.pdf. (Accessed on July 17, 2017).

Kerac, M., McGrath, M., Grijalva-Eternod, C., Bizouerne, C., Saxton, J., Bailey, H., Wilkinson, C., Hirsch, J., Blencowe, H., Shoham, J., and Seal, A. (2010). Management of acute malnutrition in infants (MAMI) project. Summary report. Available at: http://reliefweb.int/sites/reliefweb.int/files/resources/8A7E77D26B35660F492576F70010D7DF-mami-report-complete.pdf. (Accessed on July 17, 2017).

Khara, T. and Dolan, C. (2014). *Technical briefing paper; Associations between wasting and stunting, policy, programming and research implications.* Emergency Nutrition Network; London, England. Available at: http://files.ennonline.net/attachments/1862/WAST_140714.pdf. (Accessed on July 17, 2017)

Makoka, D. and Masibo, P. K. (2015) Is there a threshold level of maternal education sufficient to reduce child malnutrition: Evidence from Malawi, Tanzania and Zimbabwe, *BMC Pediatrics*,**15**(96), 1–10.

MAM Taskforce of The Global Nutrition Cluster (2012). *Moderate acute malnutrition: A decision tool for emergencies.* Global Nutrition Cluster; Geneva, Switzerland.

Morris, S. S., Cogill, B., and Uauy, R., Maternal & Child Undernutrition Study, G. (2008). Effective international action against undernutrition: Why has it proven so difficult and what can be done to accelerate progress? *Lancet*, **371**, 608–621.

Nichols, E. K., Talley, L. E., Birungi, N., McClelland, A., Madraa, E., Chandia, A. B., Nivet, J., Flores-Ayala, R., and Serdula, M. K. (2013). Suspected outbreak of riboflavin deficiency among populations reliant on food assistance: A case study of drought-stricken Karamoja, Uganda, 2009–2010. *Plos One*, **8**, E62976. Available at: http://journals.plos.org/plosone/article?id=10.1371/journal.pone.0062976. (Accessed on July 17, 2017).

Nutritionworks, Emergency Nutrition Network, and The Global Nutrition Cluster. (2011). Module 4: Micronutrient malnutrition. Part 2 technical note, in *The harmonised training package (HTP): Resource material for training on nutrition in emergencies, Version 2.* Global Nutrition Cluster; Geneva, Switzerland.

Olofin, I., McDonald, C. M., Ezzati, M., Flaxman, S., Black, R. E., Fawzi, W. W., Caulfield, L. E., Danaei, G., and Nutrition Impact Model, S. (2013). Associations of suboptimal growth with all-cause and cause-specific mortality in children under five years: A pooled analysis of ten prospective studies. *Plos One*, **8**, E64636. Available at: http://journals.plos.org/plosone/article?id=10.1371/journal.pone.0064636. (Accessed on July 17, 2017).

Salama, P., Assefa, F., Talley, L., Spiegel, P., Van Der Veen, A., and Gotway, C. A. (2001). Malnutrition, Measles, mortality, and the humanitarian response during a famine in Ethiopia. *JAMA*, **286**, 563–571.

Schaible Ue, K. S. (2007). Malnutrition and infection: Complex mechanisms and global impacts. *Plos One*, **4**, E115. Available at: www.ncbi.nlm.nih.gov/pubmed/17472433. (Accessed on July 17, 2017).

SMART Technical Advisory Group. (2006). Measuring mortality, nutritional status, and food security in crisis situations: Smart methodology. *Version 1.* Available at: http://smartmethodology.org/. (Accessed on July 17, 2017).

United Nations Children's Fund, World Health Organization and the World Bank. (2017). *UNICEF-WHO-World Bank Joint Child Malnutrition Estimates.* UNICEF; New York, USA. Available at: http://www.who.int/nutgrowthdb/jme_brochoure2017.pdf?ua=1

United Nations Children's Fund, United Nations High Commissioner for Refugees, Save the Children and Emergency Nutrition Network. (2015) *Interim Operational Considerations for the feeding support of Infants and Young Children under 2 years of age in refugee and migrant transit settings in Europe.* UNICEF; New York. Available at: www.ennonline.net/interimconsiderationsiycftransit. (Accessed on July 17, 2017).

United Nations High Commissioner For Refugees. (2011). *UNHCR Operational Guidance on the Use of Special Nutritional Products to Reduce Micronutrient Deficiencies And Malnutrition In Refugee Populations.* United Nations High Commissioner For Refugees; Geneva, Switzerland.

United Nations Office Of The High Commissioner For Human Rights. (2014). Living under siege. The Syrian Arab Republic. Available at: www.ohchr.org/Documents/Countries/SY/LivingUnderSiege.pdf. (Accessed on July 17, 2017).

United Nations System Standing Committee on Nutrition (2010). Chapter 3: Maternal nutrition and the intergenerational cycle of growth failure, in *Sixth report on the world nutrition situation.* United Nations System Standing Committee on Nutrition; Geneva, Switzerland.

Ververs, M. T., Antierens, A., Sackl, A., Staderini, N., and Captier, V. (2013). Which anthropometric indicators identify a pregnant woman as acutely malnourished and predict adverse birth outcomes in the humanitarian context? *Plos Current Disasters.* Available at: http://currents.plos.org/disasters/article/which-anthropometric-indicators-identify-a-pregnant-woman-as-acutely-malnourished-and-predict-adverse-birth-outcomes-in-the-humanitarian-context. (accessed on July 17, 2017).

Victora, C. G., Adair, L., Fall, C., Hallal, P. C., Martorell, R., Richter, L., and Sachdev, H. S. (2008). Maternal & Child Undernutrition Study, G. Maternal and child undernutrition: consequences for adult health and human capital. *Lancet,* **371,** 340–357.

Walia, I., Kalia, R., and Chopra, S. (2009). Initiation of breast feeding – the cultural factors. *Nursing And Midwifery Research Journal,* **5,** 10–18.

World Food Health Organization. (2009). *Emergency Food Security Assessment Handbook (Efsa) – 2nd Edition.* World Food Programme: Rome, Italy.

World Health Organization. (2004). *Guiding principles for feeding infants and young children during emergencies.* World Health Organization; Geneva, Switzerland.

World Health Organization. (2017a). Nutrition: Micronutrients deficiencies. Iron Deficiency anemia. Available at: www.who.int/nutrition/topics/ida/en/. (Accessed on July 17, 2017).

World Health Organization. (2017b). Nutrition: Micronutrient Deficiencies. Vitamin A deficiency. Available at: www.who.int/nutrition/topics/vad/en/ (Accessed on July 17, 2017).

World Health Organization. (2017c). Media CENTRE: Obesity and overweight. Available at: www.who.int/mediacentre/factsheets/fs311/en/. (Accessed on July 17, 2017).

World Health Organization Multicentre Growth Reference Study Group. (2006). *WHO child growth standards: Length/height-for-age, weight-for-age, weight-for-length, weight-for-height and body mass index-for-age; methods and development.* World Health Organization: Geneva, Switzerland.

World Health Organization, United Nations High Commissioner for Refugees, International Federation of Red Cross and Red Crescent Societies, and World Food Programme. (2000). *The Management of nutrition in major emergencies.* World Health Organization; Geneva, Switzerland.

Chapter 13

Food Security

Silke Pietzsch, Leisel E. Talley, and Carlos Navarro-Colorado

Introduction

This chapter provides an introduction and overview of food security in the context of humanitarian emergencies. Important concepts include a review of the current environment of global food security, the commonly used framework and concept of food security, and its four pillars, as well as considerations for interventions as part of food security during an emergency response. Nutrition and Malnutrition are discussed in Chapters 13 and 28 respectively.

Global Food Security

Food security is an important yet continually debated topic. Since its foundation in 1945, the United Nations Food and Agriculture Organization (FAO) has been responsible for the fight against hunger and food security for all. FAO has provided the globally used definition of food security for the humanitarian community. In this definition, food security exists when all people, at all times, have physical, social, and economic access to sufficient safe and nutritious food that meets their dietary needs and food preferences for an active and healthy life (FAO 1996).

This definition is widely used and sets forth the complexity of food security on the individual and household level, across cultures, gender, and different contexts. Its linkages to human nutrition, health, and livelihoods are relevant and important. Food security can be chronic, seasonal, or transitory in nature, and can affect individuals, households, communities, countries or regions, independently from each other or collectively at the same time.

The global situation of food security has made only modest progress in recent years. Preventing undernutrition – acute malnutrition, chronic malnutrition and growth failure, and micronutrient deficiencies, – is a key objective in food security.

The latest *State of Food Security and Nutrition in the World*, is the first of its kind combining food security and nutrition data since the establishment of the 2030 Agenda for Sustainable Development. The second Sustainable Development Goal (SDG 2) is defined as "by 2030, end hunger and ensure access by all people, in particular the poor and people in vulnerable situations, including infants, to safe, nutritious and sufficient food all year round" (UN, 2014). The presentation of this more holistic approach of nutrition security, combining food security and nutrition indicators to bring overall attention to the ultimate goal of nutritionally secure populations, provides a comprehensive view on the world's state of undernourishment and food insecurity.

After a decline of the total global numbers of hungry and undernourished people in the world until 2015, a significant increase has been observed in 2016. The most recent estimates indicate that global undernourishment increased in 2016 and now affects 815 million people, up from 777 million in 2015. In the spring of 2017, a number of countries reached extreme levels of hunger, with a famine declared in areas of South Sudan and warnings of high risk of famine issued for three other countries (northeast Nigeria, Somalia and Yemen) (FAO, 2017).

The term hunger is often used interchangeably with undernutrition and food insecurity. Rather than being the same concept, a causal relationship between these concepts should be established, with food insecurity contributing to hunger and undernourishment. Hunger usually refers to the discomfort experienced and associated with a lack of food. Often it is defined as food deprivation or the consumption of fewer than 2,100 kilocalories a day, the minimum that most people require to live a healthy and productive life. A number of different indicators can be used to measure hunger. To reflect the multidimensional nature of hunger, the International Food Policy Research Institute's (IFPRI) Global Hunger Index combines the three equally weighted indicators of undernourishment, child underweight, and child mortality. The multidimensional approach to hunger reflects the

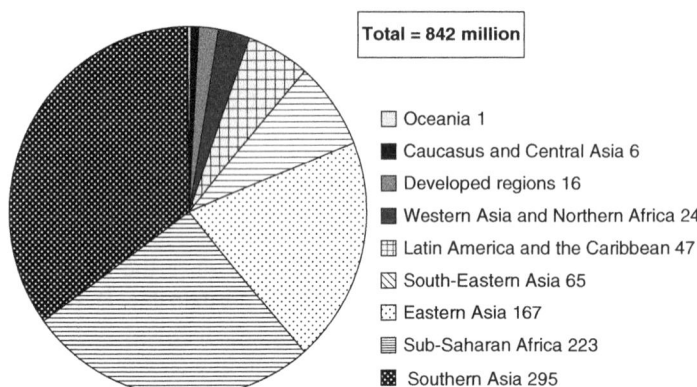

Figure 13.1 Undernourishment globally from 2000 to 2016, in millions of people (FAO, 2017)

nutrition situation not only of the population as a whole, but also of a physiologically vulnerable group, children, for whom a lack of nutrients leads to a high risk of illness, poor physical and cognitive development, or death. In addition, by combining independently measured indicators, the effects of random measurement errors is reduced (von Grebmer et al. 2016).

Food insecurity, however, is not the sole underlying cause for hunger and undernutrition, but rather a contributing factor, depending on the local context. Often, food security is oversimplified and reduced to agriculture, but in reality food security and livelihoods involve a much more complex interaction of activities, linkages, networks, productive assets, natural resources and results of human productivity. Livelihood systems of households and communities have an intrinsic contribution to their food security and the ability to provide food for all household or community members to lead healthy and productive lives. In a well-functioning livelihood system, households and communities are food secure and have sufficient and adequate food available and accessible throughout the year.

During humanitarian emergencies, livelihood can be negatively affected due to loss of productive assets such as land, animals, or equipment, or reduced access to markets, or suppliers of raw materials and inputs. Disasters can be rapid or slow onset, short- or long-term, often leading to an interruption of the local livelihood systems, resulting in food insecurity, hunger, and consequently undernutrition. Households or communities with strong resilience capacities will be better able to cope with a shock during humanitarian emergencies than those who are more vulnerable to the consequences of disasters such as floods, droughts, displacement and epidemics.

To help households and communities better cope with threats to food security, governments in many countries have established policies and systems to prevent and address food insecurity and food crises. National grain and agriculture reserves designed to provide free or subsidized grain for vulnerable and disaster affected populations are well established in most countries of the world. Social protection systems and safety nets exist to provide reliable and timely transfer of food or cash to the most vulnerable populations. These transfers are facilitated through variety of schemes for households suffering from chronic and acute emergencies. Examples of this type of social protection system and safety nets can be found in Kenya, Ethiopia, India, and Pakistan, Fiji and many more places. Often the targeted population is preregistered within the government system as part of contingency planning and emergency preparedness in order to facilitate easy access and transfers during a humanitarian emergency. These already established systems can enable a timely and comprehensive response throughout the emergency.

Four Pillars of Food Security

The concept of food security is broken down into four pillars including availability of food, access to food, utilization of food, and stability of food throughout the year (FAO 2006a). These components are detailed

Table 13.1 The 4 pillars of food security

Availability of Food [Quality & Quantity]	Access to Food (Economical & Physical)	Utilization of Food	Stability of Food
National level; Food supplies, production for the market, commercial food imports and food assistance.	Ability to acquire appropriate food for a nutritious diet through self-supply, purchase, exchange or social transfers (e.g., government).	Intra-household food behavior patterns: food choice and demand, preparation, allocation, storage, etc.	Continuity and duration of access and availability to nutritious food, through production and stocks/storage, food purchase, and social transfers/government, ideally 12 months/year.
Household level: Physical existence of adequate quantity and quality of food for all family members through production or trade	Depending on income and prices and distant and distribution of available resources (purchasing power and access to service).	Biological patterns: ability of body to take in and use food for absorption and growth, physical activity, metabolism and storage within the body, care and hygiene practices, access to water and sanitation	Hampered by the duration of the annual lean season, e.g., 3 months per year. Resilience of households to cope with shortages throughout the year.

in static and dynamic determinants. The four pillars of food security are shown in Table 13.1 and described in the following sections.

Availability of Food

This refers to the physical existence of food in sufficient quantity and quality, meaning balanced and nutritious foods providing needed proportions of carbohydrates, protein, fat and micronutrients, on either an individual, household, local market, country, or regional level. A reduction in availability of food at the household level can be caused by a loss of agricultural production that may lead to a reduction in consumption, loss of income, loss of access to markets, and bartering power. Availability of food at the household level is often seasonally influenced by production and consumption and linked to the agriculture cycle and rainy season. When availability of food in the market is not sufficient, households who do not produce food may not be able to access food in the market due to scarcity and increasing prices. Individual food availability can be influenced by a lack of food for the overall household, and prioritization of household members to eat, i.e. children and pregnant or lactating women who receive before the other household members. Individual lack of food availability can contribute to undernourishment and nutritional deficiencies in this individual.

Accessibility of Food

This refers to the economic and physical ability to obtain food from the market in sufficient quality and quantity. Economic access refers to the household's purchasing power influenced by the portion of household income that is available to purchase food from the local or national market. Economic access to food is influenced by a household's livelihood and income generating activities, and available income, and financial means. If the household loses its sources of income, such as employment, sale of produce, or exchange of produce, as a result of an emergency, their access to food is jeopardized, and with it, the household's food security. Even if food is available from the local market, a household may be food insecure if it does not have economic access to food due to high food prices. Market prices tend to fluctuate with the seasons, being lowest post-harvest with high supply, and highest in the lean- and pre-harvest season with low supplies. This is a normal market demand-and-supply-dynamic, where a high demand and low supply drives up local prices. In an emergency or a strong lean season, with a possible rupture of supply due to a halt in the agriculture production or due to a regions cut-off from transport, poor and vulnerable households may experience food insecurity due to lack of purchasing power. Physical access to food may be restricted by the local road system and distance to markets. During an emergency, roads might be impassable due to floods or conflict; therefore a household's access to food in the market might be interrupted. Similarly, physical access influenced by social norms might prevent individuals and households from going to the market, i. e. female or child headed households, displaced households, etc.

Availability and accessibility of food are intrinsically linked with one influencing the other though market linkages plus demand and supply dynamics. Both availability and accessibility occur at the household and community level linked to local, regional, national, and global markets and production dynamics scenarios. Over the last decade, particularly since 2008 with the world food price crisis, more attention is being given to the influence that market prices and subsidies have on household food security and how these can be influenced and regulated through national food trade, subsidies, safety nets and markets.

Utilization of Food

This refers to the utilization, preparation, and intake of food at the individual and household level. At the individual level, food utilization or intake may be influenced by cultural and traditional norms, gender and religious practices. Individual food utilization also includes individual digestion and absorption capacities that has an influence on the person's nutritional status. The ability of an individual's gut to absorb nutrients may be reduced by acute and chronic diseases, nutritional deficiencies and environmental factors. At the household level, food utilization includes the choice of food and its preparation, which define the macro- and micronutrient intake of an individual.

The intrahousehold distribution, feeding practices and food taboos, especially of children less than five years of age, and of pregnant and lactating women, also play a large role in utilization of food, individual food insecurity and undernourishment. Intrahousehold distribution of food and priority eating between men, women, adults, and children is well known and varies by community. It may have significant impact on the nutritional and food security status of an individual. In certain contexts, communal sharing of food on a larger level may contribute to food insecurity on the community and household level. The context, including local circumstances, are important factors that need investigation to gain a clear understanding to ensure the most appropriate food security intervention is designed and implemented during a particular humanitarian emergency.

Accessibility and availability of food as well as the knowledge of the decision maker or caretaker in the household influence the choice and preparation of food. Consumption of healthy and nutritious food is dependent on the availability of clean, safe water and sanitary systems, to prevent the transmission of food and water-borne diseases. Water, sanitation and hygiene (WASH) are discussed in Chapter 12.

Stability of Food Supply

This refers to accessibility, availability, and utilization of food focusing on their continuity throughout the year. Many food and livelihood systems exhibit seasonal variations. In the best-case scenario there are sufficient foods available throughout the year that may be substituted for one another depending on the season, including wild foods. Unfortunately, there are often seasons where the overall amount of available or accessible food is significantly reduced, resulting in seasonal hunger and undernourishment. The recognition of seasonal hunger as an important contributor to food insecurity and undernutrition has gained significant importance in contextual analysis and response planning for the mitigation of seasonal, chronic, and protracted crises (ACF 2009). Seasonal hunger, food insecurity, and undernutrition are foreseeable and preventable; therefore good food security and nutrition information and surveillance systems are of utmost importance for successful crisis prevention, mitigation, and interventionSeasonal social protection systems and safety nets can play an important role to stabilize food availability and access throughout the year.

Risks to Food Security

During a humanitarian emergency, these four pillars might be threatened to different degrees, creating food insecurity on a household level only, or on a community or country level. Conflict, natural disasters, policy failure, and epidemics may cause

Table 13.2 Risks and effect on livelihood and impact on food security

Risk	Effect on livelihoods	Impact on food security
Conflict	Restricted movements for access to fields and farms; restricted livestock movements due to insecurity and displacement resulting in reduced productivity; loss of assets or access to assets due to displacement; destruction/looting of productive assets like agriculture fields or livestock; restricted access to markets and services; increased coping to cover household needs hence increased asset depletion.	Reduced availability of food due to reduced productivity; reduced access to food due to lack of income, lack of access to markets for sale, purchase and exchange; changes in food utilization due to reduced food sources; hampered food stability due to lack of availability and access depending on length of civil thrive and displacement.
Natural Disasters (floods, droughts, volcanoes)	Loss or destruction of productive assets due to disaster itself or displacement due to disaster; resulting in reduced household productivity; restricted access to markets and services; increased coping activities to cater for household food and livelihood needs.	Reduced availability of food due to reduced productivity; reduced access to food due to lack of income, lack of access to markets or availability of food in markets; changes in food utilization; hampered food stability.
Strong or extended seasonality	Vulnerable households have low shock absorption capacity due to already depleted productive assets and livelihoods during previous and extended shocks and lean seasons; livelihood cope capacity is low.	Lack of coping capacity impacts on availability and access to food through own productivity, exchange or purchasing powers. Lack of coping capacity will expose the households to increased food insecurity, seasonal hunger and undernutrition, which may deteriorate to permanent manifestations.
Policy failure, maybe linked to a disaster	Government strategic reserves and social mismanaged or unavailable for support during emergencies or lean season; food subsidies are not well targeted and monitored; farmer insurance systems do not function appropriately.	Regular and reliable food transfers as part of a social protection safety net or subsidies are not available; insurance does not compensate for farmers' loss; therefore both are impacting on the households' coping

widespread disruption of the local food systems resulting in food insecurity at various levels from individual to country level (FAO 2013b). The severity of the annual lean season, facing food shortages every year once households' harvest and food stocks are depleted, can contribute to the risk factors for communities and households. Compared to natural disasters like floods and earthquakes, annual lean seasons are more predictable, and deterioration to a large-scale emergency level is thus potentially more easily preventablethrough systematic interventions like social protection and safety nets.

Emergencies can have different impacts on food and livelihoods systems, and will result in different productive outcomes and influences for each of the four pillars above. Similarly, different communities and households, in the same geographical area, affected by an emergency, might be affected in different ways depending on their resilience capacity, livelihood, and wealth profile. Table 13.2 shows a number of risks and their effect on livelihood and impact on food security.

Availability of Food

Conflict may prevent famers and pastoralists from accessing their fields or driving their animals to pasture grounds, which may result in a decreased productivity or even loss of their livelihoods assets including fields, plantations, and animals. This may happen due to the inability to use the asset due to household displacement, lack of safe access to the agriculture fields or plantations, or the destruction of the assets itself including killing of animals. Natural disasters (droughts, floods, hurricanes, and volcanic eruptions) can affect food availability through destruction of assets. Biological disasters such as locust swarms and epidemics of animal diseases can also affect these assets. Lastly, slow but continuous depletion of assets due to recurrent or chronic disasters such as droughts or hurricanes, and a lack of rehabilitation or recovery time in between recurrent shocks, may contribute to an overall loss or change of livelihood systems.

Accessibility of Food

Similar to availability of food, accessibility of food may be hampered by conflict through destruction of infrastructure and reduced access for farmers to bring their produce to market or households going to the market to buy food. In humanitarian emergencies populations displaced by conflict might be trapped in hiding and cut off from markets or relief provisions. Natural disaster might result in loss of harvest and subsequent unavailability of food that in turn increases the prices on the market. This will reduce the economic access for food to households, especially those with low or decreased purchasing power. The purchasing power of a household is likely to decrease with loss of productive assets and household production as a result of disaster or emergency.

Availability and accessibility to food are closely linked and threats to one often affect the other. Investment in recovery post emergency is essential to establish shock-absorptive livelihoods, which can thrive and evolve in their given environmental context. National social protection and safety nets are crucial in these situations to support recovery and protect chronically vulnerable households and their livelihoods.

Utilization of Food

Utilization of food is affected by restrictions to the availability and accessibility to food during normal and emergency situations. A reduced amount of the quality and quantity of food will influence the choice and preparation of food at the household level, and likely influence the intra-household distribution. During humanitarian emergencies there may be reduced meal intake, reduced dietary diversity and reduction of particular micro- and macronutrient intake. This will have an impact on the nutrition and health status of the population. For example, drought may reduce the available milk in pastoral households as the available grazing land and water sources for livestock are diminished. Floods or hurricanes could destroy an entire garden making fresh vegetables and fruits inaccessible to the household.

In addition, during humanitarian emergencies priorities for food allocations on household level may shift from working male members of the household, to children, the elderly, and the sick. The latter groups might be prioritized to ensure their mobility during movements associated with displacement. Displaced populations may have insufficient access to fire fuel due to insecurity, limited access to the forest, or lack of purchasing power resulting in altered preparation of food at the household level affecting the quality, quantity, and digestibility of the food.

Lastly, the breakdown in sanitary conditions often seen during humanitarian emergencies may have an impact on the safety of food consumed. For example, floods and hurricanes may have a major impact on water quality and sanitary conditions, requiring additional attention to hygiene needs, waterborne diseases, and disease control and prevention on community, household, and individual levels.

Stability of Food Supply

The stability of the food supply is often interrupted during humanitarian emergencies. As a result of threats to availability and accessibility of food, lack of stability of the food supply might result in a household not being able to meet its food needs throughout the year. Often, this affects the most vulnerable and poorest households and individuals challenged to cover their annual food needs already in a normal year. Humanitarian emergencies like influence the food security of households through reduced food availability when household and community food stocks run out, or when reduced availability on the markets leads to increased food prices, making food inaccessible for the most vulnerable households due to limited purchasing power. When this occurs, a household will struggle in its capacity to cover its food requirements and provide sufficient quality and quantity of food to the household members. In these situations, a household's productive asset base influences the accessibility and availability of food through coping activities. Coping involves

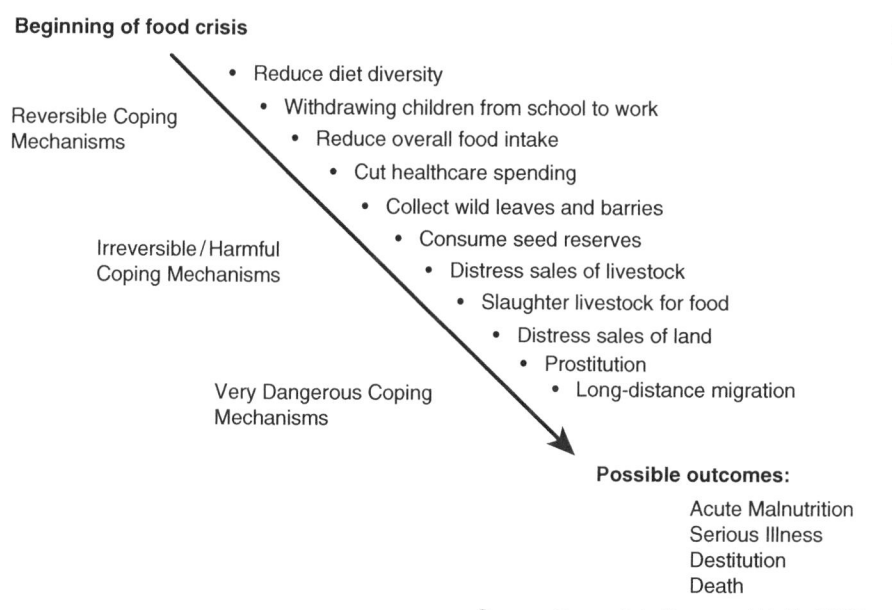

Figure 13.2 Household coping activities (ACF 2009)

selling productive assets to gain additional purchasing power to cover the food gap, as shown in Figure 13.2.

Some degree of coping is normal, integrated into livelihood strategies, and is generally reversible after a lean season, such as the selling of one goat. Most communities and households are accustomed to a gap in the stability of their food supply and have established temporary or longer lasting coping mechanisms with which they are able to provide a minimum of food to the community and households throughout the year. Other situations require additional degrees of coping, which might be irreversible due to the severity of the impact on the households' livelihood, such as selling productive land. In a situation such as a humanitarian emergency, where the household is no longer able to cope, additional external assistance is required to ensure survival.

Challenges in Food Security

Food insecurity is complex and should not be considered as a standalone phenomenon. Acute or chronic food insecurity can have long lasting impact on the livelihoods, security, level of poverty, and development at-large of individuals and the population. A household in a dire situation, unable to meet minimum food requirements, will need to make decisions on intrahousehold food allocations that can be life and death decisions.

Food Insecurity, Nutrition and Health

Food insecurity is directly linked with undernutrition and mortality. The food security of each household member and the provision of sufficient and adequate foods for intake are major challenges in humanitarian emergencies. Children under five years of age, pregnant and lactating mothers, and the elderly and chronically ill all have increased and specific food and nutritional needs. In addition, health and nutrition have an impact on people's physical well-being and productivity necessary to successfully implement livelihood strategies such as agriculture labor. These needs must be considered in any response; linkages of nutrition and health are of utmost importance in the discussion of food security.

Food Security and Livelihood Resilience

Resilience includes the ability of a household to prevent and mitigate disasters, as well as to anticipate, absorb, adapt to, and recover from them in a timely, efficient, and sustainable manner. This includes protecting, restoring, and improving livelihood systems in the face of threats that impact agriculture, food and nutrition, and related public health infrastructure (FAO 2013b).

The more resilient a household, the more likely the household has sufficient capacities, often in the form

Section 2: Public Health Principles

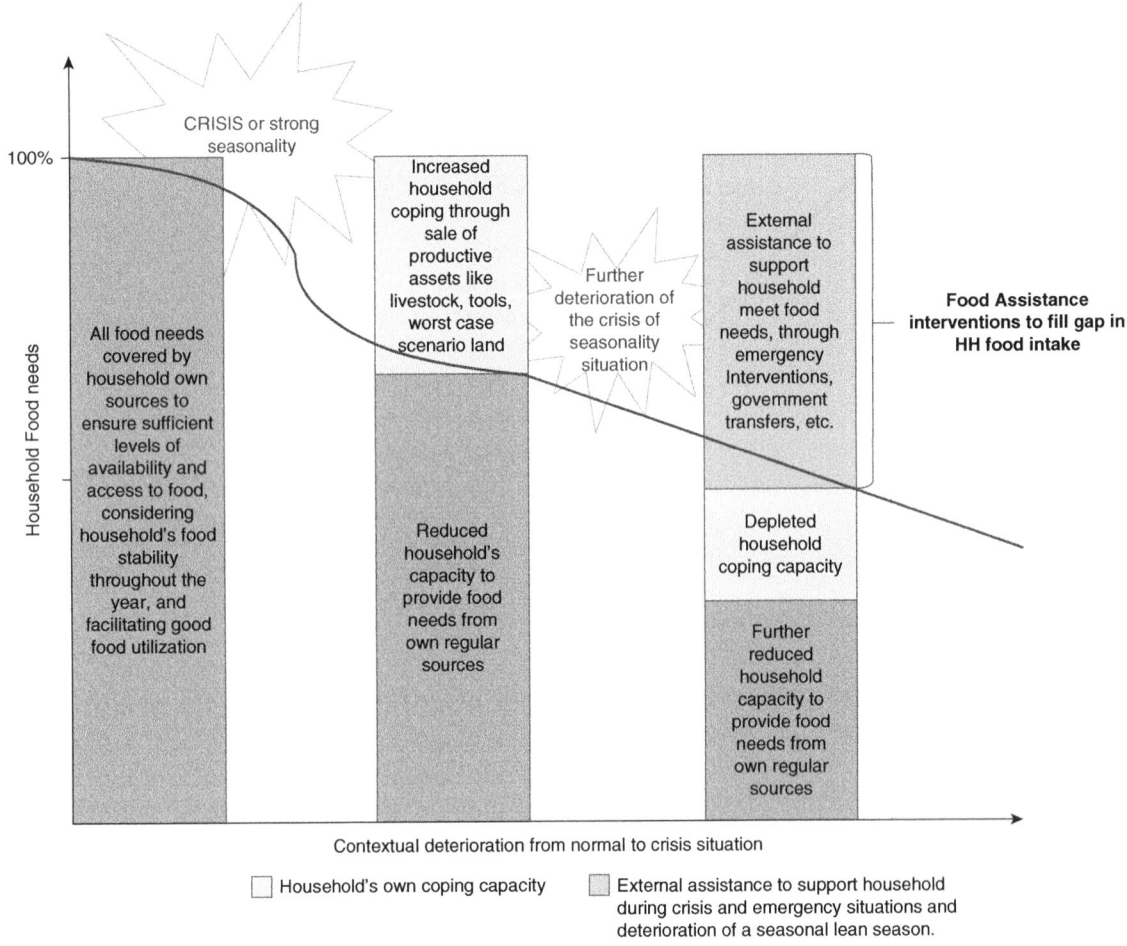

Figure 13.3 Food gaps and household coping

of productive assets and investments, to either not be affected by a disaster, or be able to cope sufficiently with the disaster and recover afterwards. In this case the household might not experience a situation where choices over scarce resources need to be made.

In households without lower resilience, and coping capacities, decisions over scarce resources at the household level might in turn expose the household to new vulnerabilities. For instance, in a short term situation the redirection of all resources to food will provide sufficient food intake, but might divert resources needed for access to clean water or health services or education. Similarly, a household might need to sell its land, which provides in return sufficient purchasing power to access food during an emergency, but the household will not be able to reverse this trend, and reacquire its land, resulting in food insecurity and hunger in the future. In the longer term, the need for children to drop out of school to search for food and create additional income to fill the food gap for the household will prevent the children from gaining the capacities and skills needed to create resilience in the form of a stable livelihood and income for their own families in the future. Food security and resilience have an intergenerational impact on households and livelihood survival and development

Food Security and Context Analysis

The complexities and interlinkages around food security require careful analysis and follow-up of the food security situation and underlying causes and effects on the household, community, or country level, on both a short-term and long-term basis. Given the potentially negative consequences of coping strategies that a household may need to employ to cope with food insecurity, early detection and prevention of food insecurity are of utmost importance not only for food security but for other needs and capacities of the household including livelihoods, social networks, education, and health. Food security plus nutrition assessments and early warning plus surveillance systems are frequently implemented in countries with recurrent potential food insecurity. Detailed analysis and understanding of the food security situation before and after the emergency through existing secondary information or new primary data collection is important to ensure that the emergency response designed to support households and communities is appropriate, relevant, and impactful.

The understanding of food security has shifted from food availability to food access. Observations have shown that market access and global and local food prices have a major influence on household food security. This shift in focus from food availability to food access during an emergency requires a modification in the approach and response to the emergency. Government policies to regulate markets or provide access to subsidies to support household food availability and accessibility are of great importance. Linking early detection and prevention of food insecurity, hunger, and undernutrition should be facilitated through national disaster risk management and mitigation strategies and policies. Services and safety nets might expand beyond food and reach into other productive livelihoods assets (e.g., farm and livestock insurance and fodder banks) as well as other complementary services (e.g., health services and school support) to prevent a deterioration of the household's and individual food security status.

Responses in food security or nutrition emergency are often handled through the provision of food assistance, but these are not always the most effective responses given the complexity of food systems. Therefore, other emergency interventions should be equally or simultaneously considered based on a thorough food insecurity cause-and-effect analysis, addressing the immediate and underlying gaps of household and individual food insecurity with appropriate measures.

Emergency Food Security Interventions

There may be a variety of appropriate responses to a food crisis depending on the context, the emergency, and the resulting degree or deterioration of household food security. The earlier a deterioration or expected deterioration in food security can be predicted or identified, the better and more cost-effective a response can be implemented to protect lives and livelihoods. Slow onset crises such as drought provide many more opportunities to protect or stabilize food security for households and communities, as compared to rapid onset crises (including earthquakes, floods, or hurricanes).

Food security emergency response interventions are based on a needs assessment and identification of the gaps in a household's food or livelihood source. Food security and livelihoods assessment are considered one of the very first interventions implemented in a humanitarian emergency, and can most successful be conducted in collaboration with the various humanitarian partners and the local government in a given context.

Food Security and Livelihoods Needs Assessments

There are multiple approaches to emergency food security and livelihood assessments. Key aspects for any assessment include (ACF 2010, Maxwell et al. 2008a):

- What are the changes in availability, access, utilization and stability of food security incurred by the affected population?
- What are the underlying causes of food insecurity and threats to livelihoods in the affected area?
- What are the local coping strategies and capacities?
- Who are the most vulnerable and affected population?
- Where are the most vulnerable and affected populations?
- How long is the situation likely to last?
- What are appropriate responses to save and protect lives and livelihoods?
- What and how much support is needed?
- What will be the logistics and security constraints?

Depending on the information available, secondary data might be used in a rapid appraisal immediately

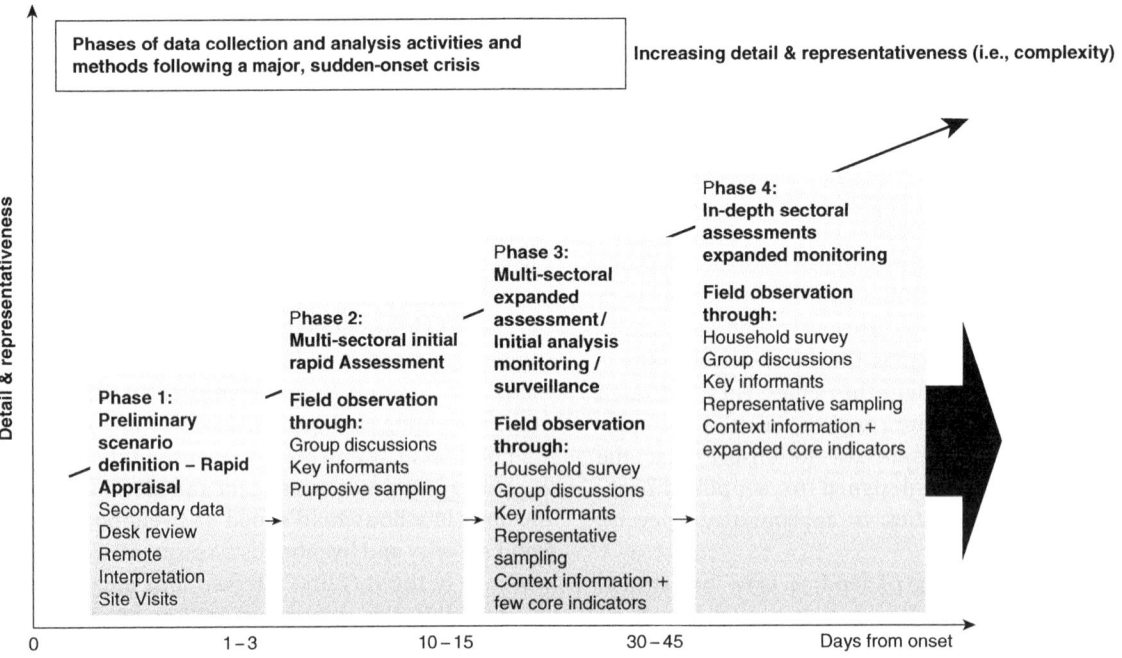

Figure 13.4 Food security and livelihoods assessments in emergencies (ACF 2010)

following a disaster and may be useful for the design of the immediate response. Additional data collection will most likely be necessary to better define the detailed food security and livelihood needs and underlying factors contributing to food insecurity and undernutrition. As soon as possible, a multisectoral assessment may be conducted to facilitate a holistic understanding of the needs of the population. Figure 13.4 shows the phases of data collection comparing rapid appraisal within the first few days of a disaster, with existing information, to different types of multisectoral assessments done in the days and weeks after the onset of the disaster.

There are a large variety of indicators and existing tools utilized in the emergency food security and livelihoods sector. A brief overview on the most common indicators is shown in Table 13.3 (Based on ACF 2010, Maxwell et al. 2008a).

There are a number of market assessment methodologies ranging from simple market price and stock data collection to discussions with customers and traders on the local market, to in-depth emergency market mapping exercises following more extensive methodologies (Albu 2011) Market assessments will be essential to define the most appropriate and effective emergency response modality, market-based or commodity-based.

The needs assessment will likely use a combination of different methodologies including household questionnaires, key informant interviews, focus group discussions, and observation exercises like transect walks. The necessary level of informant will evolve with the need for more detailed information necessary to design more comprehensive intervention to address not only immediate food needs, but immediate and recovery needs for food systems and livelihoods. Some of these methodologies are shown in Figure 13.4.

During a large-scale humanitarian emergency, the Integrated Food Security Phase Classification (IPC) process (FAO 2006b) is usually activated and applied, bringing together various partners to contribute their data and support the analysis of food security needs in a comprehensive and consultative way. Active partner and stakeholder contributions and participation in the IPC process are essential to create a common understanding and consensus about the needs and the location and size of the vulnerable and most affected population.

Table 13.3 Food security assessment indicators (based on ACF 2010, Maxwell et al. 2008a)

Food Security Pillar	Indicator	Description
Availability	Food stocks at household and market level, food imports, market prices, production estimates.	Sufficiency and diversity of household and market level food stocks, market assessments and observations for availability and prices of staple foods and basic commodities.
Access	Food sources, income sources, coping strategies.	Diversity and seasonality of food sources and income sources, range of food consumption and coping strategies through coping strategy index (Maxwell and Caldwell, 2008b)
Utilization	Dietary diversity, malnutrition prevalence, water access and availability, public health and care practices.	Household and individual dietary diversity (FANTA 2006, FAO 2010), meal frequency, global and severe acute malnutrition rates, MUAC screenings, water sources quality, quantity and cost; incidence and severity of disease outbreaks, access to health care, prevalence and changes in breastfeeding, complementary feeding and food sharing practices.
Utilization	Dietary diversity, malnutrition prevalence, water access and availability, public health and care practices.	Household and individual dietary diversity (FANTA, 2006; FAO, 2010), food consumption score (WFP, 2008); meal frequency, global and severe acute malnutrition rates, MUAC screenings, water sources quality, quantity and cost; incidence and severity of disease outbreaks, access to health care, prevalence and changes in breastfeeding, complementary feeding and food sharing practices.
Stability	Household food stocks, meal frequency, perception of hunger, food prices.	Months of adequate households food provisioning (MAHFP) (Bilinsky and Swindale, 2010), stability of number of meals eaten per day throughout the year, Household Hunger Scale (HHS) (Ballard et al., 2011) defining a continuous understanding of the perception of hunger in the household, and stability of food prices throughout the year indicating continuous access to food

Food Security and Livelihoods Interventions Responding to Identified Needs

Over the past decade there has been a shift from simply responding to food needs first with delayed consideration of any affected livelihoods damages, to early consideration of livelihoods as part of the larger, early, food security emergency response. Currently, food security emergency interventions can be structured according to three core objectives:

- Covering immediate food needs
- Covering livelihood protection needs
- Covering livelihood recovery needs

These interventions are most effective when they are complementary and occur in parallel. The earlier and more effective food systems and livelihoods can be protected and/or recovered, the sooner the affected population will be back to self-sufficiency and any risk of dependency on emergency hand outs can be reduced.

Immediate Food Needs and Food Assistance

Following a disaster, either slow or rapid onset, households may not be able to meet their immediate food requirements. Based on a situational or contextual analysis, a food gap can be calculated which needs to be filled to prevent undernutrition and loss of life as seen in Figure 13.3. The calculation of this household food ration or food basket is based on local food habits, the number of household members, and special needs of household members such as children, pregnant women, the elderly, and the sick. Sphere Project standards include a minimum of 2,100 kcal per person per day as part of a food ration, divided into carbohydrates, protein-rich foods, and fatty foods (Sphere

Project 2011). The Sphere Project is discussed in detail in Chapter 7. In the past, micronutrient requirements have been neglected, but are currently more recognized and addressed through either fortification of food aid, provision of fresh foods or supplementation of key micronutrients. Depending on the delivery modality, local markets can play a major role in the delivery of food assistance to cover immediate or longer term food needs, as well as other non-food items.

Food Assistance- In-kind Aid

Food aid is the provision of a food ration locally purchased or imported with support from partners, such as the World Food Program (WFP) to support the immediate food requirements of an individual, household, or community. Food aid primarily targets the pillar of availability of food, or the lack thereof. Immediate food needs right after the onset of an emergency may be met by high-energy biscuits or similar products distributed to local host, the displaced, and disaster-affected populations. They have a long shelf life and are appropriate for covering immediate food needs during the first few days of a disaster. Water may be needed for consumption of the biscuits and for preparation of porridge for younger children. These biscuits should not be used as a long terms response to address household food needs, in an effort to protect dignity, local food habits, environment concerns.

Following these immediate provisions, ration or food basket requirements should be calculated utilizing computer software (NutVal 2016). Rations typically include cereals, pulses/legumes, oil, and some condiments like sugar and salt. They are delivered in monthly quantities based on the average household size. Important considerations in developing a ration or food basket include: local availability of food, local food habits such as knowing if people eat sorghum or corn, acceptability of the various ration commodities, quality of the food items, access to distribution points, and hygienic storage and transport systems.

In-kind food aid is implemented when the local markets do not provide sufficient foods, are not functioning well or the population in need does not have physical access to the markets. Food aid can be provided as a free and unconditional general ration distribution or as part of a working scheme like *food for work* where the food is provided under the condition of the households' labor contribution to a communal working project. This may include such work as clearance of rubble, recuperation of agriculture fields, or rehabilitation of community buildings. Food-for-work programs expects households to actively contribute; however, exceptions may be made for the most vulnerable households without working capacities. These might include households with people with physical handicaps or other limitations, for example, the elderly.

Given the complex nature of household needs, a standalone food aid program will likely see some selling of the transferred food enabling household to acquire other immediate needs like water, access to health services, and rent. The cash, commodities, or services acquired for the food are often well below the real value of that food. This reality is an important consideration in program implementation to ensure the food aid ration has its intended effect of meeting immediate food needs, preventing undernutrition and subsequent loss of life. It is therefore important to have a clear contextual analysis and understanding of the situation as a basis for decision-making.

Special food aid programs using fortified blended foods such as corn soya blend (CSB), ready-to-use foods (RUF) or other products can be implemented for pregnant and lactating women or children under five years of age to address supplementary caloric or micronutrient needs. These programs may address prevention of undernutrition or the treatment of already existing undernutrition malnutrition is discussed in detail in Chapter 28.

Food Assistance- Cash and Vouchers

Cash and voucher programs have become a key element of emergency responses to address food and other household needs. Cash transfer programs are generally very flexible and can provide an opportunity to cater to people's needs with dignity and provide them with choices of their own in an emergency situation. To ensure individual and household food requirements are met, the contents of a food basket are calculated and a local monetary value determined based on local market prices. The calculated amount of cash is then transferred to the household through various options including cash grants (either conditional or unconditional), cash payment as part of a community work scheme similar to work schemes (except food is replaced with an equivalent cash amount), or vouchers. Cash and voucher transfers for food address economic lack of access to food, i.e. purchasing power, but require local markets to function well and provide all necessary items and for local vendors to be actively participating if the program includes vouchers. Due to its flexibility, cash can be an ideal means to provide not only food, but include additional allocations to allow other immediate needs for instance rent, medical care, water, etc., to avoid any liquidation or diversion of transfers (in kind or cash) from the food objective to other needs. These transfers are often found as Multi-Purpose-Cash grants – catering for a multitude of needs based on a minimum expenditure basket covering food, water, rent, health, education, transport, and other locally appropriate items (CaLP, 2015).

Individual and special needs including fresh foods and fruits to cover micronutrients, additional animal proteins like milk, egg, and fish for children, pregnant women, and lactating mothers to prevent undernutrition can be addressed with earmarked vouchers.

For cash transfers to be effective and appropriate, a good market assessment, careful calculations for the transfer amount and scoping of possible transfer systems and mechanisms need to be facilitated. There are many options to transfer cash and vouchers including paper-based, electronic-based, mobile phone–based and other modalities (Hutton et al., 2013).

Livelihood Protection

Food security is a result of productive livelihoods; therefore protection and prevention of livelihood and productive asset depletion is important to maintain and stabilize household food security. Ideally, in an emergency response, protection of further loss of livelihoods is still possible, as compared to everything being lost and interventions needing to focus on livelihoods recovery. The emergency response for the protection of these livelihoods might take different shapes depending on the scale and type of disaster. Food security emergency interventions often focus on the productive assets of the affected household. These may go hand-in-hand with food assistance interventions depending on the severity of the situation. Examples for the most common livelihoods responses are listed below.

Livestock Protection

In both slow and rapid onset emergencies, the protection of large and small livestock, such as poultry, goats, sheep, cattle, camels, and donkeys, is important to ensure direct availability of food or access to food through income generation for the household. Interventions ensuring the provision of livestock fodder and water are of great importance in keeping animals alive. Preventive vaccination campaigns to avoid excess loss of livestock due to epidemics are often applied. In addition, special animal shelter provisions for populations displaced by conflict or living in refugee or IDP camps might be considered.

In extreme situations, strategic destocking of livestock through humanitarian actors buying non-essential animals from herders may be necessary to reduce the pressure on scarce feeding and water resources. In these situations, the market value of the animals may be so reduced that the herder would rather keep the animal than sell it. It is therefore essential that in a destocking program, the humanitarian actors pay a fair price for the animals, which might be above the current market price. The purchased animals can be slaughtered and used for food assistance or as a supplement in nutrition programming (LEGS Project 2014).

Crop Protection

The focus of these interventions is both the protection of actual crop planting and the facilitation of crop growth until harvest. Some of these interventions might be in place prior to the emergency while others will be in response to the emergency. In contexts with recurrent strong seasonality or drought, crop insurance protection can safeguard crops during a drought or pest attack. Similar insurance can cover livestock as well.

Crop and livestock insurance is a risk management tool that farmers purchase to protect themselves against the loss of their crops due to natural disasters such as hail, drought, freezes, floods, hurricanes, fire, insects, diseases, and wildlife. Conventional agricultural insurance pays out to farmers after a poor growing season or extreme weather event, typically based on crop or animal loss, which requires verification through on-the-ground inspection; thus, it is very costly to administer for remote smallholder farmers and rural populations. Without insurance, many farmers lack a safety net and often find it hard to convince banks to give them loans to invest in better agriculture inputs. Index insurance can address these problems, as payouts are triggered not by manually accounting for observed damages such as failed crops, but rather when an index, such as wind speed or an amount of rainfall over a specified time period, falls above or below a predetermined threshold. Because payouts do not depend on demonstrating losses, administrative costs are reduced, allowing insurers to offer more affordable insurance premiums. As climate change makes weather shocks such as droughts more frequent and more intense, index insurance can help smallholder farmers and herders reduce their vulnerability and protect their assets (USAID 2013). This will ensure that the household's food security is not jeopardized during a disaster.

During civil strife or conflict, assuring safe access to agriculture land where food can be produced might be an appropriate intervention. Other interventions that can provide food during an emergency include food production in IDP or refugee camps through microsystems such as bag gardens or multistory gardens.

When the local market is inaccessible or no longer functioning as a result of the emergency, interventions to facilitate the purchase of agriculture produce from local farmers might support the income and continuous food security of the farming households. In such a situation, local produce could be part of the food assistance interventions. For instance, agricultural produce from local farmers might support a displaced population in the same community.

Livelihood Value Chain Protection

All livelihoods have a value chain structuring the life of the food from production to consumption. All along these value chains, different households create production income that ensures their household's food security. Some of these households provide services or products necessary for the preparation of food. For example, a household may provide ice for cooling fish, fire fuel, or water needed for food preparation. These households also need opportunities to maintain their livelihoods during an emergency. Hever, these households often do not benefit from interventions targeted at the primary producers of food rather than related services or products. For instance, in a situation where fishing households are provided ice through an ice delivery service, the loss of fishing capacity due to a disaster will affect both the fisherman and ice transporter. A well defined emergency intervention will address the food security and livelihood needs of both households while recovery processes will take place.

It is important to appreciate the connection and dependency of livelihoods on each other. It is therefore important to ensure an appropriate analysis of the context and how the emergency or disaster effects different livelihoods, including identifying existing gaps around access, availability, utilization, and stability of food for populations affected by the disaster.

Livelihood Recovery

The third component of food security interventions in humanitarian emergencies, livelihood recovery, addresses loss or destruction of livelihoods during the disaster or emergency, which lead to increased vulnerabilities and risk of food insecurity for the affected household. These livelihood recovery interventions are in contrast to livelihood protection interventions discussed above. Depending on the context and local livelihoods, as well as the scale and type of disaster, interventions will need to be designed and adjusted to the local needs.

Livestock Recovery

When local herders have lost a significant proportion of their animals during an emergency, it is appropriate to focus on livestock recovery. As a livelihood recovery intervention, restocking activities can facilitate to reestablish household food availability and access. As part of this process, core and breeding animals are distributed to support the quick rehabilitation of the herd. Calculations on the number of animals needed per family may be made using the tropical livestock units system, based on the number of household members and other income and food sources for the household. Similarly, livestock recovery can include the establishment of fodder storage or bank systems, and support improved vaccination and animal health services. The recovery of the quantity and quality of animals available to the household will reinforce the ability of the households to produce and access sufficient food for all family members. Careful considerations of the environmental carrying capacity must be ensured to avoid introduction of additional stress factors to pasture and water resources (see LEGS Project 2014 for guidance).

Crop Recovery

Following a drought or flood, agriculture crop production may have failed, or land made unusable, for example, as a result of salination. Due to the loss of harvest, farming households often suffer an additional loss of their potential seed inputs for the following season. In a normal year they may be able to buy new seeds, but following a major disaster without income or stocks from the harvest, this might be impossible for the most vulnerable and food insecure households. In these situations, crop recovery programs may focus on the provision of planting materials and equipment needed for agriculture production to support the household in restarting production. In cases of land inundation or salination, the recovery of agriculture land might be facilitated through support of agriculture labor or food/cash for work to recover agriculture production. The investment in agriculture production will be important to prevent further deterioration or relapse of food insecurity and malnutrition in the affected population. The promotion of improved crop varieties, for instance saline-tolerant or drought-tolerant seed varieties, might be an option in areas with recurrent shocks and for farmers who are interested to improving their crop protection and disaster mitigation

Value Chain Recovery

The effects of a disaster on value chains often include loss or damage of necessary equipment, transport and linkages to markets. Value chain recovery includes a careful analysis of the situation, restocking of equipment and transport and reestablishment of linkages to markets. This may be as simple as repairing a boat or a donkey cart or more complex like repairing a road or irrigation pumping system. Similarly, it might involve support to the local labor market to assisting other households in the recovery of their systems and infrastructures to create income and employ their laborers in the future. For example, recovery of salt pans is key to the employment of labor and production of salt, but due to loss of assets during the disaster, the salt pan owners are not able to get a loan to hire labor to recover their land. As a result, salt pan laborers remained food insecure and unemployed even after the disaster was over. In this case, support to the salt pan owner in the form of labor wages to pay the salt pan laborers would have provided immediate income to the salt laborers, giving them access to food, as well as supporting the recovery of the salt pans. This in turn ensures the future production of salt and employment of the laborers, providing food security for all now and in the future.

For any food security and livelihood interventions during a humanitarian emergency, a careful assessment of food security and local markets is necessary. Livelihoods protection and recovery interventions are designed to reinforce and foster food security for the households and communities are often facilitated through a transfer. The transfers can be in-kind such as fodder, water, animals, or seeds or in cash or vouchers. Cash and voucher transfers are often used major recovery interventions during the response to humanitarian emergencies in the food security and livelihood sector.

Notes from the Field

Pakistan (2010)

In 2010, the worst natural disaster on record in Pakistan occurred. Extraordinarily heavy monsoon rains tore through the upper part of the country and sent floodwaters rushing into the central and southern plains. In all, floodwaters inundated one-fifth of the country, destroyed 1.6 million homes, and displaced upwards of 20 million people, 14 million of whom were acutely vulnerable and in need of immediate assistance. Action Against Hunger | ACF International (ACF) responded quickly in Sindh Province, focusing not only on reaching as many people as possible with the basics (such as in-kind food assistance) but also ensuring longer-term recovery by restoring livelihoods and protecting valuable household assets.

Early in the crisis, an Emergency Market Analysis and Mapping Assessment (EMMA) was conducted and indicated that market resilience in Pakistan was uneven. Specifically, markets in Sindh Province took longer to recover due to the degree of damage and the persistence of the floodwaters. Further, the EMMA findings suggested that the distribution of in-kind food assistance for 2–3 months postflooding followed by and accompanied with the provision of market support and transition to community-based initiatives was the most appropriate approach. Thus, ACF decided to first distribute emergency in-kind food assistance comprised of a two-month ration of rice, wheat flour, beans, cooking oil, and salt for an average household of 7 people. Then, influenced by the needs and market assessment findings, ACF distributed

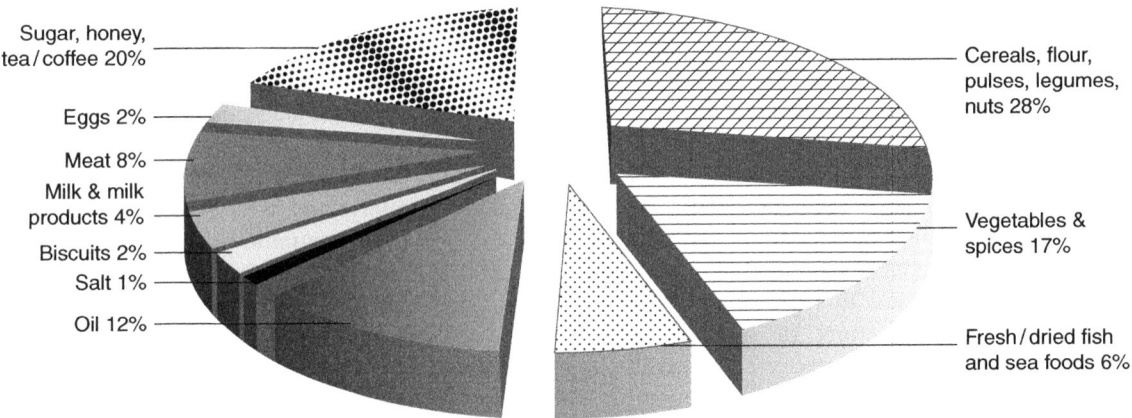

Figure 13.5 Household expenditure pattern during post distribution monitoring

small grants to local shopkeepers to provide funds for small business owners to recover their businesses and food vouchers to vulnerable households as a safety net to prevent the selling of valuable assets (oxen, cows, and buffalos) and to maintain the ability to cover their immediate food needs.

Rather than having a specific nutritional objective, food vouchers were intended to maintain minimum consumption levels as households eased out of the crisis. They were specifically implemented after the conclusion of the two-month general food ration distribution and even more importantly, after the provision of small business grants to local vendors. The sequential nature of this transition provided small business owners with the capital to restore their supplies locally and the confidence to restart their shops, since market demand would be guaranteed by the use of the food vouchers. Subsequent implementation of the voucher component ensured that there would be no supply-side constraints for beneficiaries accessing food and that shopkeepers would see a significant increase in income generating potential, leading to the eventual recovery and strengthening of local markets and supplies.

During the first phase of the program, which lasted two months, five thousand flood affected households or 34 thousand people received a general food ration (rice, wheat flour, pulse, cooking oil, salt). In parallel, business restart cash grants of US$200 were provided to 150 small business owners, including food vendors. In the second phase of the program, 5,300 flood-affected households or 37 thousand people received food vouchers worth a monthly amount of US$75 with an earmarked expenditure to food items, both staple (cereals, pulse, oil, sugar, salt, tea) and fresh (vegetable, dairy, egg, meat, fish). Out of the 150 vendors supported through the cash grants, 57 food vendors registered as suppliers for the food voucher program.

At the conclusion of the program, a Postdistribution Monitoring survey conducted by ACF showed that the Household Dietary Diversity Score among program beneficiary households improved significantly over the course of the program implementation, rising from approximately 4.8 immediately following the flood to 9 after the end of the emergency relief program. Figure 13.5 shows the expenditure pattern of beneficiary households during postdistribution monitoring. In total, the program benefited approximately 45 thousand individuals in severely affected communities, reestablishing economic activities and ensuring livelihood resilience in Sindh Province.

This example illustrates the importance and opportunity of linking relief and recovery through detailed and appropriate needs assessments. Careful analysis allowed for the design of a comprehensive and integrated intervention to address immediate basic needs and medium-term needs to enable communities and households to be self-sufficient and resilient against recurrent climatic shocks. As well, the case study demonstrates the use and application of cash transfers as a tool for various intervention objectives, covering immediate food needs through the food vouchers and recovery through the shopkeeper's cash grants.

References

ACF International Network. (2009). *Feeding Hunger and Insecurity – Field analysis of volatile global food commodity prices, food security and child malnutrition*. A Hunger Watch Publication. ACF International Network; New York, NY. Available at: www.actionagainsthunger.org/sites/defau lt/files/publications/ACF-Feeding-Hunger-and-Insecurity-Report-09.pdf. (Accessed on July 17, 2017).

ACF International Network. (2010). Food security and livelihoods assessment – A practical guide for fieldworkers. Available at: www.actionagainsthunger.org/sites/default/fil es/publications/acf-fsl-manual-final-10-lr.pdf. (Accessed on July 17, 2017).

Albu, M. (2011). Emergency market mapping and analysis toolkit - People, markets and emergency response. Available at: http://emma-toolkit.org/about-emma. (Accessed on July 17, 2017).

Food and Agricultural Organization. (1996). World Food Summit. Rome Declaration on Food Security. Available at: www.fao.org/docrep/003/w3613e/w3613e00.htm. (Accessed on July 17, 2017).

Food and Agricultural Organization. (2006a). Food security. *Policy Brief*, Issue 2. Available at: www.fao.org/for estry/13128-0e6f36f27e0091055bec28ebe830f46b3.pdf. (Accessed on July 17, 2017).

Food and Agricultural Organization. (2006b). Integrated food security and humanitarian classification tool. Available at: www.ipcinfo.org. (Accessed on July 17, 2017).

Food and Agricultural Organization. (2010). Guidelines for measuring household and individual dietary diversity. Available at: www.fao.org/3/a-i1983e.pdf. (Accessed on July 17, 2017).

Food and Agricultural Organization. (2013a). The state of food insecurity in the world: The multiple dimensions of food security. Available at: www.fao.org/docrep/018/i3434 e/i3434c.pdf. (Accessed on July 17, 2017).

Food and Agricultural Organization. (2013b). Resilient livelihoods – Disaster risk reduction for food and nutrition security framework programme. Available at: www.fao.org/3/a-i3270e.pdf. (Accessed on July 17, 2017).

Food and Nutrition Technical Assistance Project. (2006). Household Dietary Diversity (HDSS) for measurement of household food access indicator guide. Version 2. Food and Nutrition Technical Assistance Project; Washington, DC. Available at: www.fantaproject.org/sit es/default/files/resources/HDDS_v2_Sep06_0.pdf. (Accessed on July 17, 2017).

Livestock Emergency Guidelines and Standards Project. (2014). Livestock Emergency Guidelines and Standards (LEGS), second edition. Practical Action Publishing; Rugby, UK. Available at: www.livestock-emergency.net/resources/ download-legs. (Accessed on July 17, 2017).

Maxwell, D. and Caldwell, R. (2008b). The coping strategies index: A tool for rapidly monitoring food security in emergencies. Field methods manual, 2nd Edition. Available at: http://documents.wfp.org/stellent/groups/public/docu ments/manual_guide_proced/wfp211058.pdf?_ga=2.15561 7470.422400530.1500379660–1391676381.1500379660. (Accessed on July 17, 2017).

Maxwell, D., Sadler, K., Sim, A., Mytonyi, M., Egan, R., and Webster, M. (2008a). Emergency food security interventions. *Good Practice Review, Humanitarian Practice Network*, **10**. Overseas Development Institute; London, UK. Available at: http://odihpn.org/resources/em ergency-food-security-interventions. (Accessed on July 17, 2017).

NutVal. (2016). The planning, calculation and monitoring application for food assistance programs. Available at: www.nutval.net/. (Accessed on July 17, 2017).

The Sphere Project. (2011). Minimum standards in food security and nutrition, in *The Sphere Project: Charter and Minimum Standards in Humanitarian Response*. Rugby, UK: Practical Action Publishing, pp 139–238.

USAID. (2013). Index insurance: Building agricultural resilience to climate variability and change, fact sheet. Available at: www.climatelinks.org/sites/default/files/asset/ document/CCRD-IndexInsuranceFactSheet.pdf. (Accessed on July 17, 2017).

von Grebmer, K., Bernstein, J., Nabarro, D., Prasai, N., Amin, S., Yohannes, Y., Sonntag, A., Patterson, F., Towey, O., and Thompson, J. (2016). *The concept of the Global Hunger Index. In 2016 Global hunger index: Getting to zero hunger*. Bonn Washington, DC and Dublin: Welthungerhilfe, International Food Policy Research Institute, and Concern Worldwide, pp. 6–9.

Chapter 14

Reproductive Health

Barbara Tomczyk, Diane Morof, and Malcolm Potts

Introduction

In the context of humanitarian emergencies where reproductive health (RH) services may be disrupted or unavailable, public health principles and response strategies to support the collective action for RH lifesaving interventions are essential for clinical and public health practitioners designing interventions to integrate RH into the humanitarian response architecture. During humanitarian emergencies, providing a range of RH services is essential, yet deficits in supplies, commodities, and data for public health action may compromise the full capacity of responders to deliver care. The overall need for RH services is significant and humanitarian responders need to rapidly scale-up essential RH services to reduce RH related mortality and morbidity.

Over the past few decades, humanitarian emergencies have become severe and frequent. Climate change, rapid population growth, urbanization and shifting political, economic, and social trends are causing additional strains on the ability of the humanitarian community to respond effectively (OCHA 2013). Worldwide, the negative effects of these humanitarian emergencies weigh most heavily on women and children, who are disproportionately affected (McGinn 2000).

Women and children make up to an estimated 85 percent of displaced persons worldwide. Women of reproductive age (15–49 years) make up 25 percent of displaced persons worldwide, and it is estimated that on average one in five of these women is likely to be pregnant at any time (Women's Refugee Commission 2014). Lack of quality healthcare makes pregnancy and childbirth dangerous. Female head of households, widows, adolescents, and unaccompanied minors are often alone, cut off, and poor, placing them at risk for gender-based violence (GBV) and subsequently unwanted pregnancy, human immunodeficiency virus (HIV), other sexually-transmitted infections (STIs) and mental health issues (Inter-Agency Working Group on Reproductive Health in Crises 2010).

It is crucial that RH issues are addressed in humanitarian emergencies and that women are included in the early stages of the relief effort. It is necessary to collect, analyze, disseminate, and act on timely and accurate data to enhance an effective response. Interventions based on epidemiological data lead to improved RH responses that directly target the beneficiaries. A harbinger of lifesaving interventions is the use of public health activities such as rapid assessments, surveillance, surveys, and program monitoring and evaluation that will provide data to inform critical decisions and allocate resources to those who need it the most.

Epidemiology

Maternal Morbidity and Mortality

Although the absolute number of maternal deaths has fallen by 45% since 1990, many of the countries with the highest Maternal Mortality Ratios (MMR) are conflict-affected. Sierra Leone has the highest reported MMR at 1,360 per 100,000 live births. Sierra Leone and Chad report the highest adult lifetime risk of maternal mortality at 1 in 17 and 1 in 18, respectively (WHO 2015). Measuring maternal mortality in humanitarian emergencies is particularly difficult because of the relative infrequency of these events, challenges in data collection, and the difficulty applying standardized case definitions in this context. Nevertheless, it seems probable that the MMR will be highest during humanitarian emergencies especially during the acute phase (McGinn 2000, O'Heir 2004). The majority of published data on maternal mortality have been collected in postemergency refugee camp settings. One study found that the MMR is lower in stable camp settings than in the host population

(Hynes 2012). However, patterns of camp-based maternal mortality vary widely, even in the same camp, over time. Such changes over time illustrate one difficulty in measuring maternal mortality (Zimmerman et al. 2011).

Maternal deaths are due to direct causes including immediate obstetric complications and indirect causes such as preexisting diseases or conditions. Most maternal deaths are caused by direct obstetrical complications. One study of refugee camps found the same common causes of maternal death as noncamp settings including obstetric hemorrhage (31%), hypertensive disorders (25%) and pregnancy-related sepsis (12%) (Hynes et al. 2012). Indirect causes, about 20% of all maternal deaths, include conditions such as diabetes, malaria, anemia, and HIV/AIDS. Most importantly, the majority of maternal deaths that occur in these settings could be avoided with improved maternal health, adequate nutrition and health care during prepregnancy, pregnancy, delivery, and postdelivery, including postabortion care (WHO 2009a).

It is estimated that for each maternal death, 16 to 25 women suffer from illness related to pregnancy and childbirth, such as anemia, sepsis, incontinence, fistula, uterine prolapse, and infertility. Malaria during pregnancy exhibits an additional burden. One study showed that poor pregnancy outcomes were associated with the first or second pregnancy and with frequent malaria infections and the associated health impacts aggravated by pregnancy (Jamieson et al. 2000).

Neonatal Morbidity and Mortality

In 2016, 2.6 (2.5, 2.8) million newborns died, accounting for 46 percent of under five mortality with 99 percent of those found in low- and middle income countries (UNICEF 2017). Additionally, there were an estimated 2.6 million stillbirths. Two-thirds of all newborn deaths occur in 12 countries, six of which are in sub-Saharan Africa. Sixty percent of all newborn deaths occur in countries with a neonatal mortality rate of 30 or more deaths/1,000 live births. Public health interventions have led to a decrease in under-five and infant mortality at a faster pace than neonatal mortality, excluding countries affected by the HIV/AIDS epidemic. Approximately three-quarters of neonatal deaths take place in the first week of life and more than a third die within 24 hours of birth (Lawn et al. 2005, Lawn et al. 2009, Save the Children 2013).

Intensified efforts are needed to further reduce child mortality, end preventable deaths, and ensure newborn survival. As with maternal deaths, most neonatal deaths are due to preventable and treatable causes. Preterm birth complications, intrapartum-related deaths, and infections account for more than 80% of neonatal deaths globally (Liu 2012). Over two-thirds of newborn deaths could be averted worldwide if mothers and newborns receive quality care. Although efforts to improve best practices for care for newborn survival in resource-poor settings have been increasing, this movement has not translated significantly to emergency settings. Many of the countries with the highest neonatal mortality rates are currently or have recently been affected by humanitarian emergencies. However, as with the MMR, some studies on neonatal mortality in camps have also shown lower neonatal mortality rate (NMR) than the host community. One study looked at 52 camps and found that all but one had a lower NMR than the host country (Hynes 2002). Other studies, although limited, have supported these findings (Bitar 1998, O'Heir 2004).

Direct causes of neonatal mortality are usually divided into early and late, designated by less than 7 days of age and 7–28 days of age respectively. Early neonatal mortality is usually due to congenital malformations, complications of preterm birth, birth asphyxia, trauma, or infections. Late neonatal mortality is often caused by infections, including neonatal tetanus. Indirect causes of neonatal mortality include the health of the pregnant women, prevalence of endemic diseases, and availability and access to care. Studies on causes of neonatal deaths in humanitarian emergencies are very limited. Only one study, in West Bank and Gaza, found congenital disorders and intrapartum asphyxia, alone or together with neonatal sepsis, were the most common causes of full-term early neonatal deaths. Respiratory distress syndrome (RDS) was the main cause of death of preterm neonates with sepsis as a contributing factor in about a third. RDS (21%) and sepsis (16%) alone and together (11%) were also the main causes of the 19 late neonatal deaths (Kalter et al. 2008). These factors parallel what is known in other populations about causes of neonatal mortality.

HIV

Since 2002, UNHCR and its partners have conducted HIV sentinel surveillance among pregnant women in more than 20 postemergency refugee camps in Kenya,

Rwanda, Sudan, and Tanzania housing some 800,000 refugees. Refugees in three of the four countries (Kenya, Rwanda, and Tanzania) examined had lower HIV-prevalence rates than did the surrounding host communities (Spiegel 2004). Only in Sudan did the displaced and host communities have comparable rates (Lubbers 2003).

The difference in prevalence between refugee and host communities noted draws attention to the complicated epidemiology of HIV in humanitarian emergencies that varies according to many factors. HIV incidence may increase or decrease depending on some key factors, including area-of-origin HIV prevalence, surrounding host population HIV prevalence, level of interaction of the population, type and location of displaced population (e.g. urban vs. camp); phase of the emergency, length of time of conflict, and fertility plans (Dahab et al. 2013, Spiegel 2004, Spiegel et al. 2007, Woodward et al. 2014).

Factors that may lead to increased risk of HIV acquisition include behavioral change, sexual violence, transactional sex, reduction in resources and services (e.g. health, education, community services, protection, food), interaction between populations with different HIV prevalences, and desire for pregnancy (Spiegel 2007, Woodward et al. 2014). Factors that may lead to a decrease in risk include reduction in mobility or accessibility, slowing down of urbanization, and access to increase in resources and services including antiretroviral treatment (ARV) in host country (Spiegel 2007).

Although the focus in acute onset emergencies is on prevention of HIV transmission, the role of antiretroviral (ARV) treatment comes up frequently. Some studies in refugee settings have demonstrated optimal adherence prevalence at 87–99.5% (Mendelsohn et al. 2012; Mendelsohn et al. 2014b) and the provision of ARVs is increasingly seen as a human rights issue (Mendelsohn et al. 2014a). In addition, as prevention as treatment has an increasing role, it's likely this will be an area of greater interest to those involved in response to humanitarian emergencies. Additional information on HIV can be found in Chapter 23.

Gender-Based Violence

Based on research conducted globally, estimates of gender-based violence (GBV) vary by type, location, and timing in the displacement cycle, but they can be extraordinarily high. A study in Sierra Leone found that up to 94 percent of displaced women surveyed reported an incidence of GBV, including rape, torture, and/or sexual slavery (Physicians for Human Rights 2002). In Lofa County, Liberia, nearly 60 percent of women of reproductive age reported at least one sexually violent incident during the conflict, ten times greater than the postconflict period (c, 2007). In another study, 49 percent of 205 women surveyed in Liberia reported at least one act of physical or GBV by a soldier or fighter during the civil war of 1989–94 (Swiss et al. 1998). In postconflict East Timor, a survey showed levels of reported GBV by nonfamilial perpetrators decreased by 57 percent postconflict, while sexual coercion by intimate partners did not change (Hynes, 2004). Another study on urban refugees, found that Somali and Congolese female urban refugees reported a lifetime prevalence of experiencing any violence (physical and/or sexual), physical violence, and sexual violence of 77%, 76%, and 63%, respectively (Morof et al. 2014b). Sexual violence research is incredibly challenging, not only because of the sensitive nature of the topic and the need to ensure the research subject is protected, but also because methodology varies greatly (Ellsberg and Heise 2005; WHO 2009b). While population-based data provides prevalence estimates of GBV, studies can vary in their definition of terms and methodological approach that creates challenges in determining the true burden of GBV. One issue that is universally agreed upon is that GBV is underreported globally.

Fertility and Family Planning

Understanding fertility and family planning in the context of humanitarian emergencies is challenging. The Demographic and Health Surveys (DHS) provide standardized indicators that collect information on indicators such as marriage, level of education, type and place of residence, and female participation in the workforce. Additional measures include contraceptive prevalence rates, total fertility rate, crude birth rate, and fertility measures such as desired number of children. (DHS 2014). The demographic and fertility measures have well-established associations with fertility but have not been well studied in humanitarian emergency settings (Hill 2004). Some have postulated that reduced fertility during humanitarian emergencies could be due to loss of spouses/partners, increased ill health from infectious diseases such as malaria and HIV/AIDS, and increase in length of breastfeeding due to decrease in access to food. Factors that may increase fecundity include decreased access to contraception and interruption of use, and desire to replace lost family members (Hill 2004). Although each humanitarian emergency is different, effects on fertility are likely to be present and it is important for public health professionals to be aware of the possible implications on childbearing intentions.

Studies on knowledge and use of family planning in humanitarian emergencies demonstrate varying rates of contraceptive prevalence rate (CPR) among refugee populations. One study showed a CPR of 5.6% and 6.9% among Somali refugees living in Djibouti and Kenya, respectively. The CPR was 16.1% among Burundi refugees in Nakivale Camp, 31.9% among Iraqi refugees living in Amman, and 42.2% among Burmese refugees living in Kuala Lumpur. The type of family planning refugee women preferred varied by group. Iraqi women tend to use IUDs while Somali refugees use more oral contraceptive pills (UNHC 2011). Prompted levels of knowledge of family planning methods was measured in another study conducted in six conflict-affected areas in Sudan, northern Uganda, and the Democratic Republic of Congo and found 39.4%, 68.5%, and 92.6%, respectively. In the same study 30.7% to 39.8% of women stated that they wanted to delay childbirth for at least two years and 12.2% to 34.7% stated that they wanted to limit childbirth (McGinn et al. 2011). These studies also examined barriers to access and availability of contraceptives and concluded that especially for long-term family planning methods such as IUDs, referral mechanisms were limited. Procurement and maintenance of a steady supply to meet the demand was difficult to ensure.

Concepts

The number of refugees from conflict and climate change is likely to rise, especially rapidly in parts of Africa. In 1950, the population of the Sahel, defined as the ecologically vulnerable, semiarid region stretching from the Atlantic to the Red Sea, stood at 30 million. Today there are over one hundred million people and in 2050, the UN Population Division projects there will be over three hundred million people with the population still growing rapidly (Potts et al. 2011). Climatologists project that this region will suffer some of the worst impact of global warming, and crop yields will fall rapidly as ambient temperatures exceed 84°F (29°C). The UN Convention on Desertification warns that there could be 60 million ecological refugees fleeing parts of Africa as soon as 2020 (Kandji et al. 2006). The exact timing can be disputed, but what seems certain is that sometime near the beginning of the second half of the twenty-first century, more people than live in the United States will be watching their crops whither and their livestock die.

These somber projections are made more dire by several additional adverse factors. Many of the least developed countries likely to generate the largest numbers of involuntary migrants are already mired in poverty, and some have weak and corrupt governments. Rapid population growth makes it difficult for even well-governed countries to keep pace in health or education. A high ratio of young men from 15 to 30 years old, compared with the rest of the population, is one variable associated with conflict and violence (Staveteig 2005).

Reproductive health in humanitarian emergencies as a priority public health issue has experienced attention over the past few decades. For example, in 1995, over 50 governments, international nongovernmental agencies (INGOs), universities and UN agencies engaged to advance RH services to refugees resulting in the Inter-Agency Working Group on Reproductive Health in Crises (IWAG 2005). In addition, other developments have resulted in the Interagency Standing Committee/World Health Organization Global Health Cluster's guidance to include sexual and reproductive health in 2009 (IASC 2010a). There are comprehensive guidelines such as The Field Manual on RH in Humanitarian Settings (Inter-agency Working Group on Reproductive Health in Crises 2010), and The Minimum Initial Service Package (MISP 2014). In addition, the Reproductive Health Access, Information and Services in Emergencies (RAISE Initiative 2006) and Sexual and Reproductive Health Programme in Crisis and Post-Crisis Situations (SPRINT Initiative 2007) have worked consistently to develop and improve practical RH interventions in some of the most difficult humanitarian emergency settings.

Minimum Initial Service Package

The Minimum Initial Service Package (MISP) is a coordinated set of priority activities designed to prevent excess maternal and newborn morbidity and mortality, reduce HIV transmission, prevent and manage the consequences of sexual violence, and plan for comprehensive RH services (Inter-agency Working Group on Reproductive Health in Crises 2010a). The five objectives and related activities of the MISP are shown in Table 14.1. MISP activities include provision of 24/7 emergency obstetric and newborn care services, establishing a 24/7 referral system, provision of clean delivery kits to all visibly pregnant women and birth attendants, and provision of immediate care to infants after birth. Activities focused on decreasing transmission of HIV include practicing universal precautions, providing safe blood transfusion, and providing free condoms. MISP activities for the prevention and treatment of sexual violence include establishing prevention strategies, providing clinical services to care for survivors of rape, and informing the community on available services. Finally, as part of the MISP, the implementing agencies need to plan for comprehensive RH services that will include collecting background population-based data, identifying sites for future delivery of RH services, assessing staff capacity and training needs and ordering RH supplies and equipment (Women's Refugee Committee 2014).

Table 14.2 shows various health service delivery levels by Inter-Agency Kits. The kits can be ordered through UNFPA, or when appropriate, they can be produced locally. Implementing MISP and using the kits does not rely on conducting a rapid assessment first. There are a number of demographic assumptions that are used to calculate the type and number of kits needed to fulfill the needs of the population. For example, the percentage of the population that is female, the percentage of the population 15–49 years old, and the Crude Birth Rate are estimated based on epidemiological data, population profiles, and experience gained from previous emergency responses. Although these assumptions have been used globally, it is important to set up monitoring systems to identify procurement, distribution, and storage challenges that may develop and therefore prevent unnecessary delays in getting lifesaving supplies to those who need it the most.

Maternal and Newborn Health

During humanitarian emergencies, women may already be pregnant or become pregnant at any point during displacement; it is assumed that at least 4% of the total population will be pregnant at any given time (Inter-agency Working Group on Reproductive Health in Crises 2010). It is also estimated that 15 percent of pregnant women in humanitarian emergencies experience complications during pregnancy or delivery that are life threatening and require emergency obstetric care. One in three pregnant women requires an intervention during childbirth; and between 5 and

Table 14.1 List of MISP objectives and appropriate implementation activities

MISP Objectives	MISP Implementation Activities
Identify organization(s) and individuals to facilitate the coordination and implementation of the MISP	• Ensure the overall Reproductive Health Coordinator is in place and functioning • Ensure Reproductive Health focal points and implementing agencies are in place • Make available material for implementing the MISP and ensuring its use
Prevent sexual violence	• Ensure systems are in place to protect displaced populations, particularly women and girls, from sexual violence • Ensure medical services, including psychosocial support, are available for survivors of sexual violence • Ensure the community is aware of services
Reduce the transmission of HIV	• Ensure safe blood transfusion practices • Ensure implementation of universal precautions • Make free condoms available
Prevent excess maternal and neonatal mortality and morbidity	• Ensure availability of emergency obstetric and newborn care services • Establish a referral system • Provide clean delivery kits
Plan for the provision of comprehensive RH services	• Collect basic background information on the population • Identify sites for comprehensive reproductive health services delivery • Assess staff and identify training protocols • Identify procurement channels and assess monthly drug consumption

Table 14.2 Health service delivery level by appropriate Inter-Agency RH Kits

Health Service Delivery Level	Inter-Agency RH Kits
Community and primary health care level	Kit 0 – Administration
• 10,000 persons/3 months	Kit 1 – Condom (Part A: male; Part B: female)
	Kit 2 – Clean delivery (Part A: clean delivery packages individual; Part B: supplies for birth attendants)
	Kit 3 – Post-rape (Part A: ECP and STI treatment; Part B: PEP)
	Kit 4 – Oral and injectable contraception
	Kit 5 – STI treatment
Primary health care and referral hospital level	Kit 6 – Delivery kit facility level
• 30,000 persons/3 months	Kit 7 – IUD
	Kit 8 – Management of complications of miscarriage and abortion
	Kit 9 – Suture repair and vaginal examination equipment
	Kit 10 – Vacuum extraction manual delivery
Referral hospital level	Kit 11 – Referral level surgical items
• 150,000 persons/3 months	Kit 12 – Blood transfusion

15 percent of women require a caesarean section delivery (Inter-agency Working Group on Reproductive Health in Crises 2010b). Because birth complications are often unpredictable, having an emergency plan in place can mean the difference between life and death for a mother and her newborn.

Regular antenatal care (ANC) consists of four visits for uncomplicated pregnancies and is considered essential to the health of the mother and child. The main purpose of ANC is to screen for high-risk pregnancies and prevent complications, screen and treat for malaria, anemia, syphilis, HIV/AIDS, and GBV. Health education is essential to provide information on warning signs during pregnancy, information on nutrition, breastfeeding, and referral services, and to develop a birth plan. These services need to be provided as part of comprehensive RH and careful planning is needed for successful implementation of high quality and equitable services.

The three delays model developed by Thaddeus and Maine (1994) has been used to illustrate the delays between onset of a maternal complication and its efficient management in health facilities. The three delays are:

- Delay in deciding to seek care by the woman and/or her family
- Delay in reaching an adequate health care facility
- Delay in receiving care, once the women arrives at the facility

The WHO's *maternal near-miss* approach *and maternal severity index* (MSI) model are tools used for assessing the management of severe *maternal morbidity* (Souza et al. 2012). These tools have important public health implications for improving maternal and newborn health (MNH) outcomes in humanitarian emergencies. For example, emergency obstetric and neonatal care (EmONC) services must be available and of high quality to all women at the time of birth to address the unpredictable but treatable complications that arise during delivery. In addition, all providers need to be trained in the skills needed in basic or comprehensive emergency obstetric and neonatal care (BEmONC and CEmONC). Table 14.3 shows the signal functions for BEmOC and CEmOC (WHO 2009c). Signal functions are key interventions and activities that address major causes of morbidity or mortality and that are indicative of a certain type and level of care. For example, signal functions indicative of BEmOC could be provided by midwives at the level of a health center, while CEmOC signal functions indicate a higher level of care, usually at a hospital. It is important to acknowledge that no signal functions for emergency newborn care have

Table 14.3 Basic and comprehensive emergency obstetric and neonatal care services by level of facility

Basic emergency obstetric and neonatal care (BEmOC)	Comprehensive emergency obstetric and neonatal care (CEmOC)
• Administer parenteral antibiotics • Administer uterotonic drugs (i.e., parenteral oxytocin or sublingual misoprostol) • Administer parenteral anticonvulsants for preeclampsia and eclampsia (i.e., magnesium sulfate) • Manually remove the placenta • Remove retained products (e.g., manual vacuum extraction, dilation and curettage) • Perform assisted vaginal delivery (e.g., vacuum extraction, forceps delivery) • Perform basic neonatal resuscitation (e.g., with bag and mask)	• Perform signal functions for BEmOC, plus: • Perform surgery (e.g., caesarean section) • Perform blood transfusion

been defined except resuscitation. In order to maintain high quality services, periodic assessments are necessary and field staff should refer to the *Field-friendly Guide to Integrate Emergency Obstetric Care in Humanitarian Programmes* (RHRC 2005).

Early postnatal care is particularly important for reducing newborn mortality occurring on the first day of life. Good-quality postnatal care within 24 hours, on day 3, and between day 7 and 14 has a major impact on maternal and newborn health (Requejo et al. 2013). Globally, only 36 percent of infants younger than six months of age are exclusively breastfed, often owing to inadequate care that starts in the first week of a baby's life. Postnatal care at the community level should include emphasis on thermal warming, exclusive breastfeeding within the first hour, and hygienic cord and skin care, and care seeking when a newborn develops signs of illness.

Interventions at the hospital level include resuscitation with bag and mask, case management of neonatal sepsis, meningitis, and pneumonia, kangaroo mother care for preterm and for less than 2,000 gram babies, management of newborns with jaundice, and testing and treating for HIV/AIDS. At the referral level, more hospital services should be provided but are rarely available, such as surfactant to prevent respiratory distress syndrome in preterm babies, continuous positive airway pressure (CPAP) to manage babies with respiratory distress syndrome, extra support for feeding small and preterm babies, and presumptive antibiotic therapy for newborns at risk of bacterial infections (Lawn et al. 2005, 2009).

Comprehensive Abortion Care

To prevent and mitigate the consequences of hemorrhage or sepsis following a spontaneous or induced abortion, a lifesaving intervention in humanitarian emergencies may be safe abortion care and post-abortion care (SAC, PAC). Lifesaving interventions include a human rights–based approach and should be situated within a harm reduction framework, which takes the ethical high ground and emphasizes the health professional's obligation to reduce suffering even in the case of a behavior they may disapprove of (Hyman et al. 2013). In many countries where abortion is notionally illegal, legislation often includes a specific clause permitting abortion after rape as, for example, in Liberia (Inter-agency Working Group on Reproductive Health in Crises 2010). Lastly, both manual vacuum aspiration abortion (MVA) and medical abortion are procedures that can be performed safely in low-resource settings (WHO 2012).

HIV/AIDS

Effective HIV prevention requires a coordinated set of strategies across the continuum of care, which includes data collection, providing high quality HIV testing and counseling (HTC), linking persons diagnosed with HIV to HIV clinical care and treatment (hereafter "HIV care"), retaining patients in HIV care to facilitate antiretroviral therapy (ART) initiation, and supporting adherence to ART. The Inter-Agency Standing Committee Task Force on HIV/AIDS in Emergency Settings provides guidelines for the collection of baseline data related to HIV/AIDS that can be undertaken even in the minimum response phase of an ongoing emergency (IASC 2010). It is important to collect information on STIs and HIV prevalence levels in the host country and the country of origin, including the identification of specific high-risk locations such as areas of commercial sex work. The level, quality, and accessibility of local services for the prevention and treatment of STI/HIV/AIDS (including voluntary confidential counseling and testing for HIV) should be assessed. Other issues such as STI diagnosis and treatment, indicators for the prevention of mother-to-child transmission of HIV, accessibility of ART, adherence to universal precautions, and blood screening should be documented and programmatic interventions adjusted based on this information. The national and/or local protocols on STI/HIV/AIDS prevention and treatment services for both the communities of origin and hosting communities should also be reviewed and built upon to achieve quality programming (Inter-agency Working Group on Reproductive Health in Crises 2010).

Gender-Based Violence (GBV)

The term "sexual violence" covers" all forms of sexual threat, assault, domestic violence, interference, and exploitation including involuntary prostitution, statutory rape and molestation without physical harm or penetration" (WHO 2009a). In the emergency phase, rape is the form of sexual violence that receives most attention. The consequences of rape are extremely traumatic for the survivor and can cause long-term physical and emotional pain. In order to mitigate the negative consequences of rape, a public health approach based on prevention and treatment strategies can be implemented in the acute stage of an emergency. It is important to identify a team of professionals and community members who are involved in caring for people who have been raped, in order to discuss and identify critical issues that can improve programs (Inter-agency Working Group on Reproductive Health in Crises 2010). For example, a referral network that includes health, community, security, and protection sectors should be implemented based on these discussions and available resources and expanded with support from humanitarian agencies as soon as possible. As noted, even countries with restrictive abortion laws commonly have exceptions permitting safe abortion for women pregnant following rape. In most emergency settings there is a lack of appropriate treatment protocols, so they will need to be developed and implemented.

Providers, especially female, will need to be trained on how to implement clinical guidelines on the treatment of rape. Plans need to be made to ensure that the survivor is prepared for the examination in a safe and private space, which is possible even in the early stages of an emergency. In addition, a medical and incident history should be obtained and forensic evidence collected as relevant. A physical and genital examination needs to be performed and appropriate medications prescribed. Lastly, referrals for counseling and follow-up care are needed. It is important to know that each survivor will have had a unique situation and special considerations should be taken when caring for pregnant women, children, men, or elderly individuals (WHO 2005).

Designing and implementing programs that seek to respond to and prevent GBV saves lives and mitigates the consequences of such violence for survivors. With the right evidence about the scale and nature of GBV, health practitioners can improve programming, support services where they are needed, and develop policies to address GBV. Prevention strategies need to be implemented through a coordinated multisectoral approach using a gender lens through protection, food, water, shelter, camp management, health, psychosocial, and legal sectors. Each sector has a role to play in preventing and responding to GBV. Population interventions that are well planned, executed, and supported with consultation from the community are the most successful. Focusing on the underlying root causes of GBV such as issues related to gender, culture, economic, religious, and social issues take a long time to address but should be considered during program implementation (Inter-agency Working Group on Reproductive Health in Crises 2010).

Family Planning

As previously stated, millions of women in developing countries (including crisis-affected populations) are not using contraception, yet prefer to delay or space childbirth. At the onset of an emergency, it is important to make contraceptive methods, such as condoms, pills, injections, emergency contraceptive pills, and intrauterine devices (IUDs), available to meet demand. The benefits of family planning are multifold, and offering contraception can prevent unwanted pregnancies. A family planning program should be implemented once the situation stabilizes and procurement and distribution portals can be maintained (UNHCR 2011). A family planning program should include trainings and other mechanisms for retraining of clinical staff, as both are crucial for good quality services. Successful programs are responsive to the needs of the community focusing on cultural, religious, and social issues. Flexible educational outreach strategies are needed to reach the population in insecure and hard-to-reach areas (Inter-agency Working Group on Reproductive Health in Crises 2010). By examining a few basic health indicators such as unmet needs for contraception and contraceptive prevalence rate, it is possible to improve programs.

Adolescents

Adolescents are generally classified as those aged 10–19 years and include very young adolescents (10–14 years). Child soldiers, unaccompanied minors, and head of households of younger siblings are often adolescents. For war-affected adolescents, little is known about what factors contribute to resilient or positive outcomes in the face of war-related stressors such as violence, displacement, and loss (UNFPA 2009). Adolescents face multiple health challenges due to their young age, including high rates of early marriage, unintended pregnancy, HIV and other STIs, and maternal death and disability (WRC 2012).

Evidence suggests that adolescent RH services (ARH) should be "youth friendly" and take a multisectoral approach. Some sectors that can contribute are child protection, education, shelter, and health. Building programs at the beginning with multiple sectors can ensure that the needs of adolescents will be mainstreamed and avoid vertical programs. Youth friendly health services and information can be made available in formal and nonformal schools, as well as at vocational training centers that are typically set up soon after the emergency (Inter-agency Working Group on Reproductive Health in Crises, 2010).

Reproductive health entry points can be devised in existing programs, such as disarmament, demobilization, and reintegration, and nonformal education programs for those out of school. Peer educators have been shown as another source of support for helping adolescents obtain information on RH services (UNFPA 2009). Programs working with adolescents need to document and evaluate the unique needs of this population in order to prioritize and provide high quality services.

Challenges and Controversies

Research and Data Collection

RH research in humanitarian settings poses unique and complex challenges that must be addressed to ensure strict adherence to ethical principles, offers direct benefit to the research subjects, and has the potential for improving RH outcomes. Improved and consistently applied epidemiologic definitions and methods are the cornerstone for tracking the burden of RH and better addressing the multiple and often interrelated causes of morbidity, disability, and mortality. Simpler and lower cost methods are needed for measuring maternal and perinatal outcomes, especially in emergencies where the burden is not well measured (WHO 2005). More descriptive research is needed, for example, to standardize methods for diagnosing and treating prematurity and its related impairments (Lawn et al. 2005). The field needs to refine and disseminate standard definitions of exposures and outcomes of risks for morbidity and mortality and to monitor and evaluate the impact of interventions especially quality of care. It is also important to use a multidisciplinary approach and discover new strategies for prevention, related to the multiple biological, clinical, behavioral, social, infectious, and nutritional causes related to poor RH outcomes. Lastly, there is limited evidence in humanitarian emergencies on the intersection between displacement, mental health, family dissolution, and social change, yet these factors may be important to understanding the underlying causes of the burden of RH in humanitarian emergencies (Hill 2004).

Early on in the emergency, preexisting information can be used to provide vital information. For example, initial assessments include a quick "head count" of visibly pregnant women plus a quick listing and profiling that includes very basic characteristics such as language, livelihoods, family size, and the number of female head of households and unaccompanied minors. Methods include qualitative focus groups, in-depth interviews, and community-based studies that combine collection of qualitative and quantitative data. Despite these various methods, inherent and consistent problems have emerged across many humanitarian emergencies. For example, data collection is usually limited to accessible populations and not those living in insecure areas or urban setting/cities. Response agencies at the early stages of the emergency often rely on baseline RH information from UNICEF, UNFPA, and WHO websites that is typically collected at the national level that may not be reflective of the RH outcomes among the displaced population.

The collection of timely and accurate data is an important activity that should be used to achieve high-level RH program activities. Surveillance is critical to detect RH health events as early as possible and minimize or avoid negative health outcomes. Good data collection techniques need to be established early on in the emergency in order to set the stage for an effective RH response. Key challenges to this process include:

- Use of different case definitions, indicators, and methods
- Failure to capture maternal and perinatal deaths
- Lack of data sharing and communication
- Use of estimated denominators

Programs

Whether women and girls who are affected by a humanitarian emergency have access to and use RH services depends on a number of factors. Getting high-quality RH services in place during a sudden onset emergency can be difficult. For example, technically competent staff may be in short supply. The skill level of clinical providers needed to diagnose and treat RH problems includes well-trained medical staff to deliver care such as forensic exams after a rape, surgical services, and neonatal resuscitation. It is a challenge to expand specific skills to a broader cadre of workers such as midwives, nurses, and community health workers due to the length of time needed to train staff (WHO 2013a, WHO 2013b).

More information is needed on the degree to which existing RH service delivery models developed in low-resource countries may be used or adapted for emergencies. For example, there is information on the benefits of the continuum of care practices during pregnancy and implementation of bundling of those services in developing countries (WHO 2010). These packages of services are articulated in the MISP, yet implementation is not uniform within or across emergencies. There is a need to understand the barriers and challenges with MISP program implementation and make recommendations using evidence-based assessments to improve program delivery. Medical and public health professionals are needed that are trained in RH epidemiology that can standardize and harmonize data collection of MISP activities in order to describe best practices in implementation and improve RH programming.

Sexual violence, and especially pregnancy following rape, is a serious public health problem in humanitarian emergencies, yet prevention and response programs have lagged behind. A priority set of activities has been articulated in guidelines but are difficult for agencies to implement. A public health approach is important to define the scope and magnitude of the problem, identify risk and protective factors, develop and test prevention strategies, and to assure widespread adoption. In humanitarian emergencies, the burden and risk factors have not been systematically measured, case definitions vary, and population-based surveys have been difficult to implement (Moore 2014). Methods to screen potential victims have not been identified and it is unclear whether screening leads to better health, help-seeking behavior, or prevents the recurrence of violence. While the evidence of effective strategies is steadily increasing, there is a gap between knowledge that has been generated through studies and evaluations and application of these findings to improve violence prevention practices. GBV response and prevention programs are urgently needed in humanitarian settings and are crucial to implement however challenging in multi-sectoral responses.

Next Steps

Research

The public health evidence-base for RH decision-making in humanitarian emergencies has been steadily increasing over the past decade. RH research gaps exist in humanitarian emergency programs primarily due to lack of understanding of established best practices, funding, and advocacy. In order to address these issues on behalf of the IAWG, the US Centers for Disease Control and Prevention (CDC) and Columbia University, Mailman School of Public Health convened a RH in crises research workshop on June 28–29, 2011. The workshop gathered 25 experts on RH in crises settings from UN organizations, international nongovernmental organizations, academic experts, and donors. The purpose of the technical workshop was to set a research agenda for the field of RH in crises for IAWG to work on jointly over the next calendar year. The group identified priority research questions using the Child Health Nutrition Research Initiative Methodology (CHRNI, 2005). The key steps used were the following:

- A primary list of 28 research questions/gaps, collected from previous meetings, previous working groups and evaluations was collated
- This list was sent to 36 agencies, and researchers were asked to review the questions and submit any additional questions pertinent to their organizations
- Sixteen individuals from 16 agencies responded
- The expanded list included 94 research questions, divided into eight categories (adolescent RH, comprehensive abortion care, family planning, MISP, maternal & newborn health, GBV, HIV/STI, and crosscutting issues)
- The attendants of the workshop completed a prioritization exercise prior to the workshop to allow the research questions to be ranked by selected criteria
- During the workshop, the research priorities were finalized by consensus and included adolescent family planning, MISP evaluation, and global evaluation of RH

Due to the changing context of the humanitarian architecture, the current scope, coverage, quality, and impact of RH services on the populations affected by humanitarian emergencies is unknown. In order to better guide RH field programs and agency activities, an updated field review is needed to identify services, quantify progress, document gaps, and determine future directions for programs, advocacy and funding priorities. By identifying priority strategies and clear targets and by working closely with stakeholders, significant progress in reducing the overall RH burden can be achieved.

Programs

Save the Children through the Saving Newborn Lives Initiative, funded by the Bill and Melinda Gates Foundation, is working to improve and strengthen newborn health programs in 18 developing countries with the highest burden of maternal and neonatal morbidity and mortality (Lawn et al. 2005). Strategic partnerships between agencies that work in development and those that work in humanitarian emergencies have been formed. The Emergency Response Unit at Save the Children subsequently partnered with UNICEF, CDC, and IAWG partners to align neonatal health efforts for humanitarian settings using the same evidence based strategies designed and tested in developing countries:

- Identifying, implementing, and evaluating "packages" of proven strategies for reducing newborn illness and death
- Determining how resources can be used most efficiently in humanitarian settings
- Integrating newborn care into existing maternal and child health programs
- Developing and introducing new tools, such as topical antiseptics and moisturizers

Sharing information through this collaborative process provides benefit to the field of newborn survival and eliminates duplication of efforts, making the best use of scarce resources and reinforcing best practices (Morof 2014a). Similar integration of other programs including maternal health, family planning, and GBV programs is also needed if ecological and conflict driven refugees continue to increase in numbers.

Data limitations in GBV have led to an increase in the number of high profile initiatives addressing this issue in conflict. Governments, UN agencies, and INGOs have accelerated commitments, funds, and political will to fight GBV in conflict (UNSCR 1325 2000, UNSCR 1820 2008). These initiatives have already changed the course of humanitarian action on this issue and therefore it will be difficult to revert back to the standard response patterns that have most often not been effective. However, if the movement forward is to be sustained for the future, which is needed, funding and political will also need to be sustained. The collective research on GBV from the past decade has shown us that rape and other forms of violence are rampant, especially in conflict-affected populations. The negative health and psychosocial consequences leave a devastating impact on survivors for years following the assault. There are no easy solutions to addressing the issue of GBV. Next steps should address multiple-component interventions and sensitive community engagement while at the same time protecting the anonymity of women and improving access to services, including safe abortion for women who have been raped. It is a delicate programmatic balance to build and maintain these interventions building upon the local capacity and at the same time avoid increased risk and retraumatization to survivors of GBV (Spangaro et al. 2013).

Notes from the Field

Liberia (2007)

Liberia experienced many years of devastating civil war. Lofa County in particular was identified as a postconflict area and selected for an RH Survey (Tomczyk et al. 2007). This research aimed to highlight the long-term impact of civil war on RH and included multiple partners including the Ministry of Health and Social Welfare, Liberian Institute of Statistics and Geo-Information (LISGIS), the University of Liberia, and UNFPA. CDC provided technical oversight and local partners provided logistical support.

In order to better develop strategies for effective RH services in postconflict situations, UN and INGOs must question how they can build relationships with local NGOs that will enable RH to be addressed jointly in a constructive way. In postconflict Liberia, local NGOs were providing RH services but had not yet collected systematic population-based data that could provide important programmatic data to help target services and resources to the most vulnerable populations. Applied research and the activities targeting capacity building in RH epidemiology were used in this setting to improve the overall health of mothers, children, and families. The key components were to link research to action (in-country programming), build the capacity of local health staff agencies, and enhance RH programming in a postconflict setting. Working with multiple stakeholders the model went through the following phases:

- Identify local health agencies to implement programs linked to survey findings
- Conduct a reproductive health survey to identify needs
- Provide skill building opportunities as needed such as proposal writing, monitoring and evaluation, and implementation
- Make available ongoing support to the local NGOs and share program findings

The local technical counterpart from the University provided support with identifying, hiring, training, and supervising enumerators, drivers, and supervisors for the survey. They also helped secure a training site, access to vehicles, and assisted with lodging and food for the survey staff. We modified the RH survey tool based on the Liberian DHS and CDC RH surveys in order to enhance the types and numbers of RH indicators collected to be based on the following:

- Measure the most salient RH outcomes in the past five years (such as pregnancy outcomes)
- Determine unmet need for family planning
- Identify knowledge and practices of HIV/AIDS
- Document the scope and magnitude of GBV during three time periods: pre-, during, and postwar

In collaboration with our Liberian counterparts the instrument was modified to reflect the most important public health issues appropriate for action. Three issues were apparent when we developed the questionnaire for Lofa County – the need to capture the multiple perpetrators of GBV, the need to capture multiple types of sexual and physical violence, and to differentiate between two periods of time – during the conflict and after the conflict. To understand the scope of GBV in this context, it was necessary to be specific about these issues while also ensuring that the questionnaire does not become unmanageably long and complicated.

Liberia has dozens of local languages. Therefore, during training many of the questions were asked in a simpler form of "Liberian English" that interviewers could use with respondents. Other challenges of doing research in postconflict Lofa County became apparent when we started to train and deploy local staff. Most of the enumerators themselves or had known someone that had directly experienced violence during the conflict. Special counseling sessions were then provided as needed.

Population-based research was difficult but not impossible in Lofa County, employing the decision-linked research model in a postconflict setting. The Liberian civil war left buildings, entire villages, health posts, hospitals and roads, and bridges entirely destroyed. The emotional toll on the population was too enormous to comprehend. In the short term, the RH survey helped local NGOs to use data to improve programming in RH. The local agencies that had developed programs were able to strengthen and develop a consistent strategy for networking and information exchange between those working on RH issues and those working on postconflict issues in general. Agencies developed skills as trainers of trainers that strengthened the local NGOs' ability to improve RH response in their own work. It is important to distinguish between the practical difficulties of survey work and the suitability of decision-linked research in postconflict settings. This research demonstrated that a variety of agencies can work in these settings and that supporting local NGOs in RH programs can have an important role to play in a fragile postconflict setting.

Glossary

Gender-based violence is defined as "physical, sexual, and psychological violence occurring in the family and in the community, including battering, sexual abuse of female children, dowry-related violence, marital rape, female genital mutilation, and other traditional practices harmful to women, non-spousal violence, violence related to exploitation, sexual harassment and intimidation at work, in educational institutions and elsewhere, trafficking in women, forced prostitution, and violence perpetrated or condoned by the state" (Inter-agency Working Group on Reproductive Health in Crises 2010).

Infant mortality rate is the risk of a baby dying between birth and one year of age.

Maternal death is defined as the death of a women while pregnant or within forty-two days of the termination of pregnancy irrespective of the duration and site of the pregnancy, from any cause related to or aggravated by the pregnancy or its management but not from accidental or incidental causes (Inter-agency Working Group on Reproductive Health in Crises 2010).

Direct obstetric deaths include maternal deaths resulting from complications of the pregnancy, labor, or puerperium, or from interventions omissions or incorrect treatment.

Indirect obstetric deaths include maternal deaths resulting from previously existing disease or newly developed medical conditions that were aggravated by the physiologic effects of pregnancy.

Maternal mortality ratio is the number of maternal deaths in a specified time period per 100,000 live births in the same time period.

Neonatal mortality rate is the number of deaths in the first twenty-eight completed days of life per 1,000 live births in a given year or time period.

Reproductive health is a "state of complete physical, mental and social well-being and not merely the absence of disease and infirmity, in all matters relating to the reproductive system and to its functions and processes reproductive health addresses the reproductive processes, functions and system at all stages of life. Reproductive health, therefore, implies that people are able to have a responsible, satisfying and safe sex life and that they have the capability to reproduce and the freedom to decide if, when and how often to do so. Implicit in this are the right of men and women to be informed of and to have access to safe, effective, affordable and acceptable methods of fertility regulation of their choice, and the right of access to appropriate health care services that will enable women to go safely through pregnancy and childbirth and provide couples with the best chance of having a healthy infant" (WHO 2014).

Sexual violence is "any sexual act, attempt to obtain a sexual act, unwanted sexual comments or advances, or acts to traffic a person's sexuality, using coercion, threats of harm or physical force, by any person regardless of relationship to the victim, in any setting, including but not limited to home and work" (WHO 2002).

References

Bitar, D. (1998). *Reproductive health in refugee situations: Review of existing reproductive health indicators*. Geneva: UNHCR, in Krause S. K., Jones R.K., Purdin S. J. (2000). Programmatic responses to refugees' reproductive health needs. *Int Fam Plann Perspect*, 26, 181–187.

Child Health and Nutrition Research Initiative (CHNRI). (2005). About CHRNI (online). Available at: http://chnri.org/about.php (Accessed on December 12, 2014).

Dahab, M., Spiegel, P., Njogu, P., et al. (2013). Changes in HIV-related behaviors, knowledge and testing among refugees and surrounding national populations: a multicountry study. *AIDS Care*, 25(8), 998–1009.

Demographic and Health Surveys: Fertility and Fertility Preferences. (2014). The demographic and health program (online). Available at: http://dhsprogram.com/topics/Fertility-and-Fertility-Preferences.cfm. (Accessed on October 15, 2014).

Ellsberg, M. and Heise, L. (2005). *Researching violence against women: A practical guide for researchers and activists*. Washington, DC: World Health Organization.

Hill, K. (2004). War, humanitarian crises, population displacement, and fertility: A review of evidence (online). Available at: www.ncbi.nlm.nih.gov/books/NBK215696/?report=reader (Accessed on October 15, 2014).

Hyman, S., Blanchard, K., Coeytaux, F., et al. (2013). Misoprostol in women's hands: A harm reduction strategy for unsafe abortions (online). Available at: www.arhp.org/

publications-and-resources/contraception-journal/february-2013 (Accessed on September 15, 2014).

Hynes, M. et al. (2004). A determination of the prevalence of gender-based violence among conflict-affected populations in East Timor. *Disaster*, 28(3), 294–321.

Hynes, M., Sakani, O., Spiegel, P., et al. (2012). A study of refugee maternal mortality in 10 countries, 2008–2010. *Int Perspect Sex Reprod Health*, 38(4), 205–213.

Hynes, M., Sheik, M., Wilson, H. G., et al. (2002). Reproductive health indicators and outcomes among refugee and internally displaced persons in postemergency phase camps. *JAMA*, 288(5), 595–603.

Inter-agency Standing Committee. (2010). IASC guidelines for addressing HIV in humanitarian settings (online). Available at: www.humanitarianinfo.org/iasc/pageloader.aspx?page=content-subsidi-common-default&sb=66 (Accessed on June 24, 2014).

Inter-agency Working Group on Reproductive Health in Crises. (2005). Reproductive health services for refugees and internally displaced persons: Report of an inter-agency global evaluation, 2004 online). Available at: www.womensrefugeecommission.org/resources (Accessed on June 20, 2014).

Inter-agency Working Group on Reproductive Health in Crises. (2010a). Inter-agency field manual on reproductive health in humanitarian settings (online). Available at: www.iawg.net/resources/field_manual.html (Accessed on June 28, 2014).

Inter-agency Working Group on Reproductive Health in Crises. (2010b). A statement on family planning for women and girls as a life-saving intervention in humanitarian Settings (online). Available at: http://iawg.net/IAWG_%20FP%20Statement_Final.pdf (Accessed on June 28, 2014).

Jamieson, D. J., Meikle, S. F., Hillis, S. D., et al. (2000). An evaluation of poor pregnancy outcomes among Burundian refugees in Tanzania. *JAMA*, 283(3), 397–402.

Kalter, H., Khazen, Rahil, R., Barghouthi, M., and Odeh, M. (2008). Prospective community-based cluster census and case-control study of stillbirths and neonatal deaths in the West Bank and Gaza Strip. *Paediatric and Perinatal Epidemiology*, 22, 321–333.

Kandji, S., Verchot, L., and Mackensen, J. (2006). Climate change and variability in the Sahel region: Impacts and adaptation strategies in the agricultural sector (online). Available at: www.unep.org/Themes/Freshwater/Documents/pdf/ClimateChangeSahelCombine.pdf. (Accessed on June 24, 2014).

Lawn, J. E., Cousens, S., and Zupan, J. (2005). 4 million neonatal deaths: when? Where? Why? *Lancet*, 365(9462), 891–900.

Lawn, J. E. et al. (2009). Two million intrapartum-related stillbirths and neonatal deaths: where, why, and what can be done? *Int J Gynaecol Obstet*, 107 **Suppl 1**, S5-18, S19.

Liu, L. et al. (2012). Global, regional, and national causes of child mortality: an updated systematic analysis for 2010 with time trends since 2000. *Lancet*, 379(9832), 2151–2161.

Lubbers, R. (2003). In the war on AIDS refugees are often excluded (online). Available at: www.unhcr.org/3fc71f614.html; (Accessed on June 22, 2014).

McGinn, T. (2000) Reproductive health of war-affected populations: What do we know? *Int Fam Plann Perspect*, 26, 174–80.

McGinn, T., Austin, J., Anfinson, K., et al. (2011). Family planning in conflict: results of cross sectional baseline surveys in three African countries Conflict and Health (online). Available at: www.conflictandhealth.com/content/5/1/11. (Accessed on June 13, 2014).

Mendelsohn, J., Schilperoord, M., Spiegel, P., et al. (2012). Adherence to antiretroviral therapy and treatment outcomes among conflict-affected and forcibly displaced populations: a systematic review. *Confl Health*, 6(1), 9.

Mendelsohn, J., Schilperoord, M., Spiegel, P., et al. (2014a). Is forced migration a barrier to treatment success? Similar HIV treatment outcomes among refugees and a surrounding host community in Kuala Lumpur, Malaysia. *AIDS Behav.*, 18(2), 323–34.

Mendelsohn, J., Spiegel, P., Schilperoord, M., et al. (2014b). Antiretroviral Therapy for Refugees and Internally Displaced Persons: A Call for Equity. *PLoS Med*, 11(6).

Moore, J. (2014). There's good news in two decades of progress on sexual violence in war zones (online). Available at: www.buzzfeed.com/jinamoore/theres-good-news-in-two-decades-of-progress-on-sexual-violen/ (Accessed on June 26, 2014).

Morof, D. F., Kerber, K., Tomczyk, B., et al. (2014a). Neonatal survival in complex humanitarian emergencies: setting an evidence-based research agenda. *Confl Health*, 8, 8.

Morof, D. F, Sami, S., Mangeni, M., et al. (2014b). A cross-sectional survey on gender-based violence and mental health among female urban refugees and asylum seekers in Kampala, Uganda. *Int J Gynaecol Obstet*, 127 (2):138-143.

O'Heir, J. (2004). Pregnancy and childbirth care following conflict and displacement: care for refugee women in low-resource settings. *J Midwifery Womens Health*, 49(4 Suppl 1), 14–18.

OCHA (online). World Humanitarian Data. (2013). Available at: https://docs.unocha.org/sites/dms/Documents/WHDT_192013%20WEB.pdf. (Accessed on July 31, 2014).

Physicians for Human Rights. (2002). War related violence in Sierra Leone: a population based assessment. Available at:

https://s3.amazonaws.com/PHR_Reports/sierra-leone-sexual-violence-2002.pdf. (Accessed on December 1, 2017).

Potts, M., Gid, V., Campbel, M., et al. (2011). Niger too little too late. International perspectives on sexual and reproductive health (online). Available at: http://bixby.berkeley.edu/pub-author/gidi-v/. (Accessed on July 14, 2014).

Reproductive Health Access, Information and Services in Emergencies (RAISE). (2006). Available at: www.raiseinitiative.org/home/. (Accessed on July 16, 2014).

Reproductive Health for Refugees Consortium (RHRC). 2005. Obstetric care in humanitarian programs (online). Available at: www.rhrc.org/resources/emoc/EmOC_ffg.pdf (Accessed on July 1, 2014).

Requejo, J. H., Bryce, J., Victora, C., and Deixel, A. (2013). *Accountability for maternal, newborn and child survival: the 2013 update.* Geneva: World Health Organization and UNICEF.

Save the Children. (2013). Surviving the First Day: State of the Worlds Mothers (online). Available at: www.savethechildrenweb.org/SOWM-2013/#/1/ (Accessed on May 20, 2013).

Sexual and Reproductive Health Programme in Crisis and Post-Crisis Situations SPRINT Initiative. (2007). Available at: www.ippf.org/our-work/what-we-do/humanitarian/sprint-essential-services-crisis-situations. (Accessed on July 11, 2014).

Souza, J. P., Cecatti, J. G., Hadded, S. M., et al. (2012). The WHO Maternal Near-Miss Approach and the Maternal Severity Index Model (MSI): Tools for Assessing the Management of Severe Maternal Morbidity. *PLOS ONE,* 7(8): e44129.

Spangaro, J., Adogu, C., Ranmuthugala, G., et al. (2013). What evidence exists for initiatives to reduce risk and incidence of sexual violence in armed conflict and other humanitarian crises? A systematic review. *Plos One,* **8**(5).

Spiegel, P. (2004). HIV/AIDS among conflict-affected and displaced populations: dispelling myths and taking action. *Disasters.* 28(3), 322–39.

Spiegel, P., Bennedsen, R., Claass, J., et al. (2007). Prevalence of HIV infection in conflict-affected and displaced people in seven sub-Saharan African countries: a systematic review. *Lancet,* 369(9580), 2187–2195.

Staveteig, S. (2005). The young and the restless: Population age structure and civil war (online). Available at: www.wilsoncenter.org/sites/default/files/Staveteig.pdf. (Accessed on July 31, 2014).

Swiss, S. et al. (1998). Violence against women during the Liberian civil conflict. *Journal of the American Medical Association,* **279**, 625.

Thaddeus, S. and Maine, D. (1994). Too far to walk: maternal mortality in context. *Social Science and Medicine,* 38 (8), 1091–1100.

Tomcyzk, B., Goldberg, H., Blanton, C., et al. (2007). Women's Reproductive Health in Liberia: The Lofa County Reproductive Health Survey January–February 2007 (online). Available at: www.africare.org/our-work/where-we-work/liberia/Resources/5Liberia_ResourceDoc.pdf. Published 2007. (Accessed April 15, 2014).

Trends in Maternal Mortality: 1990 to 2015 Estimates by WHO, UNICEF, UNFPA, World Bank Group, and the United Nations Population Division

UNFPA. (2009). Adolescent sexual and reproductive health toolkit for humanitarian settings (online). Available at: www.unfpa.org/public/global/publications/pid/4169 (Accessed on June 14, 2014).

UNHCR. (2011). Refocusing family planning in refugee settings: Findings and recommendations from a multi-country baseline study (online). Available at: www.unhcr.org/4ee6142a9.pdf. (Accessed on June 18, 2014).

United Nations Children's Fund UNICEF, Save the Children, (2015)Newborn Health in Humanitarian Settings Field Guide (online) Available at: https://www.unicef.org/videoaudio/PDFs/NewBornHealthBook-ProductionV12A.pdf (Accessed on January 29, 2018).

United Nations Children's Fund (UNICEF), WHO, World Bank Group, United Nations – Levels & Trends in Child Mortality Report 2017 Estimates Developed by the UN Inter0agency Group for Child Mortality Estimation (online). Available at: https://www.unicef.org/publications/files/Child_Mortality_Report_2017.pdf (Accessed on January 29, 2018).

UN Security Council Resolution (UNSCR) 1325 of 31 October 2000, S/Res/1325 (online). Available at: www.un.org/womenwatch/osagi/wps/. (Accessed on June 14, 2014).

UN Security Council Resolution (UNSCR) 1820 of 19 June 2008 (online). Available at: www.securitycouncilreport.org/atf/cf/. (Accessed on June 14, 2014).

Women's Refugee Commission. (2012). Adolescent sexual and reproductive health programs in humanitarian settings: An in-depth look at family planning services (online). Available at: www.K4health.Org/Toolkits/Rh-Humanitarian-Settings/Adolescent-Sexual-And-Reproductive-Health-Programs-Humanitarian. (Accessed on July 31, 2014).

Women's Refugee Commission. (2014). Minimum initial service package (MISP) for reproductive health in crisis situations (online). Available at: http://womensrefugeecommission.org/programs/reproductive-health/emergency-response/misp (Accessed on June 28, 2014)

Woodward, A., Howard, N., Kollie, S., et al. (2014). HIV knowledge, risk perception and avoidant behaviour change among Sierra Leonean refugees in Guinea (online). Available at: www.who.int/topics/reproductive_health/en/. (Accessed on June 18, 2014).

World Health Organization. (2002). World report on violence and health (online). Available at: www.who.int/violence_injury_prevention/violence/global_campaign/en/chap6.pdf. (Accessed on July 31, 2014)

World Health Organization. (2005). The World Health Report 2005: Make every mother and child count. *Statistical annex*. Geneva: World Health Organization, 219.

World Health Organization. (2009a). Sexual violence in conflict: Data and data collection methodologies (online). Available at: www.who.int/reproductivehealth/publications/monitoring/9789241502221/en/ (Accessed on July 1, 2014).

World Health Organization. (2009b). Health Cluster guide: A practical guide for country-level implementation of the Health Cluster (online). Available at: www.who.int/hac/global_health_cluster/guide/en/. (Accessed on June 30, 2014).

World Health Organization. (2009c). Monitoring emergency obstetric care: A handbook (online). Available at: www.who.int/reproductivehealth/publications/monitoring/9789241547734/en/ (Accessed on June 28, 2014).

World Health Organization. (2010). Packages of interventions for family planning, safe abortion care, maternal, newborn and child health (online). Available at: http://whqlibdoc.who.int/hq/ 192010/WHO_FCH_10.06_eng.pdf. (Accessed on June 20, 2014)

WHO (World Health Organization). 2010. ICD-10: International Classification of Diseases and Related Health Problems. 10th Revision, Vol. 2, Instruction Manual. Geneva: WHO.

World Health Organization. (2012). Safe abortion: Technical and Policy Guidance for Health Systems, Second edition (online). Available at: www.who.int/reproductivehealth/publications/unsafe_abortion/9789241548434/en/ (Accessed on July 1, 2013).

World Health Organization. (2013a). Compilation of WHO recommendations on maternal, newborn, child and adolescent health.

World Health Organization. (2013b). Global Health Atlas of the Health Workforce (online). Available at: http://who.int/globalatlas/autologin/hrh_login.asp (Accessed on June 27, 2014).

World Health Organization. (2014). Reproductive Health (online). Available at: http://www.who.int/topics/reproductive_health/en/ (Accessed on June 27, 2014).

World Health Organization. (2015) Trends in Maternal Mortality: 1990 to 2015 Estimates by WHO, UNICEF, UNFPA, World Bank Group and the United Nations Population Division (online). Available at: http://www.who.int/reproductivehealth/publications/monitoring/maternal-mortality-2015/en/ (Accessed January 29, 2018).

World Health Organization. (2017) Infant and young child feeding fact sheet (online). Available at: mediacentre/factsheets/fs342/en/ (Accessed on January 29, 2018).

Zimmerman, L., Packer, C., and Robinson, C. (2011). Reproductive health in post-emergency refugee camps (online). Available at: http://paa2011.princeton.edu/papers/110927 (Accessed on June 28, 2014).

Protection

Wendy Wheaton, Dabney P. Evans, and Mark Anderson

Introduction

In the setting of a humanitarian emergency, protection involves more than the provision of material assistance. Protection is the concern for the safety and dignity of persons through the application of human rights, international humanitarian law, and refugee law in practical assistance programs. Over the past decade, such concerns have been increasingly integrated into the policies and practice of humanitarian agencies mandated to protect displaced populations, such as UNHCR, ICRC, and OHCHR. Protection has also become a focus for many nongovernmental organizations (NGOs) that are not mandated to provide protection (Slim and Bonwick 2005).

After some of the humanitarian emergencies in the 1990s and 2000s, such as those in Rwanda, Kosovo, Iraq, Haiti, and Pakistan, it became apparent that the response by the international relief community inadequately addressed protection concerns. It was no longer considered reasonable for humanitarian agencies to focus solely on material needs without regard to the safety, dignity, and rights of individuals and communities (Caritas Australia et al. 2008). In response, efforts have been made to develop practical programming and related tools that protect people from all forms of violation, exploitation, and abuse during humanitarian emergencies.

Protection programs most related to health in humanitarian emergencies include activities focused on gender-based violence, child protection, mental health, and psychosocial support. In each of these humanitarian response areas, steps are taken in the first days of an emergency to protect vulnerable populations from unnecessary harm. These types of humanitarian assistance program have increased significantly in recent years. Along with the groundswell of programming came a demand for better guidance and although there remains limited evidence, evidence of good practice is emerging. As a result, there has been a proliferation of interagency studies, evaluations, and guidelines.

Background

Some of the key legal instruments framing protection work in humanitarian settings include:

- International Humanitarian Law (IHL)
- The four Geneva Conventions of 1949 and Additional Protocols of 1977 that govern the treatment of combatants and civilians during times of international and internal armed conflict
- International Human Rights Law (IHRL) that outlines the fundamental rights of all human beings that must be protected at all times of peace, armed conflict, and disasters
- The Refugee Convention of 1951 that outlines the rights applicable to refugees and asylum seekers
- The Guiding Principles on Internal Displacement that provide nonbinding principles for the protection of internally displaced persons (IDPs)

The basis of these legal instruments and the underlying principle guiding protection efforts in humanitarian emergencies is the simple awareness of the inherent dignity of the human person.

Most protection actors working in humanitarian emergencies apply this principle and the associated rights through advocacy, by influencing national policies, and ensuring that humanitarian actions and activities are delivered in a way that reinforces these rights. Increasingly common in humanitarian emergencies are protection actors who deliver practical, on-the-ground protection activities and services in immediate response to violent incidents, shocks, and trauma experienced by the affected population. Whether from protection-mandated humanitarian organizations or nonmandated agencies, fieldworkers are concerned with protection and doing it more often than ever before. This also holds true also across sectors with a new emphasis on how to "mainstream" protection into the current set of humanitarian actions in the early phase of a response (Global Protection Cluster, n.d.).

Agencies working in protection are also expected to train others on how to do it and show active concern for people's personal dignity as well as for their safety and material needs (Slim and Bonwick 2005). A cautionary note amidst increased protection-related efforts in emergency response is the need for better metrics to track progress and come to an agreed definition of protection. According to a 2013 scoping study on protection, progress on these two fronts is still lagging behind (Reichhold et al. 2013). While the scope of protection has expanded to include natural disasters, there are only a few attempts to date on how to measure success, monitor practice, and evaluate protection activities and even these are far from comprehensive (Inter-Agency Standing Committee 2011, ICRC 2008).

Key Groups

There are three key groups of people protected in emergencies, namely, refugees, internally displaced persons and the stateless.

Refugees

The principle of nonrefoulement says that refugees may not be forcibly returned to a country where they have reason to fear persecution. This principle is still the cornerstone of the international system for protecting refugees. The Convention's definition of a refugee focuses on individual cases of persecution and did not address mass movements of people spilling over international borders, which characterized many refugee situations at the time. In 1967, the "Protocol Relating to the Status of Refugees" abolished the geographic and temporal restrictions on the scope of the Convention (UN General Assembly 1967). Over the most recent decade, the number of refugees of concern to UNHCR and NGOs working with refugees has fluctuated greatly. In 2015, of the 21.3 million people who were considered refugees, over half were under the age of 18 (UNHCR 2016).

Internally Displaced Persons

The second group requiring protection in humanitarian emergencies are internally displaced persons. Nearly two-thirds of the world's forcibly uprooted people are displaced within their country. The Internal Displacement Monitoring Center (IDMC), established in 1998 at the request of the Interagency Standing Committee on humanitarian assistance, has a unique function to track and estimate displacement trends globally. By the end of 2016, there were 40.3 million people living in internal displacement as a result of conflict and violence in the world (Internal Displacement Monitoring Centre 2016). This number indicates a consistently upward trend since 2001 when there were 25 million estimated IDPs. Unlike refugees, there is no legal definition for IDPs, which complicates protection assistance for this target population. A United Nations report entitled the Guiding Principles on Internal Displacement includes the definition:

> Internally displaced people are people or groups of people who have been forced or obliged to flee or to leave their homes or places of habitual residence, in particular as a result of or in order to avoid the effects of armed conflict, situations of generalized violence, violations of human rights or natural or human-made disasters, and who have not crossed an internationally recognized State border (Deng 1998).

The above definition stresses two important elements of internal displacement: coercion and internal movement. It is important to note that rather than a strict definition, the Guiding Principles offer a description of the category of persons whose needs should be addressed under the Guiding Principles. In this way, the document "intentionally steers toward flexibility rather than legal precision" (Vincent 2000). As the words "in particular" indicate, the list of reasons for displacement is not exhaustive. Thus, we have an imperfect legal measure upon which to base protection assistance.

We also need to be aware that global statistics on internal displacement count only IDPs uprooted by conflict and human rights violations. IDP protection mirrors many activities provided to refugees, yet applying this assistance requires one to navigate the intentions, capacities, and choices of governments much more directly. It also concerns only those persons remaining within a country's national borders, whether in camps or local settlements. New challenges arise with regards to national sovereignty and a government's responsibility to protect (R2P or RtoP) its people, particularly when these state actors may be directly or indirectly implicated in the humanitarian emergency itself.

The Stateless

The third group is the stateless. A stateless person is someone who is not considered as a national by any state. In other words, a stateless person has no citizenship or nationality. There are numerous causes for statelessness that include:

- Conflicting nationality laws (e.g., birth registration vs. having a national parent)
- Gender, as many countries still do not allow their female citizens to confer nationality to their children in the absence of a father
- State succession, which renders a state nonexistent
- Residing in nonstate territories (e.g., Palestinian territories are not a state, thus, individuals claiming nationality are stateless)

While statelessness has existed for centuries, the international community has only been concerned with addressing the issue since the middle of the twentieth century. In 1954, the United Nations adopted the Convention Relating to the Status of Stateless Persons, that provides a framework for the protection of stateless persons. Seven years later, the 1961 Convention on the Reduction of Statelessness was adopted, which contains provisions to prevent and reduce statelessness. A range of regional and international human rights treaties guarantee a right to nationality, with special protections for certain groups including stateless persons. For example, states bound by the 1989 UN Convention on the Rights of the Child are obligated to ensure that every child acquires a nationality.

Stateless persons may face problems accessing services such as humanitarian emergency services and protection. If individual registration is required by agencies in displacement situations, then the stateless person may not officially exist until their status can be confirmed. As a practical matter, the longer a person is undocumented, the greater the likelihood that they will end up in a situation where no state recognizes them as a national. Whether someone is stateless ultimately depends on the viewpoint of the state on the individual or a group of people. In some cases, the state makes its view clear and explicit. In other situations, the viewpoint of the state is harder to discern, which, based on *prima facie* evidence of the opinion of the state, may give rise to a presumption of statelessness.

Principles

The general principles of protection in humanitarian assistance are to ensure information (Steering Committee for Humanitarian Response 2011):

- Provision of aid does not further expose people to physical hazards, violence, or other rights abuse
- Assistance and protection efforts do not undermine the affected population's capacity for self-protection
- Agencies manage sensitive information in a way that does not jeopardize the security of the informants or those who may be identifiable from the information

In addition to these basic principles of protection and assistance delivered to local populations by protection-focused actors or agencies, there are additional principles of protection used in practice.

Human Rights and Equity

Maximizing fairness during a humanitarian response to ensure equal availability, accessibility, and nondiscrimination of humanitarian services promotes human rights across gender, age, language groups, ethnic groups, political groups, and other parts of an affected population.

Do No Harm

Humanitarian aid, a critical means of helping people affected by crises, also recognizes that the assistance can also cause unintentional harm. Protection work has potential to do harm because it deals with highly sensitive issues. Also, this work lacks the extensive evidence base that is available in other sectors. Humanitarians can reduce harm by participating in coordination groups, ensuring sufficient information is collected to inform interventions, committing to evaluation and openness to criticism and scrutiny, developing cultural sensitivity, and ensuring continuous reflection on power dynamics between outsiders and the emergency-affected populations.

Build on Available Resources and Capacities

All affected groups have assets or resources, even in the early stages of an emergency. Identifying and tapping into these already present resources will help humanitarian workers avoid inappropriate services that have limited sustainability. A key task is to identify, mobilize, and strengthen the skills and capacities of the affected groups instead of supplanting or undermining these capabilities by bringing in external skills, knowledge, and staff that may lead to unnecessary tension.

Participation

During humanitarian emergencies, significant numbers of people exhibit sufficient resilience to participate actively in relief efforts. Gaining control over decisions that affect their lives helps build a sense of ownership among the affected populations. From the outset of an emergency response, local people should be involved in the design, implementation, monitoring, and evaluation of humanitarian assistance programs.

Interventions

A comprehensive set of protection activities, methodologies, and interventions includes needs assessment, program design, evaluation, monitoring human rights, and international law (IHL), security analysis, capacity-building, advocacy, or interagency cooperation. Depending on the context, these interventions may focus on specific groups, including people in war, children, women, the elderly, minorities, the displaced, stateless, and refugees.

The focus of this chapter is specific health sector–related guidance, including information that a health worker should know about protection when responding to a humanitarian emergency. These focus areas include:

- Understanding the general frameworks and principles of protection relevant to humanitarian emergencies
- Response to gender-based violence
- Support for mental health and psychosocial well-being
- Response to child-focused protection needs.

These key measures have been agreed upon, developed by, and written into broad interagency guidelines and tools used by UN, NGO, Health, Protection, and other humanitarian response actors over the past 5–10 years. Every 3–5 years, this guidance is updated, and ongoing efforts to build evidence on best practice are underway. Each action is meant to link directly with the broader health sector, community health workers, mental health professionals, and psychosocial support priorities for programming in humanitarian emergencies.

Protection Frameworks

Since 2000, there have been some interagency initiatives taken to define a framework for thinking about protection in humanitarian emergencies. One of the first substantive frameworks was developed by ICRC in 2001 and described the so-called "egg model" of protection. This model combines overlapping actions of responsive, remedial, and environment-building activities in situations of crisis (Caverzasio 2001). Soon afterward, *The Sphere Handbook* moved to incorporate protection directly into its humanitarian standards and guidance by supporting the notion that both assistance and protection are critical pillars of humanitarian action. *The Sphere Handbook* is discussed in Chapter 4. The purpose of this integration was to further develop the protection aspect of humanitarian aid by including a set of "protection principles" to inform humanitarian practice (Steering Committee for Humanitarian Response 2011). Five years later and as a direct result of United Nations reform efforts, this process led to the establishment of what is today called the "cluster approach" to humanitarian response and the formation of the Global Protection Cluster (GPC). The Global Protection Cluster was established in 2005 as an overarching international interagency forum for standards and policy setting. It was tasked with collaboration and overall coordination of protection activities that support the humanitarian response to humanitarian emergencies. The GPC coordinates policy guidance to field-based protection actors during humanitarian responses. The Cluster Approach is discussed in Chapter 4.

The GPC recognizes the primacy of States in having the responsibility to protect all persons within their jurisdiction. However, in certain cases, such as occurred during humanitarian emergencies in Haiti and Pakistan in 2010, national authorities may become overwhelmed by the scope of the emergency and may lack sufficient capacity to ensure the effective protection of all those affected by humanitarian crises. In these instances, States are supported by humanitarian organizations to provide protection assistance to the affected population with a goal of facilitating a more predictable, accountable, and appropriate response. UNHCR is the Global Cluster Lead Agency for Protection and has the responsibility to coordinate other United Nations agencies, intergovernmental organizations and nongovernmental organizations participating in network activities. This initiative outlines areas of responsibilities for specific agencies including Child Protection (UNICEF); Gender-Based Violence (UNFPA/UNICEF); Land, Housing, and Property (UN-Habitat); and, Mine Action (UNMAS). At present, this is one of the main interagency initiatives for protection actors as a group to refine approaches, test tools and gather evidence of good practice.

Gender-Based Violence

Gender-based violence (GBV) refers to any harmful act that is perpetrated against a person's will and is based on socially ascribed differences between males and females. Some of these acts violate universal human rights protected by international instruments and conventions and many, but not all, forms of GBV are illegal under national laws and policies. Protection assistance to survivors of GBV is critical during humanitarian emergencies. GBV survivors have received unprecedented attention over the past ten years through advocacy, increased funding, and new networks to address the immediate and mitigate the long-term effects of exposure to violence. While the nature and extent of GBV in humanitarian emergencies vary across settings, examples include sexual violence (most common), sexual exploitation and forced prostitution, domestic violence, trafficking, forced or early marriage, and, harmful traditional practices such as female genital mutilation, honor killings, and widow inheritance.

In times of crisis, healthcare services are often severely affected by a notable lack of coordination, overcrowding, security constraints, and competing priorities, all of which can contribute to decreases and limitations in available and accessible health services, especially for women and children. Well-functioning and accessible health services also make a difference in women's ability to reduce risks to their health and their children's health. Being able to protect her health and her family's health will not only promote a woman's general well-being, but it will also contribute to information sharing and community awareness of prevention and response to sexual violence. Although it is known from practice that most survivors of sexual violence do not disclose the abuse to anyone, some will talk with a health provider if health services are accessible and confidential. Services able to handle sensitive information and accommodate private consultations are those most often able to receive reports of violence. Often in emergencies, health centers may serve as a "neutral" location to provide information and counseling on women's and girls' reproductive health risks. Good practice points to survivors of violence being more able to access health services and support if it is within the context of basic healthcare and not provided by specialty or separate programs targeting women. In the acute phase of an emergency, services must be available to assist survivors to minimize the harmful consequences of sexual violence, which include severe emotional and physical trauma, unwanted pregnancies, complications of abortions, complications of pregnancy due to trauma or infections, and complications of delivery and neonatal problems such as low birthweight, for which emergency obstetric care services need to be put in place (Interagency field manual on reproductive health in humanitarian settings, IAWG).

A healthcare provider's responsibility is to provide appropriate care to survivors of sexual violence, to record the details of the history, the physical examination, and other relevant information, and, with the person's consent, collect any forensic evidence that might be needed in a subsequent investigation. It is not the responsibility of the healthcare provider to determine whether a person has been raped; that is a legal determination. Healthcare services must be ready to respond compassionately to survivors of sexual violence and should ensure that all staff are sensitized to sexual violence and are aware of and abide by medical confidentiality. In early phases of an emergency, healthcare providers such as doctors, medical assistants, and nurses should establish an agreed-upon protocol for the care of rape survivors, and this protocol should be in line with relevant national protocols and accepted international standards. It is also critical to ensure that facilities have the necessary equipment and supplies. While there have been suggestions to try and recruit more female healthcare providers, a lack of trained female health workers should not prevent the provision of services for survivors of rape. Awareness of relevant laws and policies governing healthcare providers in cases of sexual violence are critical. For example, there may be legislation that permits legal abortion in cases of sexual violence. Also, healthcare providers will likely interact with the police in cases where the survivor or, in the case of a child, her family wishes to pursue legal justice.

In many countries, there are police forms that must be completed by the healthcare provider. These forms vary in name, length, and complexity from country to country. Providers need to understand how to fill out these forms. In some countries, laws mandate that providers report cases of sexual violence to police or other authorities, which present challenges regarding medical confidentiality and respect for the survivor's right to choose whether or not she wants to pursue legal action. When there are mandatory reporting laws in place, many survivors do not disclose sexual violence to healthcare providers because of fear of public scrutiny or concern for subsequent harm to the survivor, which may be commonplace in that culture. Another consideration related to legal action is that the healthcare provider may be required to testify in court about the medical findings observed during the examination. If the case may go to court, it is often prudent to have a national healthcare provider conduct the exam.

Key Actions

Healthcare providers should develop an agreed-upon protocol to care for survivors of sexual violence. In addition to protocols, providers should receive training in the use of these protocols, which should include the actions that follow.

Prepare the Survivor

Before starting a physical examination, prepare the survivor for what they will experience. An insensitive or improperly done examination could contribute to the emotional distress of the survivor. The provider should begin by introducing themselves and explain key components and procedures (e.g., pelvic exam) of the exam. Next, the survivor should be asked if she wants to have a specific support person present during the exam. Then, obtain the consent of the survivor or a parent if the survivor is a minor. This is a necessary legal step and reassures the survivor that she is in control of the examination and that she has the right to refuse any aspect she does not wish to undergo. Finally, it is important for the examiner to explain that the findings are confidential.

Perform an Examination

At the time of physical examination, acknowledge any symptoms potentially related to panic or anxiety, such as dizziness, shortness of breath, palpitations, and choking sensations that may be without an organic cause. This means explaining in simple words that these sensations are common in people who have gone through such a frightening experience and may not be due to disease or injury. Then, conduct the medical examination only with the survivor's consent. It should be compassionate, confidential, systematic, and complete, following an agreed upon protocol.

Provide Compassionate and Confidential Treatment

- Treatment of life-threatening complications and referral if appropriate
- Treatment or presumptive treatment for STIs
- Postexposure prophylaxis for HIV (PEP), where appropriate
- Emergency contraception
- Care of wounds
- Supportive counseling
- Discussion of immediate safety issues and make a safety plan
- Make referrals, with survivor's consent, to other services such as social and emotional support, security, and shelter

Collect Minimum Forensic Evidence

Local legal requirements and laboratory facilities determine if and what evidence should be collected. Health workers should not gather evidence that cannot be processed or that will not be used. Counsel the survivor about taking evidence if she may eventually want to take the case to court. Ensure her that the information will only be released to the authorities with her consent. Ideally, for all cases of sexual violence, a carefully written record should be kept of all the findings of the medical examination that could support the survivor's story, including the state of her clothes. The medical chart is part of the legal record and can be submitted as evidence if the survivor decides to bring the case to court. As such, it is important to keep samples of damaged clothing, if replacement clothing is provided, and foreign debris present on her clothes or body, which can support her story. Other options for collecting evidence include, if a microscope is available, having a trained healthcare provider or laboratory worker examine wet-mount slides for the presence of sperm, which can prove penetration took place.

GBV and Psychosocial Distress

Sexual violence involves both physical and psychological trauma. Survivors may experience an array of psychological consequences, such as sadness and depression, self-blame, physical distress, sexual problems, mood swings, anger and anxiety-related problems including sleeplessness, fearfulness, stress, and fear of "going crazy." For most survivors, these experiences are normal emotional responses to trauma. With social and emotional support, many survivors learn to cope, and the distress decreases over time. In some cases, the survivor may experience intense psychological distress and dysfunction suggesting mental disorder, which requires a referral to a health provider for evaluation and treatment when possible. Social consequences can also result in societies that tend to blame victims of sexual violence. Social stigma, isolation, and rejection, including by husbands and families, are serious consequences, often making emotional recovery difficult when survivors withdraw from day-to-day activities and social support. Emotional support and counseling includes confidential and compassionate listening; systematically providing gentle reassurance that the incident was not the survivor's fault and that the emotions they are experiencing are normal responses to an extreme event is highly recommended. This type of survivor-centered care can often be made available in communities through existing natural helpers such as traditional birth attendants, midwives, and family members. At times, religious leaders can play a major role in providing needed support for survivors. While not all survivors need or want emotional support, counseling, or help with social reintegration, access to psychological and social support should be made available, even in early stages of a humanitarian emergency.

Mental Health and Psychosocial Support

Mental health and psychosocial support (MHPSS) is a composite term, meant to describe both local and outside support that aims to protect or promote psychosocial well-being and prevent or treat mental disorders (Inter-Agency Standing Committee 2007). Humanitarian emergencies cause significant psychological and social suffering on affected populations, which may have acute short-term impacts. In fact, psychological stress that goes unaddressed can undermine the long-term mental health and psychosocial well-being of affected populations. Humanitarian workers outside the health sector speak most often about supporting psychosocial well-being while health professionals tend to speak about mental health. Psychosocial rehabilitation and psychosocial treatment are two other terms used to describe non-biological interventions for people with mental disorders. Recent guidelines for practice bring together these expressions under a unified approach, as opposed to referring to one or the other (Inter-Agency Standing Committee 2007).

Social supports are also essential to protect and support mental health and psychosocial well-being in emergencies. Organizing social support through multiple sectors, for instance, camp management, education, food security and nutrition, health, protection, shelter and water, and sanitation, is critical. Humanitarian health actors are encouraged to promote the IASC Guidelines and their key messages to colleagues in other disciplines to ensure that there is appropriate action to address the social risk factors affecting mental health and psychosocial well-being. Essential clinical psychological and psychiatric interventions need to be made available for specific, urgent problems. However, these interventions should be implemented only under the leadership of mental health professionals, who tend to work in the health sector. Including considerations of mental health and psychosocial well-being in the general health response will protect the dignity of survivors and enhance the general health response.

During a humanitarian emergency, specific psychological and social problems can occur at the individual, group, family, community, or societal level. Emergencies tend to erode existing protective support systems, increase the risk of various problems, and amplify issues related to social justice or inequality (Inter-Agency Standing Committee 2007). In humanitarian emergencies, three categories of problems emerge: those that are preexisting, those created by the event itself, and those induced by the presence of humanitarian aid.

In recent years, a community of practice has developed, containing resources, discussion groups, research, training, events, vacancies, and other information related to psychosocial support and mental health in humanitarian emergencies, that can be viewed on the MHPSS website at http://mhpss.net. In 2007, after working together for two years, over thirty agencies came to a consensus on the main actions for the psychosocial and mental health response to humanitarian emergencies. This effort resulted in the development of a checklist for the field implementation of mental health and psychosocial support activities (Inter-Agency Standing Committee 2007). A summary of those key actions for health-related workers is outlined below. The do's and don't's for good practice are shown in Table 15.1.

Community Mobilization and Support

All sectors, including the health sector, have a shared responsibility to facilitate community mobilization and support. "Community mobilization" in this context and in the IASC Guidelines refers to the effort to involve community members in all the discussions, decisions, and actions that affect them and their future. Communities tend to include multiple subgroups that have different needs that frequently compete for influence and power. Facilitating community participation requires understanding the local power structure and patterns of community conflict, working with various subgroups, and avoiding promoting the interests of one group over another. Facilitating community self-help and social support can involve identifying naturally occurring psychosocial support systems and sources of coping and resilience. When appropriate, it can involve supporting existing community initiatives, especially those that promote family and community support for all emergency-affected community members, including people at greatest risk of MHPSS problems. In addition to supporting a community's spontaneous initiatives, additional initiatives should be considered for all emergency-affected community members and specifically for people at greatest risk. Overall, a self-help approach is vital for individuals who have undergone overwhelming experiences because having a measure of control over some aspects of their lives promotes mental health and psychosocial well-being.

Psychological Considerations

Psychological considerations that should be incorporated into general healthcare include:

- Communicating to patients and giving clear and accurate information on their health status and relevant services inside and outside the health sector. A refresher on communicating could include basic knowledge on how to deliver bad

Table 15.1 The do's and don't's for psychosocial and mental health activities in humanitarian emergencies

Do's	Don't's
Establish one overall coordination mechanism or group focusing on mental health and psychosocial support.	Do not create separate groups on mental health or psychosocial support that do not coordinate with one another.
Support a coordinated response, participating in coordination meetings and adding value by complementing the work of others.	Do not work in isolation or without thinking how one's work fits with that of others.
Collect and analyze information to determine whether a response is needed and, if so, what kind of response.	Do not conduct duplicate assessments or accept preliminary data in an uncritical manner.
Tailor assessment tools to the local context.	Do not use assessment tools not validated in the local, emergency-affected context.
Recognize that people are affected by emergencies in different ways. More resilient people may function well, while others may be severely affected and may need specialized support.	Do not assume that everyone in an emergency is traumatized, or that people who appear resilient need no support.
Ask questions in the local language(s) and in a safe, supportive manner that respects confidentiality.	Do not duplicate assessments or ask very distressing questions without providing follow-up support.

Section 2: Public Health Principles

Table 15.1 (cont.)

Do's	Don'ts
Pay attention to gender differences.	Do not assume that emergencies affect men and women (or boys and girls) in the same way, or that programs designed for men will be of equal help or accessibility for women.
Check references in recruiting staff and volunteers and build the capacity of new personnel from the local and affected community.	Do not use recruiting practices that severely weaken existing local structures.
After training on MHPSS, provide follow-up supervision and monitoring to ensure that interventions are implemented correctly.	Do not use one-time, stand-alone training or very short training without follow-up if preparing people to perform complex psychological interventions.
Facilitate the development of community-owned, managed, and run programs.	Do not use a charity model that treats people in the community mainly as beneficiaries of services.
Build local capacities, supporting self-help and strengthening the resources already present in affected groups.	Do not organize supports that undermine or ignore local responsibilities and capacities.
Learn about and, where appropriate, use local cultural practices to support local people.	Do not assume that all local cultural practices are helpful or that all local people are supportive of particular practices.
Use methods from outside the culture where it is appropriate to do so.	Do not assume that methods from abroad are necessarily better or impose them on local people in ways that marginalize local supportive practices and beliefs.
Build government capacities and integrate mental healthcare for emergency survivors in general health services and, if available, in community mental health services.	Do not create parallel mental health services for specific subpopulations.
Organize access to a range of supports, including psychological first aid, to people in acute distress after exposure to an extreme stressor.	Do not provide one-off, single-session psychological debriefing for people in the general population as an early intervention after exposure to conflict or natural disaster.
Train and supervise primary/general healthcare workers in good prescription practices and basic psychological support.	Do not provide psychotropic medication or psychological support without training and supervision.
Use generic medications that are on the essential drug list of the country.	Do not introduce new, branded medications in contexts where such medications are not widely used.
Establish effective systems for referring and supporting severely affected people.	Do not establish screening for people with mental disorders without having in place appropriate and accessible services to care for identified persons.
Develop locally appropriate care solutions for people at risk of being institutionalized.	Do not institutionalize people (unless an institution is temporarily an indisputable last resort for basic care and protection).
Use agency communication officers to promote two-way communication with the affected population as well as with the outside world.	Do not use agency communication officers to communicate only with the outside world.
Use channels such as the media to provide accurate information that reduces stress and enables people to access humanitarian services.	Do not create or show media images that sensationalize people's suffering or put people at risk.
Seek to integrate psychosocial considerations as relevant to all sectors of humanitarian assistance.	Do not focus solely on clinical activities in the absence of a multisectoral response.

news in a supportive manner, how to deal with angry, very anxious, suicidal, psychotic or withdrawn patients, and how to respond to the sharing of extremely private and emotional events.
- Supporting problem management and empowerment by helping people clarify their problems, working together to identify ways of coping, highlighting choices, and evaluating the value and consequences of those choices.
- Assisting individuals with referrals to tracing, social, and legal services.
- Referring undernourished children to stimulation programs to reduce the chance of developmental disability and to enhance child development.
- Managing medically unexplained somatic complaints through nonpharmacological methods (IASC Task Team on the Cluster Approach, n.d.).
- Providing psychological first aid (PFA), which entails basic, nonintrusive pragmatic psychological support with a focus on listening, assessing needs, and ensuring that basic needs are met, encouraging but not forcing the company of significant others, and, protecting clients from further harm. PFA provides a nonclinical, supportive response to a fellow human being who is suffering and who may need support immediately after an extremely stressful event. It is very different from psychological debriefing because it does not necessarily involve a discussion of the event that caused the distress. Psychological debriefing is a popular but ineffective technique and should not be implemented. All aid workers, and especially health workers, should be able to provide very basic PFA.
- In a minority of cases, when emergency-induced severe, acute distress limits basic functioning or is intolerable, clinical management will probably be needed. Some guidance for this is available (Patel, 2003).

Essential MHPSS Knowledge

In the clinical treatment of acute distress during humanitarian emergencies, benzodiazepines are frequently greatly overprescribed. These medications may be appropriately prescribed however, for a very short time for specific clinical problems (e.g., severe insomnia).

Caution is required as the use of benzodiazepines can quickly lead to dependence. In a minority of cases, a chronic mood or anxiety disorder, including severe presentations of PTSD, will develop. If severe, the disorder should be treated by a trained clinician as part of the minimum emergency response. If the disorder is not severe, and the person can function and tolerate the suffering, then the person should receive appropriate care as part of a more comprehensive aid response. Where applicable, support may be given by trained and clinically supervised community health workers, social workers, or counselors attached to health services.

Healthcare for People with Severe Mental Illness

Serious mental illness often predates a humanitarian emergency; however, it may have been induced or exacerbated by the emergency. People with such disorders are extremely vulnerable and are often abandoned in humanitarian emergencies. Models for organizing mental healthcare in primary healthcare (PHC) include:

- Mental health professionals attaching themselves to government and NGO PHC teams
- Training and supervising local PHC staff to integrate mental healthcare into standard practice and to give it dedicated time
- Training and supervising one member of the local PHC team such as a doctor or a nurse to provide full-time mental healthcare alongside the other PHC services.

Psychotropic Medications

Adequate supplies of essential psychotropic medications must be ensured in PHC and other health services (Inter-Agency Standing Committee 2007). Humanitarian health actors should know that overall, generic off-patent medicines are recommended because, in most countries, they tend to be less expensive than patented psychotropic medications and are just as effective. Although new medications tend to have a more favorable side-effect profiles, overall adherence to these drugs is only marginally better.

At a minimum, a PHC essential drug list should include one antipsychotic, one anti-Parkinsonian medication to manage potential extrapyramidal side-effects, one anticonvulsant or antiepileptic medication, one antidepressant and one anxiolytic, for use with severe substance abuse and convulsions. The 2010 Interagency Emergency Health Kit provides these medications.

Health Information Systems (HIS)

Emergency PHC provides a significant opportunity to support people with mental health problems. PHC staff should be taught to document mental health concerns using seven categories:

- Seizures/epilepsy
- Alcohol or other substance use disorder
- Mental retardation/intellectual disability
- Psychotic disorders
- Severe emotional disorders
- Other psychological complaints
- Medically unexplained somatic complaints

Institutionalized Persons

People in mental hospitals and other institutions have been abandoned in humanitarian emergencies, often becoming victims of violence, neglect, and human rights violations. Throughout the crisis, health professionals need to check on people in institutions and address their urgent needs, ensuring that such people are cared for and protected.

Alcohol and Other Substances

The health sector, in collaboration with other sectors, may need to act to minimize harm related to alcohol and other substance use in humanitarian emergencies where the use of such substances can lead to far-reaching protection, medical, or socio-economic problems. The IASC Guidelines outline the initial steps that should be taken in a humanitarian emergency to minimize harm related to alcohol and other drugs. These steps include assessments, prevention of harmful use and dependence, harm reduction interventions in the community, and management of withdrawal.

Link with Other Healing Systems

It is often important to learn about and, where appropriate, collaborate with local, indigenous, and traditional healing systems. Whether or not traditional healing approaches are clinically effective or harmful, establishing a dialogue with traditional healers can lead to a range of positive outcomes, including increased understanding of the spiritual, psychological, and social worlds of affected people and improved referral systems, among others. Some traditional healers may avoid collaboration however. At the same time, health staff may be unsympathetic or hostile to traditional practices or may be ignorant of them. In some situations, keeping a distance may be the best option to facilitate a constructive bridge between different systems of care.

Guidance from existing "best practices" and experiences in humanitarian emergencies indicates that some psychosocial and mental health interventions are advisable while others should be avoided. A health manager should be familiar with these do's and don't's and may use them as a checklist for program development, implementation, and monitoring.

Child-Focused Needs

The Handbook on the Minimum Standards for Child Protection in Humanitarian Action (CPMS) provides guidance to deliver protection to children caught in humanitarian crises (Child Protection Working Group 2012). Over four hundred individuals from thirty agencies in over forty countries, including child protection practitioners, humanitarian actors from other sectors, academics, and policy makers, were involved in its development. The CPMS was developed to:

- Establish common principles among those working in child protection
- Improve the quality of child protection programming and its impact on children
- Improve accountability within child protection work
- Provide a synthesis of good practice and learning to date
- Enable better advocacy and communication on child protection risks, needs, and responses

While child protection strategies should contribute to and maintain a child's health, health programs must also work to reduce protection risks. This happens when health services are carried out in a protective way. Quality health interventions are a central part of the overall approach to child-focused support services when responding to major child protection risks in humanitarian emergencies.

There are several major health-related risks for children that relate to protection. Children who are survivors of violence, abuse, and exploitation, and also those exposed to explosive remnants of war (ERW) such as landmines, are of particular concern. While varying by context, certain traditional practices pose serious risks to children, and documenting these early on is very important in informing an appropriate protection response.

Key Actions

Key actions in Child Protection for health workers include:

- Include the safety of the affected population as a subobjective of each health intervention.
- Identify pediatricians and health workers specialized in working with children at risk of violence, exploitation, abuse, and neglect. This group of children may include those in residential care, children who have lost one or more caregiver, child caregivers, child heads of households, children on the street, and children with disabilities.
- Ensure minimum standards for child protection in humanitarian action including ways to strengthen, adapt, or develop child-friendly and disability-inclusive procedures for admitting, treating, and discharging unaccompanied children.
- Promote the recruitment of social workers and child psychologists where appropriate, at least during the peak of the emergency and, where possible and appropriate, use community health workers to identify and refer cases.
- Reorganize existing health services so that they are accessible and safe for children, such as through the provision of community and home-based care.
- Respond to child victims and survivors of violence, abuse, exploitation, and neglect, including GBV, links and referrals to relevant services, for example, HIV testing and reproductive health services.
- Train health staff on clinical care of children exposed to physical violence. In areas contaminated by explosive remnants of war such as landmines, put in place specialized age-appropriate emergency medical, surgical, and longer-term physical rehabilitation and orthotic-prosthetic services for child survivors and children with disabilities whenever possible.
- Ensure health workers are trained in basic child protection as is relevant to their work, including the prevention of child separation.
- Disseminate child protection messages through health workers, including community health workers, both at the health facility and the community level; for example, vaccination campaigns, treatment of diarrhea, and promotion of exclusive breastfeeding.
- Ensure access to sexual and reproductive health services for older children.
- Ensure that healthcare workers adhere to a code of conduct or other policy that covers the safeguarding of children.
- Invite child protection workers to training sessions, retreats, or workshops, particularly when their perspective and information may enhance the outcome.

Monitoring and Reporting Violations

The early 1990s brought about a new global understanding of conflict and its impact on civilians, and on children in particular. Children were clearly identified as unique victims of natural disasters and armed conflict, including recognition of child soldiers as a prominent concern. In 1996, a study on the "Impact of Armed Conflict on Children" called for the creation of a system for monitoring and reporting on grave violations of children's rights (Machel 1996). This landmark report also advocated for the active involvement of the UN Security Council, the highest decision-making body of the United Nations.

UN Security Council Resolution 1612

The UN Security Council Resolution 1612, adopted in 2005, established a mandatory framework for a monitoring and reporting mechanism (MRM) in countries with an established pattern of recruiting child soldiers. The mechanism should provide "timely, objective, accurate and reliable information on the recruitment and use of child soldiers in violation of international humanitarian law, and on other violations and abuses committed against children in armed conflict." All UN offices in countries designated by the UN Secretary-General have established a 1612 MRM, a country-level task force, and an action plan to support affected children. UNSCR 1612 also calls for establishing a Security Council working group for the regular monitoring of grave violations against children. The MRM is not intended to secure criminal prosecutions or to contribute to national or international criminal processes, although cases can be referred to organizations that support victims in pursuing legal action.

The six grave children's rights violations include:

- Killing and maiming children
- Recruitment or use of children by armed forces or armed groups

- Attacks on schools or hospitals
- Rape or other sexual violence against children
- Abduction of children
- Denial of humanitarian access to children

In 2010, there were already fourteen countries with SC Resolution 1612 Task Forces reporting bimonthly to the Security Council on the six grave violations.

UN Security Council Resolution 1882

UN Security Council Resolution 1882, which passed unanimously in 2009, established expanded criteria for selecting countries and parties that are mandated to report on such violations including killing, maiming, rape, and sexual abuse. Since 1999, the UN Security Council has issued seven resolutions related to children affected by armed conflict, which demonstrates a high-level of commitment to the protection of children.

References

Caritas Australia et al. (2008). Minimum agency standards for incorporating protection into humanitarian response. Caritas Australia, CARE Australia, Oxfam Australia, World Vision Australia. Available at: https://drc.dk/media/2113371/minimum-agency-standards-for-incorporating-protection-into-humanitarian-reponse.pdf (Accessed July 8, 2017).

Caverzasio, S. G. (2001). *Strengthening protection in war: A search for professional standards: Summary of discussions among human rights and humanitarian organizations*, ICRC: Geneva, Switzerland.

Child Protection Working Group. (2012). Minimum standards for child protection in humanitarian action; Geneva, Switzerland.

Deng, F. (1998). *Guiding principles on internal displacement*; United Nations: New York.

Global Protection Cluster, Brief on protection mainstreaming. Available at: www.globalprotectioncluster.org/_assets/files/aors/protection_mainstreaming/brief_on_protection_mainstreaming.pdf (Accessed July 8, 2017).

IASC Task team on the cluster approach, key Messages: The IASC transformative agenda. Available at: https://interagencystandingcommittee.org/system/files/legacy_files/KM%20and%20FAQ%20on%20Transformative%20Agenda%20final.docx (Accessed October 15, 2016).

Inter-agency field manual on reproductive health in humanitarian settings. New York (NY): IAWG; 2018.

International Committee of the Red Cross and Red Crescent (ICRC). (2008). *Enhancing protection for civilians in armed conflict and other situations of Violence*, ICRC: Geneva, Switzerland.

Inter-Agency Standing Committee. (2007). IASC guidelines on mental health and psychosocial support in emergency settings; Geneva, Switzerland.

Inter-Agency Standing Committee. (2011). IASC operational guidelines on the protection of persons in situations of natural disasters; Geneva, Switzerland.

Internal Displacement Monitoring Centre. (2016). Global report on internal displacement, Norwegian refugee council; Geneva, Switzerland.

Machel, G. (1996). *Impact of armed conflict on children*, UNICEF, New York.

Patel, V. (2003). *Where there is no psychiatrist: A mental healthcare manual*, Royal College of Psychiatrist Publications, London.

Reichhold, U., Binder, A. and Niland, N. (2013). *Scoping study: what works in protection and how do we know?* Global Public Policy Institute; Berlin.

Slim, H. and Bonwick, A. (2005). *Protection: an ANLAP guide for humanitarian agencies*, Overseas Development Institute; London.

Steering Committee for Humanitarian Response. (2011). *The Sphere Project: Humanitarian charter and minimum standards in humanitarian response*, Sphere Project: Bourton on Dunsmore, UK.

UN General Assembly. (1967). *Protocol relating to the status of refugees*, Treaty Series: New York.

UNHCR. (2016). Global trends: Forced displacement in 2015, UNHCR. Available at: www.unhcr.org/en-us/statistics/unhcrstats/576408cd7/unhcr-global-trends-2015.html. (Accessed July 8, 2017).

United Nations. (1951). Final act and convention relating to the status of refugees, New York.

Vincent, M. (2000). IDPs: Rights and status. *Forced Migration Review*, **8**(August), 29–30.

Chapter 16

Vaccine-Preventable Diseases

Eugene Lam, Henri Van Hombergh, Allen Gidraf Kahindo Maina, Lisandro Torre, and Muireann Brennan

Introduction

Humanitarian emergencies result in major disruptions in the delivery of health services, including routine vaccination programs. Security issues and logistic challenges often associated with humanitarian emergencies often hamper the ability of the population to access health services and receive complete routine and recommended vaccinations. Disruption of immunization services, even for short periods, will increase the number of susceptible individuals and thus the likelihood of outbreaks of vaccine-preventable diseases (VPDs). This chapter will provide a general overview of the major VPDs in humanitarian emergencies and the risk factors that may lead to an outbreak of disease. Important specific diseases are discussed later in the text in the third section.

The primary objective of vaccination in the setting of a humanitarian emergency is to rapidly reduce the risk of disease in order to protect the population during a period of extreme vulnerability (WHO 2012a). The goals of vaccination during a humanitarian emergency may differ from those of routine immunization programs. The former focuses on limiting the number of excess preventable deaths attributed to the emergency. The latter focuses on ensuring long-term protection against a given disease through the progressive increase of population immunity. In humanitarian emergencies, where routine vaccination services may not be functional, emphasis is placed on mass vaccination campaigns, expanded target age groups, and particular pathogens of epidemic potential (WHO 2012a).

Common VPDs recognized in humanitarian emergencies include measles, polio, and depending on geographical location, meningococcal meningitis, yellow fever, and cholera. Mass population movements, scarcity of safe water and sanitation, poor nutritional status, suboptimal living conditions, and overcrowding increases a population's susceptibility to VPD's (WHO 2012a). Risk factors for outbreaks in the context of emergencies will differ depending on the characteristics of each VPD. These risk factors are inextricably linked to excess risk of morbidity and mortality from VPDs, the reduction of which is the aim of public health interventions during crises (WHO 2012a).

Mitigation of risk factors is an effective way of preventing outbreaks of VPDs; however, once an outbreak does occur, swift public health interventions and access to adequate curative services can significantly reduce mortality and morbidity among the affected populations, especially during the initial phase of an emergency. Experience with measles and polio outbreaks have shown that a rapid response, even with relatively low vaccination coverage, can avert more cases than higher vaccination coverage with a later intervention (WHO 2013a).

The goal of an outbreak response immunization (ORI) is not to substitute high coverage required in routine immunization programs, but rather to rapidly interrupt transmission of the disease to prevent excess deaths. Therefore, implementation of an ORI should be done as soon as possible and ideally no later than two weeks after laboratory confirmation of the case (WHO 2013a). The magnitude and extent of an ORI may be limited by logistical challenges, budgetary limitations, security concerns, and human resource constraints, but such factors should not delay the response (Cohn 2014).

Prior to the publication of a decision framework on vaccination in humanitarian emergencies developed by the World Health Organization (WHO) Strategic Advisory Group of Experts (SAGE) on Immunization Working Group, there was minimal guidance for widely accepted decision making regarding vaccination strategies in emergencies (WHO 2012a). The WHO SAGE guideline provides a more transparent process for assessing risk of and response to VPDs during acute emergencies. The document outlines an approach for assessing epidemiological risk of VPDs, considerations for vaccine selection, and local contextual constraints, all of which are important factors to consider when decisions are made regarding the use of vaccines in emergencies.

The WHO SAGE decision-framework document is intended for use by senior-level government and partner agency officials to determine the need of one or more vaccines in a given humanitarian emergency. This chapter aims to build on the WHO SAGE framework by providing an overview of the major vaccine-preventable diseases in humanitarian emergencies, its associated risk factors for outbreaks, the role of major organizations, and general control measures related to VPDs including surveillance, outbreak response, and mass vaccination campaigns. In addition, lessons learned from a real-world example are illustrated in *Notes from the Field* later in the chapter.

Important Vaccine-Preventable Diseases

This chapter focuses on common/important VPDs encountered during the acute phase of humanitarian emergencies, including measles, polio, meningococcal meningitis, yellow fever, and cholera. This is by no means an exhaustive list; rather it illustrates the major VPDs as they pertain to humanitarian emergencies. In addition, reestablishment of routine vaccinations, including tetanus and diphtheria vaccines, using the national Expanded Program on Immunization (EPI) schedule, will be discussed in this section as it is needed once the acute emergency phase is over (WHO 2005a). Other VPDs including *S. pneumoniae* and *H. influenzae* type B, rotavirus, and typhoid fever are discussed in the chapters dedicated to Acute Respiratory Disease (Chapter 21) and Diarrheal Disease (Chapter 22).

Measles

Measles is one of the most common and serious VPDs encountered in emergencies (Toole and Waldman 1990). It is a highly communicable, acute viral disease transmitted by airborne or direct contact with nasal or throat secretions of an infected person (Heymann 2008). A suspected measles case is characterized by fever and rash and either cough, coryza, or conjunctivitis, or an illness that the clinician suspects is caused by measles virus infection (WHO 2013a). The nonvesicular maculopapular rash typically starts on the face and spreads to the core and extremities (Pickering et al. 2012). Koplik spots, which are ulcerated lesions in the buccal mucosa, is a pathognomonic sign indicative of measles virus infection but is not always seen among patients with measles. Humans are the only reservoir and the incubation period ranges between 10 to 12 days (Zenner and Nacul 2012). Common complications of measles include diarrhea and pneumonia (WHO 2005a). Acute encephalitis occurs in less than 1 percent of cases, but can lead to permanent brain damage (Pickering et al. 2012).

In humanitarian emergencies, risk factors for measles include high prevalence of malnutrition, young populations, overcrowding, insufficient sanitation, and lack of access to healthcare services (WHO 2012a). Malnourished children are especially vulnerable to severe measles infection and its complications due to vitamin A deficiency (WHO 2005a). In these children, measles infection also depletes vitamin A levels that can ultimately lead to blindness (Heymann 2008). Vitamin A supplementation is therefore critical in both case management and mass measles vaccination campaigns. In spite of being a live vaccine, children with asymptomatic human immunodeficiency virus (HIV) infection should also receive vaccinations as they are at a greater risk for a severe measles case (WHO 2009; Polonsky et al. 2015).

The measles containing-vaccine is a live-attenuated vaccine considered to be safe, effective, and inexpensive. Measles vaccination coverage of 93 to 95 percent is needed for effective herd immunity in a target population (WHO 2009). WHO recommends a first dose in a nonoutbreak setting be given to children 9–11 months old and a second dose delivered either through routine immunization services or supplementary immunization activities (SIAs) (WHO 2009). The main objective of a measles vaccination program is to boost population immunity and prevent potential morbidity and mortality associated with measles outbreaks.

The case fatality rate (CFR) due to measles is typically 3 to 5 percent in developing countries, but may reach 10 to 30 percent among displaced populations (Heymann 2008). Because of high mortality rates associated with measles in emergency settings, the measles vaccine is one of the most cost-effective public health tools (WHO 2005a). Measles outbreaks in refugee settings can lead to high rates of mortality due to the presence of risk factors, including acute malnutrition and poor access to healthcare and preventive services. For example, a survey conducted in the Tuareg refugee camps of Mauritania identified that 40 percent of childhood deaths were due to measles (MSF 1997, Paquet 1992). Emergency measles vaccination is a public health priority among displaced populations and should be initiated as soon as possible (Connolly et al. 2004, Heymann 2008, Toole and Waldman 1988).

Measles vaccination campaigns should incorporate vitamin A distribution to children aged 6 months to 5 years. During a measles outbreak in a humanitarian emergency, the target age group for vaccination is typically expanded to 6 months to 14 years, with a minimum target age range of 6 months to 59 months (Kamugisha et al. 2003). However, the target age group should be determined by examination of the epidemiology of cases and the historical vaccine coverage in the country of origin of the affected population (Salama et al. 2004). Recent measles outbreaks in displaced population suggests consideration of expanding the target age group to include adolescent and young adults if surveillance data suggest a large proportion of cases are among persons greater than 14 years of age (Navarro-Colorado et al. 2014, Kaiser 2014). Expansion of the target age group will also need to ensure additional resources required to reach older populations. Children aged 6 months to 8 months who receive vaccinations during an outbreak should be revaccinated at 9 months of age for their first dose of measles vaccination as part of the EPI schedule. Further details about measles will be discussed in Chapter 26.

Poliomyelitis

While there has been significant progress in global polio eradication efforts, outbreaks of poliomyelitis do take place in certain humanitarian emergencies. Until poliovirus transmission is stopped in all countries globally, this will continue to be a possibility. Poliomyelitis is a viral disease caused by poliovirus types 1, 2, and 3. Poliovirus is transmitted person to person through the fecal-oral route, and humans are the only reservoir (Heymann 2008). The majority of cases in susceptible children are asymptomatic, with approximately 1 in 200 infected susceptible individuals developing paralytic poliomyelitis (WHO 2014a). Minor illness, including low-grade fever and sore throat, occurs in 24 percent of cases and aseptic meningitis occurs in 1 to 5 percent of cases a few days after the minor illness has ended. Less than 1 percent of cases experiences rapid onset asymmetric acute flaccid paralysis (AFP). The incubation period for the onset of paralysis is usually 7 to 10 days but can range from 4 to 35 days (WHO 2014a).

Any of the three serotypes of poliovirus can cause AFP, which is defined as one or more limbs with decreased or absent tendon reflexes without other apparent cause and without sensory or cognitive loss (CDC 2008). Wild poliovirus (WPV) type 1 is often isolated from paralytic cases and frequently causes epidemics. Wild poliovirus type 2 has not been detected since 1999 and no new cases of wild poliovirus type 3 have been reported since November 2012 (WHO 2014a). The risk of poliovirus infection is higher in emergency settings among large susceptible populations with overcrowding and insufficient water, sanitation, and hygiene (WASH) (WHO 2012a). Population displacement during humanitarian emergencies may threaten global eradication and elimination efforts, as people move from endemic areas to nonendemic areas.

According to WHO, a suspected case of poliomyelitis is defined as any case of AFP in a person aged less than 15 years or an illness that is suspected by a physician to be poliomyelitis in a person of any age (WHO 2014a). Laboratory confirmation of poliovirus from the stools of patients with AFP is necessary to confirm poliomyelitis and to determine if the poliovirus is wild type or vaccine-related. For diagnostic purposes, two or more stool samples should be taken at least 24 hours apart (CDC 2008). Poliovirus can also be detected in specimens from pharynx, urine, and (rarely) in cerebrospinal fluid (CSF). Samples should be stored for no longer than 3 days and transported at 4 degrees Celsius (Médecins Sans Frontières 2008).

There are two types of poliovirus vaccine: inactivated polio vaccine (IPV) and live-attenuated oral polio vaccine (OPV). In developing countries, four doses of OPV are typically administered at 6, 10, and 14 weeks of age with the fourth dose given either at birth or with measles vaccination at 9 months (Heymann 2008). In emergency settings, OPV is often used in preventive vaccination campaigns and in response to polio outbreaks. For example, during a WPV outbreak in Somalia, trivalent OPV was used in mass vaccination campaign targeting 360,000 children under the age of 5 years in several districts surrounding the capital (Kamadjeu et al. 2014).

In 2012, completion of polio eradication was declared by the World Health Assembly to be a programmatic emergency for global public health. The WHO position paper on polio vaccination recommends the inclusion of one dose of IPV for routine immunization schedules in countries using only OPV (WHO 2014a). The feasibility of administering OPV and IPV simultaneously in large-scale vaccination efforts has been demonstrated in refugee camps and host communities in Kenya (Sheikh et al. 2014). The purpose of the IPV dose to all routine immunization schedules is to maintain immunity against type 2 poliovirus during and after the planned global switch from trivalent OPV to bivalent OPV against types 1 and 3 (WHO 2014a).

Meningococcal Disease

Epidemics of meningitis have been a serious public health problem for two hundred years (Bhatt 1996). In developing countries and emergency situations, the bacterium *Neisseria meningitidis* is primarily responsible for epidemic meningitis. The bacteria infect humans by colonizing the nasopharynx. There is no other known reservoir (Heymann 2008). Droplets of respiratory secretions or throat secretions from carriers usually transmit the infection from person to person.

Rural-to-urban migration and overcrowding in poorly constructed buildings in camps and slums are risk factors for increased transmission. Prolonged close contact between people or living in close quarters with an infected person can also increase transmission. Both displacement and overcrowding are common to humanitarian emergencies, increasing the risk of meningococcal disease in these settings. Bacterial meningitis outbreaks occur seasonally when conditions are dry (Heymann 2008). Therefore, disease transmission may stop with the onset of the rainy season.

Symptoms of meningococcal meningitis include sudden onset of fever, headache, stiff neck, occasional vomiting, and irritability (WHO 2005a). In fulminant cases, coagulopathy, pulmonary edema, shock, coma, and death can occur in hours, even while the patient is receiving treatment (Pickering et al. 2012). There are various serogroups of meningococcal meningitis, and the majority of invasive meningococcal infections are caused by either serogroup A, B, C, W135, or Y (WHO 2011). A suspected case is defined as a person with sudden onset of fever and neck stiffness, altered consciousness, or other meningeal signs. A suspected case is confirmed by isolation of *N. meningitides* from cerebrospinal fluid or blood. Laboratory surveillance is necessary to confirm outbreaks and determine the particular serogroup, antibiotic sensitivity, and whether the monovalent, bivalent, trivalent, or tetravalent vaccine is needed. The gold standard to meningitis diagnosis is the recovery of meningococci from a sterile site, such as CSF (WHO 2011). To collect the sample, a lumbar puncture is performed on probable cases using aseptic techniques. An experienced health worker should perform the lumbar puncture, which can be difficult to find in emergency settings.

The disease can be treated effectively with antimicrobials; however, even with appropriate treatment, the CFR in epidemics can be between 5 and 15 percent (WHO 2005a). In an outbreak of serogroup A meningococcal meningitis among Rwandan refugees in Zaire in 1994, the mortality rate was 14 percent (Heyman 1998) and in another outbreak in a Sudanese refugee camp in Northern Uganda in 1994, the mortality rate was 13 percent (Santaniello-Newton and Hunter 2000).

Meningococcal serogroups that cause epidemics of meningitis vary by geography (WHO 2011). In sub-Saharan Africa, serogroup A meningococcal disease commonly leads to periodic epidemics during hot and dry months (Heymann 2008). The meningitis belt of sub-Saharan Africa, which has the highest rates of the disease, stretches from Senegal to Ethiopia, including 26 countries in total.

According to WHO, the definition of a meningococcal outbreak varies by geography. In the African meningitis belt, the threshold for defining a meningococcal outbreak is >100 cases/100,000 population/year (WHO 2011). In areas outside the meningitis belt, an outbreak is defined as a substantial increase in invasive meningococcal disease above that which is expected by place and time in a specified population. In emergency-affected populations, however, particularly in overcrowded situations, the threshold for action may be lower and the decision to implement a vaccination campaign must be taken locally in consultation with the relevant health authorities and partners. When the epidemic threshold is reached, a mass vaccination campaign should be implemented in the at-risk population.

There are several types of meningitis vaccines, including polysaccharide vaccines that protect against meningococcal meningitis A, C, W-135, and Y, and conjugate vaccines such as monovalent serogroup A or MenA conjugate vaccine primarily intended for use in the African meningitis belt. More recently, a protein-based vaccine against serogroup B was released in 2014. Optimum protection is effective 8–14 days after vaccination with seroconversion of 90 percent of the recipients over 18–24 months of age. Meningococcal polysaccharide vaccines include bivalent vaccines for serogroups A and C, trivalent vaccine for serogroups A, C, and W-135, and tetravalent for groups A, C, W135, and Y. Trivalent vaccines have been used in response to epidemics in sub-Saharan Africa (Plotkin et al. 2013). Immunity lasts 2 years in younger children and 5 years in adults and older children (Plotkin et al. 2013).

Limitations of the polysaccharide vaccines include poor immune response for children under 2 and short-lived immunity that requires multiple doses. Children aged 2–10 years should be the priority group in campaigns during humanitarian emergencies as they are at highest risk for infection. MenA conjugate vaccine has been used in large vaccine campaigns targeting individuals 1–29 years of age in Burkina Faso, Mali, and Niger, and it is being progressively introduced in other countries of the African meningitis belt (WHO 2011). In response to meningitis outbreaks, the International Coordinating Group (ICG) on Vaccine Provision for Epidemic Meningitis Control is tasked with maintaining an emergency vaccine stockpile globally.

Yellow Fever

Yellow fever is a vector-borne viral disease that is introduced into the bloodstream of humans through the bite of an infected mosquito of the *Aedes* or *Haemogogus* species (WHO 2014b). The yellow fever virus persists in the blood for 17 days, during which transmission is propagated when a mosquito takes a blood meal from an infected human (Heymann, 2008). In urban populations, humans and *Aedes* mosquitoes are the main reservoir (WHO 2005a). Because disease transmission relies on mosquitoes, people living in emergency situations with poor vector control measures, inadequate shelters, malnutrition, and poor sanitation and hygiene are at high risk for contracting yellow fever (WHO 2012a). In addition, transmission of yellow fever increases in jungle or forested areas of tropical settings and during rainy seasons (WHO 2012a). Globally, over nine hundred million people are at risk for yellow fever, with the African region accounting for 90 percent of the burden of disease in 2013, estimated at 84,000–170,000 cases and 29,000–60,000 deaths (WHO 2014b).

The WHO suspected case definition for yellow fever is a disease characterized by fever of abrupt onset followed by jaundice two weeks after the onset of symptoms, and one of the following: (1) bleeding from the nose, gums, skin, or digestive tract, or (2) death within three weeks of the onset of symptoms. (PAHO 2005). Its clinical diagnosis is particularly difficult because its presentation is similar to other viral hemorrhagic diseases, therefore requiring laboratory testing for confirmation (WHO 2008). Confirmed cases are suspected cases that have been laboratory-confirmed or epidemiologically linked to a laboratory-confirmed case. Laboratory criteria for diagnosis include the presence of yellow-fever-specific antibodies, viral isolation, positive postmortem liver histopathology, or detection by immunohistochemistry or PCR (WHO 2008). One confirmed case of yellow fever is considered to be an outbreak (PAHO 2005).

The incubation period for yellow fever is 3–6 days, after which the infection may progress to either an acute or toxic phase (WHO 2005a). The acute phase is characterized by symptoms such as sudden onset fever, chills, headache, muscle pain with backache, and nausea and vomiting (WHO 2014b). The overall CFR is typically less than 5 percent for cases in the acute phase. However, 15 percent of cases progress to the toxic phase, which is characterized by jaundice and hemorrhagic symptoms such as epistaxis, gingival bleeding, hematemesis, and melena (Heymann 2008). In patients with jaundice, the CFR may be as high as 20–50% due to liver and renal failure. There is no specific treatment for yellow fever, but general supportive care should be provided for treatment of fever, dehydration, and respiratory failure (WHO 2014b).

Yellow fever vaccine is a highly effective live-attenuated vaccine with immunity lasting from ten years to lifelong (WHO 2005a). Seroconversion rate is over 95 percent in children and adults after one dose. The vaccine is recommended for those over the age of 6 months and in high-risk populations (PAHO 2005). Many countries provide the yellow fever vaccine concurrently with the measles-containing vaccine (MCV) as part of their national EPI program with no inhibition in serological response (WHO 2005a). Although there is no evidence that the vaccine results in abnormal effects of the fetus, vaccination of pregnant women is recommended only in emergencies and outbreaks. The vaccine is not recommended for symptomatic people living with HIV or other immunosuppressed individuals, but can be given to asymptomatic individuals with HIV.

Cholera

Cholera is an acute bacterial enteric disease caused by an enterotoxin produced by the bacterium *Vibrio cholerae*. There are several serogroups of *V. cholerae*, but only serogroups O1 and O139 lead to outbreaks, with the latter being less common and confined to South-East Asia (WHO 2014c). The environment, such as brackish water and estuaries, and humans are the main reservoirs. *V. cholera* can be transmitted through ingestion of contaminated food or water and subsequently reintroduced into the environment through defecation. The incubation period for cholera ranges from a few hours to five days (Heymann 2008). Approximately 75 percent of infected cases are asymptomatic carriers of the bacterium (WHO 2014c). Severe cases of cholera produce symptoms of sudden profuse watery diarrhea that may resemble rice water (Heymann 2008). Risk of cholera during an emergency increases in endemic areas with overcrowding and lack of access to safe water and sanitary facilities. Poor hygiene practices also increase the risk of an outbreak (WHO 2012a).

In areas where cholera is not endemic, a case of cholera is suspected when a patient aged 5 years or older develops severe dehydration or dies from acute watery diarrhea. In areas where cholera is endemic, cholera is suspected when a patient aged 5 years and older develops acute watery diarrhea with or without vomiting; dehydration or death is no longer required for the case definition (WHO 2014c).

Cholera is confirmed when *V. cholerae* O1 or O139 is isolated from the stool, with antigen identified, of patients presenting with diarrhea (WHO 2014c). Although a rapid diagnostic test (RDT) exists, WHO recommends that all samples that test positive with the rapid test be retested in a laboratory for antimicrobial susceptibility, biotyping, and serotyping (WHO 2003). The biotype and serotype of the isolate can be documented but this information should not delay an appropriate and timely outbreak response. To preserve the viability of the bacteria during transport, the sample should be kept at room temperature and preserved with Cary-Blair or Amies transport media. The alert threshold for cholera is set at one suspected case (CDC 2012). In endemic areas, the outbreak threshold is set based on data from prior years.

Proper case management, provision of safe water, and improvements in sanitation and hygiene are the primary means of containing an outbreak. Untreated cases can lead to rapid dehydration, hypokalemia, hypoglycemia, renal failure, and ultimately death. In severe cases, death can occur within a few hours with CFR exceeding 50 percent. However, given timely and appropriate rehydration treatment, the CFR can be reduced to less than 1 percent (WHO 2014c). Sick individuals should be transported to designated cholera treatment centers for supportive therapy with oral rehydration salts and/or intravenous fluids in severe cases. Antibiotics should be prescribed with caution and according to antimicrobial susceptibility profiles; they have been shown to decrease the duration of illness and bacterial shedding (Nelson et al. 2011). Although conventional measures are recommended as primary means of control, the use of cholera vaccine may be considered among high-risk populations.

There are currently two commercially available, WHO prequalified oral cholera vaccines (OCV). Dukoral^{TM}, produced in Sweden, contains recombinant cholera toxin B subunit (CTB) with O1 serogroup killed whole-cell (WCs) to be administered to the entire population over the age of 2, as a two-dose regimen. A third dose is recommended for children aged 2–5 years. Dukoral is administered in a buffer solution that requires 150 ml of clean water per adult, 75 ml for children. Overall protection is 85 percent for 2 years, with lower protection in children under 5 years of age. Shanchol^{TM}, produced in India, consists of both O1 and O139 serogroup killed WCs but no CTB (Clemens and Holmgren 2014). It is administered orally with a two-dose regimen (WHO 2014d) for the entire population over age 1. No buffer is required, making it the preferred vaccine for field administration. Overall protection is 66 percent at 5 years (Bhattacharya et al. 2013). The vaccines should be stored between 2 to 8 degrees Celsius but should not be frozen (Plotkin et al. 2013). Other vaccines either exist or are under development, but are not yet commercially available on the international market.

While demand for OCVs had been from industrialized countries for those planning travel through endemic areas (WHO 2005a), there is increasing use of OCVs in cholera control in both epidemic and endemic contexts. There have been over 3 million doses of WHO prequalified OCVs administered in more than 16 vaccination campaigns between 1997 and 2014 with costs ranging from $0.11–3.99 USD per person (Lopez et al. 2014). Use has increased significantly since the pre-qualification of Shanchol in 2011 (Lopez et al. 2014). In 2012–13, an OCV campaign conducted in four refugee settings in South Sudan was able to achieve vaccination coverage rates ranging from 70 to 104 percent (Porta et al. 2014). Since then, OCV have been used by various international NGOs in demonstration projects, outbreak response, and preventive vaccination efforts to support the possible use of vaccination as part of the overall response to areas at risk of cholera outbreaks (Ivers et al. 2013, Ivers et al. 2015, Luquero et al. 2013, Luquero et al. 2014, Médecins Sans Frontières 2014, Rouzier et al. 2013).

In 2006, WHO issued recommendations for the use of OCVs in emergency and endemic settings (Chaignot and Monti 2007). In emergency settings, use of OCVs may be considered as a strategy to control outbreaks but must be linked to other public health interventions. These include improving water, sanitation, and hygiene conditions, as well as disease surveillance. WHO recommended a three-tier approach to guide the decision to use OCV. It consists of assessing the risk of a cholera outbreak, the likelihood of timely implementation and the feasibility of conducting a vaccination campaign (Chaignot and Monti 2007). OCVs are recommended in certain endemic settings but the conditions of endemicity should be well defined (Chaignot and Monti 2007). In the Gambella region of Ethiopia where cholera is endemic, OCV vaccination campaigns were conducted among South Sudanese refugees in 2014 to prevent cholera outbreaks in camp settings (Médecins Sans Frontières 2014).

Tetanus

Tetanus is caused when the spores of the bacterium *Clostridium tetani*, which are found in human, animal, and environmental reservoirs, enter the body through a wound or a newborn's umbilical stump (Plotkin et al. 2013). The disease is characterized by painful muscular contractions usually in the jaw and neck muscles and spasms induced by sensory stimuli (Heymann 2008). There is no definition for a confirmed case of tetanus but a clinical case is recorded as an acute illness accompanied by muscle spasms or hypertonia and diagnosed as tetanus by a health care provider in the absence of a more likely diagnosis; or death with tetanus listed as the cause of death or a significant condition contributing to death (CDC 2008). There is no diagnostic test for tetanus; the diagnosis is made clinically by excluding other causes of sudden and involuntary spasms (Pickering et al. 2012).

The incubation period for tetanus is typically between 3 and 21 days, but can range from one day to several months. The elderly and young children are most at risk for tetanus. The CFR ranges from 10–80 percent depending on age and quality of care. Neonatal tetanus is often fatal and can be common in areas where deliveries are conducted under inadequate hygienic conditions (WHO 2012b). A study in Pakistan found that neonatal tetanus accounted for 9 percent of all neonatal mortality among the entire Afghan refugee population (Boss 1987).

Tetanus-containing vaccines include TT (tetanus toxoid), DT (diphtheria toxoids and tetanus toxoid), Td (tetanus toxoid and low dose diphtheria toxoid), DTP or DTwP (diphtheria, tetanus, and killed whole cell pertussis), DTaP or Tdap (diphtheria, tetanus, and acellular pertussis) and pentavalent vaccine (DTP, hepatitis B, and *Haemophilius influenzae* type A). The WHO recommends that tetanus vaccination be offered to anyone engaged in debris clean-up or construction and to internally displaced persons (IDPs) who have not yet received three doses (WHO 2013b). The Advisory Committee on Immunization Practices recommends routine booster vaccination with tetanus toxoid-containing vaccines every ten years (Chapman et al. 2008). Tetanus vaccination is typically offered to victims of emergencies on an as-needed basis due to the noncommunicable nature of the condition and because a subpopulation may have partial protection against tetanus from previous vaccinations (WHO 2013b).

Immunization against tetanus is considered important in disasters involving traumatic wounds and injuries and particularly among populations with low tetanus vaccination coverage (WHO 2012a). In 2005, 109 cases of severe tetanus associated with superficial wounds occurred following the Boxing Day Tsunami in Aceh, Indonesia, resulting in a CFR of 19 percent (Jeremijenko et al. 2007). In emergency situations, special attention is also given to preventing maternal and neonatal tetanus (WHO 2012a). There have been clusters of tetanus cases following the earthquake in Haiti and floods in Pakistan, resulting in vaccination campaigns targeting women and children under 5 years of age in IDP camps (Afshar et al. 2011, Khan et al. 2013). It is important to note that a sudden surge in the number of tetanus cases due to mass injuries, particularly in the first few weeks after a disaster, may resemble an outbreak, but this is not attributable to person-to-person transmission as there is no person-to-person transmission for *C. tetani*. In addition to tetanus vaccination, treatment of contaminated, open wounds should be combined with rapid access to appropriate medical and surgical care. In protracted emergencies, reestablishment of routine vaccination services should be the focus of tetanus prevention. Immunizing women of childbearing age will help prevent maternal and neonatal tetanus in emergencies where prior TT immunization levels have been low (WHO 2013b).

Diphtheria

Diphtheria is an acute upper respiratory disease caused by exotoxin produced by the bacterium *Corynebacterium diphtheriae* (PAHO 2005). A probable case of diphtheria is defined as an upper respiratory tract illness with an adherent membrane of the nose, pharynx, tonsils, or larynx (CDC 2008). A confirmed case is an upper respiratory tract illness with an adherent membrane of the nose, pharynx, tonsils, or larynx, and any of the following: isolation of *C. diphtheriae* from the nose or throat, histopathologic diagnosis of diphtheria, or epidemiologic linkage to a laboratory-confirmed case of diphtheria (CDC 2008).

For laboratory confirmation, a bacteriological culture is done using specimen from pharyngeal swabs. Throat swab specimens should be transported in Amies or Stuart media. After *C. diphtheriae* is isolated, the biotype can be determined. Testing for toxin production can only be done in selected reference laboratories (PAHO 2005).

Diphtheria is transmitted person to person via oral or respiratory droplets and close physical contact with an infected human (Tiwari 2014). The incubation period is usually from 2 to 5 days, but may range from 1 to 10 days (Heymann 2008). Different types of diphtheria affect various anatomic sites there by producing different symptoms (Atkinson et al. 2012). For instance, respiratory diphtheria commonly affects mucous membranes of the upper respiratory tract while cutaneous diphtheria affects the skin (Tiwari 2014). In moderate to severe cases, airway obstruction may develop and lead to death. The CFR is generally from 5-10 percent but may be as high as 20 percent among those younger than 5 years and over 40 years of age (Atkinson et al. 2012). Overcrowding and population movement can lead to outbreaks of diphtheria as can low access to preventive and curative services (WHO 2012a). Diphtheria is seasonal and most commonly occurs during cold seasons.

Diphtheria vaccines are based on diphtheria toxoid, a modified bacterial toxin that induces protective antitoxin (WHO 2006). The most common vaccines for prevention of diphtheria are DTP, DTaP, and pentavalent combination vaccines. WHO recommends three doses of diphtheria vaccine and at least one booster for children, while adults should receive boosters every 10 years (Plotkin et al. 2013). The WHO recommends the primary vaccination series to start at 6 weeks of age with two additional doses at 4–8 week intervals and the last dose completed by 6 months of age (WHO 2006).

Risk Assessment

In the emergency phase, an initial epidemiological assessment should be made to evaluate the immunity gap of the affected population and the risk of VPD transmission (WHO 2012a). Assessing the risk of an epidemic and the size of the population at risk will guide decision-making regarding the need for vaccine use during an emergency. Resources to be considered in such an assessment include administrative vaccination coverage data from routine immunization programs, which can be found on the WHO online database: www.who.int/immunization/monitoring_surveillance/data/en/. SIAs such as mass vaccination campaigns, periodic intensification of routine immunization activities (PIRI), or prior ORI activities as well as previous coverage or serological surveys conducted, if available, can provide valuable information.

Due to the challenges in obtaining accurate administrative coverage data, it is important to utilize additional complimentary data sources such as surveillance and epidemic reports, including those from

Ministries of Health (MoH), joint WHO-UNICEF estimates (WUENIC), early warning reporting systems (EWARN), and ProMed (ISID 2015, WHO 2015a, WHO 2012c).

The magnitude of, and areas affected by the previous outbreaks can provide information regarding the degree of natural immunity within a population. Proxy variables, such as child mortality ratios and burden of disease estimates among children, may also be useful information since VPDs account for a majority of postneonatal deaths among children under 5 years of age in many settings.

During humanitarian emergencies, risk assessments for VPD transmission should include the prevalence of malnutrition and chronic disease; overcrowding; insufficient water, sanitation, and hygiene; and access to curative health services (WHO 2012a). Geography, climate and season, levels of sexual violence, and incidence of injuries should also be taken into account in the overall risk assessment.

Other important issues to be considered include the feasibility of implementing high quality vaccination efforts in potentially politically unstable and insecure environments, vaccine availability, and comprehensive supply chain management attributes. Any recent changes in the routine immunization system, including cold chain management and financing of vaccine supplies and health staff, should be accounted for in the assessment. Moreover, the opportunity cost of not conducting emergency vaccination efforts needs to be examined. If any of these steps are not conducive to vaccine use, one should continue monitoring barriers for implementation as well as changes in disease patterns and key risk factors (WHO 2012a).

Control Measures

Surveillance

During humanitarian emergencies, broad public health surveillance systems for detection of VPDs and other communicable diseases may be underperforming, disrupted, or nonexistent. Efforts should focus on strengthening surveillance of priority conditions and diseases, especially diseases of epidemic potential. Additional details on surveillance during emergencies can be found in Chapter 9.

High-quality surveillance that ensures rapid identification is a key component of early outbreak detection and response. This includes formulating a case definition and an appropriate alert threshold that may be defined as the number of cases higher than expected for a specified time period and population. Distinction between immediate or weekly reporting, alert thresholds to initiate investigation, and rapid systems for reporting and response should be established before emergencies and activated as early as possible in the response phase. In addition, standard procedures for information-sharing and timely feedback of surveillance data will encourage consistent and complete reporting from relevant partners. Regular supportive supervision with feedback will improve the quality of data being reported.

According to Sphere standards, an early warning system for outbreak detection should be implemented at both health facility and community levels by engaging a network of implementing partners (The Sphere Project 2011). The early warning alert and response network (EWARN) developed by WHO to rapidly detect and respond to outbreaks of epidemic-prone diseases is an example of such a surveillance system (World Health Organization 2012). Although EWARN is not a substitute for the national surveillance system, it serves the purpose of filling in a surveillance gap while routine systems are reestablished. The network consists of two main components, including an immediate alert component that signals the early stages of an outbreak and a weekly reporting component that reports weekly data aggregated by health facilities. These complementary components ensure timely detection of outbreaks, which allows prompt case investigation and effective monitoring of morbidity patterns. Once the acute emergency phase is over, EWARN should be integrated into the national surveillance system (World Health Organization 2012).

A successful EWARN system is characterized by its ability to rapidly detect and respond to diseases of high priority. For instance, the EWARN established in Darfur, Sudan, between January and October 2009 was able to detect thirty alerts by strengthening surveillance capabilities at health clinics and respond to ten outbreaks of epidemic-prone diseases (Morof et al. 2013). In 2010, an early warning disease surveillance system was also established in Pakistan after months of extreme flooding and was able to detect 130 alerts of acute watery diarrhea (AWD), suspected measles, acute flaccid paralysis, and suspected meningitis (Centers for Disease Control and Prevention

2012); at least one sample from AWD alert was confirmed to be cholera.

Outbreak Response

Essential components of outbreak response include appropriate and timely investigation of reported cases and confirmation of suspected cases through laboratory testing of specimens. An outbreak investigation team should be established early in the response and ideally include individuals from the MoH, WHO, and UN organizations, and NGOs working in health, WASH, and other relevant sectors. The investigation should consist of descriptive epidemiological information such as the number of cases by age and sex, time period, and geographic location to guide outbreak control measures in vulnerable locations or among subpopulations. The attack rates can also be calculated if the size of the affected population is known. Additional epidemiological studies can be conducted to identify mode of transmission, key risk factors, and at-risk populations. All reported cases and respective contacts should have appropriate follow-up. The results of the investigation should be documented and disseminated to key partners along with recommended actions.

Another critical component of outbreak response is implementation of control and prevention measures specific for the disease. Interventions to control outbreaks may vary according to the disease and may range from prevention of exposure (such as rapid isolation and treatment for cholera) or prevention of infection through mass vaccination (i.e., measles or meningococcal disease) (WHO 2005a). Ensuring timely treatment of cases per national or WHO guidelines, adequate number of trained personnel, treatment supplies including medications and rehydration modalities, laboratory and treatment facilities, and resources for transportation of patients, specimens, and vaccines are all crucial components to appropriate case management. Outbreak detection and response can be maximized through effective communication and coordination between agencies involved in public health activities, clinical and laboratory services, and the community.

For certain VPDs such as measles, preemptive vaccination campaigns are often conducted before an outbreak occurs to mitigate the risk of an outbreak that may result in high mortality (World Health Organization 2012a). Other VPDs, such as yellow fever or cholera, often require lab confirmation before the vaccine can be requested from a global stockpile (World Health Organization 2013c). Subtyping of *N. meningitidis* is also needed to request the appropriate vaccine for use (ICG 2008).

Vaccination Campaigns

Based on the initial risk assessment, outbreaks requiring mass vaccination efforts will need to consider key issues in the planning of a vaccination campaign. These are outlined in Table 16.1. Organization of a vaccination campaign requires strong technical knowledge and management. Roles and responsibilities for each component of the vaccination campaign should be assigned clearly to participating organizations by the health coordination agency. The national EPI manager of the host country should be involved from the beginning of the planning stages of the campaign.

The scope and timing of vaccination campaigns, including the target age group, geographic location, and duration and dates of activities will need to be defined, along with estimates of vaccine needs, presentation, and estimate wastage rates. Mass vaccination activities can vary in scale, ranging from a community level or subnational selective approach to a nationwide nonselective vaccination strategy. In selective vaccination, the vaccination status of the child is checked and vaccine administered only to those without evidence of previous vaccination. In a nonselective approach, vaccination is given to all children regardless of their previous vaccination status. Nonselective vaccination is often preferred in a mass campaign, as it allows for a more rapid response – it is often difficult to ascertain vaccination status. Coordination with key stakeholders and development of a budgeted macroplan will help ensure political commitment. Creation of technical, logistics, and communication working groups will help to address key components of a successful campaign.

To ensure high vaccination coverage during humanitarian emergencies, vaccine administration may be conducted at screening centers or entry points on arrival of displaced populations as part of the mass vaccination strategy. This approach is feasible when the screening facility is already established and the influx of the displaced population is steady and moderate. Alternatively, mass vaccination can take place in selected areas through health facilities or by outreach teams. This approach is appropriate when individuals have already settled

Table 16.1 Key issues in the planning of a vaccination campaign

Scope and timing of the campaign	• National vs. subnational • Target population (age, numbers) • Time, place, days and duration
Macroplanning and coordination	• Develop budgeted macroplan • Ensure political commitment • Engage interagency coordination • Create working groups to address (1) technical, (2) vaccine, cold chain, and logistics, and (3) advocacy, social mobilization, and communication aspects of the campaign
Strategies to achieve high vaccine coverage	• Fixed vs. mobile posts (or combination) • Mass vaccination vs. routine vaccination • Selective vs. nonselective vaccination • Consideration of special populations and high-risk groups • Integration with other public health interventions
Microplanning and logistics	• Obtain map of site (major access routes, health facilities, schools, market places) • Estimate target population • Requirements for vaccine and supplies, cold chain, personnel, transport, waste disposal
Communication and social mobilization	• Develop communication plan and key messages, visual displays with posters, banners, pamphlets; media messaging (radio, TV, SMS, megaphones) • Announcements at community and religious gatherings • Involvement of schools and local volunteers; consideration of underserved population and high-risk groups
Training	• Training of vaccination teams • Intracampaign supervision and monitoring • Adverse events following immunization (AEFI) • Management and coordination of operations
Implementation and operations of vaccination campaign	• Organization and management of vaccination posts • Roles and responsibilities of vaccination team (vaccinator, recorder, crowd control, supervisors) • Safe vaccine administration • Waste disposal (incineration or burial pits) • Intracampaign monitoring
Postcampaign activities	• Mop-up vaccination activities • Analysis and summary of administrative coverage data • Postcampaign coverage survey

within the camp or when a screening facility has not been established due to rapid influx of the displaced population. After such mass vaccination campaigns, efforts should be placed in vaccination at entry points and establishment of routine immunization programs to ensure adequate vaccination coverage among all displaced populations.

Careful microplanning is needed to ensure that the entire target population within the catchment area is well covered. Vaccination sites should be mapped out to identify the location and capacity of all health facilities. In addition, the location of outreach teams should be determined where additional vaccination sites are needed along with the movement plans of these outreach teams for planning and monitoring purposes. Logistic requirements for a mass vaccination campaign will include the total number of vaccine doses required after taking into account vaccine wastage. The vaccine wastage factor is used to calculate how much additional vaccination should be ordered (WHO 2005c). For example, a wastage factor of 1.5 means that 1.5 times the anticipated vaccine needed for coverage should be ordered given how much vaccine wastage is anticipated. A typical vaccine wastage factor for the measles vaccine is 1.1 and for the oral polio vaccine, 1.3. The number of disposable needles and syringes required is the same as the total number of vaccine doses needed including wasted doses.

Symbol	Explanation	Stage
◯ ✓	The inner square is lighter than the outer circle. If the expiry date has not passed, **USE** the vaccine.	I
◯ ✓	As time passes the inner square is still lighter than the outer circle. If the expiry date has not passed, **USE** the vaccine.	II
◯ ✗	**Discard point:** the color of the inner square matches that of the outer circle. **DO NOT** USE the vaccine.	III
◼ ✗	Beyond the discard point: inner square is darker than the outer circle. **DO NOT** USE the vaccine.	IV

Figure 16.1 Vaccine Vial Monitor (VVM) Reading Key (WHO 2002)

All vaccines are temperature sensitive and will require vaccine specific management to ensure adequate temperature control until the time of administration; therefore, the logistic requirements for mass vaccination include assessing the number of vaccine vials required and the number of any necessary cold chain equipment such as refrigerators, freezers, cold boxes, vaccine carriers, and ice packs. The availability and procurement of vaccines and cold chain equipment should be assessed with the MOH, United Nations Children's Fund (UNICEF) or WHO.

Various types of refrigerator and freezer are available either powered by kerosene, electricity, gas or solar energy. When vaccines are placed in a cold box for any purpose, a thermometer should also be placed with the vaccine to monitor the temperature. Two major types of cold box are available: the small box allows vaccines to be stored for 24 hours, while the larger box stores vaccines safely for up to 7 days. It is crucial to check the expiration date of the vaccine and the vaccine vial monitor (VVM) to determine whether the vaccines have been exposed to heat. A vaccine vial monitor reading key is shown in Figure 16–1. Sufficient and reliable cold chain capacity remains a considerable challenge in disaster and emergency settings where infrastructure or electricity for refrigeration may be damaged or destroyed (Desai and Kamat, 2014).

An effective communication plan is crucial for conveying key messages of the vaccination campaign to the community and target population. Media messaging, visual aids, and engagement of community and religious leaders are useful for social mobilization purposes. Involvement of schools and civil society will also ensure the catchment population is aware of the vaccination campaign. In preparation of the campaign, sufficient amount of time should be allotted for training of staff. Key areas to be covered in the training of vaccination teams include the overall strategy and campaign operations, antigens to be given and safe injection techniques, accurate and timely recording and reporting of vaccinations given, guidance on vaccination contradictions and precautions, protocols on dealing with adverse events following immunization (AEFI), appropriate waste management, and intracampaign monitoring and supervision to ensure immediate corrective actions.

A joint policy statement on injection safety by WHO and UNICEF was issued to ensure that each injection is given with a sterile needle and a sterile syringe, and that single-use needles and syringes must be safely stored and incinerated after use (WHO 1999). Sufficient quantities of auto-destruct syringes and safety disposal boxes should be included in the planning and implementation of all mass vaccination campaigns. It is crucial that needles are not recapped, rather discarded immediately into a puncture-resistant container after use. Unsafe injection practices can result in complications including skin abscesses, transmission of bloodborne viruses such as hepatitis B and C as well as HIV.

Vaccination sites should be organized in such a way to ensure ease of access with protection against sun and rain. A member of the team can monitor and enforce appropriate crowd control and flow of operations at the vaccination site. The entrances and exits should be at different ends of the vaccination site. A registration point should be placed at the entrance and a supervisor at the exit point to check that the individual has been registered and received the appropriate vaccine and vaccination card.

Once the campaign is complete, evaluation of vaccination coverage of the target population is important. This can be done by immediate analysis of administrative coverage reported during the campaign, followed by a postcampaign coverage survey. Survey guidelines developed by WHO for EPI and an inter-agency initiative for nutrition surveys are available to provide reference for appropriate sampling methodology during emergencies (WHO 2012d; WHO 2005b; Smart Methodology 2013). Geographic areas that exhibit low vaccination coverage may require follow-up or mop-up vaccination activities.

Organizations

An effective vaccination campaign requires coordination with local governing bodies and cooperation from multiple agencies and humanitarian partners, especially when multiple interventions are being implemented. Roles and responsibilities should be established early to monitor and ensure tasks are carried out in an adequate and quality controlled manner by each operating partner (MSF 1997). The MoH and national EPI manager of the host country should be involved from the beginning of the campaign's planning stages as national vaccination guidelines are often applied in emergency situations (WHO 2005a). Involvement of civil society and local NGOs in the decision making process will ensure the campaign is well communicated to all beneficiaries and conducted in a manner that is accepted by the local community (Grais and Juan-Giner 2014).

Various UN agencies are involved in the planning and response to outbreaks of VPD. During humanitarian emergencies, WHO, or their designee, typically coordinates the overall response as the health cluster lead along with local governing bodies to strengthen surveillance and provides technical guidance and standards in case-management. Timely procurement of a sufficient quantity of vaccines is required during an emergency in order to adequately cover the campaign's target population. UNICEF typically leads efforts in procurement of vaccines and cold chain equipment. The MoH may choose to purchase vaccines directly from the manufacturer or to request assistance from UNICEF to purchase the vaccines through its Supply Division. For certain VPDs, such as yellow fever, meningococcal disease, and cholera, international vaccine stockpiles have been established for emergency use and are currently managed jointly by UNICEF, Doctors Without Borders (Médecins Sans Frontières [MSF]), International Federation of the Red Cross and Red Crescent (IFRC) and WHO through the International Coordination Group (ICG) (World Health Organization 2012a). To request vaccine supplies from ICG, a country should provide evidence to support the need and capacity for mass vaccination, such as laboratory confirmation of an outbreak, documentation of action plans and sufficient cold chain storage capacity.

Coordination specifically for refugees is typically provided by UNHCR (with the exception of Palestine refugees under the coordination of the UN Relief and Works Agency for Palestine Refugees [UNWRA]). IFRC and its national societies as well as international NGOs such as Médecins Sans Frontières, Save the Children International, International Rescue Committee, among others, can also strengthen efforts through social mobilization, case management, and case detection through health facility and community-based surveillance.

Civil societies, religious and community leaders, community health workers, and traditional healers also play important roles in raising community awareness and addressing concerns of families and the local community (WHO 2005a). Issues such as informed consent is an important ethical consideration for mass vaccination campaigns in emergency settings where autonomy and the right to refuse vaccination may not be absolute (Moodley et al. 2013). Involvement of all key stakeholders is critical in ensuring that the community understands the purpose and importance of the vaccination campaign.

Conclusion

Humanitarian emergencies place affected populations at risk for elevated morbidity and mortality from VPDs due to risk factors such as mass population movements, overcrowding, poor water and sanitation conditions, malnutrition, and inadequate access to health care and preventive services.

Epidemic-prone VPDs are of particular concern during acute emergencies. Enhancement of surveillance and case management is critical in outbreak response. Vaccination is one of the most basic and critical health interventions for protecting at risk, vulnerable populations during humanitarian emergencies. Therefore, successful planning and implementation of mass vaccination campaigns should consider all of the key issues presented in this chapter.

During emergencies that involve civil unrest, insecurity may prevent access to certain areas within a region or country. Rapid accumulation of susceptible populations can occur in these areas deemed unsafe to conduct vaccination activities. In periods of active conflict, high vaccination coverage for certain epidemic-prone diseases including measles and polio is difficult to achieve. Growing insecurities, as seen in the increasing number of targeted attacks on health workers in recent years during polio eradication efforts in Pakistan, can dramatically limit the ability of humanitarian players to provide the necessary vaccinations (Alexander et al. 2014, Owais et al. 2013, Riaz and Rehman 2013).

During the World Humanitarian Day in 2014, WHO called for increased protection of health workers in conflicts and disasters, stating that recent attacks in Syria, South Sudan, Gaza, Pakistan, and Nigeria have adversely impacted the treatment of patients as well as the prevention and control of communicable diseases (WHO 2014e). Possible solutions may include temporary peace negotiated to permit implementation of vaccination activities, such as the Days of Tranquility for polio campaigns in Latin America back in the 1980s and 1990s (World Health Organization, 2015). Immunization activities in limited geographic locations may also be negotiated with the local authorities. Effective coordination and collaboration between all health partners can rebuild confidence in vaccination among the affected population and ensure all susceptible persons have access to life saving vaccines.

Notes from the Field

Jordan (2013)

The conflict in Syria has resulted in over 2 million refugees living in neighboring countries including Jordan. Because of the conflict, vaccination in this population has been extremely low, and as a result, a measles outbreak among refugees was reported in 2013, with spread to Jordanians (Sharara and Kanj, 2014). The US Centers for Disease Prevention and Control (CDC) provided technical assistance in planning and implementing an emergency measles immunization campaign in two governorates bordering Syria, Irbid and Mafraq, at the request of the Jordanian MoH. A measles and vitamin A campaign targeting six hundred thousand children between 6 months and 15 years of age was implemented in June 2014. CDC provided assistance in developing microplans, tally and summary sheets, field guides, and supervisory checklists.

The planning and implementation of the mass vaccination activity was coordinated with key UN agencies including WHO, UNICEF, UNHCR, and UNWRA. Coordination efforts with NGOs working with Syrian and Iraqi refugees and schools with Syrian children ensured that those populations were also targeted. An independent local academic institution conducted the intracampaign monitoring using a rapid assessment tool. The emergency coordination resulted in the vaccination of 540,000 children against measles. Through advocacy meetings before the campaign, governorate staff at the highest level took ownership and leadership of the campaign. This was a crucial feature for the success of the campaign.

Additional lessons learned include close collaboration and coordination of MOH with NGOs and relevant partners to facilitate smooth implementation and timely decisions related to the campaign. Furthermore, both the MoH and governorate management staff were highly motivated and committed, responding swiftly to feedback from the field by taking the necessary corrective actions. A postcampaign evaluation survey was conducted shortly after the campaign to provide an external assessment of vaccination coverage for both Jordanian and non-Jordanian populations within the governorates of Irbid and Mafraq.

Acknowledgement

The authors would like to thank Anyie Li and Jennifer Head for their editorial assistance and help in review of the current literature.

References

Afshar, M., Raju, M., Ansell, D., et al. (2011). Narrative review: Tetanus-a health threat after natural disasters in developing countries. *Annals of Internal Medicine*, **154**, 329–335.

Alexander, J. P., Jr., Zubair, M., Khan, M., et al. (2014). Progress and peril: poliomyelitis eradication efforts in Pakistan, 1994–2013. *The Journal of Infectious Diseases*, **210**, S152–161.

Atkinson, W., Wolfe, S., and Hamborsky, J. (2012). *Epidemiology and prevention of vaccine-preventable diseases*, 12th edition, Washington, DC: Public Health Foundation.

Bhatt, K. M., Bhatt, S. M., and Mirza, N. B. (1996). Meningococcal meningitis. *East African Medical Journal*, **73**, 35–39.

Bhattacharya, S. K., Sur, D., Ali, M., et al. (2013). 5 year efficacy of a bivalent killed whole-cell oral cholera vaccine in Kolkata, India: A cluster-randomised, double-blind, placebo-controlled trial. *The Lancet Infectious Diseases*, **13**, 1050–1056.

Boss, L. P., Brink, E. W., and Dondero, T. J. (1987). Infant mortality and childhood nutritional status among Afghan refugees in Pakistan. *International Journal of Epidemiology*, **16**, 556–560.

Centers for Disease Control and Prevention. (2008). Manual for the surveillance of vaccine-preventable diseases (online). Available at: www.cdc.gov/vaccines/pubs/surv-manual/index.html (Accessed November 5, 2015).

Centers for Disease Control and Prevention. (2012). Early warning disease surveillance after a flood emergency–Pakistan, 2010. *Morbidity and Mortality Weekly Report*, **61**, 1002–1007.

Chaignat, C. L. and Monti, V. (2007). Use of oral cholera vaccine in complex emergencies: What next? Summary report of an expert meeting and recommendations of WHO. *Journal of Health, Population and Nutrition*, **25**, 244–261.

Chapman, L. E., Sullivent, E. E., Grohskopf, L. A., et al. (2008). Postexposure interventions to prevent infection with HBV, HCV, or HIV, and tetanus in people wounded during bombings and other mass casualty events–United States, 2008: Recommendations of the Centers for Disease Control and Prevention and Disaster Medicine and Public Health Preparedness. *Disaster Medicine and Public Health Preparedness*, **2**, 150–165.

Clemens, J. and Holmgren, J. (2014). When, how, and where can oral cholera vaccines be used to interrupt cholera outbreaks? *Current Topics in Microbiology and Immunology*, **379**, 231–258.

Cohn, J. (2014). The challenge of vaccinating in emergency settings: Policy and advocacy implications. *International Journal of Infectious Diseases*, **21**, 51.

Connolly, M. A., Gayer, M., Ryan, M. J., et al. (2004). Communicable diseases in complex emergencies: impact and challenges. *Lancet*, **364**, 1974–1983.

Date, K. A., Vicari, A., Hyde, T. B., et al. (2011). Considerations for oral cholera vaccine use during outbreak after earthquake in Haiti, 2010–2011. *Emerging Infectious Diseases*, **17**, 2105–2112.

Desai, S. N. and Kamat, D. (2014). Closing the global immunization gap: delivery of lifesaving vaccines through innovation and technology. *Pediatrics in Review*, **35**, e32–40.

Dorlencourt, F., Legros, D., Paquet, C., et al. (1999). Effectiveness of mass vaccination with WC/rBS cholera vaccine during an epidemic in Adjumani district, Uganda. *Bulletin of the World Health Organization*, **77**, 949–950.

Grais, R. F. and Juan-Giner, A. (2014). Vaccination in humanitarian crises: Satisficing should no longer suffice. *International Health*, **6**, 160–161.

Heyman, S. N., Ginosar, Y., Niel, L., et al. (1998). Meningococcal meningitis among Rwandan refugees: Diagnosis, management, and outcome in a field hospital. *International Journal of Infectious Diseases*, **2**, 137–142.

Heymann, D. L. (2008). *Control of communicable diseases manual*, nineteenth edition, Washington, DC: American Public Health Association.

International Coordinating Group. (2008). International coordinating group in vaccine provision for epidemic meningitis control: Guidelines for applying to the emergency stockpile (online). Available at: www.who.int/csr/disease/meningococcal/ICG_guidelines_2008_02_09.pdf (Accessed March 30, 2015).

International Society for Infectious Diseases. (2015). *ProMed mail* (online). Available at: http://promedmail.org/ (Accessed March 21, 2015).

Ivers, L. C., Hilaire, I. J., Teng, J. E., et al. (2015). Effectiveness of reactive oral cholera vaccination in rural Haiti: a case-control study and bias-indicator analysis. *The Lancet Global Health*, **3**, e162–168.

Ivers, L. C., Teng, J. E., Lascher, J., et al. (2013). Use of oral cholera vaccine in Haiti: a rural demonstration project. *The American Journal of Tropical Medicine and Hygiene*, **89**, 617–624.

Jeremijenko, A., Mclaws, M. L., and Kosasih, H. (2007). A tsunami related tetanus epidemic in Aceh, Indonesia. *Asia Pacific Journal of Public Health*, **19**, 40–44.

Kaiser, R. (2014). Emergency settings: be prepared to vaccinate persons aged 15 and over against measles. *The Journal of Infectious Diseases*, **210**, 1857–1859.

Kamadjeu, R., Mahamud, A., Webeck, J., et al. (2014). Polio outbreak investigation and response in Somalia, 2013. *The Journal of Infectious Diseases*, **210**, S181–1816.

Kamugisha, C., Cairns, K. L. and Akim, C. (2003). An outbreak of measles in Tanzanian refugee camps. *The Journal of Infectious Diseases*, **187**, S58–62.

Khan, A. A., Zahidie, A., and Rabbani, F. (2013). Interventions to reduce neonatal mortality from neonatal tetanus in low and middle income countries–a systematic review. *BMC Public Health*, **13**, 322.

Luquero, F. J., Grout, L., Ciglenecki, I., et al. (2013). First outbreak response using an oral cholera vaccine in Africa: Vaccine coverage, acceptability and surveillance of adverse events, Guinea, 2012. *PLOS Neglected Tropical Diseases*, **7**, e2465.

Luquero, F. J., Grout, L., Ciglenecki, I., et al. (2014). Use of Vibrio cholerae vaccine in an outbreak in Guinea. *The New England Journal of Medicine*, **370**, 2111–20.

Martin, S., Lopez, A. L., Bellos, A., et al. (2014). Post-licensure deployment of oral cholera vaccines: A systematic review. *Bulletin of the World Health Organization*, **92**, 881–93.

Médecins Sans Frontières. (1997). *Refugee health: An approach to emergency situations*. London, UK: Pan Macmillan.

Médecins Sans Frontières. (2008). Sample collection, storage and transport from field to reference laboratory (online). Available at: https://pmb.gva.ocg.msf.org/opac_css/doc_num.php?explnum_id=1291 (Accessed March 30, 2015).

Médecins Sans Frontières. (2014). Ethiopia: Tens of thousands of South Sudanese refugees receive cholera vaccine (online). www.msf.org/article/ethiopia-tens-thousands-south-sudanese-refugees-receive-cholera-vaccine (Accessed August 30, 2015).

Moodley, K., Hardie, K., Selgelid, M. J., et al. (2013). Ethical considerations for vaccination programmes in acute humanitarian emergencies. *Bulletin of the World Health Organization*, **91**, 290–297.

Navarro-Colorado, C., Mahamud, A., Burton, A., et al. (2014). Measles outbreak response among adolescent and adult Somali refugees displaced by famine in Kenya and Ethiopia, 2011. *The Journal of Infectious Diseases*, **210**, 1863–1870.

Nelson, E. J., Nelson, D. S., Salam, M. A., et al. (2011). Antibiotics for both moderate and severe cholera. *The New England Journal of Medicine*, **364**, 5–7.

Owais, A., Khowaja, A. R., Ali, S. A., et al. (2013). Pakistan's expanded programme on immunization: an overview in the context of polio eradication and strategies for improving coverage. *Vaccine*, **31**, 3313–3319.

Pan American Health Organization. (2005). Control of yellow fever field guide (online). Available at: http://new.PAHO.org/hq/dmdocuments/2009/fieldguide_yellowfever.pdf (Accessed August 10, 2015).

Paquet, C. (1992). *Rèfugiès Touaregs dans le sud-est de la Mauritanie*. Paris: Epicentre.

Perry, R. T., Plowe, C. V., Koumare, B., et al. (1998). A single dose of live oral cholera vaccine CVD 103-HgR is safe and immunogenic in HIV-infected and HIV-noninfected adults in Mali. *Bulletin of the World Health Organization*, **76**, 63–71.

Pickering, L. K., Baker C. J., and Kimberlin, D. W. (2012). *Red Book: Report of the Committee on Infectious Diseases*, 29th edition, Elk Grove Village, IL: American Academy of Pediatrics.

Plotkin, S. A., Orenstein, W. A., and Offit, P. A. (2013). *Vaccines*, 6th edition, Atlanta: Elsevier Inc.

Polonsky, J. A., Singh, B., Masiku, C., et al. (2015). Exploring HIV infection and susceptibility to measles among older children and adults in Malawi: A facility-based study. *International Journal of Infectious Diseases*, **31**, 61–67.

Porta, M. I., Lenglet, A., De Weerdt, S., et al. (2014). Feasibility of a preventive mass vaccination campaign with two doses of oral cholera vaccine during a humanitarian emergency in South Sudan. *Transactions of the Royal Society of Tropical Medicine and Hygiene*, **108**, 810–815.

Riaz, H., Rehman, A. (2013). Polio vaccination workers gunned down in Pakistan. *The Lancet Infectious Diseases*, **13**, 120

Rouzier, V., Severe, K., Jean Juste, M. A., et al. (2013) Cholera vaccination in urban Haiti. *The American Journal of Tropical Medicine and Hygiene*, **89**, 671–681.

Salama, P., Spiegel, P., Talley, L., et al. (2004). Lessons learned from complex emergencies over past decade. *Lancet*, **364**, 1801–1813.

Santaniello-Newton, A. and Hunter, P. R. (2000). Management of an outbreak of meningococcal meningitis in a Sudanese refugee camp in Northern Uganda. *Epidemiology and Infection*, **124**, 75–81.

Sharara, S. L. and Kanj, S. S. (2014). War and infectious diseases: Challenges of the Syrian civil war. *PLOS Pathogens*, **10**, e1004438.

Sheikh, M. A., Makokha, F., Hussein, A. M., et al. (2014). Combined use of inactivated and oral poliovirus vaccines in refugee camps and surrounding communities – Kenya, December 2013. *Morbidity and Mortality Weekly Report*, **63**, 237–241.

Smart Methodology. (2013). Sampling methods and sample size calculation for the SMART methodology (online). Available at: http://smartmethodology.org/survey-planning-tools/smart-methodology (Accessed March 30, 2015).

The Sphere Project. (2011). Essential health services SPHERE Handbook: Humanitarian Charter and Minimum Standards in Humanitarian Response (online). Available at: www.spherehandbook.org (Accessed March 30, 2015).

Tiwari, T. S. P. (2014). *Infectious diseases related to travel* (online). Available at: wwwnc.cdc.gov/travel/yellowbook/2014/chapter-3-infectious-diseases-related-to-travel/diphtheria (Accessed March 21, 2015).

Toole, M. J. and Waldman, R. J. (1988). An analysis of mortality trends among refugee populations in Somalia, Sudan, and Thailand. *Bulletin of the World Health Organization*, 66, 237–247.

Toole, M. J. and Waldman, R. J. (1990). Prevention of excess mortality in refugee and displaced populations in developing countries. *JAMA*, **263**, 3296–3302.

World Health Organization. (1999). WHO-UNICEF-UNFPA joint statement on the use of auto-disable syringes in immunization services (online). Available at: www.who.int/injection_safety/toolbox/Bundling.pdf (Accessed March 30, 2015).

World Health Organization. (2002). Getting Started with vaccine vial monitors (online) Available at: www.path.org/vaccineresources/files/Getting_started_with_VVMs.pdf (Accessed March 30, 2015).

World Health Organization. (2003). Manual for the laboratory identification and antimicrobial susceptibility testing of bacterial pathogens of public health importance in the developing world (online). Available at: www.who.int/csr/resources/publications/drugresist/IIIAMRManual.pdf?ua=1 (Accessed August 10, 2015).

World Health Organization. (2005a). Communicable disease control in emergencies (online). Available at: http://whqlibdoc.who.int/publications/2005/9241546166_eng.pdf?ua=1. (Accessed Nov 5, 2015).

World Health Organization. (2005b). Immunization coverage cluster survey – reference manual (online).

Available at: http://whqlibdoc.who.int/hq/2005/WHO_IVB_04.23.pdf. (Accessed July 10, 2017).

World Health Organization. (2005c). Monitoring vaccine wastage at country level (online). Available at: http://apps.who.int/iris/bitstream/10665/68463/1/WHO_VB_03.18.Rev.1_eng.pdf. (Accessed January 29, 2018).

World Health Organization. (2006). Vaccine position papers: Diphtheria (online). Available at: www.who.int/wer/2006/wer8103.pdf (Accessed March 30, 2015).

World Health Organization. (2008). WHO-recommended standards for surveillance of selected vaccine-preventable diseases (online). Available at: http://apps.who.int/iris/bitstream/10665/68334/1/WHO_V-B_03.01_eng.pdf. (Accessed August 10, 2015).

World Health Organization. (2009). Vaccine position papers: *Measles* (online). Available at: www.who.int/wer/2009/wer8435.pdf (Accessed March 30, 2015).

World Health Organization. (2011). Vaccine position papers: Meningococcal vaccines (online). Available at: www.who.int/wer/2011/wer8647.pdf (Accessed March 30, 2015).

World Health Organization. (2012a). SAGE working group on vaccination in humanitarian emergencies, vaccination in acute emergencies: A framework for decision making, revised draft (online). Available at: www.who.int/immunization/sage/meetings/2012/november/FinalFraft_FrmwrkDocument_SWGVHE_23OctFullWEBVERSION.pdf (Accessed March 30, 2015).

World Health Organization. (2012b). *Tetanus* (online). Available at: www.wpro.who.int/mediacentre/factsheets/fs_20120307_tetanus/en/ (Accessed March 21, 2015).

World Health Organization. (2012c). Outbreak surveillance and response in humanitarian emergencies (online). Available at: www.who.int/diseasecontrol_emergencies/publications/who_hse_epr_dce_2012.1/en/ (Accessed March 30, 2015).

World Health Organization. (2012d). Assessing vaccination coverage levels using clustered lot quality assurance sampling. Version edited for the Global Polio Eradication Initiative (GPEI) (online). Available at: www.polioeradication.org/portals/0/document/research/opvdelivery/lqas.pdf (Accessed August 10, 2015).

World Health Organization. (2013a). Measles elimination field guide (online). Available at: www.wpro.who.int/immunization/documents/measles_elimination_field_guide_2013.pdf (Accessed March 30, 2015).

World Health Organization. (2013b). *Should tetanus immunizations be given to survivors with injuries in emergency situations Q&A* (online). Available at: www.who.int/features/qa/04/en/ (Accessed March 21, 2015).

World Health Organization. (2013c). Guidance on how to access the oral cholera vaccine (OCV) from the ICG emergency stockpile (online). Available at: www.who.int/cholera/vaccines/Guidance_accessing_OCV_stockpile.pdf (Accessed March 30, 2015).

World Health Organization. (2014a). Vaccine position papers: Polio (online). Available at: www.who.int/wer/2014/wer8909.pdf (Accessed March 30, 2015).

World Health Organization. (2014b). Yellow fever fact sheet (online). Available at: www.who.int/mediacentre/factsheets/fs100/en/ (Accessed March 21, 2015).

World Health Organization. (2014c). Prevention and control of cholera outbreaks: WHO policy and recommendations (online). Available at: www.who.int/cholera/technical/prevention/control/en/index1.html (Accessed March 21, 2015).

World Health Organization. (2014d). Cholera fact sheet (online). Available at: www.who.int/mediacentre/factsheets/fs107/en/ (Accessed March 21, 2015).

World Health Organization. (2014e). World Humanitarian Day: WHO calls for protection of health workers in conflicts, disasters (online). Available at: www.who.int/mediacentre/news/releases/2014/world-humanitarian-day/en/ (Accessed July 24, 2015).

World Health Organization. (2015a). Disease outbreak news (online). Available at: www.who.int/csr/don/en/ (Accessed March 21, 2015).

World Health Organization. (2015b). Health as a bridge for peace – Humanitarian cease-fires project (HCFP) (online). Available at: www.who.int/hac/techguidance/hbp/cease_fires/en/ (Accessed August 10, 2015).

Zenner, D. and Nacul, L. (2012). Predictive power of Koplik's spots for the diagnosis of measles. *The Journal of Infection in Developing Countries*, **12**, 271–275.

Chapter 17

Camp Management

Paul J. Giannone, Mohamed Hilmi, and Mark Anderson

Introduction

In many ways, the management of a settlement or camp for displaced populations mimics running a small city (Montclos and Kagwanja 2000). Systems to support the provision of food, water and sanitation are required. Schools, health facilities, and roads need to be built and maintained and the population must have adequate shelter. There is one profound exception to these similarities however. While the growth of cities and the services they provide develop over hundreds, even thousands of years, displacement camps develop over several weeks or months. The Za'atari camp in Jordan for example, that houses refugees from the Syrian conflict, grew from 2,400 shelters to over 26,000 shelters between September 2012 and March 2013, representing a more than tenfold increase in size in seven months. The Za'atari camp, at its peak, housed over 150,000 residents, making it the fourth largest city in Jordan, dwarfing the nearby town of Mafraq. With this in mind, the logistical challenges of establishing and maintaining a settlement on the scale of Za'atari are profound with important implications for the health and well-being of the population.

When displaced in the setting of a humanitarian emergency, the affected population often moves to a location they consider safe, or they may be relocated by a government or international entity to an area of safety. Government or humanitarian agencies might then assist them in settling in a planned settlement or "camp." Alternatively, the displaced population may self-settle in collective centers such as public buildings and schools. Collective centers are discussed further in Chapter 18. It is becoming increasingly common for displaced persons to find their own solutions, some living with relatives, friends, or host families, while others integrate into host country cities and live independently. Consequently, humanitarian emergencies result in several different displacement scenarios for the affected population.

Displacement Scenarios

In some situations, the affected population may not be displaced from their homes or communities. Instead, they may be cut off from the outside world and not able to travel or communicate outside their communities. This was the case in Sarajevo, where the city was essentially under siege and, because it was unsafe to leave the city, residents continued to live in their homes. In another scenario, affected populations are displaced from their home communities and integrated into a host community. During the conflict in Liberia, many displaced persons were living in abandoned buildings throughout the capital city of Monrovia. In a third scenario, the displaced population resides in settlements such as transit centers or refugee camps, which may be self-settled or planned. Many refugees from Darfur for example, have been living for years in camps along the eastern border of Chad.

The two most common scenarios are integration into the host community or settlement in a camp situation. It is also possible that displaced populations can live in camps and be integrated into host communities at the same time, where camp residents work or shop in the local community.

There are advantages and disadvantages to both of these two scenarios. In camps, it is often easier to provide essential services and advocate for the needs of the displaced population. It is also easier to monitor their health status. At the same time, overcrowding in camp settings may increase the risk of disease. As shown in Table 17.1, overcrowding and poor living conditions are risk factors for three of the five leading causes of death among refugee populations. In addition, living in camps can lead to dependency, since most of the needs of the population are being provided at no expense.

The advantages of integrating displaced persons into the host community include promoting self-sufficiency, providing access to work, and encouraging

Table 17.1 Contributing factors and preventive measures for diseases among refugee populations

Disease	Contributing Factors	Preventive Measures
Malnutrition	• Inadequate food • Illness	• Food distribution • Diarrheal disease prevention
Diarrheal Illness	• Crowding • Poor sanitation and hygiene • Inadequate water	• Safe water, sanitation, hygiene • Education • ORT
Measles	• Crowding • Low vaccine coverage	• Immunization • Vitamin A
Malaria	• Exposure to vectors	• Bed nets • Indoor residual spraying • Treatment • Shelter
Acute Respiratory Illness	• Crowding • Poor living conditions	• Shelter • Adequate spacing

the use of existing services. However, there are also distinct disadvantages posed by integrating displaced persons into a host community. It becomes much more difficult to monitor the needs of the population and to provide them with essential services. It also places a significant burden on the host community, one that they may not be able to support without outside assistance.

If the affected population is nomadic, such as the Beja nomads who traverse the Red Sea Hills in Sudan, one strategy is to supply lifesaving commodities along the nomad's route. Although logistically difficult and costly, providing food, medicine, and water along migration routes may keep nomads from forming long-term camps.

Camps

Camps are sometimes called transitional camps, displacement camps, transitional settlements or, most commonly, refugee camps (Corsellis and Vitale 2005). Camps are groupings of physical shelters, often temporary in nature, that are either planned or unplanned. In this chapter, we will focus on the camp scenario, specifically the public health implications of planned settlements built for displaced populations. It is important to remember, however, that a significant number of the displaced population may live outside planned camps, living instead in urban settings or collective centers (Brookings Institution, Project on Internal Displacement 2013). Camps are often considered the least preferable solution, used when all other options are exhausted. However, in many humanitarian emergencies, camps are the only feasible solution.

Camps vary in size from a few dozen families living together in an informal settlement to hundreds of thousands of people living in a planned camp. During the acute phase of a humanitarian emergency, the urgency and complexity of the situation combined with the large number of displaced people means that decisions regarding the camp management must be made rapidly. In many cases, a camp must be established with basic services in place within a few days to a few weeks.

The displaced population is often forced to settle in some of the least hospitable locations, because more suitable areas are unavailable or restricted by local authorities. The common expectation is that displacement is temporary, which when combined with socioeconomic and cultural factors, can influence where a camp is established. For instance, in areas where agricultural land is sparse, the need to cultivate the little available land will limit where a camp can be established. Refugees and internally displaced persons (IDPs) often find themselves forced to live in barren or desert regions.

There are several key questions in determining the location of a camp including, how long is the displacement expected to last? While it is often difficult to determine the lifespan of a camp, history shows us that most camps exist longer than initial predictions. On average, a displaced person lives in a camp for about five years. The Dadaab refugee camp, now the third-largest "city" in Kenya, started in 1991 and some Palestinian refugee camps have existed for over five decades. Despite the difficulty in determining the life cycle of a camp, it is important to plan for a situation lasting five or more years. Planners should discuss this with local government officials, the host communities, and other stakeholders early in the planning process.

Another important consideration in determining the location of a camp relates to weather conditions; seasonal variations in rainfall may make campsites unusable during the rainy season. In addition, it is important to consider the legal status of the displaced population within the host country. Will the local government allow freedom of movement for the camp population or will they be restricted to camp? Will the camp residents be able to seek local employment? Will they be able to access to local services?

It is critical to estimate the population trends within the displaced population because the ultimate size of the camp will be determined by its location. Critical questions include, is there expected to be a sustained increase in the camp population? Alternatively, could there be a dramatic increase in the numbers of displaced due to an escalation of armed conflict in the area? It is also critical for the safety of the refugee population to analyze and understand the social, cultural, economic, political, and ethnic composition of arriving refugees.

It is also possible that the size of the camp population may vary due to other factors. Seasonal crop cultivation and harvesting, the movement of nomadic groups, and the return of combatants at holiday times may affect the camp population and should be accounted for in planning. Other considerations in the early planning of a camp include:

Environmental factors: Is the area prone to flood or drought?

Livelihood issues: Are there possibilities for employment in the host community?

Local health concerns: Are malaria or cholera endemic in the area?

Demographics should also be considered to assist in determining the age, gender, and religious/ethnic composition of the population. One way to collect all of this information is through a site assessment.

Initial Site Assessment

An initial site assessment is the most critical element in the setup of a displaced persons camp. This is true whether the site is already occupied or being planned for occupancy. The assessment must be multisectoral and include sector specialists in health care and nutrition, WASH, soil engineers, security, land use specialists, logisticians and experienced camp managers. Resources that can assist in conducting a site assessment include:

- The Camp Management Toolkit (CCCM 2015)
- The Rapid Health Assessment of Refugee or Displaced Populations (Depoortere and Brown 2006)
- Transitional Settlements – Displaced Populations (Corsellis and Vitale 2005)

Various methods have been employed in conducting site assessments. These include reviewing initial registration data, conducting key informant interviews, organizing group discussions, leading observational tours of the camp, and conducting surveys. In all cases, the involvement of the affected population, especially those representing vulnerable groups like women, children, pregnant and lactating women, elderly adults, and persons with special needs or disabilities, must be a priority. In the continuously changing environment of a camp setting, periodic assessments may be necessary to validate the initial assessment findings. Assessments are discussed in detail in Chapter 7.

The site selected for the camp, how the camp is organized, and how the camp is managed will have a significant impact on the physical and mental well-being of its inhabitants, the humanitarian workers employed there, and often, the host community. Important public health issues related to camp management include security and protection, the distribution of food and nonfood items, and the distribution of water.

Sphere Handbook

Some of the key indicators related to camp management from the *Sphere Handbook* are shown in Table 17.2. The Sphere Handbook is discussed further in Chapter 4.

Site Selection

Humanitarian agencies often have little choice in where displaced people can be settled, as the displaced population will frequently choose to settle in a location before humanitarian agencies arrive on the scene or the site will already have been selected by local or national authorities. In reality, it is rare that humanitarian agencies, with the approval of local authorities, will select the location of a camp. However, when given the opportunity to choose the site for a camp, it is extremely important to consider the total number of people displaced, whether there is an existing relationship between the local and displaced population, the cultural practices of the host and displaced populations, and the political and security environment including proximity of the site to dangerous border areas. Unfortunately, more often than not, decisions in site selection are influenced by

Table 17.2 Select indicators from the *Sphere Handbook* (Steering Committee for Humanitarian Response, 2011)

Sector	Indicator	Standard
WASH	Number of people per water tap	250
	Number of people per latrine	20
	Distance to water point	500 m maximum
	Water supply per person	15 L/day
	Queuing time for water	<30 minutes
	Fecal coliforms per 100 ml	0
	Residual chlorine	0.5 mg/L
	Distance between dwellings and latrine	50 m maximum
	Distance between water point and latrine	30 m
	Number of water containers per household	2 (10–20 L)
	Soap per person	250 g/month
Shelter/Nonfood items (NFI)	Area available per person	45 m^2
	Site gradient	1%–5%
	Shelter space per person	3.5 m^2
	Firebreaks	30 m every 300 m
	Clothing	2 sets/person
	Cooking pots per household (4–5 persons)	2
Food	Kilocalories per person	2,100/day
	Total energy provided by protein	10%
	Total energy provided by fat	17%
Health	Crude mortality rate	<2× baseline rate
	Under 5 mortality rate	<2× baseline rate
	Reproductive health	Access to Minimum Initial Service Package (MISP)
	Basic health unit per population	1/10,000 persons
	Number of health workers per population	22/10,000 persons
	Number of midwives per population	1/10,000 population

the precipitating event and the local political, cultural, and economic context. In most emergencies, there won't be time to select, plan, and build a camp before the displacement of refugees and IDPs.

One of the guiding principles of site selection is to provide sufficient space for living and the additional services necessary for the functioning of the camp. In general, it is preferable to maintain smaller camps as they are easier to manage and favor a return to self-sufficiency. A few small camps of less than ten thousand people are preferable to one large camp. Displaced persons should be involved and consulted in the planning process. Their social organization and opinions should be taken into account wherever possible. It is also important to consider the impact of site selection on the host community and to utilize local resources when feasible.

As mentioned, overcrowding has a significant impact on physical and mental health. The Sphere Standards recommend 45 m^2 per person in a camp setting. Using this formula, a refugee camp for 10,000 refugees will require a land mass 0.45 kilometers by 1.0 kilometer, including space for living, clinics, schools, and administrative support. This information is valuable in negotiating for land space and may clarify the need for other options. This is discussed further in Chapter 18. Often this amount of space is hard to find, especially in urban areas, and camps usually expand beyond their original design considerations. Continued growth of the affected population must be considered in the initial selection of a site.

Land Ownership and Usage

Whether refugees have self-settled or site planners are looking for land for a camp, it is critical to determine who owns or uses the land. Is the land owned by the government, corporations, or private individuals? Are there government environmental protection issues or mineral rights issues? Do nomads or animals traverse this land? Agreements need to be negotiated and documented including cost or no-cost use and how the land will be received and left after the camp is abandoned.

Security and Protection

One of the primary conditions for site selection is the security and protection of the displaced people. The site must be secure for the affected population as well as the humanitarian workers. The area should be physically safe, free from landmines, flooding, and extremes of heat and cold. The settlement must be located in a safe area greater than 50 km from the border or any conflict area. Security both within and outside the camp must be addressed. The security of women and children should be of particular concern. It is important to make sure common areas are well-lit including the camp entrance, latrines, showers, cooking areas, schools and play areas, and water points. If lighting is not available, then guards should be considered for these areas. In some situations, it may be necessary to establish a curfew in the camp and a system to escort vulnerable residents when leaving the camp for firewood or water.

Accessibility

Access to the site must be possible during all seasons to allow for the transportation of people, water, and relief items. An adequate, all-weather road network including appropriate access roads that are passable year-round is critical to allow for the transport of needed equipment, medicine, food, water, disaster victims, and staff. If this is not possible, improving access by building roads must be considered, but this will only add to the cost and time to develop the camp. Ideally, the road networks should provide easy access to local towns and cities, air or seaports, hospitals, and markets. Access to local commercial centers, health care facilities, and air or seaports will enhance the development and maintenance of the camp. Most importantly, roads should be adequate to allow for the rapid evacuation of the site in an emergency. The addition of a refugee camp in an area may hasten the deterioration of the government's road system, including bridges. It is important to understand who will be responsible for road and bridge repair. This should be negotiated ahead of time by site planners.

Topography

The camp should be located on a gentle slope of between 2% and 6% to provide natural drainage for rainwater away from the site. A natural gradient is important because it inhibits pooling, limits mosquito breeding, and allows for the channeling of polluted water into catchment areas. As an alternative, drainage channels can be built to route water. In some instances, drainage can be improved through grading to raise a flood prone zone or create terraces on a steep slope. However, these solutions can be costly and, ultimately, unsustainable.

Soil Conditions

The type of soil and level of the water table will determine how and where wells can be dug and the type of latrines that can be used. As discussed in other chapters, the number and type of latrines and wells available in a camp have important public health implications. Soil type may also affect the type of construction that can be supported in a particular camp and will have an impact on drainage. The "black cotton" soil of South Sudan, which becomes very sticky when saturated, was almost impassable during the rainy season and in many of the camps contributed to public health issues related to sanitation, vector control, and water-borne diseases. Finally, the site must be suitable for the construction of cemeteries.

Resources

The sudden influx of thousands of displaced people into an area will have a significant impact on the local environment. Demand for natural resources, including land, water, and wood for fuel and building materials may deplete the surrounding area. Buying commodities from the local market will support the local economy but may cause a rise in local prices, ultimately making these commodities unaffordable for the local residents. Care should be given in negotiating with area or regional merchants. In selecting a site, it is important that an adequate quantity of water is available year-round either on-site or close to the camp. An adequate supply of fuel or firewood and materials for shelter construction needs to be readily accessible. Considerations regarding the selection of a site must include the short- and long-term environmental impact as well as the long-term sustainability and management of natural resources.

Mitigation measures could be considered to lessen the environmental impact, such as the use of fuel-efficient stoves or community cooking facilities, environmental impact awareness campaigns, and even reforestation programs. The site planner must also consider existing local environmental regulations and laws, and work with local experts and authorities to ensure compliance.

Other factors in addition to those described above may contribute to the final decision on the site selection. Suggestions for comparing potential camp sites during the selection process are discussed in *Transitional Settlements Displaced Populations* (Corsellis and Vitale 2005).

As mentioned, it is common that the displaced population will have settled on a site before any site planning can be carried out. Usually, improvements to the site can be made without moving all the shelters. Organizing facilities, improving access to all sections of the camp, and planning sections for new arrivals will improve camp management. Sometimes it may be necessary to completely reorganize the site, although this is usually not advised. Such an undertaking is necessary when there is a legitimate threat to health from overcrowding or danger of a fire. Problems such as a lack of water, insecurity, or potential danger may also necessitate a move to a new site.

Site Planning

Once the site has been determined, a plan should be developed that details the location of living units, roads, and other facilities. A map should be used to develop a network of roads that divide the area into sections. The preferred method is to organize the site into basic community units, consisting of shelters and community facilities including latrines, water points, and washing areas. Good access by road to every section and facility in the camp is essential for the transport of staff and materials and removal of debris. Factors should be taken into account when organizing the site and locating the facilities and shelters including:

- Space required per person and for each installation
- The accessibility of services
- The minimum distance between facilities in shelters
- The cultural habits and social organization of the displaced population

Table 17.3 Selected standards for site planning

Indicator	Standard
Area available per person	45 m^2
Shelter space per person	3.5 m^2
Number of people per water tap	250
Number of people per latrine	20
Distance to water point	500 m maximum
Distance between water point and latrine	30 m
Firebreaks	30 m firebreak every 300 m

- Access to water points and sanitary facilities
- Ethnic and security factors

Table 17.3 lists select standards from the Sphere Handbook for site planning (Steering Committee for Humanitarian Response 2011).

Site planning is a complex process. Site design will depend on the environmental setting and the cultural, logistical, and legal requirements of both the resident and host communities. There is no standardized approach to camp design. Site planners will need to define the size, number, and layout of the facilities and buildings that will serve the camp population. This must involve consultation with sector specialists from health, WASH, livelihoods, nutrition, security, and protection. Displaced populations and host communities should also be consulted as to their preferences, needs, and perceived vulnerabilities during the camp planning process. A good site layout provides easy access to all services and protects basic human rights and dignity. Early decisions in site planning will impact the immediate and long-term health and well-being of the displaced population. In the end, the final site plan will likely represent a compromise between the competing needs of the resident population and available resources of the local context.

The importance of site planning to public health is highlighted by MSF in their site planning guidelines, which states:

> Although health agencies will not always be involved in organizing a site, they should nevertheless make sure that this is undertaken correctly because of its direct influence on the subsequent health situation; it

is, therefore, necessary to have an understanding of the basic principles of site planning (Médecins Sans Frontières 1997).

Many of the details of site planning and camp layout are beyond the scope of this chapter, but they have been presented in several recent publications including NRC's Camp Management Toolkit (CCCM, 2015) and Transitional Settlement: Displaced Populations (Corsellis and Vitale, 2005) and outlined extensively in humanitarian standards such as *Sphere Handbook* (Steering Committee for Humanitarian Response 2011). NRC's Camp Management Toolkit provides a detailed account of good practices for the whole life cycle of the camp (CCCM 2015).

Implementing these guidelines should provide residents with a minimally acceptable standard of living and promote a healthy environment in camp situations. However, each camp situation is unique, and will result in significant challenges, meaning that many of these standards may be difficult to meet and adaptations will have to be made. Consultations with appropriate sector specialists and stakeholders should help inform the adaptation of these standards to the local context when necessary.

Shelter

Early in the planning process, a decision has to be made on what type of shelters and facilities are necessary in the local environment. One factor that will influence this decision is whether an emergency, transitional, or permanent solution is being considered.

In the camp setting, it is necessary to provide sufficient covered space to protect camp residents from adverse climate conditions and disease vectors, and to ensure health, security, and privacy. Displaced persons should be encouraged to build their own shelter using local materials while taking measures to minimize the environmental impact. Whenever possible, original household units should be maintained. Ultimately, standards for adequate shelter depend on the local climate and the size of the household in question.

Shelter in a camp setting can take many forms, including plastic sheeting, tents, indigenous materials (trees and grass), prefabricated modular homes, and existing structures, such as unused homes, collective centers, and schools.

The following minimum standards should be met in providing shelter to displaced persons:

- A covered area that averages 3.5–4.5 m^2 per person
- Shelter that is appropriate for the local climate
- Shelters are hopefully made of material fire resistant or adequately spaced from one another.
- A 4×6 m sheet of plastic at the beginning of the crisis per average household (five persons)

Shelter and settlements are discussed in greater detail in Chapter 18.

Camp Layout

An important aspect of site planning is determining how the camp will be laid out within the physical space allotted. There is no universal layout of the ideal refugee camp; however, a comprehensive discussion of the advantages and disadvantages of various camp layouts including a conceptual layout of a well-organized camp have been published (Corsellis and Vitale 2005). Figure 17.1 shows an example of the subdivision of a camp into sectors, blocks, and communities.

Figure 17.2 shows an example layout for standards for service for the community.

There are potential advantages of a cluster layout, where roads radiate like the branches of a tree from central areas used for communal facilities, over the more traditional grid layout, which establishes roads in a grid pattern with communities, administrative facilities, and communal facilities placed in the gaps between the roads. Critics of grid planning have stated:

> Grid planning is simple to design and can be easily marked out. It provides access to all family plots within a community. But a grid plan does not fit easily on sites with disrupted topography, such as hills or gullies. In contrast, cluster planning allows roads and community layouts to "wrap" around topographic features, ideally following site contours. This approach allows roads to complement rather than disrupt natural drainage routes, reducing the drainage infrastructure required and the subsequent cost involved

It further argues that cluster planning has advantages such as

> reinforcing viable social communities, by creating 'private' areas, encouraging communally shared activities and practices, from water collection to cooking, supporting social hierarchy, which can improve the acceptance of extension programmes and the representation of the needs of the displaced population through committees
>
> *(Corsellis and Vitale 2005).*

Figure 17.3 shows grid vs. cluster planning.

Chapter 17: Camp Management

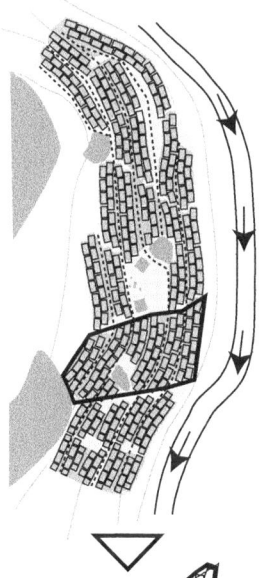

Figure 17.1 Camp subdivided into sectors, blocks, and communities
Source: Corsellis and Vitale 2005. Reproduced by the kind permission of Tom Corsellis and Oxfam GB.

Camp: approximately 20,000 inhabitants
4 sectors

- fire breaks: 30 m per built-up 300 m
- roads follow contours and lead out from centre
- run-off water also follows contours
- features used to break repeating pattern
- administrative centre located at the centre of the camp

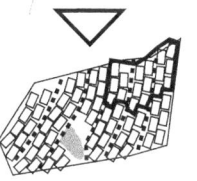

Sector: approximately 5,000 inhabitants
4 blocks

- fire breaks: 15 m between blocks
- should contain central recreational/commercial spaces

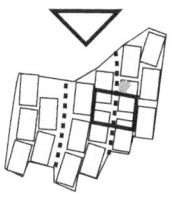

Block: approximately 1,250 inhabitants
16 communities

- fire breaks: 6 m (pathways)

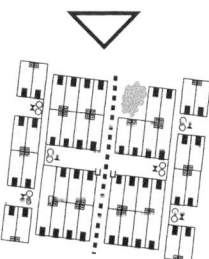

Community: approximately 80 inhabitants
16 plots with 16 shelters

- fire breaks: 2 m between dwellings
- drainage should be well planned and maintained.
- drain water must not pollute existing surface water or groundwater, or cause erosion.

Management Systems

Camps include some common facilities such as reception centers, health facilities, water and sanitation facilities, schools, feeding centers, warehouses, offices, security installations, and other infrastructure. These facilities support the camp management systems that are critical to public health and should be located within the same contiguous space as the residential areas to ensure access and utilization. Some sections of the camp may limit refuge access from areas such as warehouses, generator rooms, and senior staff administrative offices.

Camp management systems may vary based on the particular humanitarian context but should ensure that essential services are efficiently provided to the displaced population. In addition to providing essential life-saving measures such as shelter, water, food, and healthcare, there are other important

251

Section 2: Public Health Principles

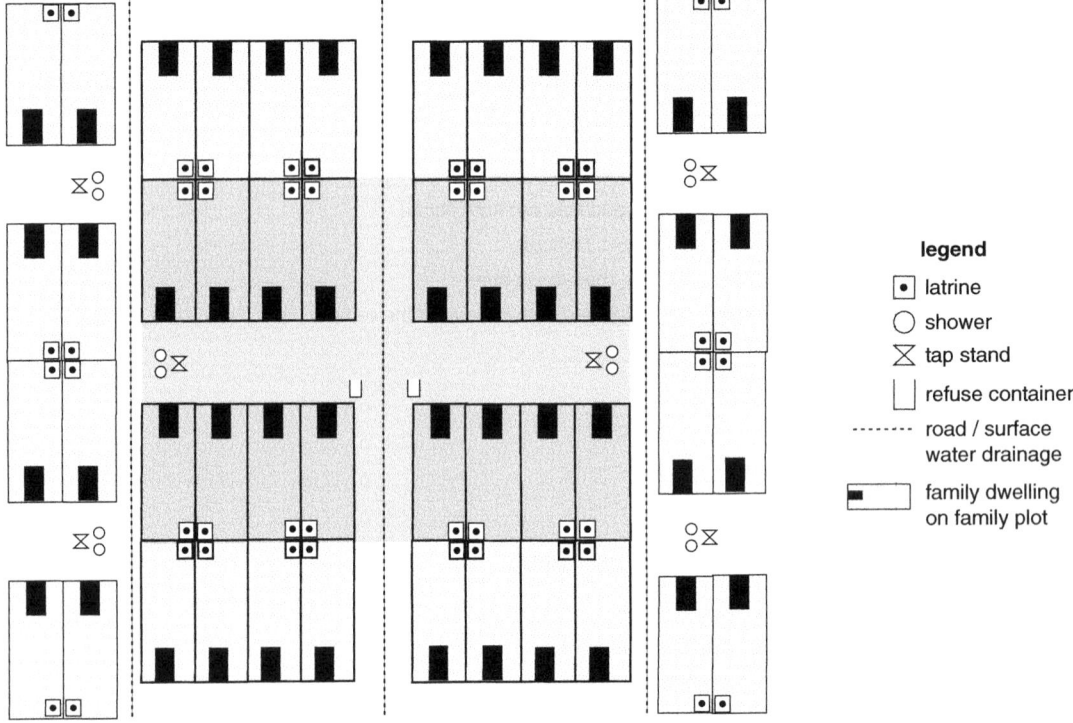

Figure 17.2 Standards for service provision for a community
Source: Corsellis and Vitale 2005.

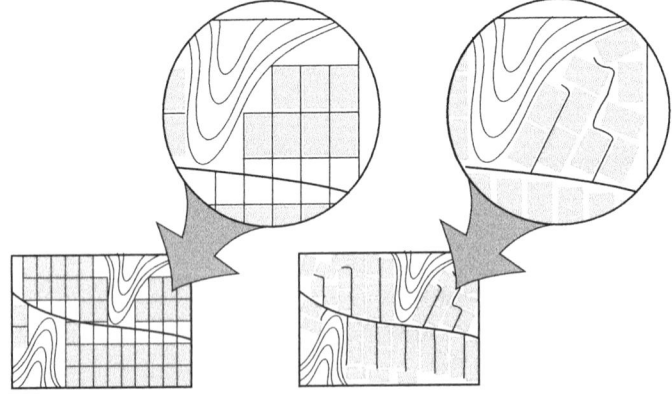

Figure 17.3 Grid vs. cluster planning
Source: Corsellis and Vitale 2005

services provided by the camp management agency. These services also contribute to the physical and mental well-being of the camp population and may include nonfood item (NFI) distribution, education programs, psychosocial services, reunification programs, livelihood programs, and women's programs. It is important that these services be delivered in a coordinated manner that includes input from the relevant sector specialists, the resident population, and the host community. It does no good, and can be harmful, for example, to deliver food if cooking utensils have not also been distributed; camp residents have been known to sell the limited food they have been provided in order to obtain these items.

The site should be well organized with easy-to-understand signage or maps that give the location of services, living sections, latrines, and food and water distribution points. The signs and maps should be in the resident's native language and include identifiable figures for illiterate residents.

Registration

Registration is the first camp management system a displaced person typically encounters. The United Nations High Commissioner for Refugees (UNHCR) Handbook for Registration identifies procedures and standards for registration, population data management, and documentation of displaced persons (UNHCR 2003). UNHCR requires a complete registration of every individual or family settled in a camp including their location. A complete registration of the camp population has several important public health and protection implications. First, registration provides information useful in the potential reunification of families separated during their displacement. Registration also provides an opportunity to identify displaced persons with the signs and symptoms of diseases with epidemic potential or life-threatening illnesses so they can be quickly isolated or referred for medical care. Finally, registration allows for the identification of vulnerable groups who might need special services.

Registration may also identify refugees who have certain important skills such as a doctor, nurse teacher, carpenter, or electrician that might be helpful to the successful management of the camp.

In addition, identification of family members in the resident's home country is important. It may allow for the notification that family members are safe and assist humanitarian agencies in identifying the best countries for resettlement.

Administration

Administrative facilities must be established in any camp, including the administrative offices for agencies managing camp programs and systems, warehouses, distribution points, maintenance workshops, parking areas and, in some cases, relief worker housing. These facilities, often operated by the United Nations (UN), the Red Cross and Red Crescent or specialist nongovernmental organizations (NGOs), serve families by providing communication, reunification, and protection services. These programs are critical to the mental health of displaced persons.

Food Distribution

Food distribution system are vitally important for the health and well-being of camp residents. Although the specific commodities included in a feeding program are discussed elsewhere, the system developed for the distribution of food should be flexible, adaptable, and culturally acceptable to the needs of the camp population. Special consideration should be given to vulnerable groups, especially the elderly, infants, and disabled, to ensure that they receive adequate rations. If there is a voucher system developed for food distribution, the status of vulnerable groups should be noted, and special consideration should be given to assisting them. The provision of food items within a camp setting requires a good supply chain, accurate population numbers, and an efficient distribution system.

Nonfood Item (NFI) Distribution

Internally displaced persons and refugees take very few personal belongings when leaving their homes. The provision of nonfood items must take into account the climate and culture of the local area as well as what people have carried with them from their homes. Providing local nonfood items is optimal, but the impact on the local population and environment must be considered before doing so. Distributions of nonfood items must be organized to provide the population with the essential goods required for daily living including:

- Water containers for the storage in households
- Cooking utensils
- Material for shelter construction
- Soap
- Tools for building latrines or waste disposal pits
- Blankets
- Clothing

As mentioned, the distribution of NFIs is just as important as that of food rations. Displaced persons will often sell or exchange part of their food ration to purchase these items unless they are freely distributed, further compromising their nutritional status.

The following minimum standards should be met when distributing nonfood items:

- Households should have a cooking pot and utensils
- Each person should be provided with 250 g of soap each month
- Households should have 5 kg of firewood (or the equivalent) per day
- People should have access to "sufficient" blankets

- Households should have two water collecting vessels of 10–20 L each, and one water storage vessel of 20 L (with cover and spigot)

There are indirect benefits from the distribution of NFIs. Tools like shovels, rakes, and hoes can assist residents in creating home gardens, which can provide greater variety in the diet and a source of livelihood. Specialized tools can provide artisans and craftsmen with the means to earn extra money or to barter their skills in exchange for other essential commodities.

Water and Sanitation

Water and sanitation systems are one of the most important public health interventions in a camp setting. As has been shown elsewhere, a wide range of infectious and vector-borne diseases, including cholera and dysentery, are directly related to contaminated water and poor sanitation. First, it is important to ensure an adequate quantity of water when locating and developing a camp. Sources of water may be limited by the camp location and alternative sources will have to be identified if the local supply is inadequate. Sanitation may also be complicated by site location and soil conditions.

Sphere Standards for the minimum drinking water needs during the emergency phase are between 2.5 and 3.5 liters per person per day, with a minimum of 15 liters per day to for drinking, bathing, cooking, and cleaning. The actual amount of water needed will depend on the local climate, cultural practices, and an individual's physiologic needs. This may seem like a trivial amount to supply but providing a sufficient quantity of water to a camp population is a constant logistical challenge. Based on 15 liters per day per person, a camp of twenty thousand inhabitants would require 300,000 liters of water per day. Transporting this amount of water to the site is both costly and logistically challenging and may be prohibitive over a long term.

The location and number of water taps or distribution points will have to be carefully designed to be convenient enough to promote their use. Sphere Standards should be followed in the development and location of each component of WASH systems to ensure easy and safe access to clean water for all camp residents. For example, for each household, the walking distance to the nearest water point should be less than 500 m, and there should be enough distribution points to keep wait times under 30 minutes (Steering Committee for Humanitarian Response 2011). Additionally, systems should be considered to ensure that the elderly or disabled can receive their daily water requirements.

All areas where WASH services are delivered, especially latrines, should be well lit at night, especially for the security of women and children. Water distribution points and latrines should be cleaned regularly and maintained to promote their use. Water points and latrines should be monitored to limit abuse or unclean practices. Camp residents can be organized into committees to monitor these sites. Refuse collection should be carried out on a regular schedule, and the disposal site should follow solid waste disposal guidelines (Steering Committee for Humanitarian Response 2011).

When planning the location of wells, latrines, and refuse disposal sites, camp planners, to reduce the possibility of contamination, should be aware of the local soil conditions, the elevation of the water table, and whether the area is subject to seasonal flooding. For a dug latrine, the base of the pit must be at least 1.5 m above the wet-season water table to prevent contamination (Harvey 2007). If the water table is high or there is seasonal flooding, then it may be necessary to construct latrines appropriate to these conditions. The Global WASH Cluster provides a number of resources to guide the construction and maintenance of latrines. WASH is discussed in detail in Chapter 11.

When providing water to affected populations, the needs of the host communities also must be taken into consideration. Site planners must avoid conflicts related to overuse of existing water sources and environmental degradation that may result from supplying the camp. Drainage of waste water must be taken into consideration to avoid unsanitary conditions and pollution to both refugee camp and host country land. Site planners must also closely follow the local/national environmental regulations on garbage disposal.

Health Systems and Facilities

Clinical health care services are a core public health component in a camp setting. Clinical health facilities may include a combination of field hospitals, health centers or clinics, health posts, mobile clinics, feeding centers, and infectious disease isolation areas. The health programs operated from these facilities or mobile clinics provide services for communicable disease control, child health, sexual and reproductive health, trauma care, mental health, and noncommunicable diseases (Steering Committee for Humanitarian Response 2011).

Community and Public Facilities

Community facilities in a camp are open to the public and include schools, cemeteries, community centers, sports fields, businesses, and worship facilities (Bakewell 2003). They may be run by camp management agencies, by camp residents, or by individuals or groups living outside the camp.

Schools

Schools are a priority in the design of any camp. The best way to support the mental health of children is to get them back into a normal routine, matching that of the home they left behind as closely as possible. Schools can be a normalizing experience for displaced children, allowing them to maintain their studies, which will ease their eventual return to their home communities. Schools can also serve as a health screening site for children with potential health issues or as an immunization site during vaccination campaigns. Schools should be incorporated into a broader camp-wide health education system, providing programs for both children and their parents. Recreational activities are another area where schools can support displaced children and provide a semblance of normality.

Markets

Private entrepreneurship should be encouraged in the camp setting because it can promote independence and self-worth among camp residents. Markets within the camp, managed by residents or members of the host community, can provide an efficient system for the distribution of food and nonfood items. Local entrepreneurs within the camp may introduce fresh fruits, vegetables, and meats into the diet of the camp population that may otherwise be lacking. In many camps, businesses are often established to sell non-food items or useful services like electronics repair, battery charging, tailoring, and barbering.

It is the responsibility of the camp management officials to ensure that unethical business practices, such as price gouging, are avoided. It also may be necessary to conduct health inspections to reduce the potential for disease outbreaks or injury due to safety hazards.

Centers of Worship

In coordination with community religious leaders, centers of worship should be established. This is an additional component essential in providing camp residents a sense of normality. Religious leaders and religious centers can be a very effective mechanism for communicating with the camp population, addressing human rights issues, and evaluating camp services. Depending on the size of the camp population, religious centers are often multidenominational, with alternating schedules established to ensure that all religious groups can worship or meet.

Recreational Facilities

Recreational facilities are extremely important for the physical and mental health of camp residents. These facilities can include sports fields, play areas for children, and community meeting places. They should be established for both children, adults, senior citizens, or those with special needs.

Self-Rule Systems

Displaced populations living in a camp setting should be seen as an equal partner to the UN, NGO, or government agencies managing the camp. In any camp setting, it is important to support the development of an elected committee of camp residents that regularly interact with camp management staff. The committee should be balanced in terms of gender, ethnicity, and cultural background to ensure equal representation. This elected committee will work with community leaders and social groups, such as women's or men's clubs, to assist in the administration of the camp. Resident committees are valuable in that they allow limited self-rule and decision-making authority to the camp population. The committees can help inform camp management of the effectiveness of public health interventions such as feeding and health care programs, and alert management officials to potential problems with camp infrastructure and security. Inclusion of members of the camp committee or other social groups in regular established assessments of camp systems can be useful in validating the findings and recommendations.

Social Groups

Generally, in camp settings, promoting political or ethnic social groups should be avoided to reduce the risk of internal camp conflict. However, membership in a group can provide individuals with a community voice, a sense of cohesion and belonging, and give members a chance to be active in a way that highlights their skills and knowledge. This can lead to the development of productive projects that support the entire community. Examples of groups that might be considered in a camp setting are in the following sections.

Women's Groups

A woman's group can be one of the most productive in a camp, especially in an area where there has been gender-based violence and gender discrimination. Women's groups can provide information on how women are being treated in various camp systems, such as feeding and reproductive health programs. They may be able to provide support to other women through self-counseling. They can also be called on to help support arriving unaccompanied minors and victims of gender-based violence.

Sports Associations

A sports association or group can be formed around particular sports popular in the community. Teams can be formed and outfitted; leagues can even be established. By creating a healthy competitive environment, these activities can be an important outlet for the resident population.

Professional Associations

Associations of particular professional groups such as electricians, carpenters, plumbers, teachers, and medical professionals can be established to help improve the camp infrastructure or social services networks (Andemicael 2011).

Summary

Developing and managing a camp for displaced persons is a complex process that involves the support of the host government and the technical expertise of numerous humanitarian actors. In many cases, factors such as the intensity of the event that caused the displacement and the political, climatic, and geographic factors that precipitated the event are outside the control of camp planners. These factors, however, may have the greatest influence on where, when and how a displacement camp is established.

The primary concern of public health professionals in a humanitarian emergency is the health and safety of the displaced population, and this concern should lead the decision-making process. Providing shelter, food, water, sanitation, and urgent medical care are the primary tasks for those who arrive first to a large scale, rapidly developing humanitarian emergency. Other systems need to be provided as soon as possible after this initial response.

References

Andemicael, A. (2011). *Positive energy: A review of the role of artistic activities in refugee camps*. UNHCR: Geneva, Switzerland.

Bakewell, O. (2003). Community services in refugee aid programs: The challenges of expectations, principles, and practice. *Praxis*, 18, 5–18.

Brookings Institution, Project on Internal Displacement. (2013). *Under the Radar: Internally Displaced Persons in Non-Camp Settings*. Brookings Institution, London School of Economics, Project on Internal Displacement: Washington, DC.

Corsellis, T. and Vitale, A. (2005). *Transitional Settlement: Displaced Populations*. Oxford. Oxfam.

Depoortere, E. and Brown, V. (2006). *Rapid health assessment of refugee or displaced populations*, Médecins Sans Frontières: Paris.

Global Camp Coordination and Camp Management (CCCM) Cluster. (2015). *The Camp Management Toolkit*. International Organization for Migration Norwegian Refugee Council, UNHCR.

Harvey, P. (2007). *Excreta disposal in emergencies: A field manual*, UNICEF; New York.

Médecins Sans Frontières. (1997). *Refugee health: An approach to emergency situations*. Pan Macmillan.

Montclos, M. A. P. D. and Kagwanja, P. M. (2000). Refugee camps or cities? The socio-economic dynamics of the Dadaab and Kakuma camps in northern Kenya. *Journal of Refugee Studies*, 13(2), 205–222.

Steering Committee for Humanitarian Response. (2011). *The Sphere Project: Humanitarian charter and minimum standards in humanitarian response*, Bourton on Dunsmore, UK: Sphere Project.

United Nations High Commissioner for Refugees. (UNHCR). (2003). *UNHCR handbook for registration*. UNHCR; Geneva.

Chapter 18

Shelter and Settlements

Charles A. Setchell, Eddie J. Argeñal, LeGrand L. Malany, and Paul J. Giannone

Introduction

When natural and man-made disasters, including conflict, result in housing damage or destruction and population displacement, people typically desire to return to their communities to rebuild or repair their homes almost immediately. Unfortunately, this return to normalcy cannot be achieved quickly, and often takes months, if not years, particularly when people are displaced far from their communities or the disaster affected a densely populated urban area, where the options to shelter people are often limited and rebuilding can take a long time. Providing shelter to those displaced, whether for a short or long period of time, is an immediate priority during humanitarian emergencies. Shelter should be a safe, secure, healthy, culturally acceptable, and habitable covered living space. Ideally, the shelter provided is part of a larger, progressive process that usually involves a range of outputs, including emergency covered living spaces, such as tents and camps, and transitional shelters, provided by humanitarian agencies, followed by permanent housing reconstruction provided by development agencies.

Affected populations typically cope with the lack of housing post-disaster by seeking accommodation with relatives and friends, occupying vacant or unfinished buildings, self-constructing basic shelters with salvaged and other building materials, or renting. The seeking of shelter after a disaster is often a spontaneous and self-resourced action on the part of disaster victims. Humanitarian actors have to understand and support these self-help coping efforts. Initially, the primary task is to support the displaced population with the minimum resources necessary for survival. For shelter, this effort involves creating a shelter responses that reflects local conditions and Sphere Project guidance, and providing, among other needs, concomitant health and sanitation measures and protocols.

The delivery of shelter during a humanitarian emergency does not happen in isolation. Rather, it is as part of a larger response framework that includes health, basic services, livelihoods, and larger economic activities, protection, environmental management, and disaster risk reduction (DRR). This linkage of shelter to related sectors is referred to as settlements. In combination, this serves as the basis for shelter and settlement (S&S) assistance. Particularly important to this text is the relationship between shelter, settlements, and health.

An important consideration for S&S programming is that every year, a larger percentage of the world's population moves to urban areas. Many of these people are poor and end up living in shantytowns or slums where they live in unsanitary conditions, exposed to hazards, and with limited access to basic services. At the same time, there has been an increase in the scale and severity of disasters, including storms, floods, and droughts that threaten cities, especially those located in coastal or low-lying areas. This combination of urbanization with larger and more frequent disasters results in an increase in the potential people vulnerable to disasters, particular the urban poor. S&S assistance in these urban areas presents unique, but increasingly common challenges for the humanitarian response community.

S&S assistance is most effective when it is based on a sound understanding of local context. This understanding is best developed through market-based assessments of damage and need, to better gauge impacts, constraints, resources, and opportunities in affected areas. The core target group of proposed actions will be the most vulnerable among affected populations, which often include households less likely to recover if unassisted, such as the elderly, disabled, orphaned/unaccompanied minors, minority groups, immigrants, foreign workers, traumatized, female-headed households, and others. Provision of support to these groups may require technical assistance and material support (e.g., construction materials and skilled labor) rather than a reliance solely on self-help capacity.

In addition to being safe, secure, healthy, and habitable, the shelter provided by humanitarian actors should be cognizant of international humanitarian and local/national guidelines. Where possible and appropriate, S&S activities should emphasize beneficiary participation and reliance on local materials and labor, as this will enhance prospects for acceptance, sustainability, cost-effectiveness, and livelihood.

Settlements Approach

The settlements approach, which includes multiple and integrated activities in socioeconomically defined spaces, such as neighborhoods, villages, towns, or cities, can serve as the much-needed spatial framework for multisector humanitarian activities. It is both a coordination tool and a means of compelling humanitarian actor accountability to affected populations living in settlements.

USAID/OFDA, for example, supports S&S sector interventions that feature a settlements approach, thereby permitting identification of, and linkages with, other sectors, particularly livelihoods, health, water, sanitation, and hygiene (WASH), and protection. This approach is becoming easier to define, depict, promote, and implement now that geobased mapping technologies are more accessible.

The goal of S&S assistance is to ensure the expeditious access to safe, habitable, and culturally appropriate living spaces and settlements, where households affected by humanitarian emergencies are able to resume critical personal, familial, social, and livelihoods activities. This assistance facilitates a process of sheltering that focuses on both immediate and short-term economic, social, and physical vulnerability reduction of disaster-affected households and their communities, while also laying the foundation for longer-term recovery.

Linkage to Health

Humanitarian emergencies undermine the health of the affected population especially in areas with insufficient resources, lack of political will, and/or know-how required to prepare and respond. This includes lack of adequate shelter and basic services for those displaced. Consequently, humanitarian S&S interventions have the potential to impact health outcomes in this context by providing healthy spaces where survivors can work, play, rest, relax, and access basic services until more permanent solutions to their needs are secured.

Universal Declaration of Human Rights

The right to adequate housing can be traced to the Universal Declaration of Human Rights, which was unanimously adopted by the world community in 1948 (Thiele 2002). Numerous international agreements since have provided further affirmation and guidance regarding this right. A core feature of the housing right is defining adequacy to include habitability and compliance with health and safety standards. The link between housing and health was recognized initially and supported subsequently.

Health Principles of Housing

The World Health Organization (WHO) forged a stronger link between health and housing in 1989 with the publication of the Health Principles of Housing, which viewed housing as the environmental factor most frequently associated with conditions for disease (Thiele 2002). The WHO identified six major principles governing the relationship between housing and health (WHO 1989):

- Protection against communicable diseases
- Protection against injuries, poisonings, and chronic diseases
- Reducing psychological and social stresses to a minimum
- Improving the housing environment
- Making informed use of housing
- Protecting populations at risk

The first two principles are particularly relevant to health, with the first focusing on basic hygiene and public services, and the second emphasizing construction materials, techniques, and safety and habitability issues.

While the international community had been contending with housing rights issues and the relationship between housing and health for decades since World War II, the international humanitarian community did not formulate a coherent and early path to addressing similar issues in emergency settings. Although numerous international, bilateral, and nongovernmental organizations had developed protocols on how to respond to humanitarian emergencies, there was no universally agreed-upon guidance for issues related to shelter and health until the adoption of the Sphere Project in 1997 (Sphere Project 2011).

Sphere identified basic levels of service to populations affected by humanitarian emergencies to improve the quality of assistance and provided guidance and accountability measures for humanitarian actors. Sphere guidance has evolved in response to new challenges and lessons learned and continues to serve as the benchmark for international humanitarian action.

The Sphere Project

Included in the 2011 *Sphere Project Handbook* is guidance on shelter, settlement, and nonfood items that strongly reflect the health concerns embodied in the WHO's Health Principles of Housing. Sphere states that the provision of 3.5 m^2 (approximately 38 square feet) of covered living space per person is a minimally adequate output of humanitarian action. Ideally, this living space is to be private, secure, safe, healthy, habitable, and linked to basic services, with reduced risk to hazards. The minimally adequate output of 3.5 m^2 of covered living space per person is not intended to replicate what was lost through disaster and crises and is often less living space than what affected populations had prior to the humanitarian emergency. The minimally adequate international humanitarian community living space for shelter is also truly minimal when compared to conditions in the US and other developed economies. The US Department of Housing and Urban Development (HUD), for example, found in 2005 that at least 99.88 percent of American households lived in dwelling units that exceeded the Sphere Project living space guidance metric of 3.5 m^2 per person (HUD 2007). This is reflective of both the modest nature of humanitarian shelter output and the significant differences in housing conditions between those living in developed economies and those receiving humanitarian assistance, largely in developing economies. Sphere Project standards are a minimum standard to be attained. In some humanitarian responses, especially those dealing with displacement of a large population, these standards may not be attainable or practical. In this event, the responding entity should carefully document why Sphere standards can't be met.

Engineering in Emergencies: A Practical Guide for Relief Workers

In 1995, at roughly the same time that the Sphere Project Handbook was being developed by humanitarian actors, *Engineering in Emergencies: A Practical Guide for Relief Workers*, was published (Davis and Lambert 2002). The Guide provides detailed information on a wide range of humanitarian activities, and includes a chapter on "Shelter and Built Infrastructure," intended to guide the provision of shelter for displaced populations. The chapter provides "how-to" level information on assessment of needs and damaged structures, and the design, procurement, and installation of needed structures to support displaced populations, including health facilities. This how-to engineering focus served as a useful complement to the more general, principle-based guidance reflected in the *Sphere Project Handbook*.

These benchmark documents and several large-scale disasters, coupled with significant increases in international and national response capacity and organization, have led to changes in thinking and practice on how to provide shelter to populations affected by humanitarian emergencies. The advent of the United Nations Cluster System in 2005, for example, changed the organizational architecture of international humanitarian response. In the emergency shelter cluster, led globally by the United Nations High Commissioner for Refugees (UNHCR) and the International Federation of the Red Cross (IFRC), there is an increasing awareness of the linkage between shelter, settlements, safety, and health. The cluster system is discussed in more detail in Chapter 4. Additional change also followed the 2010 earthquake in Haiti, which effectively introduced urban-based interventions to the humanitarian community, and generated considerable interest in revising guidelines and protocols that had heretofore been largely based on activities in rural areas.

Assistance Activities

The two main types of humanitarian S&S assistance are emergency and transitional assistance. Emergency S&S assistance is intended to meet the immediate survival needs of households who have been displaced by humanitarian emergencies. It is short-term, typically less than six months. Transitional S&S assistance often complements emergency S&S assistance and is intended to address short- to medium-term needs of disaster-affected households, typically up to three years.

Humanitarian emergency and transitional S&S assistance interventions share three main characteristics:

- Consistency with internationally recognized guidelines such as the Sphere Project, including provision of minimally adequate space, whenever possible
- Reduction of the social and economic impact of present and future disasters through integration of Disaster Risk Reduction (DRR) measures S&S activities
- Reflection of the particular needs of affected households, especially those considered most vulnerable such as the elderly, disabled, orphaned/unaccompanied minors, minorities, foreign workers, immigrants, traumatized, female-headed households, and others, in S&S activities

Traditionally, humanitarian S&S assistance often excludes linkages to longer-term needs, primarily because those needs are well beyond the mandates, expertise, and institutional practice and protocols of most humanitarian actors. Thus, humanitarian S&S assistance does not include, for example, the reconstruction of permanent housing, the development of new settlements, or efforts to resolve chronic market, policy, and institutional deficiencies related to the provision of housing and basic services, including housing financing.

However, recent humanitarian interventions, most notably in Haiti and Pakistan, have highlighted insufficiencies that need to be addressed to link humanitarian S&S assistance to the recovery of disaster-affected populations, particularly in urban areas. This includes, for example, guidance on how to incrementally improve and expand transitional shelters to turn them into permanent housing, how settlements-based interventions can bridge the gap between relief and recovery efforts, what are the political and security concerns in this region, and how a focus on DRR can inform settlements planning to create safer structures and spaces.

Which sheltering activity to pursue depends on the type and impact of a given disaster or crisis, the conditions of the affected settlements and populations, and the capacity of humanitarian and local/national agencies, which can vary greatly depending on the country or context. S&S activities can facilitate or jump-start the recovery of affected populations when they promote transitions or links to the longer-term housing development process.

High quality S&S assistance shares the following characteristics:

- **Consistency with relevant standards, guidelines, principles, and practices**

S&S assistance should be consistent with recognized guidelines such as the Sphere Project, and prioritize reliance on local building practices, regulations and building codes, and materials, to the extent possible. Whenever possible, S&S activities should include the provision of minimally adequate covered living space.

- **Integration of DRR measures**

S&S activities should integrate DRR measures to best reduce the social and economic impacts of present and future disasters. This is done by promotion of DRR mainly through the adoption of low-cost, nonstructural actions to reduce risks. For example, these actions may include watershed management, clean-up of waterways to improve management of flood waters, hazard-based site and settlements planning, locating and securing objects in homes and workplaces so they don't fall during earthquakes, as well as evacuation of buildings and settlements during earthquakes, tsunamis, and other hazardous events. In addition, technical assistance and rapid capacity building targeting local authorities can be provided, which can be linked to larger, recovery planning and DRR initiatives such as emergency urban planning. Awareness and capacity building activities can also be implemented to ensure that at-risk populations learn to live with contextual hazard risks.

- **Reflection of Beneficiary Needs**

S&S activities should incorporate the particular needs of affected households, especially those considered most vulnerable, based in part on their participation in decision-making. This is particularly true of those unable to self-build their own shelters. Use of building materials and site plans that provide adequate privacy, security, and dignity to the beneficiaries is considered a priority. Where possible and appropriate, assistance may take the form of supporting the self-recovery efforts of affected populations that commenced prior to the arrival of humanitarian actors. New settlements (camps) are constructed as a last resort only when other options have been exhausted and after a detailed market, damage, and needs assessment. When constructed, camps will be sited at an appropriate distance from areas of conflict, ecologically sensitive areas, and national borders, when possible have easy access to roads and town centers, and will be designed with consideration to promoting a sense of community, creating recreational spaces, religious services, burial sites and acceptable aesthetics, mitigating economic and environmental impacts on surrounding settlements, and minimizing threats to safety and security, including those arising from tribal, ethnic, and religious tension. If at all possible, residents and/or recognized leaders should be consulted and their ideas incorporated into the site planning, management, and upkeep process.

Emergency Assistance

In humanitarian emergencies, the purpose of emergency S&S assistance is to complement community efforts to meet urgent needs. Emergency humanitarian S&S assistance should be delivered as soon as other more immediate needs such as food and water, depending on the context, are met. The five types of emergency S&S assistance are:

- Emergency shelter kits
- Emergency shelter
- Emergency tents
- Collective shelters
- Emergency settlements/camps

Emergency Shelter Kits

Emergency shelter kits include commodities such as plastic sheeting, ropes, and tools, as well as the dissemination of basic information needed to create a temporary living space. The provision of shelter kits is recommended under the following circumstances:

- It is likely that the target population would move several times within the next 3 to 6 months
- Poor road conditions, crime or violence limit access to recipients, making it difficult to provide more substantial forms of humanitarian S&S assistance
- Most recipients have the know-how, resources, and interest to use the items included in the kits to secure a temporary space to live

Communities are responsible to assist vulnerable households to secure a space to live.

Recommendations for distribution of emergency shelter kits include:

- Securely wrap the kits to avoid losing items during transportation or distribution
- Package kits flat, in a large and enclosed space such as a warehouse or stadium, before distribution to recipients
- Use a pictorial guide to illustrate the proper use of the materials included in the kits and keep written instructions to a minimum and favor use of the local language(s)
- Assist households lacking able-bodied members to transport the shelter kits to their locations
- Organize the community before kits are distributed, making sure that each recipient knows when and where the distribution will take place and what materials will be distributed, including possibly providing fliers showing items included in the kits before distribution
- Select multiple distribution sites within the target communities to shorten the distance that households will have to carry the kits
- Develop a registration system for kit distribution to eliminate duplication of effort and double-dipping of kit supplies

Emergency Shelter

Emergency shelter includes provision of shelter materials, training, and/or technical assistance, depending on the context. Emergency shelter assistance may include customized shelters for vulnerable household with mobility or other limitations. The provision of emergency shelter is recommended under the following circumstances:

- The recipients would remain in their current location for the next 3–6 months
- The implementing agency has unrestricted access to the recipients at least during the shelter construction
- The burden on vulnerable households is reduced by keeping required contributions to shelter construction, including materials and labor, to the minimum possible as vulnerable households may be unable to secure decent living space if no additional assistance is provided
- The shelter design includes features that reduce the likelihood of death, injury or disease

Recommendations for providing emergency shelter include:

- Favor the use of local construction materials, familiar shelter designs, and well-known construction methods
- Ensure the emergency shelters are constructed in sites with low exposure to hazards and/or ensure the shelter design includes features to increase the

shelter's resistance to prevalent hazards, thus reducing the risk of death and injury caused by the sudden collapse or damage of the shelter
- Select target recipients based on their social, physical, and economic vulnerability to future disasters
- Anticipate the need for the shelter to be adapted to changing climate conditions

Emergency Tents

The provision of emergency tents for emergency, short-term sheltering in the aftermath of disasters should be considered a last resort. Experience has shown that deployment of tents and/or prefabricated structures should not be considered as a default response, as these forms of shelter often perform poorly, are too small for typical families, too expensive, and logistically demanding. Many humanitarian agencies will only deploy tents and prefabricated structures after a field-based determination that no other shelter resources are available in affected areas, affected populations are willing to accept tents and/or prefabricated structures, and sufficient financial and technical resources are available to support purchase and deployment costs. Given these shortcomings, the provision of tents is recommended under the following circumstances:

- The recipients will change their location often during the coming weeks or months
- Extreme heat, cold, or other climate conditions such as wind and rain that may threaten the health of vulnerable recipients
- Good quality tents are locally available, at a reasonable price, and can be distributed to vulnerable households within hours or days
- The tents are large enough to provide a living space to the typical household in compliance with the minimum standard set forth by the Sphere Project
- The supply of construction materials both new or recycled is limited

Recommendations for providing emergency tents include:

- Tightly package all components before distribution
- Provide additional shaded areas to allow families to play or relax comfortably during hot days, unless specifically designed for hot climates
- Provide a means to protect valuables inside the tents from thieves or fire
- Ensure unaccompanied minors are under adult supervision day and night, especially in camp settings
- Ensure cooking and heating stoves are safe to avoid carbon monoxide poisoning and fires
- Provide well-lit and/or guarded latrines, pathways, and common areas to protect vulnerable groups, especially women and children
- Make sure space between tents is at least twice their height to avoid easy spread of fires

Emergency Settlements

Creation and management of emergency shelter in identified geographic areas, whether spontaneously or developed programmatically, should include site improvements and support services where needed. These emergency settlements should be promoted when:

- The disaster-affected households are unable to return to their communities for a variety of reasons including, but not limited to, insecurity or hazardous conditions, and have limited access to basic services
- The affected population will remain living in the camp for only a few weeks unless the premises were originally designed for residential use (or could easily be repurposed) by providing needed access to private spaces for households, basic services, and livelihoods opportunities
- An organization will be responsible for the operation and closing of the settlement
- The land must be restored to its original condition after the displaced households leave the premises
- The site has low exposure to hazards such as floods, storms, and violence

Recommendations for providing emergency settlements include:

- Understand that emergency settlements often last longer than planned as the provision of basic services free of charge creates an incentive for households to remain
- Register all residents and document any special needs they may have such as chronic diseases and disabilities.
- Registration should include occupations: doctors, dentists, carpenters, electricians, etc. may

need to be identified to optimize the functioning of the camp.
- Restrict entry of nonresidents to the settlements to reduce crime and violence
- Understand the host government local policies on use of social services, employment, burial, and marriage regulations
- Include assistance to strengthen provision of services in the host community to avoid potential conflict between displaced population and host community
- Ensure that special needs of unaccompanied minors are adequately satisfied including in the areas of education, protection, and health
- Provide households with access to sources of income that fit their needs and lifestyle where possible
- Consult the residents on issues that impact them and include them in the design process, camp management, and upkeep
- Determine the need for an elected internal governing council to provide information on resident's needs and expectations and to the general population

Collective Centers

Collective centers provide short-term relocation assistance and maintenance or upgrading of structures and facilities where multiple households are sheltered in large buildings. In most cases, public buildings such as stadiums and schools can serve as collective shelter until displaced populations return to their homes, or can be relocated safely to other locations. Collective centers should be promoted when:

- Disaster-affected households are unable to return to their communities and homes due to insecurity, hazardous conditions, limited access to basic services, or government guidance
- They are structurally sound and able to sustain common hazards without the risk of collapse
- The affected population will remain displaced for a few days unless the premises were originally designed for residential use or they could be easily repurposed by providing heating, cooling, electricity, toilets, showers, kitchens, etc.
- The use of the building for residential purposes will not limit the provision of critical services to the host community such as education, health, security

- Organizations are identified to be responsible for operating and closing collective centers when the displaced leave, and to ensure that centers are restored to their original condition

Recommendations for providing collective centers include:

- Develop an exit strategy from the beginning to prevent collective centers from remaining occupied for longer than appropriate, to avoid creating an unnecessary burden for its residents or the host communities
- Register all the residents and document any special needs they may have such as treating chronic diseases or assisting with disabilities
- Restrict entry of nonresidents at least during the night to reduce crime and violence
- Strengthen basic services in the host community to provide adequate supply and equitable access to all
- Address the special needs of unaccompanied minors
- Ensure households have access to sources of income that fit their needs and lifestyle where possible
- Provide enough privacy and security to the residents
- Consult residents on issues that affect them

Transitional Assistance

Transitional humanitarian S&S assistance is intended to support the disaster-affected population until more durable solutions can be derived. Transitional S&S assistance contributes to the recovery of disaster-affected households and communities by providing the foundation for more permanent solutions. The main forms of transitional shelter and settlement assistance include:

- Transitional shelter
- Hosting support
- House repairs
- Technical assistance
- Transfers
- Transitional settlements
- Transit Centers (TC)

Transitional Shelter

Transitional shelter assistance includes the provision of inputs, sometimes including salvaged materials, construction, technical advice, and oversight, which may be needed to create shelter in compliance with the minimum Sphere Project standards for living space. In addition, it is intended to reengage disaster-affected households in the longer-term incremental housing development process disrupted by the disaster, thereby accelerating the transition to recovery and reconstruction. It should be promoted when:

- Recipients will remain in their current location longer than 6 months
- The implementing agency has unrestricted access to the recipients at least during the shelter construction
- Locations have low exposure to hazards such as floods, strong winds, and landslides
- Most households would be able to contribute to the construction of their shelters through the provision of labor or construction materials
- Sufficient skilled labor is available in the target communities

Recommendations for providing transitional shelter include:

- Design the shelter to fit the local context including cultural practices, climatic conditions, local labor availability, and skills
- Utilize familiar construction techniques and materials to ensure that recipients are able to maintain, repair, and/or upgrade their units with minimal or no external assistance
- Ensure shelters will be able to withstand common hazards such as earthquakes, strong winds, or floods with minimum risk of injury to occupants
- Provide technical assistance to ensure the quality and safety of the shelters
- Encourage the use of salvaged and/or recycled construction materials
- Ensure local materials are extracted in a sustainable way to avoid irreversible environmental damage

Hosting Support

Hosting support assistance aims to sustain hosting arrangements and reduce strain on relations and finances through a range of activities such as creation of new shelter space, improvement of existing space, and livelihoods-based assistance. It should be promoted when:

- Recipients have spontaneously moved in with host families
- It is critical to preserve hosting arrangements to avoid secondary displacements

Recommendations for providing hosting support include:

- Allocate enough time and resources to find recipients and provide the hosting support, including identifying and vetting host families, especially in large urban areas
- Provide assistance that will benefit displaced individuals, their host families, and communities
- Allow recipients to decide how best to use assistance provided at the household level, such as upgrading shelters, paying for basic services including water, education or health, or buying needed commodities such as tools
- Track the evolution of the arrangement to ensure good use of resources
- Provide assistance in tranches to ensure use for specific purposes
- Ensure that local markets are able to provide good and services when cash is provided
- Develop alternate hosting solutions for vulnerable groups and unaccompanied minorities, possibly with local host country social service agencies

House Repairs

House repair assistance includes minor repair and improvement of existing, damaged housing to facilitate occupancy that is safe, secure, and private. This might include creation of "one dry, warm room" outputs. It should be promoted when:

- Most resources used are local, including labor
- Repairs are to be performed on residential buildings
- Repair cost is typically less than 10 percent of the replacement cost

Recommendations for providing hosting support include:

- Aim housing repairs at securing a living space that meets Sphere standards
- Ensure access to sanitation and drinking water, heating, and cooling where needed
- Understand that repairs may be time consuming and require custom design interventions and extensive supervision to ensure high quality

- When making repairs, minimize changes to the original design of the home unless for safety reasons

Technical Assistance

Provision of technical assistance including training on improved construction techniques and humanitarian settlement planning, facilitate rapid recovery and the creation of safer settlements. Technical assistance should be provided when:

- Recipients lack the knowledge and/or skills required to perform an activity, such as being unable to build their shelters without the help of skilled builders provided by humanitarian actors
- An untested technology or new approach to something is introduced during the disaster response

Recommendations for providing technical assistance include:

- Verifying that experts providing technical assistance are well versed in the local language and social and cultural practices of the recipients
- Ensuring experts are familiar with the technologies to the deployed and the local environment structure

Transfers

Transfers assistance include the provision of cash-grants vouchers, rental support, and in-kind materials to disaster-affected households to help them secure shelter in compliance with minimum Sphere Project guidelines for covered living space. Transfers are recommended under the following conditions:

- Markets are functioning and there is availability of products and services on a local, regional, and/or national level and within a reasonable distance from the affected communities
- There are available delivery mechanisms including secure methods to deliver transfers to beneficiaries in the program area
- Political acceptance. Host governments must agree that transfers are appropriate solutions to help disaster-affected communities

Recommendations for the use of transfers include:

- Develop customized bills of quantities and designs
- Train local builders to enhance local construction practices
- Address potential bottlenecks in accessing high-quality materials and other construction inputs
- Provide technical assistance to ensure a high-quality construction process

Transitional Settlements

Transitional settlements assistance supports the improvement of existing neighborhoods, including informal settlements to permit provision of shelter and basic services while reducing hazard risks and the need to relocate affected populations to new locations. These settlements-based interventions can also serve as platforms for subsequent recovery and reconstruction.

Transit Centers

When there are large numbers of displaced persons, they may pass through Transit Centers (TC) to facilitate safe and organized passage from one country or region to another. During this rapid movement of refugees, the host country and responding agencies are responsible for the provisions of services. Transit Centers are recommended under the following conditions:

- Refugees will remain at a TC less than 24 hours
- Host governments and UN agree on expedited movement of refugees through countries and across borders
- Mechanisms are available to safely and economically transport large numbers of refugees
- International and local NGOs are allowed to work in assisting the UN and host government in the provision of services
- There are mechanisms in place to monitor health, welfare, and security

Recommendations for providing rapid transitional shelters include:

- TC must be in an area that is easily secured and ideally next to transportation hubs such as bus, train, and air terminals
- Site must be well lit and guarded 24/7 and access to the site must be restricted to government and nongovernment relief workers with proper identification
- Movement of refugees outside the site is restricted
- There is clear signage (written and pictorial) with translators available depicting the steps to be taken for transit arriving refugees

- There needs to be a system of registration at the food and clothing distribution points ensuring that only one visit of the distribution point is allowed
- Embarkation and disembarkation of refugees onto trains and buses needs to be organized, managed, and monitored to protect vulnerable groups and line jumping
- Agreements should be reached with hospital, clinics, and airports for the rapid evacuation and care of critically sick refugees
- Contingency planning for refugees staying longer than anticipated in event the transit pipeline is halted
- Develop evacuation plans for staff and refugees in case of natural or man-made disaster

Healthy Shelter and Settlements

As discussed previously, the link between shelter, settlements, and health has long been understood. S&S assistance and activities are important for human health and well-being in the setting of humanitarian emergencies. They contribute to emotional and mental recovery of disaster-affected populations by providing conformable and dignified spaces where households play, rest, relax, and perform cultural activities. In addition, humanitarian S&S activities reduce exposure to hazards including tropical storms, floods, and earthquakes and other environmental stressors such as cold temperatures, rain, and snow, thus preserving the health of the recipients, especially the most vulnerable. To maximize the benefits of shelter and settlements interventions during humanitarian emergencies, it is important to control stressors including:

- Overcrowding
- Poor ventilation
- Pest infestations

Overcrowding

Humanitarian S&S assistance provided during a humanitarian emergency should minimize overcrowding in both shelter and settlements to preserve the health and well-being of the recipients of assistance. Overcrowding is associated with various adverse mental and physical health outcomes, including impaired social relationships and other mental health morbidities, as well as increased vulnerability to infectious diseases including respiratory tract infections and diarrhea.

Shelter and settlements are considered overcrowded when occupancy exceeds the maximum occupancies rates defined by standards and good practices. The Sphere Project defines overcrowding in humanitarian settings for shelter when the ratio between available indoor space expressed in square meters and the number of people living in a shelter is lower than 3.5 (Sphere Project 2011). For settlements, overcrowding in humanitarian settings is present when the ratio between gross settlement area, including streets, parking lots, recreation areas, schools, clinics, etc., expressed in square meters and the total number of people living in it is less than 45 (Sphere Project 2011). Simplified, a shelter is considered crowded when indoor space available per person is less than 3.5 square meters, and a settlement is considered overcrowded when each resident has access to less than 45 square meters of land where they live, including parks, roads, schools, clinics, etc.

Neighborhood Approach

Preventing overcrowding during a humanitarian emergency is often challenging unless suitable land for new settlements are identified. If land cannot be obtained, or if land can be reconfigured more efficiently after a disaster, an alternative is the provision of multistory transitional sheltering solutions accompanied by land redevelopment as part of a process known as the Neighborhood Approach: integrated, multisector programming in socially defined spaces. Multistory transitional shelters create additional living space within a fixed building footprint, thus freeing up land that could later be redeveloped to accommodate future population growth or the provision of recreation facilities, basic services, evacuation routes, and DRR infrastructure.

Poor Ventilation

Adequate ventilation provides psychological and physical health benefits by regulating indoor temperatures/humidity and managing contamination. Ventilation can be provided to shelter using either natural or mechanical means. Mechanic ventilation systems such as fans are rarely used during the response to humanitarian emergencies as they are often more expensive to operate and maintain than natural ventilation systems. Mechanic ventilation systems often require more specialized knowledge and tools to be installed, maintained, and operated compared with most natural ventilation systems. More importantly, they often require a reliable energy source to operate that is rarely available during humanitarian emergencies. Natural ventilation systems are better suited than mechanical ventilation in the setting of humanitarian emergencies.

Natural ventilation systems work like a conveyor belt moving air through shelters powered by differences in air pressure and/or humidity. Either way, the amount of ventilation is directly related to the size and locations of the shelter openings including doors and windows. Larger and well-positioned shelter openings and increased unrestricted air flow result in better natural ventilation of the shelter.

Typical ventilation rate (outdoor fresh air inflow) for sedentary people is between 5 and 25 liters/second/person. When designing shelter, the desired rate of ventilation depends on how much heat, moisture, and pollution need to be removed.

In hot climates, natural ventilation relies on pressure differences created by the wind. Wind pushes air through the shelter openings on the windward side and sucks it out through openings in the roof and leeward side of the shelter. Properly-sized openings should be provided in three walls and the shelter roof to ensure proper cross-ventilation. In cold climates, chimneys ventilate shelters by flushing out contaminated air and sucking in fresh air. Openings are generally not required in cold climate humanitarian shelters, which are seldom air tight.

Pest Infestations

Depending on the context, it is important to control rats and other rodents, mosquitoes, and other indoor pests as they can spread a variety of diseases. Malaria, dengue, yellow fever, and Zika are examples of mosquito-borne disease while rats and rodents may spread leptospirosis, plague, and some hemorrhagic fevers.

There are other important considerations for provision of healthy shelter and settlements.

Relative Humidity

High levels of indoor relative humidity (RH) are caused by several factors, including high environmental humidity, daily activities such as sweating, cooking, and bathing, and defective construction materials and techniques that lead to infiltrations through roofs, walls, and foundations.

High RH makes shelters uncomfortable and potentially unhealthy. High RH causes thermal discomfort by making it difficult to sweat and, in turn, cool the human body off. The sweat is not evaporated fast enough to allow the body temperature to drop. In addition, high indoor RH leads to water condensation, creating an environment where mold, mildew, and other biological growth occurs. This may precipitate health problems such as allergic reactions and asthma exacerbations. RH that is too low can cause irritation of the eyes and airway.

In addition to health problems and uncomfortable environments, water condensation contributes to structural decay, increasing the risk of injury when common construction hazards strike the buildings.

The RH in shelters should remain between 30 and 70 percent under normal activity conditions. It is challenging to maintain RH in this range during humanitarian emergencies, especially during the heating season in colder climates or in hot and damp climates. Often, the affected populations have limited access to resources and know-how required to maintain the RH within the desired range.

During humanitarian emergencies, the RH in shelters is managed using a combination of measures including proper ventilation, use of the sun to dry moist objects, sealing off roofs, walls, floors, and foundations to prevent humidity infiltration, and limiting physical activities, cooking, and bathing indoors.

Temperature

The temperature inside a shelter is directly related to the rate it loses or gains heat to its surrounding environment. The more heat a shelter gains or losses, the warmer or cooler its indoor temperature. A shelter will lose heat when the temperature outside is lower than inside and it will gain heat when the outdoor temperature is higher. A shelter loses or gains heat until both the indoors and outdoors temperatures are the same, a phenomenon called thermal equilibrium.

The rate of heat that is exchanged in a shelter depends on its location, design, construction, and activities performed inside. Shelter design and orientation to the sun play a role in thermal comfort. Shelters with larger sides and openings facing south, in the northern hemisphere, are normally warmer that those facing north. The opposite is true in the southern hemisphere. Construction and materials also determine shelter thermal performance. Shelters with concrete walls are more comfortable than those with timber walls in colder climates. The opposite is true in warm conditions. Activities such as indoor cooking increase the temperature within a shelter. These are all important considerations when planning shelter activities.

Extremes in temperatures are associated with a variety of health problems. Extreme cold can result in hypothermia, frostbite, and related cold illness. Extreme heat can lead to health complications including heat cramps, heat exhaustion, heat syncope, and heatstroke. People with heart or respiratory disease may be especially vulnerable to health-related compilations due to extremes in temperature.

During a humanitarian emergency, the goal is to maintain the shelter temperatures as comfortable as technically and economically feasible by regulating the rate at which the shelter gains or loses heat. This is best done by reducing heat loss or gain by conduction through walls, doors, windows, floor, and the roof, often through the use of low thermal conductivity materials, such as timber or soil, and to fabricate structural shelter elements, such as the roof, walls, windows, doors, and floors, that are in constant contact with the external environment.

Commercial insulation products are available in many countries to reduce heat conductivity in structural elements, especially roofs. Cellulose-based products are often the most environmentally friendly insulation available.

Managing indoor temperatures during humanitarian emergencies is challenging in both hot and cold humid climates. Hot and humid climates are especially challenging as it is extremely difficult to cool shelters through natural ventilation. When the outdoor temperature is higher than the indoor temperature, it is impossible to cool off shelters using natural ventilation. Consequently, in places where using ventilation to control indoor temperatures is limited, shelter designs should minimize thermal loads. In hot climates, this may necessitate that the natural ventilation systems be assisted by low-powered mechanical means to ensure proper ventilation.

Contaminants

Depending on the context, S&S interventions should be designed to prevent or at least minimize exposure to contaminants. For example, in places where indoor cooking or heating stoves are used, poor ventilation may increase the risk of carbon monoxide poisoning. If a shelter contains lead-based paint, children are particularly vulnerable to exposure and subsequent lead poisoning, and measures should be taken to minimize this potential.

Conclusion

Current humanitarian S&S assistance often overlooks linkages to longer-term needs, mainly because those needs are well beyond the mandates, protocols, expertise, and institutional memories of most humanitarian actors. Thus, humanitarian S&S assistance does not include, for example, the reconstruction of permanent housing, the development of new settlements, or efforts to resolve chronic market, policy, and institutional deficiencies related to the provision of housing and basic services, including housing finance.

Recent humanitarian interventions, however, most notably in Haiti, Pakistan, and the Philippines, have highlighted a number of emerging issues that need to be more coherently addressed to appropriately link humanitarian S&S assistance to the recovery of disaster-affected populations, particularly in urban areas. This may include guidance, for example, on how to incrementally improve and expand transitional shelters to turn them into permanent housing, how settlements-based interventions can bridge the gap between relief and recovery efforts, and how a focus on DRR can inform settlements planning to create safer structures and spaces. Humanitarian actors will continue to improve S&S practice so that the long-standing gap between relief and recovery does not continue to undermine efforts to assist populations affected by humanitarian emergencies.

To address this gap, some argue that transitional shelter should be viewed and promoted as both an appropriate humanitarian response and permanent housing reconstruction, thereby facilitating the recovery of disaster/crisis-affected settlements more rapidly and at lower cost than conventional housing reconstruction programs (Setchell and Argenal 2014). This is not a trivial matter, for humanitarian and reconstruction budgets are not inexhaustible, even as the frequency of humanitarian emergencies is increasing. Further, as the global population continues to increase at a notable pace, this growing population is becoming increasingly urban and becoming more vulnerable through occupation of hazard-prone areas, with low-lying coastal cities subject to sea-level rise and climate change being an ominous example.

Thus, it appears that there has never been a greater need for safer, healthier shelter and settlements. The link between shelter, settlements, and health forged in the past, and strengthened in the humanitarian community in recent years, will thus serve as a strong conceptual and experiential basis to inform responses to the shelter and settlements needs generated by future humanitarian emergencies.

References

Davis, J. and Lambert, R. (2002). *Engineering in emergencies: A practical guide for relief workers.* London: ITDG Publishing.

Setchell, C. A. and Argenal, E. (2014). Under one roof: Promoting transitional shelter as both humanitarian response and permanent housing reconstruction. *Monthly Developments*, 32 (1/2), 19–21 and 27 (online). Available at: http://reliefweb.int/report/world/handouts-usaidofda-shelter-and-settlements-training-workshop (Accessed July 15, 2015).

Sphere Project. (2011). Sphere handbook: Humanitarian charter and minimum standards in disaster response (online). Available at: www.sphereproject.org (Accessed June 16, 2015).

Thiele, B. (2002). The human right to adequate housing: A tool for promoting and protecting individual and community health. *American Journal of Public Health*, 92 (5), 712–715 (online). Available at: www.ncbi.nlm.nih.gov/pmc/articles/PMC1447150/ (Accessed June 17, 2015).

United States Department of Housing and Urban Development. (2007). Measuring overcrowding in housing (online). Available at: www.huduser.org/publications/pdf/measuring_overcrowding_in_hsg.pdf (Accessed July 2, 2015).

World Health Organization. (1989). *Health principles of housing.* World Health Organization; Geneva, Switzerland.

Chapter 19

Logistics

Rebecca Turner, Travis Vail Betz, George A. Roark, and Darrell Morris Lester

Introduction

The basic goal of logistics in the setting of humanitarian emergencies is to plan, implement, and control the storage and delivery of commodities, that may include products, services, and human resources, in a quality, timely, and effective manner. This includes provision of lifesaving aid for the relief and recovery of those made vulnerable by disaster. Public health and healthcare related supplies, equipment, and personnel are critical to lifesaving aid in the setting of humanitarian emergencies. The consequences of poor logistical services in humanitarian emergencies can mean the difference between life and death. It is thus essential to provide what is needed quickly and efficiently to save lives. At a minimum, it is important to reestablish normal logistical services as quickly as possible; however, a more robust system than existed in the country or region preemergency may be necessary to provide the logistical support required for the situation. The focus of this chapter is logistics as it applies to support for public health and healthcare in the context of humanitarian emergencies.

While logistics has been defined in several ways, simply put, logistics might be defined as:

- Logistics = Supply + Materials Management + Distribution (WFP 2013)

Logistics, managed by professional logisticians, is a critical component of emergency response. Lack of coordination in timing and transport of public health and medical equipment, supplies, and human resources will cause delays and ultimately result in greater loss of life. An adaptable system managed by professional humanitarian aid logisticians is critical to the success of a humanitarian response. "A multidisciplinary perspective [is required] to overcome the unique challenges of emergency logistics, characterized by: (1) large volumes of critical supplies to be transported; (2) short time frames of response to prevent loss of lives and property; and (3) major uncertainties about what is actually needed and what is available at the site" (Holguín-Veras et al. 2007).

Commercial vs. Humanitarian Logistics

Commercial and humanitarian logistics are built around the customer and the beneficiary respectively. A supply chain is a system that facilitates the movement of commodities from production to distribution to the customer or beneficiary. As such, lessons learned from commercial logistics have application in humanitarian emergencies.

Both humanitarian and commercial supply chains will have many of the same key components including that they:

- Are dependent on professional relationships including effective contracting mechanisms with suppliers
- Must be cost effective and will not work without appropriate funding
- May break down due to poor communication and inadequate flow of information
- Require effective human resource management and timely response
- Have logistics serving as the main link between the main organization and forward locations and distribution points
- Utilize a tracking system that not only tracks items from the procurement/manufacturing point to the required location, but also uses this data to provide feedback on ways to improve overall logistical operations and effectiveness (Fritz 2013).

Predictably, there are important differences between humanitarian and commercial supply chains. First, "[t]he stark difference lies in simple economics; the cost of transporting a commodity in a commercial system must be less than the value of the commodity" (WFP 2013). For example, a commercial pipeline will fail if shipping a liter of bottled water costs more than the profit of selling that bottle in its ultimate destination. If a bottle of water costing $1 (US) is put into a logistics pipeline that costs $5 (US) to ship that water, one will have to sell that bottle for more than $6 (US) to profit. For this reason, commercial systems clearly define the value of shipping and the conditions that make shipping a reasonable option.

In contrast, in a humanitarian supply chain there is a responsibility to seek solutions of best value and not best bottom line. This humanitarian imperative will require, at times, spending considerably more on transport than the value of the commodity. Cost should not be ignored in the humanitarian supply chain and logisticians should strive to utilize the most efficient means for both cost and expediency, still ultimately prioritizing assured delivery of commodities.

The logistician can mitigate waste and improve efficiency while meeting the requirement for delivery of commodities by calculating and manipulating the variables included in the Total Logistics Cost (TLC), which may be expressed by the following equation (de Villiers et al. 2008):

- TLC = TC + DC + FC + CC + SC + IC + HC + PC + RC + MC + XC where:
- TLC = Total logistics costs
- TC = Transport cost – primary or long distance including trucking
- DC = Transport cost – secondary or short distance including local delivery
- FC = Facility cost (warehouse, etc.)
- CC = Communication cost (invoicing, etc.)
- SC = Information system cost (tracking and tracing, etc.)
- IC = Inventory cost
- HC = Materials handling cost
- PC = Protective packaging cost
- RC = Cost of reverse logistics
- MC = Logistics management cost
- XC = Direct and indirect taxes

A second difference is that commercial logistics and supply chains are often highly efficient operations based on a fairly accurate forecast of demand, stable, known locations and other constant or predictable factors. In the interest of maximizing profits, commercial logistics and supply chains are monitored on a continuous basis to optimize the operational efficiencies of every function.

This relatively stable platform for commercial logistics and supply chains is in contrast to humanitarian logistics and supply chains that are often characterized by (WFP 2013):

- Not knowing the exact requirements ahead of time including the type and amount of supplies, equipment, and services needed
- A greater sense of urgency for humanitarian supplies, equipment, and services
- Potential public scrutiny by the entire world including donors with a critical eye, in contrast to the private nature of commercial logistics and supply chains, often closed to the public
- Funding challenges compared with commercial logistics and supply chains that can influence the flow of funding and accurately tailor this to historical demands

Effective humanitarian logistics relies on the flow of information through the humanitarian supply chain. It is often necessary for logisticians to be proactive in achieving lines of communication for each phase of the response. Communication in humanitarian logistics can be more complicated than in the private sector because, unlike traditional logistics that have unidirectional lines of communication, humanitarian logistics includes communication between the donor, the internal requestor, the supplier, and the system or party taking action to support the request. Managing all of these lines of communication can prove challenging. Humanitarian logisticians who leverage the power of effective communication and manage it well in the field can make huge impacts on the overall response. There are several tools humanitarian logisticians can use to improve informational workflow including MedLog, LOGIC, LSS/SUMA, and the Log Cluster's D-LCA.

Professionalization

Over the past 20 years, the humanitarian aid community has become more credentialed and professional. This has been the result, in part, of investment in the development and codification of the humanitarian architecture led by the UN and OCHA.

In addition, the academic community has contributed to this by offering coursework, graduate level degrees, and certification programs in the area of humanitarian aid and logistics. Specifically, in the area of logistics, the Fritz Institute and the Chartered Institute of Logistics and Transportation (CILT), funded by the donor community, created a Certification in Humanitarian Logistics. Georgia

Tech University offers Health and Humanitarian Logistics as an executive learning experience targeted at the humanitarian aid community. Associations including the Humanitarian Logistics Association (HLA) and the International Association of Public Health Logisticians (IAPHL) have formed communities to foster dialogue on professionalization and innovation within the sector. The exponential increase in telecommunication capacity and real-time reporting has supported decision-making theory and professional skill development within the logistics community.

All of these efforts, combined with an emphasis on effective human resources by humanitarian organizations, will continue to increase the number of professional humanitarian logisticians.

Coordination

Coordination of delivery of aid in the setting of humanitarian emergencies, including commodities, that includes products, services, and human resources, can prove very challenging. Logistics is by nature very structured and it may be challenging for organizations to work within an existing logistics infrastructure that may be unfamiliar and coordinate with colleagues from other organizations. It is often the case that there is competition to be the first organization to deliver aid to the most vulnerable. Being the first organization to deliver aid not only meets a humanitarian imperative but also positions the organization to gain additional funding to do even more work. While it is important to deliver aid to the most vulnerable as quickly as possible, coordination is critical to reduce duplication of efforts. In addition, delivery of aid should be carried out with efforts to minimize any negative impact on the local economy.

Often the requirement to move commodities outpaces capacity of the existing supply chain. A common emergency logistics pipeline, initially implemented by the local or national authorities, is a potential solution. As the response to the humanitarian emergency grows, the logistics pipeline may increase from a few agencies to a large international response.

In a large, international, humanitarian response, the UN commonly serves as the coordinating entity operating at the request of the host nation. Specifically, the United Nation's Office for the Coordination of Humanitarian Affairs (UN OCHA) may coordinate the response through technical cluster coordination cells. It was formed to coordinate major international disaster response and serves as the UN focal point in this capacity. Its mandate includes the coordination of humanitarian response, policy development, and humanitarian advocacy.

Logistics Cluster

UN OCHA often utilizes the Cluster Approach; therefore, it is important for humanitarian logisticians to understand UN system. UN OCHA has additional responsibility to ensure intercluster communication at a field-based, operational level. This may be especially pertinent to the Global Logistics Cluster as it interacts with all of the other clusters.

The World Food Program (WFP) leads the Logistics Cluster. The Logistics Cluster has the means and the mandate to provide the structure for the commodity pipeline. In a large response, the pipeline allows for multiple agencies to prioritize the commodity flow based on the needs of beneficiaries. Commodities flowing through the shared pipeline have different priorities, storage, and transport requirements, and may be delivered to different points of distribution.

It is important that the cluster coordinator work closely with medical logistics professionals to ensure a proper and adequate supply chain for medical commodities. It is imperative that stakeholders (the host nation, militaries, UN organizations, international organizations, local and international nongovernmental organizations, commercial logistics companies, and freight forwarders) communicate and cooperate within the humanitarian architecture, including the Cluster Approach, to prevent both duplication of efforts and gaps in coverage. Since the clusters do not operate as traditional command and control structures, this collaboration is required for be effective. It is important for key stakeholders to meet and share information, identify resources, target the most vulnerable populations, and work together to quickly and effectively save lives and deliver aid. The UN Cluster Approach is discussed in detail in Chapter 4.

Host Nation

Along with UN OCHA and the clusters, at the center of coordination is the host nation. Delivery of aid through the humanitarian logistics pipeline is subject

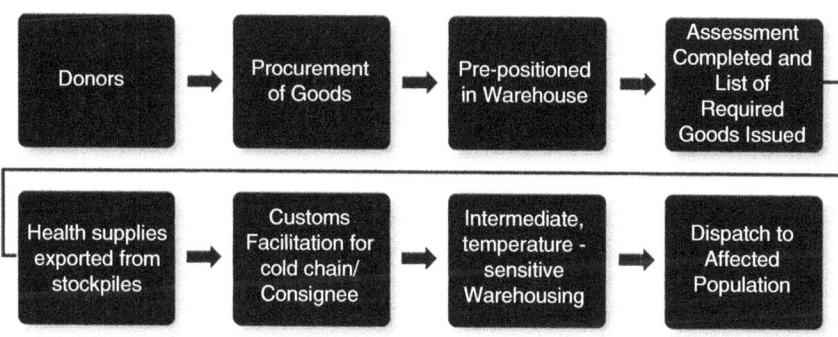

Figure 19.1 Components of the Humanitarian Supply Chain

to the laws and regulations of the host nation. Organizations delivering aid must be granted permission and access to operate in the host country, often granted only after the host nation makes a formal request for international humanitarian assistance.

As a sovereign nation, the laws, regulations, and systems of the host nation must be adhered to by humanitarian aid organizations. Rule of law is not suspended during a disaster. While it may seem more efficient to bypass local systems, working through local entities helps to build their capacity to respond. In some cases, local authorities may themselves be traumatized by the disaster, potentially compromising their effectiveness. In these situations, the humanitarian logisticians may try to offer objective courses of action and provide additional support.

If the host nation does not support the plans, processes, and participants involved in the response, logistics efforts, no matter how efficient, may fail. Consideration should be given for advocacy to local government bodies from the standpoint of process ownership.

Humanitarian Supply Chain

The humanitarian supply chain facilitates the movement of commodities from production to distribution to beneficiaries. Components of the humanitarian supply chain are shown in Figure 19.1. The humanitarian supply chain may be in support of the overall response or a specific program or project. Each situation requires efficient systems managed by professional logisticians.

In humanitarian emergencies, there is an affected geographic region. For natural disasters, the affected region may be based on the physical boundaries of the destruction. For disasters resulting from civil unrest or armed conflict, the boundaries may be defined by political, cultural, or ethnic factors. In these settings, logisticians are responsible for developing a humanitarian supply chain, often needing to overcome various obstacles. For example, destroyed or insecure roads may require the logistician to be creative in considering possible solutions, from repair of the road to use of alternate transport such as by air, water, animal, or foot.

Depending on the type and state of the emergency, the affected population may be at risk of physical insecurity, famine, drought, disease, illness and injury, lack of shelter, and breakdown of basic infrastructure. In countries where these basic needs are already compromised by economic and political factors, an emergency can quickly and significantly worsen the situation making the effectiveness of the response mechanism, including the humanitarian supply chain, critical both to the immediate situation as well as for the country working to stabilize when the disaster ends.

The humanitarian supply chain may include, for example, delivery of food, potable water, NFIs, healthcare services, and cash. Ultimately, the goal of humanitarian assistance is to provide commodities and services until they can be provided through other mechanisms and then scale back as needs are met, eventually transitioning out of supplying these commodities and services. Since response efforts and the funds that support them are theoretically and often actually time-limited, emphasis should be placed on implementing solutions, including supply chains that can be transitioned and subsequently operated and maintained by the host nation. This transition may be especially challenging in civil unrest or conflict settings.

In contrast to many of the food and nonfood items (NFIs), medical commodities are usually routed in a more controlled way. Since medical commodities are routed to healthcare providers rather than directly to beneficiaries, the humanitarian medical supply chain begins with production and ends with delivery to the healthcare facility or provider. Humanitarian logisticians need to be compliant with local rules, laws, and regulations for the handling and distribution of medical commodities, including their waste and disposal. In many countries, controlled items will require a locally licensed medical provider or institution to maintain possession. These commonly include pharmaceuticals, surgical instruments, and medical devices. Security and chain of custody for medical commodities must be compliant with local laws and appropriate for the context.

Donors

Donors are a key component of the humanitarian supply chain as they help fund the humanitarian response. Donors include governments, international organizations, companies and corporations, foundations and institutions, and individuals. Donors may provide funding, commodities, or other deliverables directly to implementing partners, coordinating organizations, governments or to a pooled appeal for funding. Donors may allow partners to utilize funding, commodities, or other deliverables based on their working knowledge of a specific country and context. Many times, however, donors earmark for highly specific mandates. This can result in disaggregated and inefficient supply chains as donors are often not on the ground and may not fully understand needs of the population and the challenges in fulfilling them.

Procurement

Procurement is part of the supply component of logistics as all commodities must be procured either through the purchase of those items or through donation.

In the context of a humanitarian emergency, it is almost always better to procure items locally when possible. This is especially true early on in the emergency when time is critical and early procurement may save lives. Local sources, for both donations and purchases, may include local hospitals, corporations, businesses, and government. The logistics coordinator should work with a host nation representative and all logistics coordination should filter through them.

Depending on the situation, local procurement may include not just the host country but surrounding countries if they have available resources. Procuring commodities locally not only saves on shipping and transportation costs and lead times, but may also support the local market. It is important to consider local capacity before looking to an international supplier, always being aware not to create false demand in the local market. In a situation where large quantities of staple commodities are needed, it may still be wiser to procure regionally to minimize volatility in the local market.

During a humanitarian emergency, especially early on, it can be very difficult to forecast demand, as there is a degree of uncertainty and instability. As part of procurement, it is necessary to account for potential inaccuracies in demand forecasting. Considering this variability in demand and clarifying exactly what is needed with the program officer can save time that would be spent later on correcting order qualities and specifications. For example, a logistician may be tasked to procure a centrifuge and simply orders the centrifuge that the supplier recommends, only to find out that there are multiple types of centrifuges and that a bench top centrifuge was ordered when a hematocrit centrifuge was needed. This concept may seem oversimplified; however, this occurs frequently in the field when effective communication is not emphasized on the front end of the procurement.

Important questions to consider before procuring a commodity include:

- What are the exact specifications of the item requested?
- How important is the brand of the item?
- How many of the items are required?
- Where will the item need to be delivered?
- What is the contact information for the person who will receive the item?
- What is the exact date that the item needs to be delivered to ensure timely response?

As part of the procurement process, it is often necessary to enter into contracts. Since contracts are legally binding agreements, it is important to solicit legal contracting expertise before entering into such agreements. Many organizations have clear procurement processes from a legal standpoint. For instance, US Government Agencies are required to follow specific procurement polices found in the Federal Acquisition Regulation (FAR). This is a complicated process requiring all US Government Agencies to have contract specialists and contract officers in order to ensure compliance with the statutory requirements of the FAR during the procurement process.

During a major humanitarian response in which the US Government has pledged support, contracting officers can use a caveat found in the FAR to bypass many of the constraints of the FAR by using the justification that the need is "urgent and compelling" indicating that lives will be lost if certain actions are not taken immediately. Therefore, during the early days of a humanitarian response, some of the time-consuming requirements can be mitigated by pushing an urgent and compelling contract through the system.

Prepositioning

There are several different strategies for the prepositioning of commodities and it is the role of the logistician to help determine which is best for a given situation. One option is to buy a certain number of commodities such as kits and store them in a primary warehouse facility until the time healthcare providers call them forward. A second option is to procure the kits and move them to regional logistics hubs in proximity to disaster-prone countries for deployment regionally when they are called forward. A third option, becoming more common, is to have the provider hold the kits until they are called forward, then ship them directly. While this may be the costliest option upfront, having the supplier maintain the stock of kits containing items with finite shelf life such as medications may ultimately be cost effective. These contracts with suppliers are sometimes referred to as framework agreements. Many large humanitarian aid agencies and donors procure and store medical kits in this way.

Many agencies maintain stockpiles of commodities in multiple locations, often regional, logistic hubs, as a way of prepositioning and thus decreasing the response time to a humanitarian emergency. Deployment of commodities can be done sequentially, locally, regional, then globally.

The UN Humanitarian Resources Depots (UNHRD) act as logistics and storage facilities that allow the United Nations to respond rapidly to crises. The depots are important resources strategically located around the world in prime international logistics hubs to leverage proximity to airports, seaports, and storage. The Italian government supports the operational costs of the UNHRD. Commodities maintained in these facilities belong to WFP, WHO, the Italian Government, and various INGOs. These commodities include emergency food aid, various types of NFIs, mobile cooking facilities, rapid response equipment, medicines, and medical kits (OCHA 2014). The UNHRD are open to the humanitarian logistics community as a cost-effective means of prepositioning through regional stockpiling.

Assessments

After the onset of a disaster, assessments are often performed to determine the scale and scope of the impact. This includes quantifying loss of life, injuries and illness, and destruction of property and infrastructure. It also includes determining needs and the capacity to respond locally, regionally, and globally. When there is a deficit in capacity to respond to the needs assessed, various actors step in to ensure proper response coverage. Depending on the context, the needs may be met locally, but if there is a gap between the needs and the local capacity to respond, regional and international actors may provide assistance. Experience has shown that assessments are inherently imperfect but humanitarian logisticians should never let this uncertainty inhibit their ability to respond to the affected population. Assessments are discussed in detail in Chapter 7.

Movement of Commodities

Once the initial or rapid assessment has been completed, commodities that cannot be sourced locally are often imported from stockpiles under the direction of a logistician. For medical commodities, healthcare professionals provide the logistician with their requirements. Emergency logisticians must balance what is needed with what can be supported. They have advocated for standardization of medical commodities to facilitate delivery of goods specifically tailored to the needs of the affected population. Kits or push packages and essential medicines lists are one way to address both clinician preference and logistics standardization. By identifying essential medicines and kits prior to the onset of a humanitarian emergency, establishing a humanitarian supply chain (including procurement, export of commodities from stockpiles, and delivery) can be done more quickly and efficiently, resulting in saving lives. This is especially important early on in the response to a humanitarian emergency.

Kits

Designing kits before a humanitarian emergency facilitates shipping commodities that will meet the needs of the emergency. For example, during Hurricane Katrina, humanitarian aid sent from the US Medical Materiel Agency, part of the US Army, was shipped to New Orleans. This set, or kit, contains very basic medicines, potable water, blankets, body bags, tents, tarps, diapers, and trash bags to cover immediate needs.

Particular to medical commodities, multiple standardized kits have been developed in conjunction with clinicians to meet specific needs of healthcare providers in different situations. These prepackaged kits can now be purchased from multiple providers internationally. Some organizations prefer to build their own. Ideally, kits are packaged in such a way that they can be used in one location or easily broken down to service multiple locations. The WHO, the International Red Cross and Red Cross Movement, and Médecins Sans Frontières (MSF) have set the standard for emergency health kits.

The most common kits utilized during humanitarian emergencies are often the most general. The Interagency Emergency Health Kit (IEHK) is a multicarton package of common pharmaceuticals and medical devices intended to support the medical needs of ten thousand people for three months. More specialized kits include surgical kits such as the Italian Trauma Kit and the Red Cross Surgical Trauma Kit, both examples of specialty kits focused on trauma patients in conflict settings. There are also specialized kits for the treatment of diarrheal diseases including cholera. Examples of additional specialized kits include those for reproductive health and mental health.

Essential Medicines

WHO maintains Model Lists of Essential Medicines from which the IEHK was derived. Other organizations have essential medicines as well. The Office of Foreign Disaster Assistance (OFDA) within the United States Agency for International Development (USAID) maintains an essential medicines list (EML) or emergency formulary called the OFDA EML.

The OFDA EML was derived from a collaboration of clinicians, pharmacists, and public health professionals. Essential medicines lists and recommendations from various organizations were referenced for its development, including the WHO Model List of Essential Medicines, the WHO Interagency Emergency Health Kit (IEHK) 2011, the United Nations Population Fund (UNFPA) Post-Exposure Prophylaxis (PEP) recommendations and kit, and the United Nations High Commissioner for Refugees (UNHCR) Essential Medicines and Medical Supplies: Policy and Guidance (UNHCR 2011). Its contents are a subset of the WHO Model List of Essential Medicines. The OFDA EML is intended to streamline procurement and delivery of medicines by identifying those most commonly needed by beneficiaries and used by implementing partners (USAID 2013).

Deployment of Personnel

Similar to movement of commodities, deployment of personnel is a critical part of the response to a humanitarian emergency. The types of professionals deployed in response to humanitarian emergencies come from a wide range of experts, including healthcare and public health sector. This might include individuals from volunteers to highly paid consultants. It may be the responsibility of the logistician to verify the credentials and specific skills of personnel being deployed. This is extremely important as sending the right, qualified people makes an enormous difference in the quality of the response effort. For an organization, rapid deployment of personnel requires an investment in readiness, including having preparedness protocols in place outlining how to get the human resources needed to the affected region. The management of personnel is commonly done via rosters and readiness checklists. Logisticians often work in collaboration with their colleagues in human resources, travel health, and transportation services to develop deployment checklists. It may ultimately be the responsibility of the logistics team to manage rosters and readiness checklists.

Many organizations that regularly respond to humanitarian emergencies have rapidly deployable teams that can provide immediate relief, perform rapid assessments, and provide technical assistance. Logisticians may be a part of these teams and/or receive critical mission information from them. Two examples of these rapidly deployable teams are the UN Disaster Assessment and Coordination (UNDAC) and the International Federation of Red Cross (IFRC) and Red Crescent Society Field Assessment and Coordination teams. These teams may include a public health

Chapter 19: Logistics

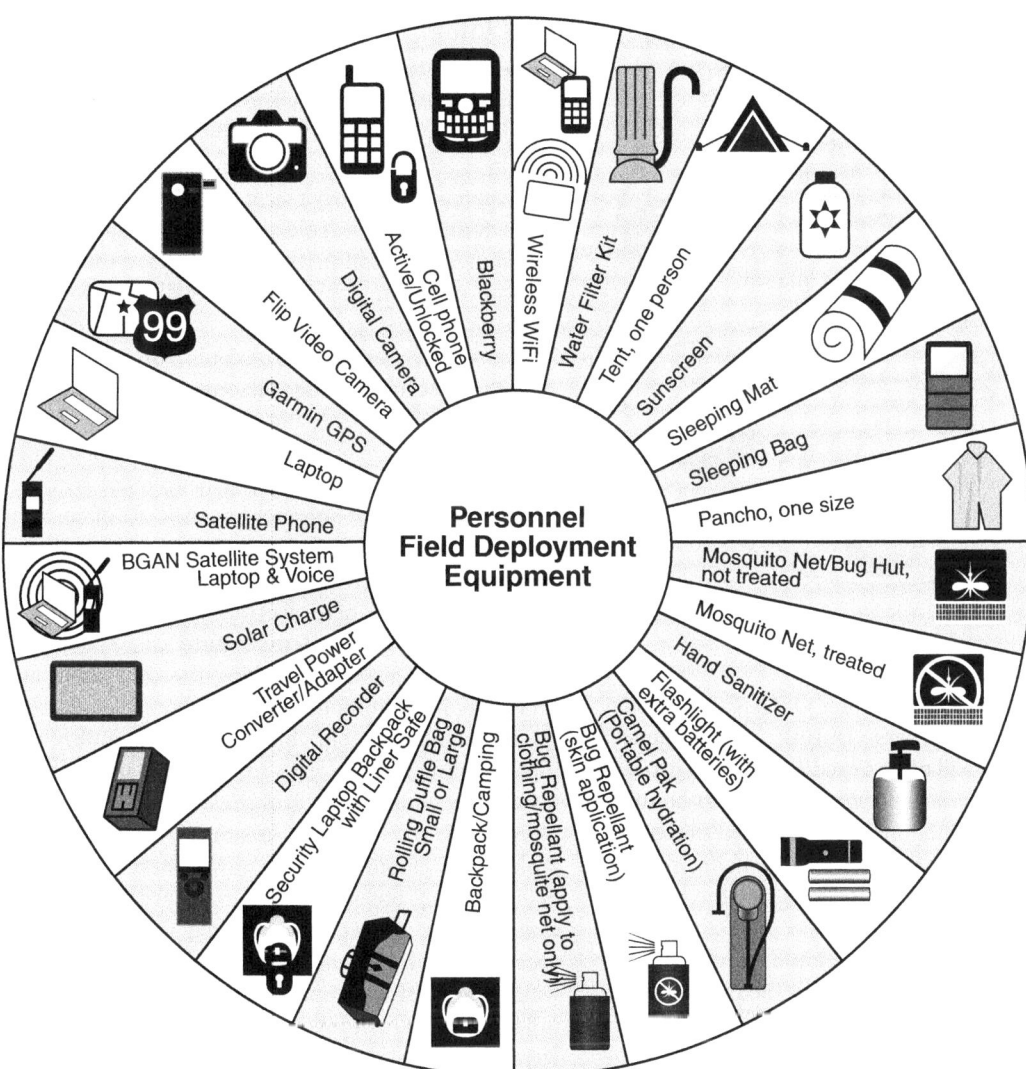

Figure 19.2 Personal field deployment equipment (created by CDC)

or medical officer and a logistics officer who will likely be key contacts early in a disaster response.

Predeployment Processing

As part of the deployment process it may be necessary to conduct predeployment briefings and/or trainings to prepare personnel. In addition to being equipped to perform their job, it is important for deployed personnel to have the necessary personal equipment and supplies to ensure their own well-being. Recommendations and requirements may be covered in the predeployment briefings and trainings. Common things to consider include visas and other necessary travel documents, vaccinations and prophylaxis, personal medications, key contact information, and plans for shelter, transportation, and communication. Examples of personal field deployment equipment are shown in Figure 19.2. Depending on the context, it may be necessary for personnel to have personal protective equipment (PPE). This may be important for healthcare and public health personnel. Examples of PPE are shown in Figure 19.3.

In-country Processing

Often, part of the deployment process is in-country processing at an in-country processing station. This may be the Embassy or Chief of Mission for foreign government personnel and through the UN On Site

277

Section 2: Public Health Principles

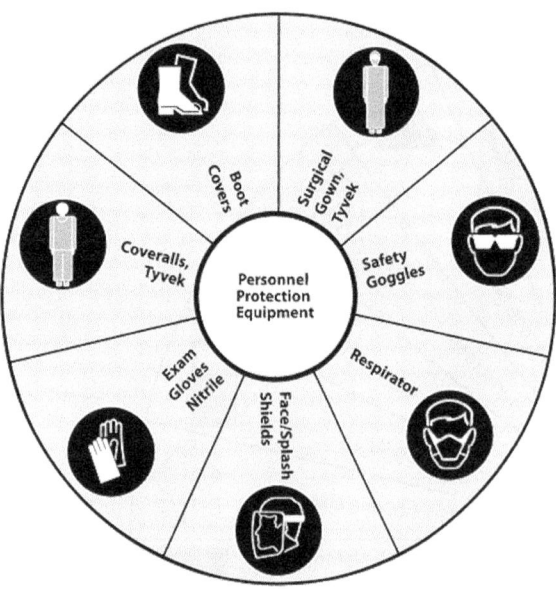

Figure 19.3 Personal protective equipment (PPE) (created by CDC)

Operations Coordination Center OSOCC for foreign humanitarian aid workers. During an emergency, affected countries will often expedite the entry processing for humanitarian personnel. This in-country processing may include briefing deployed personnel on the current situation including coordination, security, and standard protocols within the affected area.

At a minimum, processing should include recommendations and requirements for medical, shelter, security, equipment, human resources, training, cultural competency, and legal. Ideally, in-country processing stations should share information and may in fact create an in-processing zone to foster common strategies and better situational awareness, hopefully reducing errors, mistakes, and confusion by deployed personnel.

Safety and Security

Ensuring that deployed personnel have safe accommodations is critical to a successful mission. Selecting hotels or other accommodations that are known for having safety measures already in place such as guards on the premises may prevent a security incidence from occurring. Security briefings should be done prior to arrival in-country; however, additional security briefings may be done as part of the in-country processing.

Cold Chain

One of the most important challenges specific to health sector logistics is ensuring the controlled temperature standards through the entire supply chain necessary for certain medical commodities including certain vaccines, certain laboratory reagents and laboratory specimens. Maintaining a "cold chain" is especially difficult in resource poor countries where delays in transportation are common, supply chain distribution for non-cold commercial commodities is complicated, and infrastructure is inadequate. A cold chain requires special attention to shipping, customs clearance, storage, inventory management, and distribution.

In a cold chain, temperatures must be maintained within a specified range from procurement and pre-positioning through shipment to the port of customs entry in the country, through the customs approval process, to the in-country warehouse and on to intermediary depots. There are many points along this process at which the temperature can exceed the designated range, thus breaking the cold chain and rendering the commodities unusable.

To maintain a cold chain, logisticians utilize various shipping options. This may include using freight forwarders who have existing relationships with, and knowledge of, customs clearance procedures in a particular country. In this way, customs delays can be minimized, potentially avoiding a break in the cold chain. There are well-documented situations where vaccines have been properly shipped, only to be ruined waiting for customs approval because the proper documentation was not presented and customs personnel were unaware of the temperature requirement.

Warehousing

During the response to a humanitarian emergency, storage or warehousing of commodities in the pipeline is an important consideration. Considerations for warehousing of commodities include (de Villiers et al. 2008):

- Accommodating buffer stock of long production runs
- Accommodating response stock
- Allowing for consolidation of loads
- Preparation for dispatching
- Ensuring security of stock
- Facilitating high service levels by being closer to beneficiaries

As discussed in the previous section on cold chain, many medical commodities must be maintained within a specific temperature range. Once these medical commodities clear customs, they need to be both transported and warehoused in such a way as to maintain this cold chain.

For transport of temperature sensitive medical commodities, refrigerated trucks may not be readily available nor easy to contract for hire. One possible solution is to use cold boxes that can be powered through a vehicle cigarette lighter. For storage of temperature sensitive medical commodities, there are multiple cold storage options depending on the size of the shipment and the budget. Cold room storage is ideal for the central level depot or first point of receipt after customs approval. For intermediary depots, gas and electric-powered refrigerators have been used; however, more recently, standards have shifted to the use of solar-powered refrigerators in order to address difficulties maintaining and running gas and electric-powered refrigerators, especially in places where propane stock-outs and electrical shortages are common.

When warehousing perishables or items with an expiry date, such as medications, the logistician should employ a first-in-first-out (FIFO) storage method so that items closer to the date of expiry are dispatched first. For most commodities, preventing them from being exposed to harsh weather is critical. Even old abandoned warehouses or discarded tarps can offer basic protection. Food storage facilities commonly have some excess capacity that could be used for protected storage when the need arises.

Inventory Management

During the response to a humanitarian emergency, the logistics team may have to set up a temporary warehouse. In many situations, they will be inundated with all sorts of donated items, supplies, and equipment that may, or may not be useful to the response effort. Effective inventory management is critical. "Whether you are utilizing an existing, well established warehouse or starting from scratch, there are certain elements of an inventory system that must be followed" (Clearly Inventory 2011). Key elements of an inventory system include (Clearly Inventory 2011):

. Location
The storage facility should be dry and well lit. A facility with even these minimum requirements may not be readily available. For example, in Port-au-Prince, Haiti, after the earthquake in 2010, most of the warehouse-type buildings were destroyed or damaged so badly that they were not safe to use. Faced with thousands of pallets of supplies and materials, the relief logistics workers used the airport tarmac as their temporary warehouse. Items on pallets were organized by general categories such as medical supplies, food, clothing, tarps, etc. After a few days, these were broken down further into smaller units of issue with the most critically needed items sorted first.

During the response to the earthquake in Haiti in 2010, one logistician reported that while working on a warehouse modernization project with a Ministry of Health National Lab, there were "boxes on boxes without shelving or lighting, corrosives next to flammables next to propane gas, and medical supplies not stocked according to use, making inventory control extremely challenging" (personal communication, Rebecca Turner, CDC-Haiti).

Labeling
Even in a temporary situation, it is important to take time to diagram the location areas and names within the warehouse as part of inventory management. Areas may be marked with placards or labels, including an easy to read and understand alphanumeric system. For example, the first row of shelving is given number 1, the second-row number 2, etc. and the first section of shelving letter "A" with the shelves numbered 1, 2, 3, etc. from top to bottom. Utilizing this type of system, an item with a location of 3-C-4 would located be on row 3, shelf unit C, on the 4th shelf from the top.

Units of Measure
It is important to specify on the label the unit of measure, such as each, box, crate, case, liter, or ampoule etc.

Inventory Software
For a small inventory of items, less than approximately one hundred line items, a manual system of receiving, storing and issuing may be used. For inventories greater than one hundred line items, inventory software should be considered. Ideally, this software should track all inventory activity and transactions, including generating a receipt of any issue or transfer of goods.

Good Policies
Taking the time to outline procedures early in inventory management planning will decrease the confusion later especially as new staff come on board. At a minimum, these written procedures should

describe the process for receiving supplies, entering data into the software, distributing the items to their proper warehouse location, and issuing items from the warehouse.

Chain of Custody

One of the basic principles of logistics is to handle the shipper's property through a systematized and documented chain of custody. From initial pick up to final delivery, the custodian of the shipper's goods should account for every minute of the transport, detailing dates, times, names, and other key chain-of-custody information.

Each step of the supply chain should have a point of contact (POC) to ensure accountability in handovers from the central warehouse to the distribution centers and onto the use facilities. These POCs should be notified before goods are distributed to allow them to prepare their storage facility to accommodate the incoming order.

Medical commodities including pharmaceuticals require a strict chain of custody. Temperature sensitive items require proof that adequate temperature has been maintained throughout the shipment. Local or regional laws for possession of controlled pharmaceuticals must be adhered to. Many of the laws regarding controlled substances are in place to ensure that quality pharmaceuticals are being imported. The humanitarian aid community, donors in particular, require that the standards for pharmaceutical procurement meet the International minimum standards. These are somewhat similar to receiving FDA approval.

In some circumstances, pharmaceuticals may only be received and carried by licensed medical professionals. This may be restricted to medical professionals licensed to practice in the affected country. Often, the Ministry of Health website or POCs can provide this type of information prior to shipment.

During the influenza outbreak in Mexico in 2009, agencies based in the US tried to ship packages containing treatment doses of oseltamivir (Tamiflu®) to their employees and their families living in Mexico. Most of these packages were returned to their international sender because the Mexican Ministry of Health placed strict requirements on the importation of prescription pharmaceuticals. The reason was to prevent importation of counterfeit drugs. Many of these shipments lacked the extensive documentation required.

Dispatch

The movement or dispatch of commodities to the affected population is the final component in the humanitarian supply chain. As has been discussed previously, for medical commodities dispatch might be to the health facility or professional health worker instead of the affected population. Careful record keeping, including tracking of waybills and airway bills, and information management are critical to this process. Additionally, security must be sufficient to prevent theft and maintain safety of those delivering commodities.

Theft prevention should include locks and/or tamperproof seals placed on commodity storage units such as cold boxes, warehouses, trucks, and smaller depots. Adequate lighting both inside and outside storage depots can also help prevent theft. Theft prevention should be considered, especially when expensive equipment is stored in the warehouse or there are otherwise valuable items such as solar panels on the roof. In some situations, a physical security presence in the way of armed guards and patrols may be necessary. Determining the best option for each situation may need to be discovered by trial and error.

During dispatch, emblems or symbols indicating neutrality or delivery of humanitarian aid may be utilized. The use of the Red Cross and Red Crescent emblems, in particular, may only be used when certain conditions are met, as defined in Article 44 of the First Geneva convention. As a humanitarian logistician charged with dispatch of medical commodities, it is critically important to understand the rules governing the use of this emblem, in part, that it is "a protective device, which aims to confer the protection stipulated by international humanitarian law in situations of armed conflict, is reserved primarily for the medical services of armed forces and, with the express agreement of the State authorities, for hospitals and other civilian medical units" (Layover 1996). Appropriate discretion should be exercised based on the context and situation.

Challenges

Unsolicited Donations

It is the logisticians' responsibility to prioritize shipments and ensure that life-saving materials get pushed to the front of the pipeline during the response. A common impediment to this process is unsolicited donations. Procedures for vetting donations need to be established so that unsolicited donated supplies do not impede the ability of logisticians to manage the humanitarian supply chain. Unsolicited donations may not meet standards set for content, quality, nomenclature, expiration dates, and cold chain requirements. There may not be adequate storage facilities, security, transportation, and distribution capacity. Making sense of a mix of solicited donations, unsolicited donations, and purposefully procured shipments can prove very difficult, especially in a resource poor setting during a humanitarian emergency where time is of the essence.

Damaged Infrastructure

Damaged or insufficient infrastructure is perhaps the greatest logistical challenge in terms of communication and transportation during the response. Strategic planning for transportation type and route, in anticipation of the impact from the disaster, is of utmost importance. Doing so might avoid delays resulting from utilizing damaged infrastructure such as roads or ports. With respect to communication, diversifying the options available and building in redundancies can save significant time during the response. For example, instead of expecting to have access to mobile phones and the internet, packing two-way radios and extra batteries may be more effective.

Limited Resources

Often, in the chaos that ensues after a disaster, logistics personnel operate with limited resources. Flexibility is crucial to maximize efforts using limited resources. Bulk packing and bundling, as well as reverse transport are two ways logistics personnel use flexibility to aid in addressing resource challenges. Using bundling, for example, if a truck is earmarked for one type of commodity, any additional space available should be capitalized upon for other needed supplies going in the same direction. Additionally, the logistician should inquire before the truck returns to the intermediate depot as to whether or not the field facility has any items which need to be returned to the main location, so that reverse transport or back-loading can save on transportation costs.

Language and Cultural Differences

During a large international response, organizations and individuals from many countries and cultures, speaking many languages are likely to be part of the response. The role of the field logistician includes serving as an intermediary for both headquarter-level and field-level requests. Managing and facilitating effective communication despite language and cultural barriers is key to the response effort. In this regard, it is important to ensure that staff are aware of cultural events or national holidays that may impact the response efforts.

Neutrality

Neutrality is one of the emphasized principles of international humanitarian law (IHL). In responding quickly to immediate needs, logisticians must consider whether the interventions they are managing will be considered neutral. Lack of attention to this may have a negative impact on security. For instance, if a truck delivering life-saving commodities has diplomatic license plates and enters territory controlled by oppositional rebel groups, this could potentially create an international incident. Attention to this type of detail is critical. Understanding the potential consequences beforehand while weighing the principle of neutrality can help avoid costly mistakes.

Conclusion

The basic goal of logistics in the setting of humanitarian emergencies is to plan, implement, and control the storage and delivery of commodities, which may include products, services, and human resources, in a quality, timely, and effective manner. The basic functions of logistics (planning, deployment, communication, procurement, transportation, and inventory management) are all important. Without clear and accurate communication, however, none of these functions can be accomplished.

In preparing logistics requirements for future operations and unknown humanitarian emergencies, response organizations would serve the field well by advocating to have logistics expertise on their projects. More emphasis should be placed on developing, seeking, hiring, and retaining public health logisticians, as effective logistics is critical to the success of the response to humanitarian emergencies.

Notes from the Field

Indonesia (2009)

In September of 2009, Sumatra, Indonesia experienced a magnitude 7.9 earthquake. More than 1,000 people were killed and an estimated 250,000 families were in need of assistance from the humanitarian aid community. I had been with USAID OFDA for a month or so, coming from the Red Cross Movement. I joined the USAID Disaster Assistance Response Team (DART) as the Logistics Officer in Padang. The DART Team Lead had called forward 45 metric tons of USAID/OFDA emergency relief commodities and it was my job was to ensure that it arrived and was delivered into the hands of the Indonesian Red Cross for distribution.

This was my first time receiving an aircraft on behalf of the USG. Padang International airport is a small but capable airport that had seen a fair share of disaster response. I was anxious about getting the commodities off the aircraft and out of the gates of the airport before anything complicated could happen. USAID OFDA Logistics has been doing this kind of move for years. The Freight Forwarder had a good reputation and had been providing detailed updates of the loading and clearing from Dubai. It seemed that all was in place for a smooth delivery.

I made a point to get to know the airport ahead of time. The consignee's representative from the IFRC was an old friend. Keeping in mind that the airport was small and busy with the earthquake response, I was cautious and looked for things that might not work out as they should.

Here's what happened: scheduled arrival was delayed and ended up arriving in the wee hours of the a.m. next day. The aircraft was a Russian Ilyushian 76 retrofitted for cargo. It seemed like it dropped out of the sky, taxied, and came to a rolling screeching stop in front of us. It was just myself and our communications and press officers to greet the aircraft. The contracted ground handler never showed up. The aircraft crew dropped out of various hatches and approached me with furrowed brows and said, "We need GPU" (Ground Power Unit).

I still believed the ground handler was going to show up so I welcomed the crew and told them to stand by. After thirty minutes I was convinced we were on our own. I searched the ground handler's offices finding them mostly unoccupied and found a handler who agreed to help.

Our small team stepped into the aircraft to discover that every centimeter of the 400 cubic meters of cargo volume had been utilized. I could see warehouse pallets at the base of the load. I climbed to the top of the pile and found the loading crane. The boxes were stacked into the shape of the airframe. By this time, the newly hired ground handler had found us a forklift and an operator. Our team of three unloaded half of the aircraft ourselves with one pallet jack and one forklift. Then, two Australian airmen lent us a hand. About that time, the ground handler informed us we had 3 hours to unload the aircraft and clear the apron. Five hours later we were standing inside an empty aircraft.

At the end of the unloading I was confronted by a member of the crew demanding money for fueling. He presented a compelling case, initially approaching me from a pity angle, stating that their main office did not give them enough money for the return journey. He stated they "could not even move the aircraft they were so low on fuel" as he poked my chest a couple of time insisting that I had no choice. Understanding that I did actually have a choice, I wished him and his crew well and we departed. We had completed the mission and the commodities were moving out of the airport toward the beneficiaries who needed them.

References

Clearly Inventory. (2011). Inventory basics – All about inventory management, 2–3. Available at: (Accessed June 14, 2014).

De Villiers, G., Nieman, G., and Nieman, W. (2008). Strategic logistics management, logistics channels and network Design, 212–228.

Fritz Institute. (2013). Humanitarian logistics: Enabling disaster response, 2–3. Available at: www.fritzinstitute.org/pdfs/whitepaper/enablingdisasterresponse.pdf (Accessed June 2, 2014).

Holguín-Veras, P. E., Pérez, N., Ukkusuri, S., Wachtendorf, T., and Brown, B. (2007). Emergency logistics issues affecting the response to Katrina: A synthesis and preliminary suggestions for improvement, 1–2. Available at: http://transp.rpi.edu/~HUM-LOG/Doc/Vault/katrina1.pdf (Accessed June 25, 2014).

Lavoyer, J. P. (1996). National legislation on the use and protection of the emblem of the red cross or red crescent, ICRC Legal Division, 1–3. Available at: www.icrc.org/eng/resources/documents/misc/57jn8j.htm (Accessed June 25, 2014).

OCHA. (2014). Global mapping of emergency stockpiles, 1. Available at: www.unocha.org/what-we-do/coordination-tools/logistics-support/emergency-stockpiles (Accessed June 25, 2014).

UNHCR. (2013). UNHCR's Essential medicines and medical supplies policy and guidance 2011. Available at: http://www.unhcr.org/4f707faf9.pdf (Accessed June 25, 2014).

USAID. (2013). OFDA essential medicines list (OFDA EML), 1–15. Available at: www.usaid.gov/sites/default/files/documents/1866/Final%20OFDA%20Essential%20Medicines%20List%20Aug2013.pdf (Accessed June 25, 2014).

World Food Program. (2013). Global logistics cluster support cell and World Food Programme (WFP) Logistics Operational Guide (LOG), 1–3. Available at: log.logcluster.org/mobile/preparedness/logistics/index.html (Accessed June 10, 2014).

Disaster Risk Reduction

Lise D. Martel, Qudsia Huda, Kimberly M. Hanson, and Ali Ardalan

Introduction

The frequency of reported natural disasters and the total population affected by disasters has increased dramatically in the last five decades (CRED 2012). Since 1992, 4.4 billion people have been affected by natural disasters with over $2 trillion USD in economic losses (UN General Assembly 2013). Factors such as an increase in the world's population, urbanization, and climate change have played a role in increasing the global population's exposure and vulnerability to disasters and emergencies. Disasters disproportionately affect the poor in any nation and can particularly devastate developing nations with limited resources for recovery and resiliency (United Nations 1994). In these settings, disasters may result in humanitarian emergencies.

While large disasters receive the greatest visibility, extensive risk from low-severity, high-frequency disasters continue to represent one of the greatest challenges, especially for low- and middle-income countries (UN General Assembly 2013). From 1970 to 2007, the extensive risks accounted for 79 percent of affected people, and 65 percent and 57 percent of loss related to hospitals and schools respectively (UNISDR 2009a). For example in Iran, from 1970 to 2010, about five thousand people were killed due to extensive risk from disasters alone (Ardalan et al. 2012).

Disaster risk reduction (DRR) has its roots in the international disaster relief movement of the late 1960s. In 1965, the UN General Assembly requested all member states to "inform the Secretary-General of the type of emergency assistance they are in a position to offer" in the case of a large natural disaster (UN Office of Disaster Risk Reduction 2014). Throughout the 1970s and 1980s, the focus remained on managing international assistance in postdisaster settings with increasing focus on preparation and early warning systems. In 1987, the conversation changed from managing the response resources to minimizing the impact of disasters (UN General Assembly 1987). There was a general understanding that while the disasters themselves could not be prevented, their impact on economies and individuals could be reduced with proper preparation and understanding of the underlying risk factors.

The 1990s was declared by the UN General Assembly as the International Decade for Natural Disaster Reduction. In 1994, the first World Conference on Disaster Reduction was held in Yokohama, Japan. The conference resulted in the Yokohama Strategy for a Safer World: Guidelines for Natural Disaster Prevention, Preparedness and Mitigation. The Yokohama Strategy outlined activities for disaster impact reduction at local, national, regional, and international levels, and formally recognized that "disaster response alone is not sufficient," bringing the concept of disaster risk reduction to the forefront of the disaster response community (Briseño et al. 2005). The implementation of the International Strategy for Disaster Reduction (ISDR) by the UN General Assembly in 2000 sent a clear message that focus had shifted to minimizing disaster impact and would be considered a global priority.

Concepts

Definition

UNISDR defines disaster risk reduction as "the concept and practice of reducing disaster risks through systematic efforts to analyze and reduce the causal factors of disasters" (UN Office for Disaster Risk Reduction 2014b). The concept of disaster risk reduction can be broken down into four overarching phases (UN Office for Disaster Risk Reduction 2014a):

- Disaster risk preparedness, or the effort to identify risks and vulnerabilities beforehand and develop

plans or action steps to minimize their potential impact
- Disaster response
- Disaster recovery
- Disaster risk mitigation, or the effort to rebuild in a way to reduce risk from future disasters

These phases combine to meet the ultimate goal of disaster risk reduction that is to minimizing the impact of disasters, both in terms of economic and human elements.

Development

Disaster risk is not equally distributed throughout the world's population. The impact a disaster has on a community is determined by both the degree of exposure to the disaster as well as the community's ability to mitigate and recover from it. However, the ability to mitigate and recover relies on a variety of factors including political, structural, and economic conditions (Schipper and Pelling 2006).

In 2010, Haiti and Chile experienced earthquakes of magnitudes 7.0 and 8.8, respectively. Each earthquake caused considerable damage; however the differences in accumulated risk and its effect on the nations' ability to recover was drastically different. Strictly enforced building codes earthquake preparedness efforts including hospital training and community education, and resilient public works all contributed to Chile's ability to recover (Kovacs 2010). In the five years after the two earthquakes, Chile moved into the mitigation phase of the emergency management cycle and undertook preparedness efforts for the next earthquake. In the same amount of time, Haiti remained in the recovery phase and even faced additional emergencies, including an outbreak of cholera, due to the nation's underdevelopment at the time of the earthquake (International Council for Science 2015).

It is clear that disaster risk reduction and sustainable development are intimately connected. "Development cannot be sustainable if the disaster risk reduction approach is not fully integrated into development planning and investments" (UN General Assembly 2013). At the same time, disaster risk reduction cannot be achieved without a sustainable development approach integrated into all elements of a society. Yet, while this connection is well understood, the integration of disaster risk reduction and international development is still in its early stages.

The Millennium Development Goals (MDGs) introduced in 2000 by the United Nations Millennium Declaration have become the international standard for sustainable development. However, because each goal focuses on a specific sector, issues that span all sectors, such as disaster risk reduction, are not specifically included (Schipper and Pelling 2006). As the 2015 deadline for the MDGs approached, much of the focus was on creating a post-2015 set of goals developed in conjunction with the disaster risk reduction community that included common targets and measures. However, the challenge of focusing on preventative measures as well as immediate developmental needs remain. "When disasters are seen as the outcome of accumulated risk produced by years of vulnerability and underlying hazard, the case for preventative action can be made more plainly" (Schipper and Pelling 2006). It is the shift in how disasters are viewed that will become essential for the full integration of disaster risk reduction and sustainable development approaches. The impact of accumulated risk is well documented in the West Africa Ebola virus epidemic of 2014–15 where years of vulnerability resulting from deforestation, civil unrest, weak medical, public health, and road infrastructure, shortage of medical staff, laboratory capacity and surveillance systems, made it difficult to identify and control the disease (Bausch and Schwarz 2014, Chan 2014).

The multifactorial nature of disaster risk reduction requires multisectoral risk assessment and an analysis methodology to determine the nature and extent of risk by analyzing potential hazards and evaluating existing conditions of vulnerability that together could potentially harm exposed people, property, services, livelihoods, and the environment on which they depend (UNISDR 2009b). Hence, the risk assessment should take account of foreseeable and long-term risks, as well as those from continuing disasters and emergencies. This provides the necessary information to manage disaster risks as well allude to multisectoral interventions to best address the challenges on the ground.

Global Initiatives

International Strategy for Disaster Reduction

The International Strategy for Disaster Reduction (ISDR) was established in 2000 through the United

Nations General Assembly. ISDR originally included two mechanisms for implementation:

- Inter-Agency Task Force on Disaster Reduction

The Task Force consisted of 14 UN System representatives and up to 16 representatives from regional partners and stakeholders who formed working groups to identify courses of action and best practices for ISDR implementation (UNISDR 2004).

- Inter-Agency Secretariat of the ISDR

The Secretariat of the ISDR, or more commonly known by the acronym UNISDR, was mandated "to serve as the focal point in the United Nations system for the coordination of disaster reduction and to ensure synergies among the disaster reduction activities of the United Nations system and regional organizations and activities in socio-economic and humanitarian fields" (UN General Assembly 2001).

The essential function of UNISDR is to coordinate global efforts across various platforms and ensure that disaster risk reduction strategies and activities are planned and implemented in a harmonious manner. In order to achieve this, ISDR has identified four strategic objectives within their Work Programme 2012–15 (UNISDR 2011):

- Lead and coordinate
- Produce credible evidence
- Advocacy and outreach
- Deliver and communicate results

Hyogo Framework for Action (HFA)

In January of 2005, ISDR hosted the second World Conference on Disaster Reduction in Kobe, Hyogo, Japan. It was held in the wake of the 2004 Indian Ocean Tsunami as a means to review global progress on disaster risk reduction initiatives established at the Yokohama Conference of 1994 (Briseño et al. 2005). The result of the conference in Kobe was a 10-year strategic framework that built upon the gaps of the Yokohama Strategy and is known as the Hyogo Framework for Action 2005–2015: Building Resilience of Nations and Communities to Disasters, or the HFA.

The objective of global implementation of the HFA is "substantial reduction of disaster losses, in lives and in the social, economic, and environmental assets of communities and countries" (UNISDR 2005). The HFA identified five priorities for action:

- Ensure that disaster risk reduction is a national and a local priority with a strong institutional basis for implementation.
- Identify, assess, and monitor disaster risks and enhance early warning.
- Use knowledge, innovation, and education to build a culture of safety and resilience at all levels.
- Reduce the underlying risk factors.
- Strengthen disaster preparedness for effective response at all levels.

These priorities for action were intended as guidance for the development of HFA implementation activities specific to local contexts, including "cultural diversity, age, and vulnerable groups" (UNISDR 2005).

The structure of implementation is outlined within the Framework with three distinct levels including local/national, regional and global. The specific implementation activities and responsible parties vary by each level. Individual nations are encouraged to develop and complete a baseline assessment, determine a "national coordination mechanism," monitor activity implementation, and report periodically to their regional or international counterpart (UNISDR 2005).

Global Platform for Disaster Reduction

In order to support and coordinate the global implementation of the HFA, UNISDR has established a network of Platforms, or "forums for information exchange" at both the global and regional levels. These Platforms have replaced the original Inter-Agency Task Force on Disaster Reduction to expand participation in the discussion of disaster risk reduction ideas and practices to all stakeholders at each level of implementation. The Global Platform for Disaster Reduction, established in 2007, is held every two years as a means for stakeholders in disaster risk reduction across all sectors to convene to raise awareness, share best practices, and assess HFA implementation on a global scale (Holmes 2007).

Participation in the biennial Global Platform has grown, both in size and composition each year. Delegations to the Global Platform include Ministerial, NGO, and private sector representatives. The inaugural Global Platform in 2007 hosted 1,150 total participants, representing 124 countries (Holmes 2007). The Global Platform in 2013 hosted 3,500 participants, representing 172 countries

(Dahinden 2013). The increase in attendance, both in number and scope, indicates that the importance of disaster risk reduction is being recognized and made a priority by more and more nations worldwide.

Regional Platforms for Disaster Reduction

Regional Platforms for Disaster Reduction offer the same opportunity for disaster risk reduction stakeholders to meet and discuss awareness, best practices, and HFA implementation, but on a regional scale. UNISDR has established six regional offices, each of which oversees a Regional Platform held on an ad hoc basis. These Regional Platforms allow for more diverse participation of stakeholders and emphasis on regional strategies to "implement and oversee disaster risk reduction" for issues that transcend national boundaries (UN Office for Disaster Risk Reduction 2014).

Regional Platforms have been established for Africa, the Americas, the Arab States, Asia, Europe, and the Pacific. The frequency with which these Platforms are held is left to the UNISDR Regional Office and varies widely from region to region. In 2014, both the Regional Platforms for Asia and the Pacific hosted their sixth conferences, while the Arab States Platform held its second (UN Office for Disaster Risk Reduction 2014). Regardless, each Regional Platform convened in 2014 in order to begin to address post-2015 planning.

Post-2015 Framework for Disaster Reduction

As the end of the HFA period approaches, much of the international discussion turned to the development of a post-2015 framework that has been called Sendai Framework for Disaster Risk Reduction following the third World Conference on Disaster Reduction in March of 2015 in Sendai, Japan. Much like the process at the second World Conference on Disaster Reduction, the intention was to maintain the guiding principles of the Yokohama Strategy and the HFA, but expand on existing gaps.

The primary issues identified for the post-2015 framework include the need for further attention in the HFA Priority 4: reduce underlying disaster risk factors. As was indicated in the 2012–2013 Implementation of the ISDR Report, the HFA served to help build foundational policies and garner qualitative success. However, what are needed now are standardized, quantitative targets and indicators that can truly identify progress towards risk reduction (UN General Assembly 2013). For this purpose, scientific evidences are highly required, and investment on disaster research should be considered.

With the development of the HFA, much global attention has been paid to disaster risk reduction, but translating that attention into actionable progress cannot be done at the global level. The implementation of disaster risk reduction strategies will vary among regions and among countries within each region. Therefore, special attention is needed at both levels to ensure strategies are prioritized among all implementing partners.

In an effort to address the specialization needed at the regional level, each of the Regional Platforms has developed a strategic plan for disaster risk reduction implementation. Each strategic plan uses the HFA as a model but examines regional priority hazards, challenges, and highlights, and ultimately identifies how the five HFA priorities for action can be applied to the regional context.

While political support for disaster risk reduction approaches can be garnered through participation and lessons learned at Regional and Global Platforms, actual implementation of those approaches falls to national governments. Several nations have taken on the challenge of disaster risk reduction implementation, but it still remains an issue of priority for many others. "The low visibility of disaster risk reduction work in comparison to emergency relief has made it unattractive for governments chasing votes and international recognition" (Schipper and Pelling 2006). It will be up to the Global and Regional Platforms to help shift the thought process of national governments and help them understand how prioritizing disaster risk reduction approaches can result in long-term benefits.

Health Care Systems

All types of disasters have the potential to affect the health of a population. Yet, both the Yokohama Strategy and HFA (under Priority Action 4) are very limited in their inclusion of health-related language and goals. While there is specific mention of disaster risk reduction for health facilities in disaster situations, many of the more general development practices listed in the Yokohama Strategy and the HFA can be translated directly to the health sector. Moreover, invaluable experience and capacities of health systems can be leveraged for DRR at the community level. Considering the disaster as a health problem, the health systems can participate in assessing and monitoring of disaster risks and health consequences in line with HFA Priority Action 2 and building a culture of safety for disasters under public health education and health promotion programs, according to HFA Priority Action 3.

Health Facilities

Disasters can result in substantial physical injuries and increased disease transmission, but more often contamination of water sources and limited ability to practice good hygiene result in increased severity of otherwise minor health issues (Noji 2000). All of these may increase the number of patients needing medical care that can easily overwhelm health facilities in good working condition and cause even greater problems for areas where facilities are damaged or destroyed by the disaster. For example, the response to the 2010 Haiti earthquake was complicated by the lack of safe water sources for hygiene needs, postoperation care, and camps for the internally displaced population. The lack of proper water and sewer systems also allowed for the rapid spread of cholera, resulting in over four hundred thousand infections, six thousand deaths within Haiti, and its spread into the neighboring Dominican Republic (Tappero and Tauxe 2011).

In an effort to address this element of risk reduction, the HFA does include under Priority Action 4: Reduce underlying risk factors, the following development practice:

- Integrate disaster risk reduction planning into the health sector; promote the goal of "hospitals safe from disaster" by ensuring that all new hospitals are built with a level of resilience that strengthens their capacity to remain functional in disaster situations and implement mitigation measures to reinforce existing health facilities, particularly those providing primary health care (UN 1994).

While the idea of ensuring that health care facilities are structurally sound is important, it can be extremely difficult in low- and middle-income countries with little to no enforced building codes. In an effort to raise awareness and advocate for policy changes as well as funding, the World Health Organization (WHO) and UNISDR launched the 2008–2009 World Disaster Reduction Campaign: Hospitals Safe from Disasters. This two-year campaign ultimately emphasized the message that "the most expensive hospital is the one that fails," in an effort to rally social and political support to ensure the "physical and functional integrity of health hospitals and facilities in emergency conditions" (WHO 2009a).

The campaign resulted in the creation of the Hospital Safety Index (HSI), a qualitative score based on an assessment of structural, nonstructural, and functional capacity of a hospital including the environment and the health services network to which it belongs. As a rapid diagnostic tool, HSI provides a "snapshot of the probability that a hospital or health facility will continue to function in emergency situations" (WHO 2009b). The index has been used throughout various regions of the world and has helped identify key elements for improvement among health facilities (WHO/Europe 2012, Ardalan et al. 2014). One of the most important factors of the HSI is the emphasis on elements beyond the facility structure that account for the functionality of hospitals after disasters. These factors include resilient nonstructural elements, proper maintenance, prepared workforce, contingency plans, etc. (WHO 2009a).

While hospitals are among the central components of the health care system, there are functions that are specific to primary health centers that cannot be replaced by hospitals. These functions include community disaster preparedness before a disaster and providing public health services afterwards. Furthermore, a functional primary health center minimizes the number of nonseriously injured people who might utilize hospitals for care (Ardalan et al. 2013a). There are many examples in less-developed nations that demonstrate the importance of assessing and monitoring the safety of primary centers for disasters, and integrating DRR to primary health center systems (UNISDR 2014).

The Overseas Development Institute (ODI) has taken a strong interest in the creation of measurable targets, indicators, and goals in preparation for the HFA2. In regard to resilient health care systems, ODI supports specific target areas of surge capacity, flexibility, and planning (Mitchell et al. 2013). Preparing to handle large numbers of patients, prioritizing health services, and developing plans to ensure functionality are challenges for the most developed health care systems. These are even bigger challenges for those countries with limited health care resources (Mitchell et al. 2013). National and local health care systems should be able to quickly assess and adapt their capacity to the current needs of the disaster situation and limit the possibility of overwhelming their ability to respond by emphasizing these areas in their training programs and funding.

Risk Management

Health in emergency and disaster situations cannot be addressed by the health sector alone. The multisectoral collaboration and lessons learned from previous disaster risk management situations are necessary to ensure the protection of the population's health. This approach requires a focus beyond health facilities. It must emphasize capacity building at the community level and the development of resilient health care systems.

Community-level approaches have the potential for the greatest impact. Prepared and resilient communities that can respond to and recover from disasters with limited outside help can ensure the best use of limited resources. With that understanding, many countries are pushing community education and training in disaster-prone areas. This is especially true in low- and middle-income countries where disaster response resources may not be able to reach many isolated communities. For example, Honduras suffers from extreme poverty and is highly prone to disasters. Within the country there are extremely isolated rural areas. In 2008, in an effort to strengthen Honduras' health systems, the Swiss Red Cross implemented a multisector disaster risk reduction campaign in two remote areas. This campaign focused on community member training, water, and sanitation education, reforestation efforts, and early warning system integration (Swiss Re 2014). This ultimately resulted in the two communities having a better understanding of their existing resources, letting them more effectively leverage resources in the event of a disaster (Swiss Re 2014).

Public Health

The capacities of public health systems should be leveraged for enhancement of community disaster resilience. By definition, a public health system encompasses "all public, private, and voluntary entities that contribute to the delivery of essential public health services within a jurisdiction" (CDC 2014). While hospitals, clinics, and primary health care centers are at the frontline of the public health service delivery, the public health system is beyond only health facilities. It encompasses all sectors that impact on the health of populations including housing, agriculture, economy, etc. While DRR is a multidisciplinary field that involves environmental studies, engineering, security studies, and economic development, public health remains an underutilized partner in this effort. However, there are examples on how a public health approach has been effective in community DRR while collaborating with other sectors or disciplines such as meteorology, civil societies, and local/national disaster management governments. Examples include the establishment of a community-based early warning system for flash floods and enhancement of community preparedness for earthquakes and floods in Iran (Ardalan et al. 2013b). Both examples were initiated by the health system of Iran and mobilized the resources of other sectors. The Los Angeles County Community Disaster Resilience (LACCDR) project is another example that is led by the Los Angeles County Department of Public Health as a collaborative effort to promote community resilience in the face of public health emergencies, such as pandemics and disasters (LACDPH 2011).

Implementation

National Governments

Ultimate responsibility for implementation of any disaster risk reduction strategy falls to the national government. Interventions and trainings may be aimed at the local level, but given that disaster risk reduction crosses all sectors, government coordination and political support is needed to ensure cooperation. It is essential that representatives of all government ministries participate in disaster risk reduction planning and implementation.

While disaster risk reduction strategies may target actions at the local level, transferring authority for implementation to that level has not made a significant impact on disaster risk reduction (UN General Assembly 2013). The HFA calls for the formation of National Platforms, in addition to Global and Regional Platforms, to formally coordinate the national implementation of the framework. Between 2005 and 2013, 191 countries established national disaster risk reduction focal points, 86 countries established National Platforms, 146 countries submitted at least one HFA progress report, and 121 countries enacted legislation aimed at disaster risk reduction strategy implementation (UN General Assembly 2013).

Several intergovernmental organizations, nongovernmental organizations, and private-sector companies support national governments in their disaster risk reduction efforts. The World Bank Group, International Monetary Fund, and Red Cross and Red Crescent are a few of the global organizations that have worked directly with national governments through their regional or national offices (United Nations 2014).

Since the launch of the HFA in 2005, many countries around the world have taken the lead in implementing various aspects of disaster risk reduction. In 2012, in an effort to unite disaster risk reduction and development efforts, the national governments of Bolivia, Cameroon, India, Jordan, Nepal, Pakistan, Republic of Moldova Sri Lanka, Sudan, and Togo approved UN Development Assistance Frameworks that incorporate disaster risk reduction approaches into development planning (UN General Assembly 2013). The United Kingdom became the first nation to voluntarily submit their HFA progress report to peer review, helping to ensure accountability in the self-report mechanism and encouraging other nations to do the same (UN General Assembly 2013). As much of the implementation of disaster risk reduction falls to national governments, several National Platforms have convened a Working Group to review the progress and challenges specific to that level. The volunteer National Platforms of Ecuador, Germany, Indonesia, Mexico, Philippines, Senegal, and Sweden facilitated the review with support from a broader reference group of National Platforms and coordination from UNISDR (Sanahuja 2013).

Private Sector

The theme of the 2013 Global Platform, "From Shared Risk to Shared Value: The Business Case for Disaster Risk Reduction," highlighted the cost benefit for private sector companies to invest in disaster risk reduction strategies. As a result, the first annual general meeting on "Private sector for disaster risk reduction" was held at the 2013 Global Platform with over 150 attendees from whom the Private Sector Partnership (DRR-PSP) and the Private Sector Advisory Group (PSAG) were created (UN General Assembly 2013).

Local Communities

While disaster risk reduction implementation is the responsibility of the national government, actions for implementation are ultimately decentralized and fall on local communities. Decisions on where and how structures are built, operated, and overseen are done at the local level. Ensuring that safety regulations exist and are being followed is the responsibility of the local government. Early warning systems and emergency planning must be undertaken and maintained at the local level. Communities that are unaware or unable to manage these responsibilities accumulate disaster risk each and every day. In 2010, the World Disaster Reduction Campaign "Making cities resilient: my city is getting ready" was launched to increase awareness and commitment from local communities to enhance their disaster risk reduction capacities (UN General Assembly 2013). Between 2010 and 2013, more than 1,400 communities in 90 countries signed on to the campaign and have "prioritized disaster risk reduction as a key determinate for sustainable urban development" (UN General Assembly 2013).

The first step in ensuring a nation's ability to respond to and recover from a disaster is to ensure the resiliency of its local communities. Strengthening the capacities of civil societies is a key strategy to ensure community participation and to monitor the DRR progress at community level. Global Network of Civil Society Organizations for Disaster Reduction is a global platform that has been established for these purposes (GNDR 2014).

Challenges

Limited Resources

Disaster risk reduction has been widely accepted conceptually as a priority for national governments around the world; however, implementation of disaster risk reduction measures has made limited progress. This is often simply due to limited resources. While national governments have bought into the fact that disaster risk reduction measures are needed, they have not necessarily been able to commit the financial or physical support to implement these measures. This lack of resources is not limited to low- and middle-income countries, but is being faced by countries at "all income levels" (UN General Assembly 2013).

Because disaster risk reduction is crosscutting, the lack of resources leads to stunted progress across all sectors. In an effort to increase budgetary allowances and technical expertise, many countries have integrated disaster risk reduction elements into their existing United Nations Country Program. By leveraging existing relationships and creating United Nations Development Assistance Frameworks, these countries can include disaster risk reduction elements within development planning and ensure that they are undertaken from the inception of already-planned projects (UN General Assembly 2013).

As political support for disaster risk reduction continues to increase and the impetus to implement is undertaken, there is increased need for standardized, qualitative measures in order to measure progress towards risk reduction. It is not enough to simply report that approaches are being used without any means to determine their effectiveness. The ODI has developed possible goals, targets, and indicators across various aspects of disaster risk reduction, including the health sector. Ultimately, ODI aims to help create indicators that are coherent between the HFA2 and the successors to the Millennium Development Goals, which were also slated for release in 2015 (Mitchell et al. 2013).

Coordination and Implementation

Coordination and implementation of disaster risk reduction activities at the local level is another potential challenge. While there may be support from the national government, that does not ensure support from the local government. At the local level, governments and communities may see disaster risk reduction strategies as a burden, especially when not provided with the financial, technical, or human resources for successful implementation. The World Disaster Reduction Campaign "Making cities resilient: my city is getting ready" has increased public awareness and support for disaster risk reduction at the local level, but there is still much work to do.

Conclusion

The third World Conference on Disaster Risk Reduction held in 2015 addressed gaps in the HFA2 and helped solidify the post-2015 global framework. The development of standardized, quantitative measures including strong monitoring and evaluation, increased coordination between regional, national, and local implementation partners, and increased financial and human resources for implementation, reflects the increased priority of disaster risk reduction.

Improved coordination between disaster risk reduction and development sectors will ensure that communities that can least afford it do not accumulate risk. "The implementation of disaster risk reduction is a long-term open-ended process," and maintaining support over the course of implementation will be difficult at times (Sanahuja 2013). Additionally, strong disaster research based on tested methodologies is needed to support the continued implementation efforts. With concrete actions at the global, regional, national, and local levels and means to measure progress, enthusiasm can be maintained, vulnerability to disasters reduced, and global outcomes improved.

References

Ardalan, A., Kandi, M., Osooli, M., et al. (2012). Profile of natural hazards in *I. R. Iran., Disaster and Emergency Health Academy.* Iran's National Institute of Health Research and SPH of Tehran University of Medical Sciences.

Ardalan, A., Kandi, M., Talebian, M. T., et al. (2014). Hospitals safety from disasters in Iran: the results from assessment of 224 hospitals (online). Available at: http://currents.plos.org/disasters/article/hospitals-safety-from-disasters-in-i-r-iran-the-results-from-assessment-of-224-hospitals/ (Accessed April 20, 2015).

Ardalan, A., Mowafi, H., Malekafzali, H., et al. (2013b). Effectiveness of a primary health care program on urban and rural community disaster preparedness, Iran: A community intervention trial. *Disaster Medicine and Public Health Preparedness* (online). Available at: www.researchgate.net/publication/258920823_Effectiveness_of_a_Primary_Health_Care_Program_on_Urban_and_Rural_Community_Disaster_Preparedness_Islamic_Republic_of_Iran_A_Community_Intervention_Trial (Accessed April 20, 2015).

Ardalan, A., Mowafi, H., and Yusefi, H. (2013a). Impacts of natural hazards on primary health care facilities of Iran: A 10-year retrospective survey (online). Available at: http://currents.plos.org/disasters/article/impacts-of-natural-hazards-on-primary-health-care-facilities-of-iran-a-10-year-retrospective-survey/ (Accessed April 20, 2015).

Bausch, D. G. and Schwarz, L. (2014). Outbreak of Ebola virus disease in Guinea: Where ecology meets economy (online). Available at: http://journals.plos.org/plosntds/article?id=10.1371/journal.pntd.0003056 (Accessed 20 April 2015).

Briseño, S., Horekens, J., and Egeland, J. (2005). *Review of the Yokohama strategy and plan of action for a safer world, Proceedings of the second World Conference on Disaster Reduction*. Kobe, Japan (online). Available at: www.unisdr.org/192005/wcdr/wcdr-index.htm (Accessed April 20, 2015).

Centers for Disease Control and Prevention. (2014). The public health system and the 10 essential public health services (online). Available at: www.cdc.gov/nphpsp/essentialservices.html (Accessed February 11, 2015).

Centre for Research on Disaster Epidemiology. (2012). *The International Disaster Database, Emergency Database*. Brussels, Belgium.

Chan, M. (2014). Ebola Virus disease in West Africa – No early end to the outbreak. *New England Journal of Medicine*, 371, 1183–1185.

Dahinden, M. (2013). *United Nations International Strategy for Disaster Reduction, 4th Global Platform for Disaster Risk Reduction*. Geneva, Switzerland (online). Available at: www.scribd.com/document/218556954/34330-proceedingsenversionfinaleupdatecou (Accessed February 11, 2015).

Global Network of Civil Society Organizations for Disaster reduction. (2014). *About Global Network for Disaster Reduction* (online). Available at: www.globalnetwork-dr.org (Accessed February 11, 2015).

Holmes, J. (2007). United Nations international strategy for disaster reduction, 1st global platform for disaster risk reduction. Geneva, Switzerland (online). Available at: www.preventionweb.net/globalplatform/2007/first-session/docs/session_docs/ISDR_GP_2007_6.pdf (Accessed February 11, 2015).

International Council for Science. (2015). *Disaster risks research and assessment to promote risk reduction and management* (online). Available at: www.icsu. Org/news-centre/insight/science-for-policy/disaster risk/documents/DRRsynthesisPaper_2015.pdf (Accessed April 23, 2015).

Kovacs, P. (2010). *Reducing the risk of earthquake damage in Canada: Lessons from Haiti and Chile*, Ontario, Canada. (online). Available at: http://0361572.netsolhost.com/images/Reducing_earthquake_risk.pdf> (Accessed April 23, 2015).

Los Angeles County Department of Public Health. (2011). The Los Angeles County Community Disaster Resilience (LACCDR) project. (online). Available at: www.laresilience.org/about.php (Accessed February 11, 2015).

Mitchell, T., Jones, L., Lovell, E., and Comba, E. (2013). Disaster risk management in post-2015 development goals: potential targets and indicators (online). Available at: www.odi.org/sites/odi.org.uk/files/odi-assets/publications-opinion-files/8354.pdf (Accessed February 11, 2015).

Noji, E. (2000). The public health consequences of disasters. *Prehospital and Disaster Medicine*, 15(4), 147–157.

Sanahuja, H. (2013). *Findings of the review of National Platforms for Disaster Risk Reduction 2012–2013*. Geneva: United Nations (online). Available at: www.unisdr.org/we/inform/publications/35266 (Accessed February 11, 2015).

Schipper, L., and Pelling, M. (2006). Disaster risk, climate change and international development: Scope for, and challenges to, integration. *Disasters*, 30(1), 19–38.

Swiss Re. (2014). *Honduras disaster preparedness and prevention program* (online). Available at: www.swissre.com/corporate_responsibility/disaster_prepardness_programme_honduras.html. (Accessed August 25, 2014).

Tappero, J. and Tauxe, R. (2011). Lessons learned during public health response to cholera epidemic in Haiti and the Dominican Republic. (online). Available at: http://dx.doi.org/10.3201/eid1711.110827 (Accessed April 20, 2015).

United Nations. (1994). Yokohama strategy and plan of action for a safer world: guidelines for natural disaster prevention, preparedness, and mitigation. *Proceedings of the first World Conference on Disaster Reduction* (online). Available at: www.ifrc.org/Docs/idrl/I248EN.pdf (Accessed August 14, 2014).

United Nations. (2014). Development of the Post-2015 Framework for Disaster Risk Reduction: Co-Chairs' pre-zero draft (online). Available at: www.wcdrr.org/preparatory/post2015 (Accessed August 14, 2014).

United Nations General Assembly. (1987). *Resolution 42/169: International decade for natural disaster reduction.* (online). Available at: www.un.org/documents/ga/res/42/a42r169.htm (Accessed August 13, 2014).

United Nations General Assembly. (2001). *Resolution 56/195: International Strategy for Disaster Reduction* (online). Available at: www.un.org/en/ga/search/view_doc.asp?symbol=A/RES/56/195&Lang=E (Accessed August 13, 2014).

United Nations General Assembly. (2013). *Implementation of the International Strategy for Disaster Reduction: Report of the Secretary-General* (online). Available at: www.unisdr.org/we/inform/resolutions-reports (Accessed August 13, 2014).

United Nations International Strategy for Disaster Reduction. (2004). *Living with risk, A global review of disaster reduction initiatives; Volume 1*. Geneva, Switzerland.

United Nations International Strategy for Disaster Reduction. (2005). *Hyogo framework for action 2005–2015: Building the resilience of nations and communities to disasters* (online). Available at: www.unisdr.org/192005/wcdr/intergover/official-doc/L-docs/Hyogo-framework-for-action-english.pdf (Accessed April 20, 2015).

United Nations International Strategy for Disaster Reduction. (2009a). *2009 global assessment report on disaster reduction* (online). Available at: www.unisdr.org/we/inform/publications/9413 (Accessed April 20, 2015).

United Nations International Strategy for Disaster Reduction. (2009b). *UNISDR terminology on disaster reduction* (online). Available at: www.unisdr.org/we/inform/publications/7817 (Accessed April 20, 2015).

United Nations International Strategy for Disaster Reduction. (2011). *Strategic framework 2025: Work programme 2012–2015* (online). Available at: www.unisdr.org/we/inform/publications/23291 (Accessed August 14, 2014).

United Nations International Strategy for Disaster Reduction. (2014). *Evidence-based integration of disaster risk management to primary health care, the case of Iran* (online). Available at: www.preventionweb.net/files/workspace/7935_ardalanirancasestudy.pdf (Accessed February 11, 2015).

United Nations Office for Disaster Risk Reduction. (2014). *Regional platforms* (online). Available at: www.unisdr.org/we/coordinate/regional-platforms (Accessed August 13, 2014).

United Nations Office for Disaster Risk Reduction. (2014a). *History* (online). Available at: www.unisdr.org/who-we-are/history (Accessed August 13, 2014).

United Nations Office for Disaster Risk Reduction. (2014b). *What is disaster risk reduction?* (online). Available at: www.unisdr.org/who-we-are/what-is-drr (Accessed August 13, 2014).

World Health Organization. (2009a). *Hospitals safe from disasters* (online). Available at: www.unisdr.org/2009/campaign/wdrc-2008–2009.html (Accessed August 13, 2014).

World Health Organization. (2009b). *The WHO safety index* (online). Available at: www.paho.org/disasters/index.php?option=com_content&view=article&id=964&Itemid=911 (Accessed February 11, 2015).

World Health Organization. (2012). *WHO's hospital safety index and emergency checklist rolled out in Europe, 2012* (online). Available at: www.euro.who.int/en/health-topics/emergencies/disaster-preparedness-and-response/news/news/2012/10/whos-hospital-safety-index-and-emergency-checklist-rolled-out-in-europe (Accessed February 11, 2015).

Section 3 Illness and Injury

Chapter 21

Acute Respiratory Infection

Nina Marano and Jamal A. Ahmed

Introduction

Acute respiratory infections (ARIs) account for the majority of excess avoidable deaths in the context of humanitarian emergencies in resource poor settings (WHO 2007). However, the data for the attributable risk for specific infectious diseases in these settings are scarce (Bellos et al. 2010). Identification, prevention, and treatment of diseases with epidemic potential including those causing diarrhea, acute respiratory infections, measles, and malaria are often a priority in the response to humanitarian emergencies (Bellos et al. 2010). Worldwide, lower respiratory tract infections were the third leading cause of death in 2011 (WHO 2014b) and the leading cause of burden of disease as measured by disability-adjusted life-years (DALYs) (WHO 2004).

ARIs are divided into upper respiratory tract infections (URTI), often affecting the nose, sinuses, middle ear, larynx, and pharynx, and lower respiratory tract infections (LRTI), often affecting the trachea, bronchi, and lungs. Examples of URTIs include the common cold and pharyngitis, while examples of LRTIs include bronchitis and pneumonia (Simoes et al. 2006). ARIs may be mild, moderate, or severe. The vast majority of ARIs are mild and patients recover spontaneously.

The etiology is commonly viral or bacterial with the majority of URTIs attributed to viral infection. LRTIs are more likely due to bacteria, some of which are a secondary bacterial infection of an acute viral process such as measles, influenza, or respiratory syncytial virus (RSV) (Rudan et al. 2008). While treatment of ARIs can mitigate the severity of the infection and reduce mortality, many LRTIs do not respond well to therapy, largely because of the lack of highly effective drugs. The vast majority of deaths caused by ARIs are due to LRTIs, primarily pneumonia.

Children under five suffer a high incidence of and disproportionate mortality due to LRTIs. The incidence of pneumonia in this age group is estimated to be 0.29 episodes per child-year in developing countries (Rudan et al. 2008). In 2012, 1.1 million childhood deaths worldwide were attributable to pneumonia (WHO 2014b). Some of these deaths are from respiratory complications of vaccine preventable diseases such as pneumococcus, *Hemophilus influenzae b (Hib),* pertussis, and measles. In 2008, of the 8.8 million deaths in children under five, nearly 17 percent were due to vaccine-preventable diseases (Figure 21.1). Vaccine preventable diseases are discussed in detail in Chapter 16.

Populations affected by humanitarian emergencies are often at high risk for LRTIs because of malnutrition, vitamin A deficiency, low birthweight in infants, indoor fires, and inadequate shelter and blankets, especially in cold climates (WHO 2007). In addition, overcrowding, common during humanitarian emergencies, can amplify the risk of further transmission among the affected population. As a result, LRTIs are among the leading causes of death in complex humanitarian emergencies (Brennan and Nandy 2001 and Checchi et al. 2007).

Complicating the management of ARIs in the context of humanitarian emergencies is the fact that they are frequently treated with unnecessary antibiotics and other drugs, especially in the outpatient setting (Jong and Stevens 2011). It has been approximated that 75 percent of all outpatient antimicrobial use is for ARIs. While some ARIs require antimicrobial therapy, most respiratory infections managed on an outpatient basis are of viral etiology, for which antibiotic use is not warranted. Also, specific antiviral agents may not be available in the setting of humanitarian emergencies (Jong and Stevens 2011).

The WHO and UNICEF strategy for combatting ARIs focuses on reduction of mortality, especially in children, through early detection, diagnosis, correct case management and immunization, reduction in household air pollution, and improved breastfeeding

Section 3: Illness and Injury

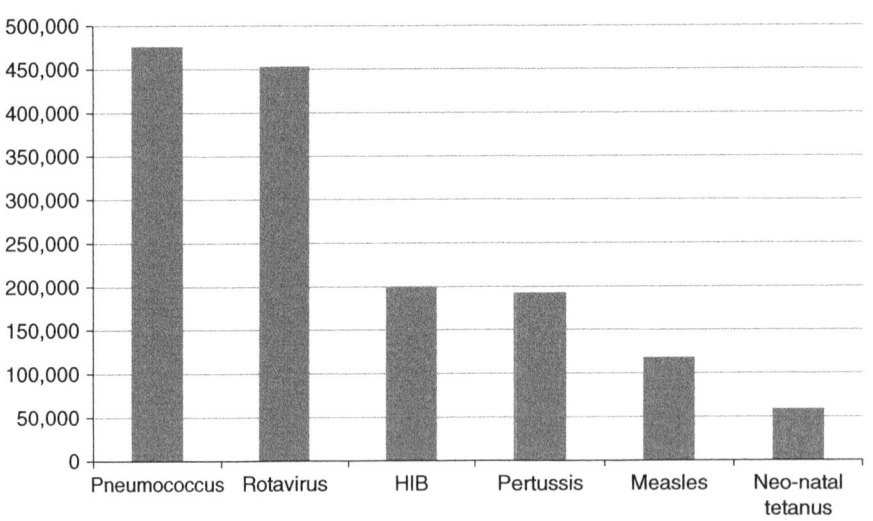

Figure 21.1 Estimated number of deaths due to vaccine preventable diseases in children under age 5 in 2008
Adapted from World Health Organization, Estimates of Disease Burden and Cost Effectiveness: www.who.int/immunization/monitoring_surveillance/burden/estimates/en/

practices (WHO 2013). Strategies for management of ARIs in humanitarian emergencies must be adaptable for refugees, internally displaced persons, and non-displaced populations in a variety of both secure and insecure settings. The burden of ARIs in these populations will vary depending on the level immunization coverage, nutrition, and access to these populations for delivery of humanitarian aid. Critical to the appropriate management of ARIs in these settings is an understanding of their epidemiology, detection, diagnosis, and treatment. This chapter reviews the concepts of ARIs in the context of humanitarian emergencies with the goal of reducing morbidity and mortality associated with these infections.

Epidemiology

In 2010, ARIs were estimated to have caused 2.8 million deaths worldwide (Lozano et al. 2012). In developing countries, pneumonia is responsible for an estimated 10–25 percent of all deaths among children under 5 (Williams et al. 2002). ARIs are the leading single cause of morbidity and mortality in this age group. Of the 6.6 million children under the age of five who died in 2012, 1.1 million (17%) of these deaths were attributable to pneumonia (WHO 2014b).

A systematic review of the literature of ARIs found an estimated 11.9 million episodes of severe and three million episodes of very severe ARIs resulting in hospital admissions in children less than five years of age, worldwide in 2010. The review also estimated 265,000 in-hospital deaths in young children, with 99 percent of these in developing countries. While 62 percent of children with ARIs were treated in hospitals, 81 percent of deaths occurred outside hospitals (Nair et al. 2013).

Approximately half of ALRTIs are caused by viral pathogens. Influenza and RSV are important pathogens in childhood pneumonia (File 2003, Iwane et al. 2004, Rudan et al. 2004, Weber et al. 1998). Infection with either of these viruses predisposes children to secondary bacterial pneumonia, especially in children less than 2 years of age (Iwane et al. 2004). RSV has been identified in up to 40 percent of cases in hospitalized children, while human metapneumovirus (hMPV) and parainfluenza viruses (PIV) are associated with a substantial proportion of ALRTIs in infants and young children (Khan 2006, Weinberg et al. 2009).

Recent studies in refugee camps in Kenya and Thailand have corroborated the significant contribution of RSV and adenovirus to severe acute respiratory illness (SARI) requiring hospitalization, especially among children. In a study conducted in two refugee camps in Kenya from 2007 to 2010, the percentage of people who tested positive for adenovirus virus and RSV was 21.7% and 12.5%, respectively. The annual rate of hospitalization due to SARI was 57/1,000 child-years and was highest in children less than one year of age (156/1,000 child-years) (Ahmed et al. 2012). An analysis of the epidemiology of pneumonia in Mae La refugee camp in Thailand conducted from 2009 to 2011 identified 708 episodes of pneumonia

Table 21.1 Risk factors for transmission of ARIs among displaced populations in humanitarian emergencies

Host Related	• Malnutrition (acute and chronic) • Vitamin A deficiency • Poor breastfeeding practices • Low birthweight and prematurity • Psychological stress • Exhaustion • Concurrent illness • Anemia
Environment Related	• Poor ventilation in shelters • Inadequate shelter/lack of blankets • Excessive exposure to dust • Exposure to cold temperatures causing hypothermia • Indoor air pollution from use of solid fuels • Overcrowding living and sleeping conditions • Exposure to environmental contaminants, toxic weapons, and airborne particulates
Pathogen Related	• Decreased coverage of routine vaccinations (measles, pertussis, Hib) • Lack of personal hygiene and infection control • Lack of or delay in diagnosis and treatment due to insecurity and breakdown in health services • Inappropriate drug treatment causing microbial resistance

Adapted from Gayer 2012.

among 698 patients who sought care. A high proportion of the episodes 702/708 (99%) required hospitalization. The median patient age was 1 year of age with 90.4 percent less than 5 years of age. RSV was detected in 176/708 (24.9%) of the episodes and was more likely to be detected in children less than 5 years of age. Adenovirus was detected in 133/708 (18.8%) episodes (Turner et al. 2013).

At least half of all ALRTI cases are due to bacteria, with some indicating a secondary infection of a viral infection such as measles, influenza, or RSV (Rudan et al. 2008). Infections with *Streptococcus pneumoniae* and *Hemophilus influenzae* type B (HiB) are the most common causes of bacterial pneumonia in children and together are responsible for about half of pneumonia deaths (O'Brien et al. 2009, Watt et al. 2009). HIV infection greatly increases the risk of death from infections with *Streptococcus pneumoniae* and *Haemophilus influenzae* type B (Nathoo et al. 2001, McNally et al. 2007). Fungal pathogens such as *Pneumocystis jiroveci* are also responsible for pneumonia deaths, especially among immunocompromised persons (Rudan et al. 2008, Thomas and Limper 2004).

A review of ARIs in humanitarian emergencies compared rates of ARIs in humanitarian emergencies with more stable populations. Thirty-six studies were included in the review including 25 studies of populations affected by armed conflict and 11 studies of populations in the immediate aftermath of natural disasters. The published evidence, mainly from refugee camps, surveillance or patient record review studies, suggests case-fatality rates (CFRs) up to 30–35% due to ALRTIs in crisis settings compared with CFRs of approximately 14% in more stable settings (Bellos et al. 2010).

Transmission

There are numerous risk factors for the transmission of ARIs among displaced populations during humanitarian emergencies. Many of these also contribute to transmission in stable settings, but are exacerbated in emergencies. In terms of control and prevention it is important to understand the risk factors for transmission. Factors for transmission are divided into host, environmental, and pathogen related risk factors in Table 21.1.

Respiratory pathogens may be transmitted through direct contact or inhalation of airborne droplets, or by indirect transmission through contact with the hands or other articles contaminated by nasal or oral secretions of an infected person. Contaminated hands can carry rhinovirus, RSV, and other viruses to the mucous membranes of the eye or nose. Transmission of enteric pathogens, including enteroviruses, may be by the fecal-oral route (Heymann 2004).

Prevention

A key component in preventing ARIs during humanitarian emergencies is planning and carefully designing facilities and services to house and care for the displaced population. Good site planning and providing basic clinical services, adequate nutrition, clean water, safe shelter, and sanitation are essential factors in reducing the incidence and severity of ARIs (Connoly et al. 2004). During the emergency phase of a humanitarian emergency, vaccinating against measles, improving the nutritional status or children, addressing vitamin A deficiency, reducing overcrowding in shelters, limiting hypothermia in infants, distributing blankets, and emphasizing handwashing with soap and water all help prevent the spread of ARIs (WHO 2005a).

Since early detection is critical to prevention of ARIs, all children with cough should be carefully assessed and referred to a health facility for further evaluation. In the nonemergency phase, focus should be on vaccination against vaccine-preventable diseases such as diphtheria, whooping cough, Hib, and streptococcal pneumonia. In addition, educating healthcare providers about infection control practices and encouraging them to avoid indiscriminate use of antibiotics is essential.

To prevent transmission of ARIs among displaced populations within reception centers, efforts should be made to identify ill persons and implement appropriate infection control measures as soon as possible. Ill persons should be referred for medical evaluation to ensure that they receive appropriate evaluation, diagnosis, and treatment. Visual alerts should be posted both at the entrance and within reception centers instructing residents to 1. report symptoms of respiratory infection and 2. practice good respiratory hygiene and cough etiquette. Screening of displaced populations for respiratory illness upon arrival at the reception center is also recommended. As part of registration, new arrivals should be asked about the presence of typical symptoms of respiratory illness. Persons meeting one of the following criteria should be referred for medical evaluation:

- Respiratory symptoms accompanied by fever, wheezing, or shortness of breath
- Chronic cough persisting for weeks or months
- Respiratory symptoms accompanied by fever, night sweats, or weight loss
- Respiratory symptoms in the setting of asthma or chronic obstructive pulmonary disease

New arrivals that do not have symptoms of respiratory illness upon arrival at the reception center should be instructed to report any new respiratory symptoms to staff when the symptoms first occur (CDC 2016).

Surveillance

To determine the burden of respiratory illness in crisis-affected populations, surveillance should be implemented according to the stage of the humanitarian emergency as shown in Table 21.2. At the initial stages of the emergency, conducting rapid health assessments of the affected population, ascertaining the number of deaths, and determining the population size and structure are critically important. After the first few months, surveillance can become more formal, using population-based surveys in addition to passive data collection as well as laboratory confirmation if it is locally or regionally available. In the more stable setting, data on severity (hospitalization vs. outpatient status), signs and symptoms, and risk factors for illness are useful to assess burden and causes of illness, and should inform prevention and control measures.

Case Definitions

To properly track the incidence of ARIs, it is important to utilize standard surveillance and/or clinical case definitions. This is essential for comparison across all sites where data are being collected and for comparison with data collected during other humanitarian emergencies. It is important to distinguish between upper and lower respiratory tract infections, but this may be difficult during the emergency phase with untrained staff. Depending on the geographic location and population affected by the emergency, case definitions for emerging respiratory diseases such as Middle East Respiratory Syndrome (MERS) coronavirus should be utilized for outbreak detection if laboratory confirmation is locally or regionally available (Abdallah and Panjabi 2008). Examples of case definitions used for ARIs are shown below.

The WHO surveillance case definition for severe acute respiratory illness (SARI) is an acute respiratory infection with (WHO 2014a):

- **A history of fever or measured fever of $\geq 38C°$ (100.4F°)**
- And cough
- With onset within the last ten days
- And requires hospitalization

A case definition for pneumonia in hospitalized children and adults that was used in a refugee camp in Thailand is shown in Table 21.3.

Table 21.2 Comparison of surveillance systems in the emergency and postemergency phase

	Emergency Phase	Post-emergency Phase
Duration	1–4 months	From the first month(s) onward
Method of data collection	Screening initial assessment, simple surveys, observation by walking around	Regular population-based surveys, ongoing health information system
Main priority	Reduce mortality rates	Detect disease outbreaks, design and monitor programs, monitor quality of programs
Types of data collection	Mostly active collection, largely qualitative	Both passive and active collection, more quantitative
Defining population size	Sample survey methods	Census and supplemental surveys
Case definition	Simple clinical signs and symptoms, a few common conditions	May include laboratory confirmation, more in number
Outbreak investigation	Informal, syndromic	Formal with process in place, reportable disease list
Surveillance and use of data	Simple, data needed for immediate actions	Comprehensive, used to assess quality, for longer-term health needs, addresses less urgent issues, emphasis on public health approach

Source: Abdallah and Panjabi 2008.

Table 21.3 Case definition for pneumonia in children and adults used in a refugee camp in Thailand

Age Group	Definition
≤ 5 years	Pneumonia: Cough or difficulty breathing and increased respiratory rate*
≤ 5 years	Severe pneumonia: Cough or difficulty breathing and at least one of: lower chest wall indrawing; nasal flaring; grunting
≤ 5 years	Very severe pneumonia: Cough OR difficulty breathing AND at least one of: central cyanosis, inability to feed or vomiting everything; convulsions, lethargy, or unconsciousness
> 5 years	Fever ≥ 38°C (100.4°F) OR history of fever AND cough OR difficulty breathing AND abnormal chest examination (e.g., crepitus, asymmetric breath sounds, or dullness to percussion)

Measured over 1 minute: > 60 if < 2 months of age; > 50 if 2–11 months of age; > 40 if 11–59 months of age.
Source: Turner et al. 2013.

Case definitions for AURTI and ALRTI used by the United Nations High Commissioner for Refugees (UNHCR) are (WHO 2005b):

- Cough or breathing difficulty
- And breathing 50 or more times per minute for infants aged 2 months to 1 year or breathing 40 times or more per minute for children aged 1 to 5 years
- And no chest indrawing, no stridor, no general danger signs

And for severe pneumonia:

- Cough or difficulty breathing
- And any general danger sign such as unable to drink or breastfeed, vomiting everything, convulsions, lethargy, unconscious, or chest indrawing in a calm child

Data Collection

Respiratory infection associated morbidity and mortality data can be collected from healthcare facilities or from the community. Surveillance systems that utilize only data from healthcare facilities can be biased as they focus on people who use health care services. These may include those who are the most ill and those with fewer barriers to access care. It is important to include community-based surveillance for tracking respiratory illnesses and deaths occurring outside existing facilities.

In community-based surveillance, community health workers gather health data directly from the community. For example, mortality data can be obtained by interviewing the patient's family or community leaders. Broad case definitions can help train community outreach workers to recognize and refer all possible cases of respiratory illness to health facilities. More highly trained healthcare personnel can then apply more specific, but less sensitive, respiratory case definitions, which may include a requirement for laboratory confirmation. This will ensure that the surveillance system does not miss any person who meets a probable or definite case definition for respiratory disease.

Outbreak Detection

An outbreak of ARI may be detected when there is an increase in the incidence of disease. For example, an RSV outbreak may be detected if the incidence of RSV at a point in time is much greater than expected.

Outbreaks of this type are fairly common in humanitarian emergencies, especially in the early months. The large influx of newly displaced populations from multiple places raises the risk that the incoming population will be immunologically naïve to pathogens circulating among the local population.

Effective disease surveillance systems are the best way to detect these types of outbreaks. The UNHCR Health Information System (HIS) used in refugee camps and the Early Warning and Response Network (EWARN) system developed by WHO and used in many countries have been configured in such a way that weekly data can be aggregated and reviewed. Once surveillance is in place, an alert threshold for outbreak detection should be determined. Outbreak alert thresholds vary according to the disease of concern and may need to be adapted for the particular context.

An alert threshold for ARIs, suggested by WHO, is a weekly case count that is 1.5 times the baseline, with the baseline defined as the average weekly number of cases of ARIs calculated over the past three weeks (WHO 2005a). Figure 21.2 shows how this type of surveillance is used to detect an unusual increase in the incidence of disease.

An ARI outbreak can occur if a new pathogen or a new strain of a pathogen is introduced into the population. There have been recent instances of new respiratory viruses affecting mobile populations including the 2009 H1N1 influenza pandemic, the SARS outbreak in Asia, and the MERS outbreak in the Middle East.

Depending on the pathogen and its transmissibility, there is a potential for a larger, more devastating outbreak because almost the entire population will have no prior immunity. Thus, surveillance systems that are designed to be flexible enough to incorporate laboratory testing for novel pathogens will result in early outbreak detection.

Challenges

There are challenges in setting up surveillance for ARIs among displaced populations in the setting of humanitarian emergencies. Epidemiologists from Médecins Sans Frontières (MSF) analyzed the strengths and weaknesses of the sentinel site/community-based surveillance system implemented after the Haiti earthquake in 2010. The results showed that showed that ARIs were one of the predominant causes of morbidity among displaced persons. During surveillance, there was a steady increase in weekly reported cases of ARI over a 4-month period. However, this increase did not trigger a formal alert in the system, suggesting that the surveillance system was more sensitive to outbreaks of immediately notifiable diseases, such as measles, leptospirosis, and diseases with relatively high CFRs such as typhoid, than to more common diseases with lower CFRs such as ARIs. The authors concluded that greater emphasis should be placed on detecting and responding to slower, steady increases in diseases with lower CFRs that nevertheless account for large proportional morbidity and mortality, due to their high incidence. The authors also found that it was difficult to calculate ARI incidence rates because the total population in the catchment areas of each clinic was unknown and subject to substantial and rapid change. In addition, the ARI case definitions used by MSF differed from those used by the Ministry of Health, resulting in differences in reported rates of ARI (Polonsky et al. 2013).

Chapter 21: Acute Respiratory Infection

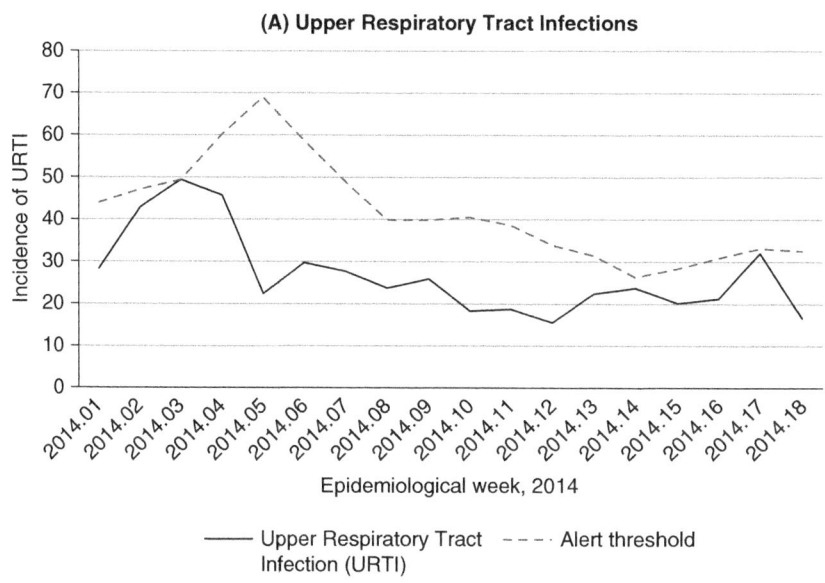

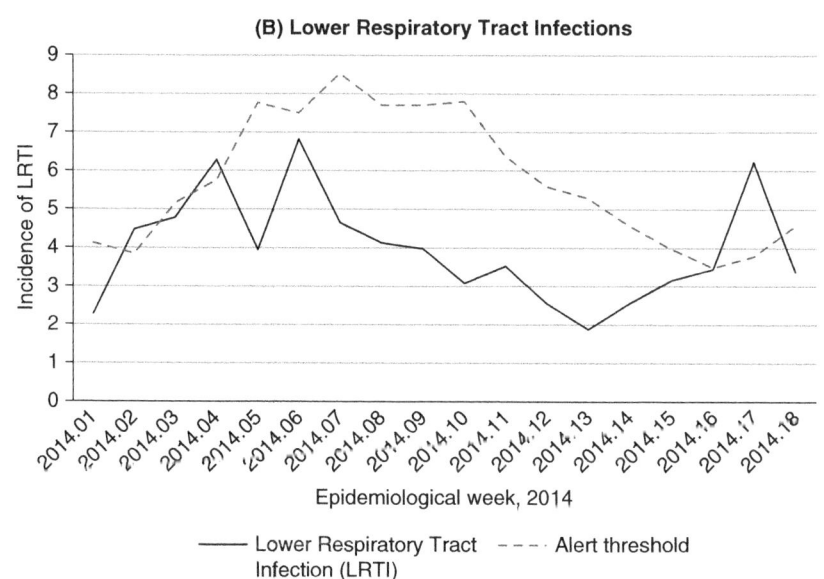

Figure 21.2 Rates of, and alert thresholds for, upper (A) and lower (B) respiratory tract infections by epidemiologic week, Kawergosk camp, Iraq, January–April 2014
Courtesy of UNHCR

Outbreak Response and Control

In 2009, an influenza strain that originated in North America quickly spread across the globe. Within four months of identifying this new strain, scientists detected it in two refugee camps in Kenya. This example highlights how quickly infectious diseases can spread in the twenty-first century.

This section will focus on how to respond to an ARI outbreak within a camp setting. Influenza will be used as an example, because most respiratory viruses are transmitted in a similar way and many aspects of response are similar for most respiratory viruses. In addition, because viral strains are unique and vary widely, the response will always have to be tailored depending on what is known about the causative agent at that point in time. There are some key items, however, that may make the difference between an effective outbreak response and an unmitigated disaster:

- There should be an outbreak control team (OCT) in every humanitarian response effort. If there isn't one in a given refugee camp, it should be created immediately.
- A common feature of humanitarian responses is the multitude of actors present. The public health officer (PHO) liaises with various governmental, nongovernmental, and intergovernmental agencies and organizations all trying to respond to the same event. Without adequate coordination and leadership, the response will likely be ineffective. Planning a response to a disease outbreak in a humanitarian setting is often an emergency within an emergency, and the importance of coordination, teamwork, and leadership cannot be overstated. An effective response needs an "all hands on deck" approach. An effective response to an outbreak requires a frequently-updated, well-accepted preparedness plan. The PHO must ensure that there is an established, detailed outbreak preparedness plan in which the roles and responsibilities of every actor are clearly defined. For example, as the risk of an influenza outbreak increases from the possible to the probable, all actors must come together, go through the outbreak preparedness plan, and review it in detail, ensuring that all that's known of the new strain is incorporated into the response plan. Consultation with subject matter experts may be necessary.
- Once the preparedness plan is in place, it is important not to let it be another paper on the shelf. Implementation of the plan is crucial. A good preparedness plan specifies tasks to be done at various stages of an outbreak. Use the plan at every stage of the outbreak.
- Using all available avenues including community leaders, youth groups, women's groups, and houses of worship, ensure that the population is kept well informed. This helps avoid unnecessary panic and mitigates the fear that's naturally aroused during infectious disease outbreaks. An important part of a PHO's duty during an outbreak is sometimes being the "soother-in-chief." Part of the PHO's job, therefore, will be to avoid the unnecessary social and economic disruption that feelings of panic, fear, and helplessness can bring.
- As mentioned earlier, a key difference between an outbreak of a new virus or a new strain of a virus, and that of an endemic pathogen is that a high proportion of the population have never been exposed to the new pathogen and are therefore susceptible. Using available data, one must estimate the probable impact including estimating the expected incidence over time, attack rates over time, hospitalization requirements, needed bed capacity, and needed drugs, supplies, and equipment. This exercise will help the OCT identify gaps and prepare for possible shortfalls as well as come up with solutions. For example, if there is a potential need for additional hospital beds, the OCT should identify space in which tents can quickly be put up for additional bed capacity. It is usually difficult to identify additional needed staff during an outbreak, and even more difficult during an epidemic that affects a whole country. The OCT can put measures in place to train healthcare workers within the camp in order to have the surge capacity that might be needed during a response.
- Vaccination is an important tool in responding to an outbreak of a vaccine-preventable disease. In the influenza example, if available and accessible, an influenza vaccine may be utilized to mitigate the impact of the outbreak. However, often vaccines are not available in country or to refugees when they are most needed.
- Strengthening disease surveillance is important, as early detection of cases can make a difference in whether the response affects the epidemic curve, lowering the attack rate. The OCT should develop or adapt case definitions specific for the particular setting and ensure that cases meeting this definition are reported and investigated. Early detection of an outbreak should trigger a series of actions outlined in a preparedness plan. Together, these actions mitigate the impact of the outbreak and ensure that resources are utilized where they are most needed. Early initiation of contingency plans ultimately means less mortality and morbidity than would otherwise have occurred. The response should not wait for laboratory confirmation.
- It is important to protect healthcare workers. If few vaccines are available, they should be prioritized for healthcare workers and other frontline workers. In addition, all healthcare workers should be given adequate personal protective equipment if appropriate. Hand

Chapter 21: Acute Respiratory Infection

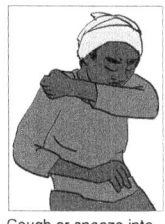
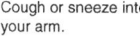
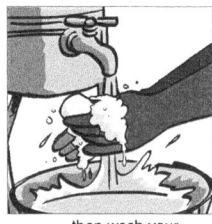

Figure 21.3 An example of a "cover your cough" poster
Source: Yoshunda Jones, CDC Division of Communication Services, Graphic Services Branch

sanitizers or handwashing facilities should be readily available.
- Health education is important. Influenza and other respiratory viruses are spread through direct inhalation of droplets (aerosols) in the air after a person coughs or sneezes or indirectly from fomites. The OCT should communicate with the public, making them part of the process.
The public should be aware of the symptoms and signs of the disease, how it spreads, and how to protect themselves and their loved ones. Health education should focus on how to cover coughs, keep social distance, and the importance of handwashing with soap. An example of a simple health education message about respiratory disease prevention is shown in Figure 21.3.
- The public should learn why it is important that some people be treated away from health facilities and at home. They should be told how to take care of the ill at home, and if necessary, provided with supplies to care for their sick family members. They should be issued adequate soap and antifever medicine. Continuous guidance on what to do should be provided. Additional water and food should be provided if needed. Caretakers should be advised that the ill person must stay in bed until he or she recovers. Caretakers should also be made aware of signs and symptoms of severe disease that may necessitate additional medical support.
A process for the continual dissemination of information throughout the outbreak should be put in place.

- Trust in governmental and nongovernmental authority may be difficult to come by for many refugees. Through communications and interactions, the PHO shows his or her trust in the public's capacity to be part of the response, and in return, the public begins to trust authority. In humanitarian emergencies, whenever the trust is broken between authority and health officers, there is often a conflict between agencies and the population they serve.
- At all times, the OCT should listen to the community and reassure them. Jargon should be avoided as it makes whoever uses it sound unempathetic and aloof. Use everyday language. Messages should be repeated and reinforced and the OCT should lead by example.
- While isolation may be an understandable and even desirable response, especially if there is no evidence of within-camp transmission, it is not an appropriate response in most instances. It is often better to have the mildly ill safe at home than to bring them together in one place, where they will attract many visitors from across the camp and act as foci of transmission. Hospital bed spaces are valuable and gain in value during an outbreak. While in some instances isolating all infected persons is necessary, in most instances, it is important to hospitalize only persons with severe disease.
- If a laboratory is available, specimens should be appropriately collected in accordance with established procedures, and sent to the laboratory.

The receiving laboratory should be notified that specimens are on the way so that they can ensure that personnel are available to receive and promptly process the test them.
- OCT meetings should be held regularly during an outbreak. The OCT should continuously use all available data and if necessary reevaluate the needs of the population, the resources available, and what can be done. For purposes of tracking the impact of the outbreak, the OCT should count cases and deaths and monitor resource utilization. The camp cannot afford to run out of antibiotics for children or bed space in the middle of an outbreak.

All measures listed above may be summarized by: prepare, prevent, and support. That is, prepare in advance, prevent as many people as possible from getting sick, and support the sick so that as many as possible regain their health. In most respiratory disease outbreaks, that balance is achievable. In major influenza outbreaks, that balance becomes very important but may be easier said than done. Infection prevention and control should be prioritized. This puts downward pressure on the epidemic curve and decreases the number of new cases seen every day. It decreases the total number of cases seen within the crucial initial weeks and months of the outbreak, and alleviates some of the strain on the health system. It increases the chance that any severely ill person gets the care that he or she needs.

To achieve this, the goal is to control infections at the source, the sick person. Teach everyone how to cover coughs and sneezes and how to wash hands. Teach people that even at home, they should separate the sick from the well. If possible, only one person should act as the caretaker. At health facilities, separate patients with cough, fever, and other respiratory symptoms from others. Ensure that there is adequate space between hospital beds and that handwashing facilities are available.

Clinical Presentation and Course

In assessing the patient with an ARI, it is important to obtain a thorough history to help differentiate between URTIs and LRTIs. It may also help the clinician differentiate between different types of URTIs.

In the setting of humanitarian emergencies, diagnostics including radiology and laboratory services may not be readily available, making a good history and a thorough physical examination even more important in making the right diagnosis and giving appropriate treatment.

In general, signs and symptoms from viral URTIs last approximately seven days in children less than five years old and nine days in older children and adults, depending on the exact etiology and host factors (Levin and Weinberg 2009).

Symptoms lasting more than two weeks may indicate a nonviral etiology and may require additional investigations and a broader differential diagnosis (Chow et al. 2012). Cough, a common symptom of URTIs, usually begins 3–4 days after the onset of symptoms and has been associated with postnasal drip. A cough lasting more than two weeks may be suggestive of pertussis infection or tuberculosis and thus requires additional investigation (WHO 1999). Nasal congestion and obstruction is common symptom in all age groups. In infants, it can lead to poor feeding. Nasal secretions often start clear and watery but due to shedding of epithelial cells and infiltration of neutrophils usually change to greenish-yellow within three days. Therefore, the color of the nasal discharge is not a good predictor of etiology unless the symptoms persist beyond 10–14 days and the patient is not having symptomatic improvement. Sore throat and difficulty eating or swallowing are also common presenting symptoms and are usually present from the onset of illness. If the sinuses are involved, viral infections may cause congestion, headache, and pressure. Fever is usually mild or not present or in older children and adults; however, in children under five, temperatures can be 39°C (100.4°F) or higher (Levin and Weinberg 2009). Influenza infections can cause fevers as high as 40°C (104°F) in all age groups. Diarrhea, while very unusual, has been observed in children with influenza (Levin and Weinberg 2009). Fatigue, general malaise, and muscle aches are other presenting symptoms, especially in adults.

Identifying patients with URTI caused by bacteria is important because of the potential need for antibiotic therapy. Of special importance are group A streptococcal infections as these are associated with long-term complications, including rheumatic fever and acute glomerulonephritis (AAP 1998). A history of rheumatic fever within the patient's household increases the probability that the patient will be infected. Sore throat and difficulty swallowing are common presenting symptoms. Fever in older children may suggest bacterial infection, especially in the absence of a runny nose, cough, and itchy eyes, which are more common in viral infections.

Acute sinusitis presents similar to other URTIs but localized symptoms should increase suspicion of sinus involvement. According to the American Academy of Pediatrics guidelines, the diagnosis of acute bacterial sinusitis in children is made when a patient with URTI presents with persistent nasal discharge and/or daytime cough for ten days or longer or a worsening course after initial improvement, and severe onset such as fever of 39°C (102°F) or higher and purulent discharge for at least three days (Wald et al. 2013).

In adults, the triad of headache, facial pain, and fever is considered a classic presentation of sinusitis, but it is not common, and persistent symptoms such as prolonged nasal discharge or postnasal drip are more frequent (Chow et al. 2012). Infections may descend and involve the larynx or the trachea. Common symptoms indicating laryngeal involvement include loss of voice or change in tone of voice. In children, a barking cough is a common feature of laryngotracheitis (Levin and Weinberg 2009).

Viral causes of LRTI are many and vary with the patient's age. Common symptoms include fever, cough (often nonproductive), fatigue, and muscle aches. Patients are likely to present with difficulty breathing. Transmission of viruses is generally cyclical, even in refugee camps in tropical countries, and it's important that clinicians understand the local seasonal patterns (Ahmed et al. 2012).

Patients with community-acquired bacterial pneumonia often present with fever, productive cough, and chest pain. Sputum is usually purulent. If there is consolidation, bronchial breathing and tactile fremitus may be observed. Pleural effusion will lead to dullness on the affected side on percussion.

Whether caused by viruses or bacteria, lower chest wall indrawing has been identified as a sign of severe disease in children.

Diagnosis

During many humanitarian emergencies diagnostic capacity is very limited. This further emphasizes the importance of obtaining a thorough history and performing in these contexts. Most children with ARI have mild illness and can be managed without hospitalization. It is important to differentiate between those with mild LRTIs and those with severe disease that may require hospitalization. Fast breathing and lower chest wall indrawing have been associated with severe disease and are used as signs for the diagnosis of severe pneumonia according to the Integrated Management of Childhood Illness (IMCI) guidelines (WHO 2005a).

Even where diagnostics are available, most patients with URTIs will not require additional workup unless targeted treatment is being considered. This is uncommon as many URTIs cause mild illness and are associated with viral infections. In some cases however, a workup may be required. Examples include children suspected of having an infection with group A streptococcus or pertussis, or if there is an outbreak alert.

Investigations may also be needed if LRTI is suspected. It is important to remember that for both URTIs and LRTIs, even when viruses are identified, coinfections with bacterial pathogens are frequent. In many humanitarian emergencies, especially in remote areas of Africa or parts of Asia, there may be no opportunity further diagnostics. In these contexts, empiric treatment is the norm. In humanitarian emergencies where reliable diagnostic and laboratory support is available they should be utilized appropriately. This is the current situation for many Syrian refugees in Turkey, Lebanon, Jordan, and Iraq.

One advantage of utilizing diagnostic tools is to ensure that patients receive the right diagnosis and treatment, hopefully limiting inappropriate use of antibiotics. Clinicians should always consider how a given test would change the management of a particular patient prior to ordering that test. Utilizing a test just because of availability is not a rational use of finite resources.

Some of the common diagnostic modalities utilized include:

Nasopharyngeal and Oropharyngeal Swabs

Throat swabs are used to culture organisms and are very useful in confirming group A streptococcal infections, including during humanitarian emergencies. Sampling should be from the oropharyngeal and nasopharyngeal walls. Nasopharyngeal (NP) and oropharyngeal (OP) sampling is especially important in outbreak detection and response. The emergence of local and global networks for disease surveillance includes internationally recognized laboratories capable of receiving specimens and testing them without additional costs to the humanitarian agencies. The laboratories are usually just a few hours' flight away (Fields et al. 2013 and Castillo-Salgado 2010).

Transport media vary depending on the targeted organism but generally, appropriately handled samples can be stored in the field before they are shipped to appropriate laboratories. These methods have been used successfully in remote refugee camps for multiple pathogens including viruses, atypical bacteria, and pertussis (Kim et al. 2011).

Group A streptococcus infections require special attention because they are associated with long-term sequelae including rheumatic fever and acute glomerulonephritis (Shulman et al. 2012). If available, throat swabs and testing by either rapid antigen detection or culture are recommended, especially for children two years or younger who are at higher risk of developing complications (Shulman et al. 2012).

Complete Blood Counts

Complete blood counts (CBC) with white blood cell differentials may help a clinician determine severity and possible etiology but will not identify pathogens. They are generally less useful in URTIs but may be helpful in LRTIs, especially in identifying patients with severe disease. During humanitarian emergencies, depending on the location and context, local laboratories may not have the right equipment or expertise to conduct CBCs.

Blood Cultures

Blood cultures are rarely available in humanitarian emergencies especially during the emergency phase. Where available, patients with severe pneumonia may benefit from blood cultures collected immediately upon the patient's presentation as they may guide antibiotic therapy.

Imaging

Imaging is rarely needed for URTIs, but may be needed in certain circumstances conditions and in suspected LRTIs. Chest radiography is indicated if pneumonia, pleural effusion, tuberculosis, or other LRTIs are suspected. Bilateral lung involvement may be a sign of viral pneumonia compared to lobar pneumonia that is more common in bacterial infections. In most humanitarian emergencies, the equipment and expertise may not be available in the field but referral opportunities to secondary and tertiary healthcare centers are almost always present and should be adequately utilized.

Understanding the healthcare seeking behaviors and health utilization habits of affected populations is extremely important. In many communities, herbal medicine is very common and can complicate diagnosis and treatment (Graham et al. 2000 and Ernst 2003). For example, among the Somali community in East Africa, cuts on the chest or burn marks may indicate a history of recurrent chest infection or prolonged pneumonia. In the Kurdistan region of northern Iraq, the use of herbal medicine for the treatment of pneumonia is common (Mati and de Boer 2011). Humanitarian workers must keep local practices in mind when they are in the midst of a response effort.

Treatment

It is important to consider that most URTIs are caused by viral pathogens. Clinicians should avoid the use of antibiotics unless they suspect a bacterial infection. Antibiotics available may vary depending on location and context. Some formulations, especially those for children may not be available. The population's acceptance of antibiotics or specific formulations may also vary. In some communities, capsules are widely accepted as better medicine compared with tablets, and injections may be viewed even more favorably. Clinicians should be aware of these factors that can influence compliance of medicines at home. This process should include reassuring and educating patients on the signs of improvement or decline in clinical status.

In infants, a blocked nose can result in difficulty feeding. Mothers should continue breastfeeding their infants throughout the infant's illness. In URTIs, antibiotics should be used judiciously and only if bacterial infection is strongly suspected or confirmed. If signs of bacterial infection are present, especially in older children and adults, antibiotics are indicated. If bacterial pathogens are suspected in a URTI, amoxicillin or amoxicillin-containing drugs are the primary treatment (Simoes et al. 2006). Amoxicillin covers the most common causes of illness and is effective against beta-lactamase-producing bacteria. Penicillin, especially long-lasting injectable penicillin, may be a way of improving compliance, especially if pharyngitis is suspected. For patients allergic to penicillin and related antibiotics, erythromycin or azithromycin may be considered. These are also treatment choices for pertussis.

Notes from the Field

Kenya (2006)

In Hagadera Refugee Camp, Dadaab, Kenya in 2006, a mother presented her 2-year-old daughter with what surveillance officers classified as a severe acute respiratory infection. The child was seen at a health post that is about a 40-minute walk from the main hospital. On arrival, the child was seen by a clinician and was admitted because of fast breathing and severe chest indrawing, indicative of severe pneumonia.

Unfortunately, no one consulted with the mother or asked for her consent. The clinician did not speak the same language as the mother, so information may have been lost during translation. About an hour after the child's admission, the mother asked that her daughter be discharged from the hospital and given medicine to take home, thus going against the clinician's judgment.

Why did the mother disregard the opinion of the physician? Did she not understand the severity of her child's illness or was she willing to gamble with her daughter's life? When faced with such scenarios, humanitarian health workers often rush to speculation and pseudoexplanations that make it easier for them to cope.

The pain-filled determination of that mother was obvious and understandable given her story. She had just fled one of the worst conflicts in Mogadishu since the start of the civil war in Somalia. She arrived as the head of household in the camp only two months earlier with her children including the patient, a young male infant still being breastfed, a 4-year-old girl, and a 6-year-old boy. The 6-year-old suffered from a mental health condition after seeing his friends mutilated by a stray mortar that landed near their local school. This event was why she decided to flee Somalia.

Her husband was still in Somalia, weighing whether to join her or continue living amidst the currents of war. She did not have immediate relatives, siblings, parents, or in-laws. When she brought her 2-year-old daughter to the health post she left her three other children in the care of a good neighbor. She had been in the queue all morning at the health post and hospital without eating any food. She didn't know how her other children were doing and didn't want to abandon her ill daughter in the hospital, but could not afford to stay away from home. One can imagine the multiple burdens she was bearing as she made her way to the health post and then the hospital.

With support from several healthcare workers who were refugees themselves, the staff voluntarily took on the responsibility of caring for her child while she rushed home and checked on her other children. The local block leadership was contacted. With their help and through community support her children were taken care of whenever she was expected at the hospital. Her daughter was discharged from the hospital as soon as possible, and follow-up home visits and visits at the nearest health posts were arranged.

Humanitarian health workers must remember that the major challenge may not be running short of antibiotics or not having diagnostic services. Rather, it is the burden borne by the afflicted population. The situation described is not uncommon in humanitarian emergencies. The people affected by humanitarian emergencies have sustained enormous trauma. They bear the significant burdens of daily living in a crisis-affected setting. It is essential that when humanitarian health workers encounter something that differs from what is normally expected, he or she must remember to take a step back and reassess the situation.

References

Abdallah, S. and Panjabi, R. (2008). Epidemiology and surveillance, in ICRC. eds., *Public health guide to emergencies*. Baltimore, MD: John Hopkins University Press.

Ahmed, J. A., Katz, M. A., Auko, E., Njenga, M. K., Weinberg, M., Kapella, B. K., Burke, H., Nyoka, R., Gichangi, A., and Waiboci, L. W. (2012). Epidemiology of respiratory viral infections in two long-term refugee camps in Kenya, 2007–2010. *BMC Infect Dis*, **12**(1), 7.

American Academy of Pediatrics. (1998). Committee on Infectious Diseases. Severe invasive group A streptococcal infections: a subject review. *Pediatrics*, **101**(1 Pt 1), 136.

Bellos, A., Mulholland, K., O'Brien, K., Qazi, S., Gayer, M., and Checchi, F. (2010). The burden of acute respiratory infections in crisis-affected populations: a systematic review. *Conflict and Health*, **4**(1), 3.

Brennan, R. J., and Nandy, R. (2001). Complex humanitarian emergencies: a major global health challenge. *Emergency Medicine*, **13**(2), 147–156.

Castillo-Salgado, C. (2010). Trends and directions of global public health surveillance. *Epidemiologic Reviews*, **32**(1), 93–109.

Centers for Disease Control and Prevention. (2016). Emergency preparedness and response, infection control, disaster recovery fact sheet. Infection control recommendations for prevention of transmission of respiratory illnesses in disaster evacuation centers. Available at: http://emergency.cdc.gov/disasters/disease/respiratoryic.asp (Accessed July 10, 2017).

Checch, F., Gayer, M., Grais, R. F., and Mills, E. J. (2007). Public health in crisis-affected populations: a practical guide for decision-makers. Available at: www.odi.org/publications/1223-public-health-crisis-affected-populations-practical-guide-decision-makersHumanitarian practice network. (Accessed on July 10, 2017).

Chow, A. W., Benninger, M. S., Brook, I., Brozek, J. L., Goldstein, E. J. C., Hicks, L. A., Pankey, G. A., Seleznick, M., Volturo, G., and Wald, E. R. et al. (2012). IDSA clinical practice guideline for acute bacterial rhinosinusitis in children and adults. *Clinical Infectious Diseases*, **54**(8), e72–e112.

Connoly, M. A., Gayer, M., Ryan, M. J., Salama, P., Spiegel, P., and Heymann, D.L. (2004). Communicable diseases in complex emergencies: impact and challenges. *Lancet*, **364**, 1974–1983.

Ernst, E. (2003). Serious adverse effects of unconventional therapies for children and adolescents: A systematic review of recent evidence. *European Journal of Pediatrics*, **162**(2), 72–80.

Fields, B. S., House, B. L., Klena, J., Waboci, L. W., Whistler, T., and Farnon, E. C. (2013). Role of global disease detection laboratories in investigations of acute respiratory Illness. *J Infect Dis*, **208**(suppl 3), S173–S176.

File, T. M. (2003). Community-acquired pneumonia. *Lancet*, **362**, 1991–2001.

Gayer, M. (2012). Infectious disease control, in N. Howard, N. E. Sondorp, and A. ter Veen, eds., *Conflict and health*. First ed. London, UK: McGraw-Hill.

Graham, S. M., Mtitimila, E. I., Kamanga, H. S., Walsh, A. L., Hart, C. A., and Molyneux, M. E. (2000). Clinical presentation and outcome of Pneumocystis carinii pneumonia in Malawian children. *The Lancet*, **355**(9201), 369–373.

Heymann, D. L., ed. (2004). Control of communicable diseases manual, *Twentieth ed*. Washington DC. APHA Press.

Iwane, M. K., Edwards, K. M., Szilagyi, P. G., Walker, F. J., Griffin, M. R., Weinberg, G. A., Coulen, C., Poehling, K. A., Shone, L. P., and Balter, S., et al. (2004). Population-based surveillance for hospitalizations associated with respiratory syncytial virus, influenza virus, and parainfluenza viruses among young children. *J Pediatr*, **113**, 1758–1764.

Jong, E. C., Stevens, D. L. (2011). *Netter's infectious diseases*. Philadelphia, PA: Elsevier Health Sciences.

Khan, J. S. (2006). Epidemiology of human metapneumovirus. *Clin Microbiol Rev*, **19**(3), 546–557.

Kim, C., Ahmed, J. A., Eidex, R. B., Nyoka, R., Waiboci, L. W., Erdman, D., Tepo, A., Mahamud, A. S., Kabura, W., and Nguhi, M. (2011). Comparison of nasopharyngeal and oropharyngeal swabs for the diagnosis of eight respiratory viruses by real-time reverse transcription-PCR assays. *PLoS ONE*, **6**(6), e21610.

Levin, M. J. and Weinberg, A. (2009). Infections: Viral & rickettsial, in W. Hay, M. Levin, J. Sondheimer, and R. Deterding, eds., *Current Diagnosis and Treatment Pediatrics*. Columbus, OH: McGraw-Hill.

Lozano, R., Naghavi, M., Foreman, K., Lim, S., Shibuya, K., Aboyans, V., Abraham, J., Adair, T., Aggarwal, R., and Ahn, S. Y., et al. Global and regional mortality from 235 causes of death for 20 age groups in 1990 and 2010: A systematic analysis for the Global Burden of Disease Study 2010. (2012). *The Lancet*, **380**(9859), **2095**–2128.

Mati, E. and de Boer, H. Ethnobotany and trade of medicinal plants in the Qaysari Market, Erbil, Kurdish Autonomous Region, Iraq. (2011). *J Ethnopharmacol*, **133**(2):490–510.

McNally, L. M., Jeena, P. M., Gajee, K., Thula, S. A., Sturm, A. W., Cassol, S., Tomkins, A. M., Coovadia, H. M., and Goldblatt, D. (2007). Effect of age, polymicrobial disease, and maternal HIV status on treatment response and cause of severe pneumonia in South African children: A prospective descriptive study. *The Lancet*, **369**(9571):1440–1451.

Nair, H., Simões, E. A. F., Rudan, I., Gessner, B. D., Azziz-Baumgartner, E., Zhang, J. S. F., Feikin, D. R., Mackenzie, G. A., Moïsi, J. C., Roca, A., et al. (2013). Global and regional burden of hospital admissions for severe acute lower respiratory infections in young children in 2010: A systematic analysis. *The Lancet*, **381**(9875), 1380–1390.

Nathoo, K. J., Gondo, M., Gwanzura, L., Mhlanga, B. R., Mavetera, T., and Mason, P. R. (2001). Fatal Pneumocystis carinii pneumonia in HIV-seropositive infants in Harare, Zimbabwe. *Transactions of The Royal Society of Tropical Medicine and Hygiene*, **95**(1), 37–39.

O'Brien, K. L., Wolfson, L. J., Watt, J. P., Henkle, E., Deloria-Knoll, M., McCall, N., Lee, E., Mulholland, K., Levine, O. S., and Cherian, T. (2009). Burden of disease caused by Streptococcus pneumoniae in children younger than 5 years: Global estimates. *The Lancet* **374**(9693), 893–902.

Polonsky, J., Luquero, F., Francois, G., Rousseau, C., Caleo, G., Ciglenecki, I., Delacre, C., Siddiqui, M. R., Terzian, M., Verhenne, L., et al. (2013). Public health surveillance after the 2010 Haiti earthquake: The experience of medecins sans frontieres. *PLoS currents*, **5**, 459–471.

Rudan, I., Boschi-Pinto, C., Biloglav, Z., Mulholland, K., and Campbell, H. (2008). Epidemiology and etiology of childhood pneumonia. *Bull World Health Organ*, **86**, 408–416B.

Rudan, I., Tomaskovic, L., Boschi-Pinto, C., and Campbell, H. (2004). Global estimate of the incidence of clinical pneumonia among children under five years of age. *Bull World Health Organ*, **82**, 895–903.

Shulman, S. T., Bisno, A. L., Clegg, H. W., Gerber, M. A., Kaplan, E. L., Lee, G., Martin, J. M., and Van Beneden, C. (2012). Clinical practice guideline for the diagnosis and management of group A streptococcal pharyngitis: 2012 Update by the Infectious Diseases Society of America. *Clinical Infectious Diseases*, **55**(10), e86–e102.

Simoes, E. A. F., Cherian, T., Chow, J., Shahid-Salles, S., Laxminarayan, R., John, T. J. (2006). Acute respiratory infections in children, in D. Jamison, J Breman, A Measham, G Alleyne, M Claeson, D Evans, P Jha, A Mills, and P Musgrove, eds., *Disease Control Priorities in Developing Countries*. 2nd edition. Washington: Oxford University Press / World Bank.

Thomas, C. F. and Limper, A. H. (2004). Pneumocystis pneumonia. *New England Journal of Medicine*, **350**(24), 2487–2498.

Turner, P., Turner, C., Watthanaworawit, W., Carrara, V., Cicelia, N., Deglise, C., Phares, C., Ortega, L., and Nosten, F. (2013). Respiratory virus surveillance in hospitalised pneumonia patients on the Thailand-Myanmar border. *BMC Infect Dis*, **13**(1), 434.

Wald, E. R., Applegate, K. E., Bordley, C., Darrow, D. H., Glode, M. P., Marcy, S. M., Nelson, C. E., Rosenfeld, R. M., Shaikh, N., Smith, M. J., et al. (2013). Clinical practice guideline for the diagnosis and management of acute bacterial sinusitis in children aged 1 to 18 years. *Pediatrics*, **132**(1), e262–e280.

Watt, J. P., Wolfson, L. J., O'Brien, K. L., Henkle, E., Deloria-Knoll, M., McCall, N., Lee, E., Levine, O. S., Hajjeh, R., Mulholland, K., et al. (2009). Burden of disease caused by Haemophilus influenzae type b in children younger than 5 years: global estimates. *The Lancet*, **374** (9693), 903–911.

Weber, M. W., Mulholland, E. K., and Greenwood, B. M. (1998). Respiratory syncytial virus infection in tropical and developing countries. *Trop Med Int Health*, 3:268–280.

Weinberg, G. A., Hall, C. B., Iwane, M. K., Poehling, K. A., Edwards, K. M., Griffin, M. R., Staat, M. A., Curns, A. T., Erdman, D. D., Szilagyi, P. G., et al. (2009). Parainfluenza virus infection of young children: estimates of the population-based burden of hospitalization. *J Pediatr*, **154** (5), 694–699.

Williams, B. G., Gouws, E., Boschi-Pinto, C., Bryce, J., and Dye, C. (2002). Estimates of world-wide distribution of child deaths from acute respiratory infections. *Lancet Infect Dis*, 2(1):25–32.

World Health Organization. (1999). *Recommended surveillance standards*, 2nd ed. World Health Organization; Geneva Switzerland.

World Health Organization. (2004). The global burden of disease. Available at: www.who.int/topics/global_burden_of_disease/en/ (Accessed on July 10, 2017).

World Health Organization. (2005a). *Communicable disease control in emergencies: A field manual*. World Health Organization; Geneva, Switzerland.

World Health Organization. (2005b). Handbook: 2005 IMCI Integrated Management of Childhood Illness (online). Available at: http://whqlibdoc.who.int/publications/2005/9241546441.pdf (Accessed on July 10, 2017).

World Health Organization. (2007). Public health in crisis-affected populations. Available at: www.odihpn.org/documents/networkpaper061.pdf (Accessed on July 10, 2017)

World Health Organization. (2013). United Nations Children's Fund: Ending preventable child deaths from pneumonia and diarrhoea by 2025: The integrated Global Action Plan for Pneumonia and Diarrhoea. Available at: http://apps.who.int/iris/bitstream/10665/79200/1/9789241505239_eng.pdf (Accessed on July 10, 2017)

World Health Organization. (2014a). Influenza WHO surveillance case definitions for ILI and SARI, 2014. Available at: http://who.int/influenza/surveillance_monitoring/ili_sari_surveillance_case_definition/en(Accessed on July 10, 2017)

World Health Organization. (2014b). The top ten causes of death. Available at: www.who.int/mediacentre/factsheets/fs310/en/ (Accessed on July 10, 2017)

Chapter 22: Diarrheal Diseases

Ciara O'Reilly, Kathryn Alberti, David Olson, and Eric Mintz

Introduction

Diarrheal diseases and other infections of the gastrointestinal tract contribute significantly to the global burden of morbidity and premature mortality and are a major public health threat in the setting of humanitarian emergencies.

An estimated 1.7 billion episodes of diarrhea occurred in children under 5 years old in low- and middle-income countries in 2010, leading to an estimated 751,000 deaths (Fischer Walker et al. 2012, Liu et al. 2012). Diarrhea is the primary clinical manifestation of infection with a broad range of bacterial, parasitic, and viral pathogens. The clinical and epidemiologic features of common enteric diseases are shown in Table 22.2. Other infections of the gastrointestinal (GI) tract may manifest as hepatitis or systemic illness, for example, enteric fever. The most important agents of diarrheal diseases in children include rotavirus, *Cryptosporidium*, enterotoxigenic *Escherichia coli*, and *Shigella* (Kotloff et al. 2013).

Diarrheal diseases with epidemic potential, such as cholera and bacillary dysentery caused by *Shigella dysenteriae* type 1, are of particular concern in humanitarian emergencies. Virtually all of these infections are transmitted through ingestion of water or food, or contact with animals, people, or objects that have been contaminated with feces. The paths of disease transmission are shown in Figure 22.1.

Primary prevention is therefore achieved through promoting and assuring access to adequate quantities of potable water, safely prepared food, sanitation facilities for the safe disposal of human waste, and facilities for handwashing with soap. For some enteric infections, including rotavirus, cholera, typhoid fever and hepatitis A, vaccines are available and may play a role in primary prevention.

Treatment is essential to prevent the secondary complications of diarrheal disease, particularly in the young and elderly. Oral rehydration therapy, or intravenous rehydration, is lifesaving treatment for patients with severely dehydrating diarrheal diseases such as cholera. Properly chosen antibiotics, if administered in a timely and appropriate manner, may be lifesaving, for certain enteric infections including bacillary dysentery and typhoid fever.

Epidemiology

In mid-July 1994, between five and eight hundred thousand Hutu refugees fled violent ethnic conflicts in Rwanda for the North Kivu region in neighboring Zaire (now the Democratic Republic of the Congo). According to the Goma Epidemiology Group (1995), the first case of cholera among refugees was diagnosed on July 20, and a peak of over six thousand cases of diarrhea was reported within a single day on July 26. Shortly thereafter, *Shigella dysenteriae* type 1 resistant to most commonly used antibiotics was identified in a stool sample from a refugee with bloody diarrhea. By early August, reported cases of bloody diarrhea outnumbered cases of watery diarrhea, with over 15,500 cases of dysentery reported during the week of August 8–14. In total, over 62,000 cases of diarrheal disease were reported from health facilities between July 14 and August 12; the overall attack rate for cholera during the first month after the influx was estimated to be between 7.3 percent and 16 percent, based on an estimated 58,000 to 80,000 cases among five to eight hundred thousand refugees. During this time period, 48,347 bodies were collected for burial by trucks for an estimated average crude mortality rate between 19.5 and 31.2 per 10,000 refugees per day. Crude mortality rates for unaccompanied children and infants were as high as 120 to 800 per ten thousand per day in some facilities. Surveys revealed that 85%–90% of all deaths were associated with diarrheal diseases.

The events in Goma in 1994 are a powerful reminder of how rapid, widespread, and deadly diarrheal

Chapter 22: Diarrheal Diseases

disease can be during a humanitarian emergency. Most refugees drank untreated water from Lake Kivu; the rocky, volcanic soil made it impossible to dig pit latrines or bury the dead on site, and soap and facilities for hygiene and handwashing were woefully absent. Crowding and the debilitating effects of malnutrition further increased the vulnerability of the population to infection. As health workers arrived and facilities for rehydration treatment were established, the case fatality rate fell from 22 percent on July 23 to 4 percent on July 26. Most deaths thereafter are believed to have occurred among refugees who never reached a health facility.

Epidemics of watery and bloody diarrhea, also known as dysentery, associated with high rates of morbidity and mortality in refugee and displaced populations have been well documented (Moore et al. 1993, Yip and Sharp 1993, CDC 1994). While cholera and dysentery caused by *Shigella dysenteriae* type 1 are of greatest concern (and will be the focus of this chapter) epidemics of other enteric infections, including hepatitis E (Boccia et al. 2006) and norovirus (Yee et al. 2007) also contribute to morbidity and mortality among refugees and displaced persons. While the infectious agents may vary, strategies for the prevention, surveillance, treatment, and control of diarrheal disease outbreaks in the setting of humanitarian emergencies are essentially the same. Key elements of these strategies are described in the remaining sections of this chapter.

Risk Factors and Transmission

Diarrheal diseases, including cholera, are primarily transmitted through the fecal-oral route. Pathogenic microorganisms excreted in the feces of an infected individual, who at the time may be acutely ill, convalescent, or asymptomatic, are ingested by another individual, usually through consumption of contaminated food or water.

Understanding the pathways through which an individual can become infected helps target interventions to reduce the spread of disease. The "F-diagram" shown in Figure 22.1 illustrates the main pathways via which diarrheal pathogens are transmitted from an infected person to another individual and the barriers or interventions that can impede transmission. Different pathogens favor different transmission pathways, and a combination of barriers provides maximal protection from epidemic disease. The F-diagram is also shown in Chapter 11.

While the F-diagram provides a good overall representation, the principles presented are general. A person's fingers can become contaminated from many different sources, such as contacting the person's own infected stool, caring for a sick person, touching the body of person who died from cholera, or using an unclean latrine. With the exception of certain low-dose pathogens, such as *Shigella spp.*, a fly will probably not carry enough fecal bacteria to directly infect an individual, but if a small inoculum is

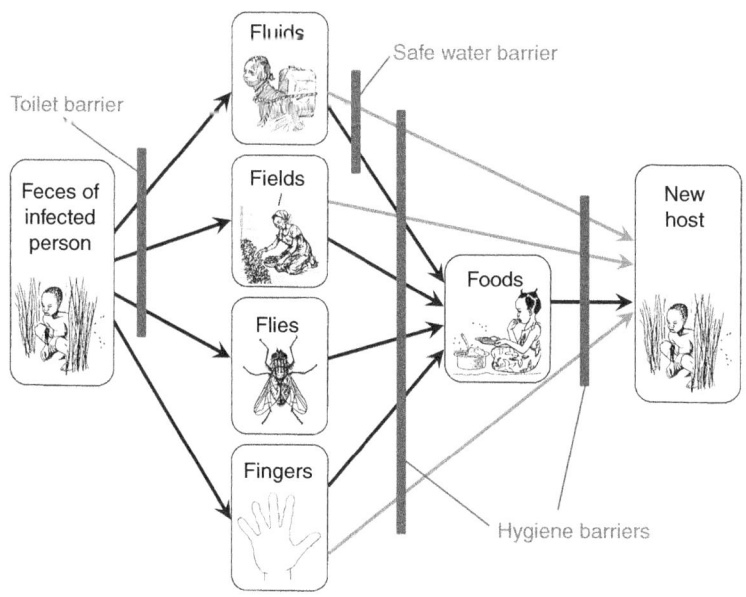

Figure 22.1 The F-diagram of routes of fecal oral transmission and barriers to them
Reproduced by the permission of Water First international (http://water1st.org/the-problem/ accessed 23 May, 2014)

deposited on food, the bacteria may multiply sufficiently to infect those exposed, particularly if the food is not adequately heated before consumption (Levine et al. 1999). Food can either be a primary source of human infection, such as seafood contaminated with *Vibrio cholerae* in the aquatic environment or a secondary source that was contaminated by an infected person during food handling or preparation. Food eaten from roadside stalls, at markets, and eaten raw are a known risk factor for transmission of cholera and other diarrheal diseases. Seafood, raw fruit and vegetables, and cooked foods that have subsequently been contaminated and inadequately reheated have all been associated with cholera transmission (Estrada-Garcia and Mintz 1996). While in different contexts different foods pose higher or lower risks for transmission of diarrheal disease, the general rule of eating only cooked food while it is still hot will always apply.

In a humanitarian emergency, infrastructure or systems that provide barriers and protect a population from diarrheal disease epidemics may be broken or disrupted. During population displacement, a large population may arrive in an area where there is no infrastructure, immediate safety potentially being the only criteria for selecting an area for settlement. Provision of, and access to, adequate clean water and sanitation are among the top priorities in this type of setting (MSF 1997). Creating at least a basic sanitation system, even if temporarily in the form of open defecation fields and provision of clean water are priorities (Sphere Project 2004) until more durable systems can be put in place. Water, sanitation, and hygiene (WASH) are discussed in detail in Chapter 11.

In more stable emergencies, risk factors may be more nuanced and a more detailed evaluation, such as a case-control study, may help identify specific risk factors. In Kakuma refugee camp in Kenya, a long-established camp where a cholera outbreak was recorded as part of a much larger national outbreak, a case-control study helped identify that new arrivals in the camp were more at risk for cholera than more established residents. Sharing a latrine with three or more households was also identified as a risk factor (Shultz et al. 2009).

In addition to the problems of lack of access to clean water and sanitation as described, the population may have moved from an area where cholera is rare to an area where cholera is endemic. In this context, in addition to lacking immunity to the disease, the displaced population may not have developed behavioral practices that would reduce their risk of cholera infection, such as treating drinking water, covering food, or washing fruits and vegetables. They may not recognize the signs of cholera or know to seek care immediately once symptoms appear. Actively educating the community through hygiene and health messaging is essential to reducing risk in these contexts.

In stable urban contexts, the risk of cholera transmission is not equal across a city. Some areas may be well-served with access to clean water and sanitation; other peri-urban or slum areas may be built with insufficient or no water and sanitation infrastructure and have a high population density, putting them at high risk of cholera transmission. These areas may also have little access to health services. There may also be cultural barriers that deter the population in these areas from going to other more central areas of a city, reducing access to health care and increasing the risk of dying in the community. Decentralizing care into these areas may be an important part of a strategy for control of epidemics of diarrheal disease.

Flooding is a specific natural disaster that can increase the risk of transmission of cholera and other enteric diseases such as enterotoxigenic *Escherichia coli* (Qadri et al. 2005). Latrines may be flooded, surface water may be contaminated by feces, and open defecation practiced by necessity. In a review of reported cholera outbreaks worldwide from 1995 to 2005, heavy rains or floods, along with water contamination and population displacement were the most common risk factor categories reported (Griffith et al. 2006).

There is a perception that any natural disaster is a risk for a cholera outbreak. This is not necessarily true. In an area with endemic cholera, it is true that a natural disaster may disrupt the water and sanitation infrastructure and the risk of cholera in the population will increase. However, many natural disasters will have no impact on the potential risk of cholera. If the causative agent is not present in the environment, disruption in services will not increase the risk of a cholera outbreak. In a recent study, no significant association between earthquakes and cholera epidemics was seen (Sumner et al. 2013). In fact, anecdotal evidence suggests that in Haiti, those displaced by the earthquake and living in camps where water, hygiene, and health promotion were provided were among the least affected by the epidemic (Schuller and Levey 2014).

Individual factors may also play a role in risk of infection or death. Young children are often at higher risk of dying from diarrheal disease than others and the same has been reported for the elderly. Malnourished patients are also at higher risk of mortality from diarrheal disease. Although other individual factors such as gastric acidity and blood type are also involved in individual risk of infection and disease, during an emergency they are rarely useful in epidemic control.

Special Considerations

Funerals

Attending a funeral or eating at a funeral of a person who died of cholera are known risk factors for cholera in West Africa (Gunnlaugsson et al. 1998). Bodily fluids excreted from a person who has died of cholera are highly infectious. In some cultures, the person who prepares the body for burial may also be involved in food preparation for those attending the funeral. Cultural rituals may also include touching the defunct as part of burial rites.

Prisons, Orphanages, Military Barracks and Other Enclosed Quarters

During an epidemic, specific populations warrant special attention. Due to the crowded living conditions in most prisons, and the difficulties prisoners face in accessing emergency medical care after hours, one case of cholera or any diarrheal disease of epidemic potential in a prison may have devastating effects (Guevart et al. 2005). Children living in orphanages and soldiers in military barracks may also be at higher risk of cholera infection and transmission for similar reasons.

Prevention

This section will focus on measures to prevent cholera and other epidemic-prone diarrheal diseases during an outbreak. While effective at reducing the risk of epidemic cholera and most other infectious diseases transmitted through the fecal-oral route, some measures may only be sustainable in the short term. Programs targeting cholera elimination will require sustainable water, hygiene, and sanitation projects, which will not specifically be addressed here.

Once a diarrheal disease outbreak has started, provision of adequate safe drinking water, soap, and hygiene messages to promote handwashing (especially after going to the toilet and before eating) are priorities. These measures can be put in place quickly. Measures to improve sanitation and solid waste management are also important but may take more time to put in place (Oxfam 2012).

When designing and implementing water, sanitation, or hygiene programs, it is important to recognize that provision of services alone is not sufficient; the population must have the information, understanding and motivation to use the provided services, which may require behavior change. Community participation in program design can help inform services that are adapted to the population and improve the likelihood that the services will be used (Sphere Project 2004).

When planning the provision of clean water in emergency settings, it is important to think of the whole chain of water supply from the source through the distribution system to the final steps of an individual accessing, transporting, storing, and drinking the water. Contamination of the water can occur at any step along this chain.

The type of water system to be established will depend on the context and on available water sources. In areas where multiple water sources are used, distribution of household water treatment products and safe water storage containers or campaigns to clean or retrofit existing water storage containers may be the simplest, quickest, and most cost-effective measure.

Household water treatment products commonly used in emergencies are chlorine tablets composed of sodium dichloroisocyanurate (NaDCC) or dilute 1%–2% liquid sodium hypochlorite, also known as bleach, manufactured and sold commercially for water treatment. If these are unavailable, 3%–6% sodium hypochlorite sold for cleaning and laundry may be substituted (Lantagne 2008, Lantagne and Clasen 2012). If the water to be treated is turbid, the dosage of chlorine products must be doubled or a combined flocculant and chlorine product must be used (Colindres et al. 2007, Lantagne 2008).

The distribution of combination kits that contain chlorine tablets, soap for handwashing and oral rehydration salts (ORS) to treat diarrhea has also become common practice. Regular monitoring of household water quality, often done through the proxy of free residual chlorine levels in treated water, should also be established. In the setting of a humanitarian emergency, household water treatment products will likely need to be distributed more than once during an epidemic. Distribution needs to be accompanied by teaching materials and demonstrations, especially in communities that have not previously used this type of water treatment (Colindres et al. 2007, Lantagne and Clasen 2012).

The use of locally available liquid chlorine may decrease the population's dependency on distributions during a humanitarian emergency. Alternative methods of water disinfection, such as ceramic or slow sand filters, or solar disinfection, are less practical than chemical methods in the emergency context because the materials needed are bulkier and more difficult to import and distribute locally (Lantagne and Clasen 2012). Boiling is also an effective method of disinfection, but requires cooking fuel, most often wood or charcoal that can be difficult to obtain in quantity. Deforestation for firewood can cause conflict especially if it is perceived by a resident population to be the result of refugees or internally displaced persons living in camps or settlements.

In areas with fewer water sources such as urban areas or camps, engaging "bucket chlorinators" at water collection points may be a more cost-effective measure. The dosage of chlorine can be empirically calculated based on source water quality and chlorine demand. Chlorination teams can be taught to adapt the dose to the size of the container (Robertson and Pollitzer 1939). Bucket chlorination is also discussed in Chapter 11.

In urban areas with municipal piped water treatment and distribution systems, it may also be appropriate to support the central water supplier(s) to ensure that adequate chlorine and other necessary supplies are available. Minor repairs or provision of parts may also be a rapid and effective way to restore adequate safe water supply to a large number of people. Urban centers may also use tanker trucks as part of the distribution system. Whatever the source of the water (surface water or municipal water system) used to fill the tanker, it should be monitored and properly chlorinated. This should be done collaboratively with the municipal water authorities.

In some settings, such as camps, water may initially be provided via water tanker trucks from a source at some distance from the site; however, this can be expensive and is usually unsustainable secondary to both the cost and availability of trucks. When it is done, efforts should be made to ensure that the trucked-in water is properly chlorinated. More commonly in camps, surface water is collected and treated centrally before distribution. Whatever system is used, water must be readily accessible. If it takes too much time or is too difficult to access treated water, people will use alternatives such as untreated surface water.

As described earlier, it is important that local water collection and storage practices be evaluated and that steps are taken to prevent contamination or recontamination events. Distribution of jerry cans or other safe water storage containers (e.g., Oxfam buckets) at the beginning of a humanitarian emergency is often important to ensure that the population has adequate and clean water storage capacity. In more established settings, educational campaigns on safe water handling, and on cleaning containers used for water collection and storage can be a useful part of seasonal cholera prevention (Oxfam 2012).

Food Handling

Food is infrequently identified as the initial source of a diarrheal disease outbreak in an emergency setting, but is frequently a significant risk factor in continued transmission. Ensuring safe food handling and preparation in general, and particularly in areas with mass food preparation such as markets, can play an important role in preventing the spread of disease. Providing hygiene promotion and ready access to latrines with handwashing stations can be an effective and rapidly implemented intervention. The cleanliness of the latrines and continued provision of clean water and soap for handwashing must be maintained through market committees and through other efforts by authorities or implementing agencies. Special messaging around food preparation is available from the UNICEF Cholera Toolkit (UNICEF 2013).

Sanitation and Solid Waste Management

Safe excreta disposal is an important part of diarrheal disease prevention. In a camp setting, the provision of latrines and the elimination of open defecation are important prevention measures. One latrine per family will be the long-term goal of sanitation programs as this minimizes the risk of diarrheal disease transmission. Shared latrines for up 50 persons, reducing as quickly as possible to 20 persons (Sphere Project 2004) with handwashing points, are an important step towards disease prevention in the short to medium term. Latrines are also discussed in Chapter 11.

As with other measures, for optimal adoption and utilization, latrine design and placement should be informed by population and community involvement and accompanied by health messaging on the importance of safe sanitation and handwashing practices.

In open or urban settings, provision of sanitation once an outbreak has begun may be more challenging. Initial energy may be better spent on provision of sufficient quantities of safe drinking water and on handwashing promotion.

Hygiene Promotion

Handwashing with soap after defecation or handling of feces from a child or a patient, and before handling, preparing, or eating food is essential to prevent diarrheal diseases from spreading. The behaviors are often not practiced because of a lack of knowledge, understanding, or easy access to handwashing facilities, soap, and water. To change human behavior, strategies that increase hand washing awareness and motivation are as important as increasing access to facilities and supplies. As a general rule, interactive approaches that include community or family leaders are more effective than passively providing health education messages. Many countries that are prone to diarrheal disease outbreaks will have long-term behavior change programs including "WaSH in Schools" that can be leveraged in the emergency setting. A vast literature is available on social mobilization, though little of it is directed towards the humanitarian emergency setting. It is important that messages be harmonized across all agencies that are doing social mobilization. If no soap is available, in cultures where ash is used for handwashing, it can be distributed and promoted instead. Hygiene promotion is also discussed in Chapter 11.

Special Considerations

During cholera outbreaks, special attention must be paid to the handling of dead bodies. Bodily fluids of cholera decedents are highly infectious. Funerals have played an important role in the spread of cholera epidemics, most likely through cultural practices of the same individuals touching or washing the body of the deceased in preparation for burial and also preparing food served at the funeral (Gunnlaugsson et al. 1998). Community leaders must be involved in discussions on how to prevent the spread of disease while still respecting the most important rituals around death and burial. For example, it may be acceptable to have a family member present or help in the preparation of a body with chlorine in a mortuary area of a health facility; food may be excluded temporarily from funerals and handwashing can be included in ceremonial practices.

Cholera Treatment Centers and other Health Facilities

Hygiene and disinfection practices in facilities that treat patients with cholera or noncholera diarrhea are critical to preventing nosocomial disease transmission. Guidelines on the specific chlorine concentrations recommended for different uses including handwashing, disinfection of excreta and vomit, or cleaning, and on wastewater disposal are readily available and should be respected (MSF 1997). If health facilities are well managed, nosocomial cholera transmission is unlikely to occur. They can be good places to demonstrate and share information on disease prevention practices with families, caregivers, and patients. Hygiene kits (water treatment products, soap, and other commodities) can be provided to families so that they can share prevention messages with household members and neighbors. More extensive kits that contain materials for disinfecting latrines and areas or belongings that came into contact with a patient's excreta may also be distributed. All staff working in a treatment structure will also benefit from training on the prevention of diarrheal disease. Not only do they need the information to protect themselves and others at work, but also, they can become good sources of information on prevention for their neighbors, friends, and families. Hygiene kits are also discussed in Chapter 11.

Household Disinfection

The previously common practice of household disinfection or spraying where teams went to the houses of patients and disinfected by spraying with chlorine, is no longer recommended (UNICEF 2013). There is no evidence for the effectiveness or lack thereof of this practice and it requires significant human and logistic resources. In addition, it may stigmatize those whose homes are disinfected. Other solutions, such as providing instructions and materials to the families of patients admitted for treatment, or group demonstrations of how to disinfect homes along with messages on cholera prevention, are currently being tested.

Antibiotic Chemoprophylaxis for Prevention of Cholera

With some specific exceptions such as prisons, provision of antibiotics for asymptomatic family members or contacts of cholera patients is not recommended as it may lead to antibiotic resistance (UNICEF 2013).

Targeting Prevention Programs

As mentioned in the previous section, local risk assessments can be very useful for targeting prevention activities. Epidemiological mapping of cholera cases and deaths can be a rapid and effective way of identifying priority areas for intervention. If many patients are coming from particular areas of a city, targeting hygiene promotion and provision of clean water to those areas may be more effective for outbreak control than a less targeted approach (Luquero et al. 2011, Azman et al. 2012).

Vaccination

Three oral cholera vaccines, Dukoral® (Crucell, Stockholm, Sweden), and Shanchol™ (Shantha Biotechnics, Hyderabad, India), and Euvichol® (EuBiologics, Chuncheon, South Korea) are commercially available and prequalified for use by the World Health Organization. All require two doses given at a minimum interval of two weeks. Due to simpler logistics of transport, storage, and distribution, Shanchol™ and Euvichol® are currently the preferred vaccines for prevention in the field. The eligible population for Shanchol™ and Euvichol(R) includes children as young as 1 year old and adults, including pregnant women. Short-term effectiveness is 85 percent (Luquero et al. 2014) with an overall five-year efficacy of 65 percent (Bhattacharya et al. 2013).

Current strategies include preventive vaccination in areas with regular seasonal peaks or outbreaks, preemptive vaccination in areas at high risk, including certain humanitarian emergencies, and, when conditions permit, reactive vaccination during an ongoing outbreak. Oral cholera vaccines should never be used alone, but as a part of a coherent strategy that includes all the other preventive measures described above.

Surveillance and Outbreak Detection

Diarrhea is such an easily recognized and important cause of epidemic disease that it is included in virtually all public health surveillance systems. Information collected by these systems varies according to available resources, and can include detailed clinical, epidemiologic, and laboratory data. In the setting of a complex humanitarian emergency, or in any population at high risk for epidemic diarrheal disease with limited resources and surveillance capacity, diarrheal disease surveillance is imperative. Surveillance information on only a few essential, easily gathered, variables is needed to detect diarrheal disease outbreaks and inform immediate actions for limiting further spread, but the information needs to be collected and reported in a timely, consistent, and representative manner. Sentinel health facilities serving the target population are logical points for gathering and reporting information on diarrheal diseases. By tailoring the surveillance system to the situation, and keeping it simple, one avoids overburdening limited human and logistical resources and thereby compromising data quality or utility. Simple case definitions are best: diarrhea is commonly defined as three or more loose or watery stools in a 24-hour period, and dysentery is commonly defined as stools with visible blood. This is most commonly by report from the patient or family member, or alternatively by observation at the health facility. It is useful to collect data from as many clinical sites as possible, though formal reporting may need to be limited to strategically located sentinel sites that see sufficient patients and have sufficient staff to reliably comply with reporting requirements. To ease the workload for clinic staff, diarrheal disease surveillance should be integrated with other clinic-based public health surveillance when possible. Diarrheal disease outbreaks may begin from a common contaminated food or water source, and most diarrheal diseases have an incubation period from a few hours to a few days. Therefore, epidemics of cholera, dysentery or other diarrheal diseases can emerge dramatically within 24 hours, and can spread rapidly through a population through many routes. For this reason, in all high-risk situations, diarrheal disease surveillance data should be collected, reported, and analyzed daily. The minimum site-specific information required on a daily basis includes the number of patients presenting to the health facility each day with diarrhea broken down by age group, most commonly <5 years old vs. ≥5 years old, and by the type of diarrhea, watery or nonbloody vs. bloody diarrhea, and the number of deaths by age group attributed to watery and to bloody diarrhea among patients at the health facility each day. Reporting can be done electronically or through the use of paper forms according to local capacity. If electronic reporting is used, it is recommended that an electronic backup and a paper copy be maintained at the reporting site. Most clinics maintain a patient register or logbook that collects the same information as surveillance forms to facilitate data collection for surveillance. An example of a daily diarrheal disease surveillance reporting form is shown in Figure 22.2. Sample forms are also available from MSF (MSF 1997). In camps for refugees or internally displaced persons, and in civil society, community health workers may be given responsibility for detecting and reporting cases of diarrheal diseases and other conditions observed outside health facilities. Data from this source may be incorporated into overall surveillance for diarrheal diseases, with the caution that some cases may be counted twice, once in the community and once at a health facility.

Daily analyses of surveillance information at sites and at the central level will allow early detection of worrisome increases in the numbers of cases and or deaths attributed to diarrheal diseases by site, age group, and type of diarrhea. The results of these analyses should be shared on a weekly basis or more frequently with all reporting sites and with agencies involved in humanitarian response, particularly the Ministry of Health, local government agencies, and

Figure 22.2 Example format for daily diarrheal diseases surveillance from health facilities

Health Facility:

    Name of Surveillance Reporter:

    Reporting Date: MONTH___ / DAY___ / YEAR___

    Case Definitions

    Diarrhea: Three or more loose or watery stools in a 24-hour period

    Bloody diarrhea (dysentery): Stools with visible blood by report from patient or guardian

All Cases of Watery Diarrhea			
<5 years old	≥5 years old	Unknown age	Total

Deaths from Watery Diarrhea			
<5 years old	≥5 years old	Unknown age	Total

All Cases of Bloody Diarrhea			
<5 years old	≥5 years old	Unknown age	Total

Deaths from Bloody Diarrhea			
<5 years old	≥5 years old	Unknown age	Total

nongovernmental organizations responsible for public health and for water, sanitation, and hygiene. An increase in cases or deaths due to diarrhea at one or more sites may represent an increase in the catchment population, a seasonal trend related to climate or other environmental or social factors, or a true outbreak of a particular diarrheal disease. This determination may require a more in-depth field and laboratory investigation, but hypotheses can be generated by comparing the results across reporting sites looking for either geographic, demographic, or temporal clustering, requesting data from other clinical sites not captured by existing surveillance, and consulting with local health care providers within and outside the surveillance area. If denominators for the catchment population are known or can be estimated, crude incidence rates can be calculated and used for comparison purposes. Site-specific case fatality rates can be estimated from the number of deaths divided by the number of patients presenting over a specified time such as daily, weekly, or monthly. In addition to routine site-based daily surveillance, it is essential to maintain a 24/7 hotline for emergency notification of suspected outbreaks of diarrheal disease, other diseases spread by contaminated food and water, such as typhoid fever and hepatitis E, and other emergencies, including sudden increases in diarrheal disease deaths in health facilities or communities. Further investigations of suspected outbreaks or other untoward events detected through analyses of routine surveillance data or through emergency notifications must be undertaken urgently and may include laboratory testing, field investigations in affected communities, and implementation of preliminary preventive measures and treatment recommendations.

In areas not endemic for cholera, an increase in cases of acute watery diarrhea in children ≥ 5 years old or in adults should signal an alert for possible cholera. For surveillance purposes where cholera has not been confirmed, WHO defines suspected cholera as death or severe dehydration due to acute watery diarrhea in a child ≥5 years old or an adult. Once an epidemic of cholera has been confirmed, all cases of acute watery diarrhea in persons ≥5 years old may be considered cholera for surveillance purposes. Similarly, a fatal case of bloody diarrhea is highly suspect for infection with *Shigella dysenteriae* type 1 (Sd1). Once an epidemic of *Shigella dysenteriae* type 1 has been confirmed, all cases of bloody diarrhea may be considered Sd1 infections for surveillance purposes.

Outbreak Response and Control

In the humanitarian emergency setting, acute watery diarrhea (and to a lesser extent, dysentery) is among the most frequently reported causes of illness in affected populations. Attention to clean water, adequate sanitation, proper hand hygiene, and access to simple therapeutic measures are universally applicable for controlling diarrheal illnesses in emergency conditions. Some diarrhea-causing pathogens, like *Vibrio cholerae* and *Shigella dysenteriae* type 1, can cause large epidemics with significant mortality and require a disease-specific, multipronged operational response.

Initial Investigation

With a surveillance system in place, early reports of an increase in cases of acute diarrhea that clinically resemble or meet established case definitions for cholera or dysentery should trigger an alert. If formal surveillance is not yet instituted or fully functional, notification may come from alternative sources, such as district health supervisors, managers of local health facilities, community health workers, or even local media. Typically, in a cholera- or *Shigella*-endemic region, a sudden increase in the number of suspect cases above typical seasonal background rates or a weekly doubling of cases over 2–3 weeks will trigger an alert. However, in regions where these illnesses are infrequent or unknown or in emergency contexts characterized by densely populated congregate settings such as refugee camps, even a single suspected case should trigger an alert and subsequent investigation. Ideally, alerts will be investigated within 24 hours.

An investigation will:

- Assess the likely etiologic agent by clinical signs and symptoms and/or rapid diagnostic testing
- Assist in collecting and sending stool specimens to a reference laboratory for confirmation of the etiology by bacterial culture or other means
- Determine, refine, or establish a surveillance case definition
- Assess the capacity for case management such as human resources, medical supplies, bed space, means of nutrition, any fee-for-service, the quality of care currently being provided, and the adequacy of hygiene practices
- Describe the affected and at-risk population, including the number of people in the immediate

zone where the outbreak is occurring and total number of people in the city, administrative area, or district, as well as population density, sanitary conditions, etc.
- Review and reinforce the system being used to collect and report case information at the facility level
- Establish a register or line list if necessary
- Obtain any locally available historical data of previous outbreaks
- Construct a basic epidemiologic curve and map, by neighborhood or village, of the affected areas using register, line list, or other available data
- Evaluate the suitability of existing or proposed treatment sites in terms of
  - Sufficient water that is properly chlorinated
  - Functional sanitation facilities and infrastructure such as number of latrines, waste water management, isolation from noncholera patients and general public, crowd control, etc.
  - Accessibility including location, modes of transportation, security, etc.
- Perform a rapid assessment of the principal means of water access and the water quality within the affected community, as well as the predominate modes of sanitation such as household or public latrines, or open-air defecation
- Note any sites capable of potentiating transmission, such as active markets with food and drink vendors, congregational settings, or communal use of surface water for drinking and/or bathing.

The investigation team should bring basic medical supplies that may include intravenous fluids, catheters and tubing; ORS, antibiotics such as doxycycline for cholera, ciprofloxacin for dysentery, zinc; rapid diagnostic test (RDT), materials to collect and transport stool samples for lab testing; and chlorine, to donate to existing facilities or to initiate treatment in a provisional setting, as dictated by the initial assessment. Visiting or contacting several surrounding villages or health posts will help determine the current extent of spread or risk factors that could be addressed by preventive measures.

Pending microbiologic confirmation of the causative agent, a report detailing the results of this investigation will form the initial basis for a response.

Organizing a Response

The principle objective in responding to a diarrheal disease outbreak in any context is to limit morbidity and mortality in the affected and at-risk population through the implementation of activities within four main objectives:

- Case management
- Disease prevention
- Community mobilization, information, education, and communication
- Outbreak surveillance and monitoring and evaluation

An outbreak in the context of a humanitarian emergency will also invoke this multimodal response, but disruptions in local institutions, damaged or absent infrastructure and supply routes, and mobile populations may limit standard deployment options and require greater adaptability of field staff to devise effective implementation of the essential elements in a sometimes chaotic and rapidly changing situation.

The first step in organizing a response is collecting the basic epidemiologic data of person, place, and time.

- Date of first suspected case
- Number of suspected cases (and deaths in suspected cases) per day for each reporting facility, using a standard epidemic curve
- Origin of suspected cases (village, neighborhood, camp, sector) to be used for creating a spot map
- Population figures for communities from which cases are originating (total population number) and breakdown by age (below 5 years and 5 years or above is usually sufficient)
- Qualitative description of affected communities (urban, rural, IDP or refugee camp)

To assure an accurate ongoing account of the caseload, a uniform case definition must be agreed upon. This case definition may differ from that used for routine surveillance purposes.

Case Management

Both cholera and *Shigella* are highly infectious and the total caseload, the level of illness of severe cases, and the need to isolate infectious cases from other patients make most typical health structures a poor choice for case management. Instead, disease-specific, usually temporary, structures have been developed which address the particular outbreak-driven needs for rapid triage, optimized patient flow, and infection control.

For shigellosis caused by Sd1, isolation units have been used successfully to isolate and provide a full course of antibiotic therapy to high-risk cases under direct observation (Guerin et al. 2003), while providing rehydration therapy and hygiene and sanitation education to lower-risk patients who return home.

For cholera, three types of structures have been devised to efficiently manage large numbers of patients based on the severity of illness and evolving access needs during the course of an outbreak.

Cholera Treatment Center (CTC)

This is a fully autonomous treatment site, typically with 50–300 beds, best suited for treating large numbers of the most severely affected patients, operating 24 hours a day. A CTC should have the capacity to include dedicated latrines, showers, laundry, kitchen, and morgue. Space may permit separate treatment areas for special patient populations such as pediatric and pregnant women.

Cholera Treatment Unit (CTU)

These are typically 10–20 beds, as patient load or space constraints dictate. The most severely ill are also treated here, but support services and specialty care are either not essential or provided elsewhere. Open 24 hours a day.

Oral Rehydration Point (ORP)

These are intended for decentralized care of patients with no or some dehydration requiring only oral rehydration therapy. The capacity to begin IV rehydration and stabilize severely dehydrated patients before transfer to a CTC or CTU is an added benefit. ORPs are usually open during daylight hours only. ORPs are an essential feature of any cholera response as they can manage a large majority of patients with symptomatic cholera, can be set up or taken down in a day for deployment elsewhere if access to care needs shift to other areas over time, and thereby free up resources of CTCs and CTUs to focus on more severely affected patients.

Determining Expected Number of Cases

Data from previous epidemics in the same locale will provide valuable information as to the expected number of patients, or the attack rate, and duration of the current outbreak. The attack rate is the cumulative number of clinical cases divided by the total population considered "at risk." In practical terms, the denominator is usually the total population of the village, city, camp, or district being affected.

If historic data are not available, context-specific characteristics of a cholera outbreak can be used for initial estimates and planning. Major characteristics of cholera outbreaks by environment are shown in Table 22.1.

For example, in a town of one hundred thousand people, an attack rate of two to three percent could be used to estimate that two to three thousand clinical cases could be expected during a typical outbreak. The results may be more accurate and more useful if the smallest at-risk administrative areas are used as units of estimation. For example,

Table 22.1 Typical cholera outbreak characteristics by environment

	Open setting (Rural, large scale)	Urban settings and slums	Closed setting (Refugee/IDP camp)
Population density	Low	High	High to very high
Population number	High	High	Small
Population mobility	Mobile, scattered	Mobile	Not very mobile
Attack rate (%)*	0.1–2	1–5	1–5
Peak reached after	1–3 months	2–8 weeks	2–4 weeks
Proportion of cases seen before the peak (%)	40	40	40
Epidemic duration (months)	3–6	2–4	1–3
Expected CFR*	< 5	2–5	< 2

Source: MSF
*The expected CFR and AR figures in the table are based on treatment being available.

in cities, estimating attack rates based on at-risk neighborhoods (if the population is known) rather than on the whole city can help differentiate "hot spots" from areas that have had little cholera in the past and lead to better informed resource allocation.

It is important to note that these figures are derived largely from treatment facility data and do not necessarily account for all cases in a community, where not all individuals can or need to seek medical attention. Of all patients who do present for care during an outbreak, approximately 35 percent are severely dehydrated, 30 percent have some dehydration, and the remainder diagnosed as having no dehydration. The proportion of patients with severe dehydration at the beginning of an outbreak may be higher.

Estimation of Bed Requirements

Approximately half of cholera patients seeking medical care will require admission to a CTC or CTU for at least one night for closely supervised rehydration and is essential for those needing intravenous fluid resuscitation. The length of stay in a CTC or CTU is usually from one to three or more days, depending on the severity of illness. Experience has shown that the number of beds required at the *peak* of the epidemic can be reasonably estimated using the following assumptions:

- The average length of stay is approximately 2.5 days
- At the peak of the epidemic, 15 percent of the total expected cases for the outbreak will present over a seven-day period
- 50 percent of all cases will need a bed, including all those with severe dehydration and about half of those with moderate dehydration

Using these parameters and the example above of two to three thousand expected cases, the number of beds required for the busiest week would be:

$$5\% \times (2{,}000 \text{ to } 3{,}000 \text{ patients}) \times 50\% \times (2.5 \text{ days}/7 \text{ days}) = 50 \text{ to } 80 \text{ beds required}$$

These beds could all be in a single CTC or divided between smaller CTU's strategically located for easier access by the affected communities. In practical terms, particularly when hundreds of beds might be required, peak bed capacity does not need immediate implementation, but can be built into the planning of CTC's that have space and materials for expansion.

Estimation of Fluid Requirements

While individual fluid needs can vary widely based on severity of disease, age, and body weight, the following estimates can be used for supply purposes:

- 8 liters of Ringer's Lactate (RL) and 8 liters of oral rehydration solution (ORS) for each expected patient with severe dehydration
- 8 liters of ORS for each expected patient with some dehydration
- 2 liters of ORS for each expected patient with no dehydration

ORS should not be limited to treatment facilities. Providing each patient with two to four sachets upon discharge permits both completion of treatment at home and early therapy for others in the household who become symptomatic. Community health workers or outreach teams can also distribute ORS more widely during the current outbreak or for future cases of isolated acute watery diarrhea that are so common in children. WHO and MSF recommend estimating ORS needs by counting on 10 liters per person for the entire cohort of expected patients calculated.

Community Information, Education, and Communication

Dissemination of information is a vital component of outbreak response. Regardless of the context, control efforts are likely to fall short or even be compromised within an uninformed community. Key messages include:

- The cause of the illness, such as bacteria, and its mode of transmission such as contaminated water, food, and dirty hands
- How to avoid infection and transmission through interventions including handwashing with soap, using treated water for drinking and cooking, avoidance of open defecation, and avoidance of uncooked or undercooked food
- Symptoms of infection including large volume diarrhea and vomiting or visible blood in stool and the necessary course of action if these symptoms appear
- Where to access ORS and how to use it

- Location of ORPs and higher level treatment centers including CTUs and CTCs

Disseminating information can be achieved in a multitude of ways and is most effective if several modalities are used and congruent messages are repeated regularly. Some common modalities used include:

- TV and radio spots
- Newspapers, posters, or fliers
- SMS-text messaging
- Information sessions at schools, houses of worship, or public squares
- Drama (street theater), dance, and song

Community leaders will advise on which methods, modalities, and language are most appropriate for the target audience.

Outbreak Surveillance, Monitoring, and Evaluation

Data Collection

Data collected from treatment sites and the community are used to:

- Follow the evolution of the outbreak over time
- Anticipate the needs of medical equipment and supplies and human resources
- Adjust the scale and location of curative and preventive activities as the outbreak evolves through the peak to its terminal phase
- Evaluate the performance of current preventive measures and treatment sites

The minimum requirements for the data set collected includes the number of cases, based on an agreed-upon case definition, and the number of cases who die from the illness over a 24-hour or 7-day period or epidemiologic week. Of similar importance is case origin or the number of cases domiciled in each administrative area, and age group, usually < 5 years and ≥5 years old. Each CTC, CTU, ORP or other treatment facility should be provided with a patient register, or "line list" on which to record this information for each patient diagnosed with cholera. Daily and/or weekly aggregate totals from all facilities are then provided to health authorities monitoring the global evolution of the outbreak. Collection of data on community cases and deaths may also be organized by local health authorities or by outreach workers in camp settings.

Data Analysis

Commonly used indicators for outbreaks are Weekly Incidence Rate (WIR), Attack Rate (AR), and Case Fatality Rate (CFR). The denominator for the WIR and AR is the total population of the geographic area of the outbreak such as a camp, settlement, city, district, or state/province. The denominator for the CFR is the total number of reported or confirmed cases.

Weekly Incidence Rate (WIR)

The weekly incidence rate provides information on the current intensity of the outbreak in the given population and may wax and wane as the epidemic peaks and subsides. It is described as the number of new cases during one week per one hundred or one thousand members of the population.

Attack Rate (AR)

The attack rate is the total number of cases to date since the start of the outbreak per one hundred or one thousand members of the population. The AR indicates the overall impact of the epidemic and will rise rapidly as the peak is reached before reaching a plateau. The AR can be used to compare different epidemics and for planning purposes. For example, the AR in *Shigella* epidemics tend to be higher than those typical for cholera, particularly in the camp setting (Guerin et al. 2003, Kerneis et al. 2009).

Case Fatality Rate (CFR)

The case fatality rate is the percentage of cases who die of the disease. For example, the CFR of untreated severe cholera can reach 50 percent or more, while the expected CFR for cases receiving medical care should be under one percent. The CFR can be calculated for individual treatment facilities as a measure of the quality of care. In addition, a significant number of deaths counted in the community can indicate that access to care and/or education on the disease is less than optimal.

Analyzing cases by patient origin or case mapping is also very useful for managing an evolving outbreak response. Resources such as treatment facilities and water and sanitation activities can be prioritized or reallocated to locations reporting a high number of cases. Epidemic extension can be detected as cases from new areas begin to be reported in existing facilities.

Clinical Presentation and Course

A complex humanitarian emergency may exacerbate diarrheal disease. In these settings, prompt identification and treatment of diarrheal disease is especially critical when it occurs among young children, those who are immunocompromised, and vulnerable persons who are displaced or living in refugee camps or conflict situations (Connolly et al. 2004, Das 2004, Burki 2013). Diarrheal disease deaths in humanitarian emergencies often occur in the setting of malnutrition.

Enteric diseases, many of which cause diarrhea, may be classified as endemic or epidemic prone. Diseases that are not considered to have epidemic potential are nonetheless very important to prevent, as they may occur widely among the population and be major contributors to mortality. As covered in the previous section, having surveillance in place to rapidly identify disease trends is of paramount importance.

The enteric diseases that have high epidemic potential and high mortality include cholera (*Vibrio cholerae* infection), shigellosis (particularly *Shigella dysenteriae* type 1 infection), and typhoid fever (*Salmonella* typhi infection). These pathogens are especially important in the context of complex humanitarian emergencies and in many cases are the specific causes of humanitarian emergencies (Swerdlow et al. 1997, Rosborough 2009, Shikanga et al. 2009, Barzilay et al. 2013, Morof et al. 2013). The potential for these pathogens to cause high case fatality rates in these settings has been well documented (Cartwright et al. 2013, Loharikar et al. 2013).

Endemic diarrheal diseases, by definition, are commonplace in the general population in developing countries. They may also occur in the setting of a humanitarian emergency. Diarrheal diseases may follow natural disasters or occur at increased rates because of the emergency conditions. Important endemic pathogens include rotavirus, other *Shigella spp.* such as *Shigella flexneri Cryptosporidium*, diarrheagenic *Escherichia coli*, and non-typhoidal *Salmonella*, among others.

The clinical and epidemiological features of common enteric diseases are shown in Table 22.2.

Epidemic Prone Enteric Diseases

Cholera

Cholera is an acute, diarrheal illness caused by infection with the toxigenic bacterium *Vibrio cholerae* serogroup O1 or O139. Though sporadic cases of cholera may result from ingestion of fish or shellfish from marine or riverine environments, where free-living *Vibrio cholerae* can survive in the absence of human hosts, epidemic transmission is always via the fecal-oral route. Infection results from ingestion of contaminated food and water or indirect contamination from person-to-person. Cholera causes watery diarrhea often flecked with mucous, referred to as "rice water stool," sometimes accompanied by vomiting. The signs and symptoms of cholera are produced by cholera toxin with a typical incubation period of 1–3 days. The infection is most often mild or asymptomatic, but between 5% and 10% of infected persons will have severe disease characterized by profuse watery diarrhea and vomiting that results in profound loss of fluid and electrolytes. In these people, loss of body fluids leads rapidly to leg cramps, dehydration, and shock, and death can result within hours. Cholera should be suspected when any patient over 5 years old develops severe dehydration or death from acute watery diarrhea. For surveillance purposes, in an area where there is a confirmed, ongoing outbreak of cholera, WHO and UNICEF recommend considering any patient over 5 years old with acute watery diarrhea as a suspected cholera case (UNICEF 2013). It is important to note that children under 5 years old are susceptible to cholera and must receive appropriate medical care and be recorded in health facility line lists; however, they are generally not included in surveillance.

In 2016, a cumulative total of 132,121 cases of cholera including 2,420 deaths, resulting in a CFR of 1.8 percent, were reported to WHO from 38 countries in all regions of the world (WHO 2016). Recent cholera outbreaks in Haiti, Zimbabwe, Kenya, and Cameroon have been large and protracted, with high CFRs (Barzilay et al. 2013, Cartwright et al. 2013, Loharikar et al. 2013, Morof et al. 2013). The attack rates in displaced populations can be as high as 10 to 15 percent whereas in normal situations, it is estimated at 1 to 2 percent. CFRs are usually around 5 percent but have reached 40 percent in large outbreaks in refugee camps (WHO 2003a). Cholera epidemics have occurred amid wars, conflicts, postelection violence, and natural disasters.

It is often impossible to distinguish a patient with cholera from a patient infected with other enteric pathogens that commonly cause outbreaks of acute

Table 22.2 Clinical and epidemiologic features of common enteric diseases

Category	Typical Clinical Syndrome	Epidemiologic Features
Bacteria		
Enterotoxigenic *Escherichia coli* (ETEC)	Acute watery diarrhea, afebrile, occasionally severe. Incubation: 10–12 hours. Duration: several days.	Common in developing countries, more so in children. Transmission via contaminated food (often weaning foods) and water.
Enteropathogenic *Escherichia coli* (EPEC)	Severe acute watery diarrhea, bloody diarrhea. Incubation: several hours. Duration: several days but may be persistent.	Common cause of infant diarrhea in developing countries.
Campylobacter species	Diarrhea (sometimes bloody), abdominal pain, fever, nausea, and vomiting. Incubation: 1–7 days. Duration: 1–5 days.	Small food or waterborne outbreaks or sporadic cases.
Nontyphoidal *Salmonella* species	Diarrhea, abdominal pain, chills, fever, vomiting, dehydration. Incubation: 6–72 hours. Duration: several days.	Typically foodborne.
Salmonella Typhi	Insidious onset of fever, marked headache, malaise, anorexia, abdominal pain, relative bradycardia, splenomegaly, nonproductive cough, rose spots on trunk, diarrhea (particularly in young children) or constipation (more common in adults). Incubation: 3–30 days, commonly 8–14 days.	Acquired through ingestion of food or water contaminated with feces or urine of an acutely ill person, or a convalescent or silent (chronic) carrier. Waterborne outbreaks can be very large and foodborne outbreaks are common.
Shigella species	Variable, with mild to severe symptoms. Fever common, watery stools (frequently containing blood) Incubation: 1–7 days. Duration: several days.	Main mode of transmission person-to-person, also waterborne. Transmitted easily via unwashed hands, poor hygiene.
Vibrio cholerae	Acute, profuse watery diarrhea; "rice water stools"; abdominal pain; vomiting, muscle cramps, and dehydration in severe cases; fever rare. Incubation: 2–3 days. Duration: 3–5 days untreated.	Waterborne epidemics or large foodborne outbreaks.
Viruses		
Rotavirus	Vomiting, fever, and watery diarrhea. Incubation: 1–3 days. Duration: 4–6 days.	Illness limited to young children.
Norovirus	Prominent nausea and vomiting; fever sometimes present. Incubation: 24–48 hours. Duration: up to 48 hours.	Food or waterborne or person-to-person transmission in all age groups.
Parasites		
Giardia intestinalis	Diarrhea, gas, greasy stools, abdominal cramps, bloating, nausea, dehydration; asymptomatic infections occur. Incubation: 1–3 weeks. Duration: 2–6 weeks.	Can cause waterborne, foodborne, or person-to-person outbreaks.
Cryptosporidium species	Watery diarrhea, abdominal cramps, nausea, vomiting, fever. Incubation: 1–12 days. Duration: 1–2 weeks, may be persistent/intermittent/chronic.	May cause waterborne or foodborne outbreaks; secondary person-to-person transmission common; persons with HIV/AIDS at high risk.

Source: CDC

watery diarrhea as shown in Table 25.2. While a review of the clinical and epidemiologic features of multiple patients who are part of a suspected diarrheal outbreak is always more informative than data from a single patient, laboratory confirmation of cholera is required and should be sought for other etiologies as well.

Shigella dysenteriae type 1

Shigellosis is an acute invasive enteric infection caused by bacteria belonging to the genus *Shigella*. It is clinically manifested by diarrhea that is frequently bloody. Shigellosis is endemic in many developing countries and can also occur in epidemics causing considerable morbidity and mortality. Among the four species and many serotypes of *Shigella*, *Shigella dysenteriae* type 1 (Sd1) is especially important because it causes the most severe disease and may occur in large regional epidemics.

Patients with shigellosis typically present with diarrhea characterized by the frequent passage of small liquid stools that contain visible blood, with or without mucus. Abdominal cramps and unproductive, painful straining, called tenesmus, are common. Fever and anorexia are also common, but are nonspecific. Patients may, however, present only with acute watery diarrhea without visible blood or mucus and without the other symptoms described above, especially at the beginning of their illness. If dehydration occurs, it is usually moderate in degree. In addition to transmission via the fecal-oral route through contaminated food and water, *Shigella* has a very low infectious dose and can easily be transmitted from person to person. *Shigella dysenteriae* type 1 causes bloody diarrhea often associated with fever, abdominal cramps and rectal pain. The incubation period is usually 1–3 days, but may be up to one week. Complications include sepsis, rectal prolapse, haemolytic uraemic syndrome, and seizures. Absent proper treatment, death may occur in 15 percent of hospitalized patients (WHO 2005a).

Refugees and internally displaced persons are at especially high risk for shigellosis. In the past two decades major outbreaks have occurred in Africa, South Asia, and Central America. Between 1993 and 1995, outbreaks were reported in several central and southern African countries. In 1994, an explosive outbreak among Rwandan refugees in Zaïre caused approximately twenty thousand deaths during the first month alone. Between 1999 and 2003, outbreaks were reported in Sierra Leone, Liberia, Guinea, Senegal, Angola, Burundi, the Central African Republic, and the Democratic Republic of Congo. In 2000, outbreaks of bloody diarrhea due to Sd1 strains that were resistant to fluoroquinolones occurred in India and Bangladesh (Ries et al. 1994, Guerin et al. 2003, Guerin et al. 2004, Naheed et al. 2004, Kerneis et al. 2009).

Typhoid Fever

Typhoid fever is an acute, life-threatening, febrile illness caused by the bacterium *Salmonella enterica* serovar Typhi. The incubation period is usually 8–14 days, but may be from three days to over one month. Transmission is via the fecal-oral route, mainly from ingestion of organisms in food and water contaminated by feces or urine of patients and carriers, or indirectly from person-to-person. Typhoid fever has an insidious onset characterized by fever, headache, constipation, malaise, chills, and myalgia (Parry et al. 2002). Many patients cough for the first few days of illness, and some report sore throat or joint pain. Splenomegaly, leukopenia, and abdominal distention and tenderness are generally present. Early in the illness, small, discrete, rose-colored spots caused by bacterial emboli in the skin capillaries may appear on the trunk. In adults, diarrhea is uncommon, and vomiting is not usually severe. In children, the disease presentation is often atypical, and respiratory symptoms and diarrhea are often present. Complications of typhoid fever include confusion, delirium, intestinal perforation, neurologic features, and death (Lutterloh et al. 2012, Neil, et al. 2012, Sejvar et al. 2012). Chronic carriage of *S*. Typhi, defined as fecal shedding of the organism for greater than one year after acute illness, occurs in 1–4 percent of patients.

Typhoid fever should be suspected when a patient has acute or insidious onset of sustained fever, headache, malaise, anorexia, relative bradycardia, constipation or diarrhea, and nonproductive cough. However, many mild and atypical infections occur.

Examples of recent typhoid fever outbreaks which have led to international emergency responses and severe complications occurred in Uganda in 2009 with a high rate of intestinal perforation, on the Malawi-Mozambique border with neurologic findings in 2009 (Lutterloh et al. 2012, Neil et al. 2012, Sejvar et al. 2012), and in Zimbabwe in 2011 (Imanishi et al.

2014). Typhoid fever outbreaks are not as common as other epidemic prone enteric diseases during complex humanitarian emergencies, but have been reported (Sutiono et al. 2010), and often in themselves cause an emergency state.

Diagnosis

Stool specimens should be collected in the early stages of any enteric illness, when pathogens are usually present in the stool in highest numbers and before antibiotic therapy has been started. Collect stools from patients in clean containers without disinfectant or detergent residue, with tight-fitting, leak-proof lids. Stool specimens should be refrigerated if possible and processed for culture within a maximum of 2 hours after collection. Specimens that cannot be cultured within 2 hours of collection should be placed in transport medium and stored at ambient temperature. Unlike other organisms, *Shigella* will die, even in transport media, if they are not refrigerated. It is generally recommended to place two rectal swabs containing the patient's stool into the same tube of transport medium for transport to the laboratory. Cary-Blair transport medium can be used to transport many enteric pathogens, including *Shigella, V. cholerae, S.* Typhi, *Escherichia coli,* and non-typhoidal *Salmonella*. Cary-Blair medium is stable and can be stored before use at room temperature for up to one year in tightly sealed containers. A manual for the laboratory identification and antimicrobial susceptibility testing of bacterial pathogens of public health importance in the developing world, including *Shigella, V. cholerae,* and *S.* Typhi is available online from the World Health Organization (WHO 2003b).

Diagnosis of cholera is confirmed by isolating *Vibrio cholerae* serogroup O1 or O139 from a stool specimen. Although *V. cholerae* will grow on a variety of commonly used agar media, isolation from fecal specimens is more easily accomplished with specialized media. Alkaline peptone water (APW) is recommended as an enrichment broth, and thiosulfate citrate bile salts sucrose (TCBS) agar is the selective agar medium of choice for isolating *V. cholerae*. Reagents for serogrouping *V. cholerae* isolates are available, whereby the strains are further characterized by O1 and O139 specific antisera. Strains that agglutinate in O1 antisera are further characterized as serotype Inaba or Ogawa. Enterotoxin assays such as PCR, EIA, or DNA probing are complex and beyond the scope of this chapter. Few laboratories are capable of doing these tests, and they are performed mainly by international reference laboratories. For clinical purposes, a quick presumptive diagnosis can be made by darkfield or phase microscopic visualization of the vibrios moving like "shooting stars," inhibited by preservative-free, serotype-specific antiserum. In areas with limited to no laboratory testing, *V. cholerae* rapid test kits can provide an early warning to public health officials that an outbreak of watery diarrhea is due to cholera. However, the sensitivity and specificity of available rapid tests is not optimal, and they provide no information on antimicrobial susceptibilities. Therefore, it is recommended that fecal specimens that test positive for *V. cholerae* O1 and/or O139 by rapid test kits be confirmed using traditional culture-based methods for the isolation and identification of *V. cholerae*. Commercially available rapid test kits are useful in epidemic settings but should not be used for routine diagnosis (Dick et al. 2012, Page et al. 2012). Following identification of the agent, it is appropriate for the laboratory to commence antimicrobial susceptibility testing to inform treatment recommendations. In cholera epidemics, once laboratory confirmation and antimicrobial susceptibility have been established, it is unnecessary to confirm all subsequent cases. Individuals presenting with clinical features corresponding to the clinical case definition are considered, and registered, as cholera cases. However, monitoring an epidemic should include laboratory confirmation and antimicrobial susceptibility testing of a small proportion of cases on a regular basis.

When an outbreak of dysentery occurs, laboratory analysis of a small number of adequately collected clinical specimens is sufficient to provide the diagnosis. The key is to collect the specimens properly and to transport them rapidly to a fully equipped clinical laboratory. Ten to 20 cases should be selected for sampling at each investigation site, and cases should meet all of the following criteria:

- Currently having bloody diarrhea
- Onset of illness less than 4 days before sampling
- Have not received antibiotic treatment for this illness
- Consent to give a specimen

Refrigeration during transport can be achieved for up to 36 hours by shipping in a well-insulated box with frozen refrigerant packs or wet ice.

No enrichment medium is suitable for *Shigella*. A general-purpose plating medium of low selectivity and one of moderate or high selectivity should be used. MacConkey agar is recommended as a medium of low selectivity. MacConkey agar with 1 µg/ml of potassium tellurite has been reported to be particularly useful for *S. dysenteriae* type 1. Xylose-lysine-desoxycholate (XLD) agar is recommended as a medium of moderate or high selectivity for isolation of *Shigella*. Desoxycholate citrate agar (DCA) is a suitable alternative. Salmonella-shigella (SS) agar often inhibits growth of *S. dysenteriae* type 1. Outside the body, Shigella remains viable only for a short period, so it is critical that stool specimens are processed rapidly (WHO 2005a, APHA 2015).

The most commonly used diagnostic methods for typhoid fever are bacterial culture of blood and stool, and serologic assays. *S.* Typhi is most frequently isolated from blood during the first week of illness, but it can also be isolated during the second and third weeks of illness, during the first week of antimicrobial therapy, and during clinical relapse. Bone marrow cultures may be positive in up to 90 percent of cases and are more likely to yield *S.* Typhi than are cultures from any other site, especially when the patient has already received antimicrobial therapy (APHA 2015). Because of limited sensitivity and specificity, serological tests based on agglutinating antibodies such as the Widal test, are generally of limited diagnostic value (Levine et al. 1978). Several rapid serodiagnostic assays are commercially available (Keddy et al. 2011). Serodiagnostic methods may facilitate initial clinical management of patients with suspected typhoid fever; however, they do not provide any information about antimicrobial resistance since the pathogen is not isolated. Rapid tests can be useful in evaluating the likelihood that an outbreak of febrile illness is due to typhoid fever, but follow-up cultures to isolate the strain and characterize antimicrobial susceptibility will be needed.

In the event of an epidemic of enteric disease, it is advisable to have the following supplies available at the health facility or prepositioned at the district level to facilitate diagnostic testing:

- Stool cups or other specimen containers
- Specimen transport medium
- Rectal swabs
- Gloves
- Rapid test kits

In addition, the official lines of communication with respect to where specimens should be sent for confirmation should be established before an outbreak occurs to avoid delays in testing. It is also important to ensure that reference laboratories report back the testing results to the health facility, including the antimicrobial susceptibility testing results if carried out, so that appropriate treatment decisions can be made. The principles of diagnostic preparedness for epidemics of typhoid fever are generally the same but would also require supplies for collecting blood for bacteriologic culture and serologic testing.

Treatment

Good case management for diarrhea can save many lives. Appropriate treatment for diarrheal disease should begin in the home; thus, training caretakers in home-based management and in recognizing the danger signs of diarrhea that mandate a visit to the health facility, can be lifesaving. Community health workers (CHWs) can play a significant role in detecting, assessing, and treating diarrheal disease in the community and in individual households. As CHWs often live in the community where they work, they are the frontline health workers. They are the first to notice any trends and to influence early case management of patients. They can be essential in saving lives in an emergency, such as a cholera outbreak, where time is critical. CHWs can see patients through their routine services, including integrated community case management (iCCM) through house-to-house visits or during an outbreak. Two recent advances in managing diarrheal disease can drastically reduce the number of child deaths: the newly formulated ORS solution, containing lower concentrations of glucose and salts to prevent dehydration and the need for intravenous therapy; and, zinc supplementation to decrease the duration and severity of diarrhea and the likelihood of future diarrhea episodes in the two to three months following supplementation. For children under 5 years old, diarrhea causes loss of zinc that must be replaced. As the first point of contact in areas where treatment facilities don't exist or are very far away, CHWs can identify acute watery diarrhea and signs of dehydration, and treat mild forms of cholera and other diarrheal diseases by rehydrating the patient with ORS and providing zinc. In addition, CHWs can save lives by starting rehydration early and transferring critically ill patients in need of higher level medical attention to a referral treatment facility (UNICEF 2013).

Recent declining trends in ORS use in some countries highlights the need for commercially available ORS to be promoted widely in the community and for caretakers and health care providers to be trained in its use, as it is one of the simplest and most affordable public health innovations for saving lives.

The most important components of diarrheal disease treatment are to prevent dehydration from occurring, to treat dehydration quickly if it does occur, to give zinc supplements for 10–14 days depending on the availability of supplies and national policy, and to continue feeding children who have diarrhea. The best treatment for dehydration is oral therapy with a solution made with commercial ORS. In the past, homemade sugar salt solutions may have been used in the community for rehydration; however, this practice should be discouraged. This is because preparing the correct ratio of sugar to salt in the appropriate volume of safe water is often not feasible, especially in the context of a complex emergency, and if incorrect quantities are mixed it can cause worsening of symptoms.

For children under 5 years old, the recommendations for treating dehydration from diarrhea are according to Integrated Management of Childhood Illnesses (IMCI) guidelines (WHO 2014b). Under the IMCI guidelines, children are treated for dehydration based on the severity of their dehydration, with specific treatment plans for children with diarrhea and no dehydration, some dehydration defined as two of the following: restless/irritable, sunken eyes, drinks eagerly/thirsty, skin pinch goes back slowly, and severe dehydration defined as two of the following: lethargic/unconscious, sunken eyes, not able to drink or drinking poorly, skin pinch goes back very slowly. ORS, zinc supplements for age 2 months to 5 years, and continued feeding are recommended, with intravenous (IV) fluid started immediately for children with severe diarrhea.

Antibiotics are not effective against most diarrhea-causing organisms, and many enteric pathogens are resistant to commonly used antimicrobials. Antibiotics are only recommended for treatment of bloody diarrhea, episodes of cholera with severe dehydration or moderate progressive dehydration, and typhoid fever as shown in Table 22.3 (WHO 2005a, WHO 2005b). Bloody diarrhea is a clinical diagnosis that refers to any diarrheal episode in which the loose or watery stools contain visible red blood. All cases of bloody diarrhea should be treated promptly with an antimicrobial that is known to be effective against *Shigella*. This lessens the risk of serious complications and death, shortens the duration of symptoms, and hastens the elimination of *Shigella* from the stool. The choice of antimicrobial should, if possible, be based on recent susceptibility data from *Shigella* strains isolated in the area. Ciprofloxacin is now the drug of choice for all patients with bloody diarrhea, irrespective of their age, although ciprofloxacin-resistant strains of *Shigella* have occasionally been reported. Adsorbents such as kaolin, pectin, and activated charcoal are not useful for treatment of acute diarrhea, and antimotility drugs such as tincture of opium or loperamide may be harmful, especially in children under five years of age (WHO 2005a, WHO 2005b). Some common antibiotic choices for selected enteric diseases are shown in Table 22.3.

Cholera

Most persons infected with cholera have mild diarrhea or no symptoms. Less than 10 percent of persons infected with *Vibrio cholerae* O1 have illness requiring treatment at a health center (Swerdlow et al. 1994,

Table 22.3 Antibiotic treatment choices for selected enteric diseases

Indication	Agent	Antibiotic of Choice for Empiric Treatment*
Bloody diarrhea	*Shigella dysenteriae* type 1	Ciprofloxacin (irrespective of age)
Cholera	*Vibrio cholerae*	Doxycycline (adults)
		Azithromycin (children and pregnant women)
Typhoid Fever	*Salmonella* Typhi	Fluoroquinolones (e.g. ciprofloxacin)
		Alternative: third-generation cephalosporins (e.g., ceftriaxone, cefotaxime), a monobactum beta-lactam (aztreonam) and a macrolide (azithromycin).

*Where possible, use antimicrobial susceptibility testing to inform treatment choices.

Jackson et al. 2013). Rehydration is the first priority in the treatment of cholera. Early detection and management of cases at the community level can ensure rapid initiation of rehydration therapy and save lives. It is critical to identify and treat all those with symptomatic cholera. With appropriate case management, with ORS in most cases, the CFR from cholera should remain below 1 percent. At the beginning of an outbreak, when care-seeking may be delayed and before appropriate treatment facilities are established, the CFR may be higher. However, within a very short time, the CFR should be reduced to less than 1 percent, which is the well-established target standard for cholera control, although for some groups, such as those compromised by underlying conditions such as HIV/AIDS or malnutrition, it might remain higher (UNICEF 2013). Patients with severe dehydration, stupor, coma, uncontrollable vomiting, or extreme fatigue that prevents drinking should be rehydrated intravenously. The best option for IV fluids for cholera treatment is Ringer's Lactate Solution. Normal saline is acceptable in an emergency but will not correct acidosis and may worsen the electrolyte imbalance. Plain glucose (dextrose) solution is unacceptable (MSPP/CDC 2010).

Antibiotics can reduce the volume and duration of cholera-related diarrhea and decrease the period of shedding. They are indicated in all cholera patients with severe dehydration, may be given to patients with moderate dehydration and progressive fluid losses, and should be administered in the first four hours (Nelson et al. 2011). The administration of antibiotics to cholera patients with moderate or severe dehydration can help reduce the patient load in health facilities or cholera treatment centers which may be overtaxed during an epidemic. The choice of antibiotic should be based on drug-resistance patterns from cholera cultures performed early in an outbreak. While awaiting results of drug sensitivity testing, patients may receive doxycycline. If drug sensitivity testing shows tetracycline resistance, these patients do not need to be offered another course of a different antibiotic; however, the results of drug sensitivity testing should be used inform future empiric treatment choices. In the context of a cholera epidemic, the usual contraindications for certain antibiotics such as doxycycline in children and pregnant women are relative, particularly if administered as a single dose. It is important to check the national recommendations. Antibiotics are not recommended for mass prophylaxis. Preventive therapy for contacts of cholera patients is also not recommended, except in specific contexts, such as outbreaks in prisons or orphanages. In the context of a cholera epidemic, zinc is indicated for all patients under 5 years old presenting with diarrhea, regardless of dehydration status. For breastfed infants, breastfeeding should continue even during the rehydration phase. Older children and adults can continue an unrestricted normal diet. For pregnant women, young children, and children with severe malnutrition, the principles of cholera management are in evolution (Ververs and Narra). Some groups may have recommended alternative regimens for these special populations. Common antibiotic choices are shown in Table 22.3.

Typhoid Fever

Typhoid fever is treated with antibiotics. Resistance to multiple antibiotics is increasing among *Salmonella* that cause typhoid fever. Reduced susceptibility to fluoroquinolones including ciprofloxacin and the emergence of multidrug-resistance has complicated treatment of infections, especially those acquired in South Asia. Antibiotic susceptibility testing may help guide appropriate therapy. Choices for antibiotic therapy include fluoroquinolones for susceptible infections, ceftriaxone, and azithromycin. Common antibiotic choices are shown in Table 22.3. Persons who do not get treatment may continue to have fever for weeks or months, and as many as 20 percent may die from complications of the infection (APHA 2015).

The prepositioning of emergency stocks of critical treatment supplies for epidemic prone enteric diseases at the health facility or district level can assist in saving lives at the onset of an outbreak. Treatment supplies should be monitored at health facilities via inventories, with the key principle of avoiding supply shortages. Having adequate emergency stocks of ORS, zinc, IV fluids, needles, and tubing for pediatric and adult patients, and appropriate antimicrobials is advisable. In addition, chlorine for water treatment or other means of making water safe for mixing ORS, and soap for handwashing are essential in all treatment facilities. Guidelines for the contents of treatment kits to treat one hundred patients with cholera and *Shigella dysenteriae* type 1 are available (WHO 1993, WHO 2005a). Oral rehydration therapy corners should be established in health facilities for use during routine and emergency diarrhea case management.

Notes from the Field

Zimbabwe (2008)

Cholera was first reported in Zimbabwe in 1992. Since 1998, when over 5,500 cases were seen, cholera was reported annually in the country. A common feature of these outbreaks was their occurrence in communities bordering neighboring cholera-endemic countries. Concurrently, Zimbabwe entered into a period of marked economic hardship that left clinics and hospitals with poorly paid staff and severe material shortages. By 2006, in the capital region of Harare, parts of the municipal water system began to fall into disrepair. Chlorine shortages, damaged pipes, and periods of low pressure caused cross-contamination of water and sewage lines, while some neighborhoods relied on hand-dug shallow wells for domestic water supply.

In August 2008, a concentrated cholera outbreak was reported in Chitungwiza, a high-density "dormitory" suburb 30 kilometers to the south of Harare. Over four weeks, 118 patients were treated before the outbreak subsided. However, by November, cases began appearing in Harare City and again in Chitungwiza, with case fatality rates of ≥ 15 percent, while new foci of cholera arose in rural areas to the north and south. As the year came to an end, cholera had spread to all ten provinces of Zimbabwe, with nearly thirty thousand cases and 1,561 deaths. By the end of the epidemic in June 2009, more than 98 thousand cases and 4,288 deaths had been reported, one of the largest and deadliest cholera outbreaks ever recorded in Africa. This outbreak is shown in Figures 22.3, 23.4, and 22.5.

By the time we arrived in Harare, the city was experiencing approximately five hundred cases per week, down from the nearly four thousand cases reported during the first two weeks of the epidemic. For the country at large, however, the situation was far from under control, with the weekly caseload rising from nearly four thousand to over eight thousand during the month, including over three hundred deaths.

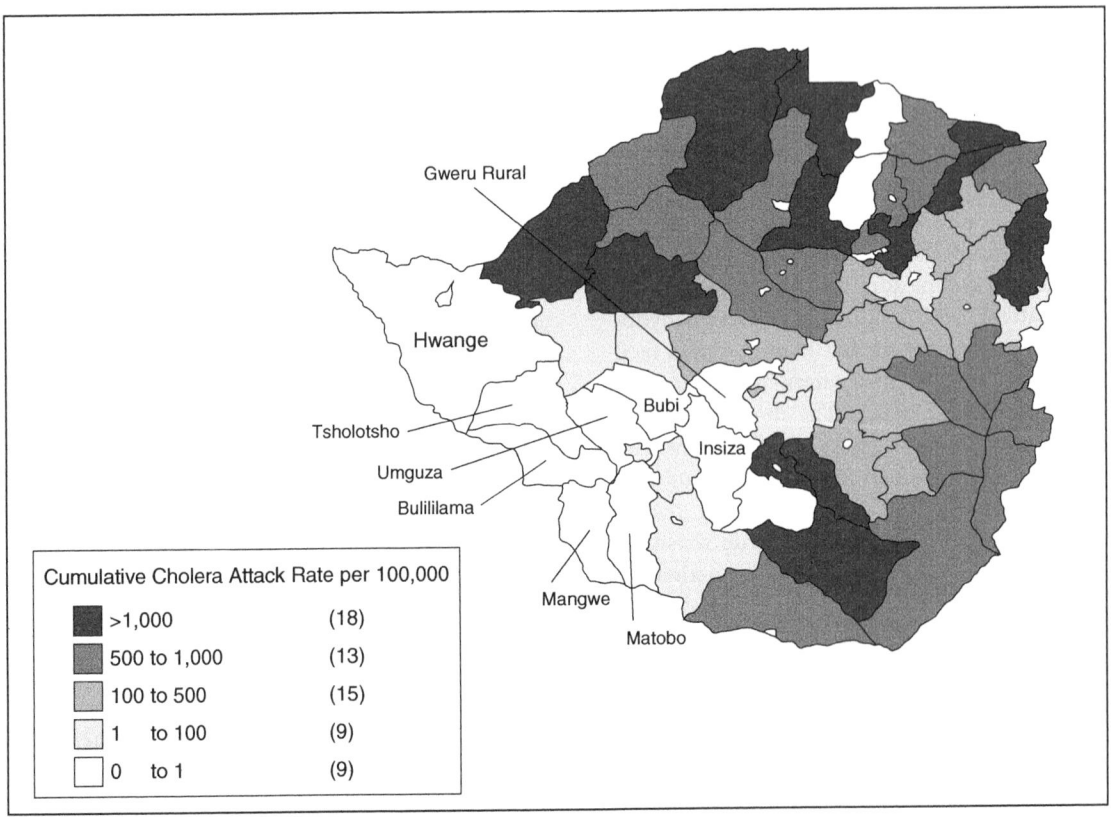

Figure 22.3 Cholera attack rates by district, Zimbabwe, August 17, 2008–May 23, 2009
Source: WHO. Reference: Epidemiological Bulletin Number 24 – Week 21 (17–23 May 2009)
Source: Epidemiological Bulletin Number 24 – Week 21 (17–23 May 2009)

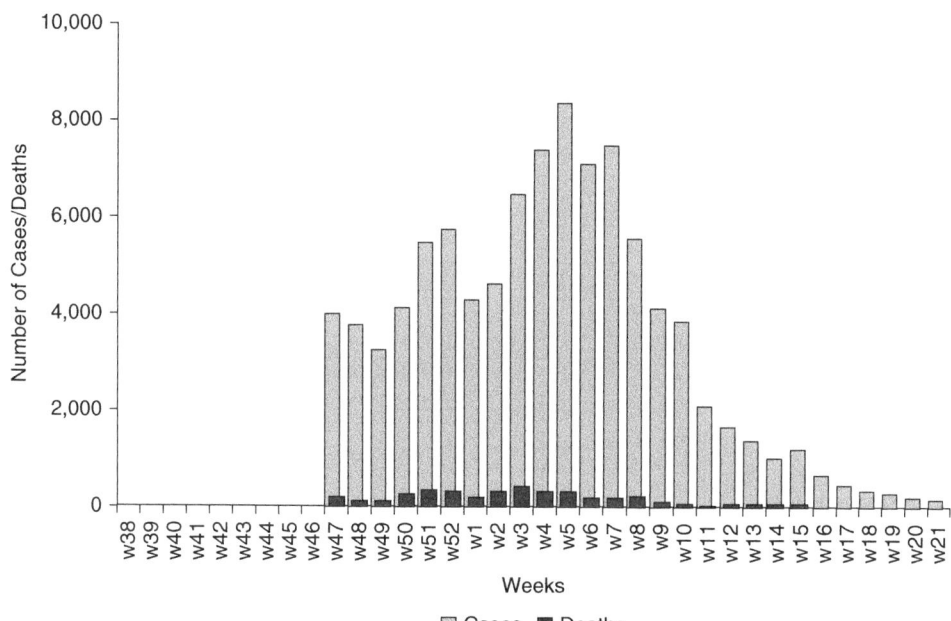

Figure 22.4 Cholera cases and deaths by epidemiologic week, Zimbabwe, August 17, 2008–May 23, 2009
Source: WHO

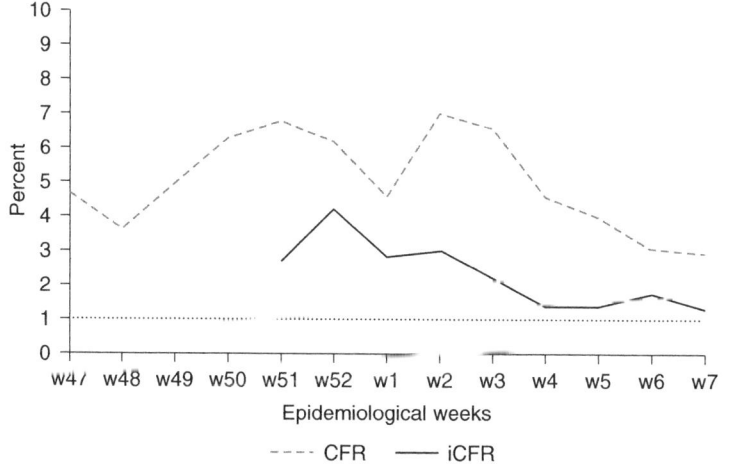

Figure 22.5 Institutional case fatality rate (iCFR) and overall case fatality rate (CFR) by epidemiologic week, Zimbabwe, November 16, 2008–February 14, 2009
Source: WHO

Harare itself exemplified several of the realities of cholera epidemics in an urban setting. First, the risk of cholera transmission is quite heterogeneous from one neighborhood to the next. In a city of nearly two million people, the final global attack rate was approximately ten per one thousand inhabitants. A postepidemic analysis revealed that individual neighborhood attack rates varied from 1 to 90 per 1,000 (Luque Fernandez et al. 2011), with most cases arising from the high-density, poorer southern sections. As planning a response to an outbreak involves estimating the number of cases that might be expected, for bed capacity, staffing needs, and treatment supplies, and their location, to maximize accessibility for the most affected population, prediction is important, but not always easy. Historic data is especially helpful here, particularly if broken down by city section or neighborhood and applied to the most current population data, but the city of Harare had been cholera-free for many years. In the end, one can estimate best-case and worst-case scenarios, and build Cholera Treatment Centers (CTCs) that are expandable to provide more bed space; extra supplies can be held in reserve and deployed at short notice.

Fortunately, two of the three existing hospitals that served as CTCs in Harare were located in or near the hardest hit neighborhoods, easing access for those patients. Erecting CTCs in a city often entails substantial negotiations with local government and communities. Space for a typical CTC of 50–300 beds that is not too close to dwellings or waterways may be difficult to find. Sports fields have been used but people don't like the idea of cholera being in a place they will subsequently use socially even if it poses almost no risk. Angry protests have occurred. School grounds have also been used, but closing schools to treat cholera is in general not a good policy. By default, existing hospitals are sometimes temporarily converted to CTCs, as occurred in this outbreak. While logical, it also can be problematic for several reasons. First, it often means that patients needing treatment for other conditions are displaced or no longer admitted and the majority of healthcare providers are shifted to only cholera care, with obvious consequences. Second, hospitals are fixed structures that are often not configured to best cope with handling the demands of a CTC: high-volume patient flow from triage to acute care to exit, while managing large quantities of contaminated waste on floors, beds, and in buckets, avoiding inadvertent infection of staff and visitors (one visitor per bed please!), and keeping controlled-entry "clean areas" for ORS and food preparation, supply storage, and staff changing rooms.

These challenges were also observed as we headed east toward the border with Mozambique. Few communities were spared the reach of the epidemic and they were coping with any means at their disposal. Given the extent of the outbreak, there was neither the manpower nor materials to construct cholera-specific treatment facilities with their special beds, waste management, and intensive hygiene practices. From small health posts to rural hospitals with in-patient wards, health staff was doing the best with what they had.

Other challenges were faced in coping with the epidemic. Commercial ORS in powder form, packaged in sachets for dilution in 1 liter of water, had been put on a list of drugs requiring prescription in Zimbabwe, meaning that ORS could only be obtained from medical or paramedical personnel. Household use of sugar-salt solution for rehydration had been high, but due to the economic collapse these commodities were either not available or affordable to most Zimbabweans. It took weeks for ORS to be taken off the medication list so that it could be made widely available for immediate use in homes and communities at the first sign of cholera.

Additionally, as is the case in countries across the world, Zimbabwe is home to certain communities whose beliefs prohibit them from accepting health care. Many patients died of cholera in these communities and it is believed that they may also have contributed to cholera transmission. Some mothers, against the community leader's orders, would bring their children for treatment under cover of the darkness and then return back to their communities.

The Zimbabwe epidemic was not confined to its borders. Cholera cases appeared in Zambia, South Africa, and Mozambique as well, though the extent of spread in these neighboring countries was fortunately limited. Due to the economic crisis, many Zimbabweans were trying to migrate to neighboring countries. At many border-crossing points, people were delayed and small, informal groups of people accumulated, without access to any water, sanitation, or hygiene facilities. Cholera attack rates in these areas were often very high. In one example, on the border with South Africa, the local epidemiological office identified at least seven people who were infected by one person with cholera who was selling fruit at a border crossing market. Great efforts were made by the government of South Africa and other countries to provide drinking water, handwashing points, and sanitation at these locations, especially at bus stations and markets.

In the end, the cholera epidemic coursed through virtually all of Zimbabwe over the better part of a year, resulting in one of the largest single-country outbreaks ever recorded on the continent. Humanitarian emergencies are vulnerable to the arrival of devastating diarrheal disease outbreaks. But sometimes the epidemic *is* the humanitarian emergency, and the context in which it was born was not rendered vulnerable by the sudden strike of an earthquake, hurricane, or tsunami, or the social collapse of armed conflict. This cholera epidemic was years in the making as political and economic chaos slowly chipped away at infrastructure and services until only the right spark was needed.

References

APHA. (2015). *Control of communicable diseases manual: An official report of the American Public Health Association.* American Public Health Association, Washington, DC.

Azman, A. S., Luquero. F. J., and Rodrigues, A., et al. (2012). Urban cholera transmission hotspots and their implications for reactive vaccination: evidence from Bissau city, Guinea Bissau. *PLoS Neglected Tropical Diseases* 6, e1901.

Barzilay. E. J., Schaad. N., and Magloire. R., et al. (2013). Cholera surveillance during the Haiti epidemic–the first 2 years. *New England Journal of Medicine* 368, 599–609.

Bhattacharya, S. K., Sur D., and Ali, M., et al. (2013). 5 year efficacy of a bivalent killed whole-cell oral cholera vaccine in Kolkata, India: a cluster-randomised, double-blind, placebo-controlled trial. *The Lancet Infectious Diseases* 13, 1050–1056.

Boccia, D., Guthmann, J. P., and Klovstad, H., et al. (2006). High mortality associated with an outbreak of hepatitis E among displaced persons in Darfur, Sudan. *Clinical Infectious Diseases* 42, 1679–1684.

Burki, T. (2013). Infectious diseases in Malian and Syrian conflicts. *The Lancet Infectious Diseases* 13, 296–297.

Cartwright, E. J., Patel, M. K., Mbopi-Keou, F. X., et al. (2013). Recurrent epidemic cholera with high mortality in Cameroon: persistent challenges 40 years into the seventh pandemic. *Epidemiology and Infection* 141, 2083–2093.

CDC. (1994). Health status of displaced persons following Civil War–Burundi, December 1993–January 1994. *Morbidity & Mortality Weekly Report* 43, 701–703.

Colindres, R. E., Jain, S., Bowen, A., Mintz, E., and Domond, P. (2007). After the flood: An evaluation of in-home drinking water treatment with combined flocculent-disinfectant following Tropical Storm Jeanne – Gonaives, Haiti, 2004. *Journal of Water and Health* 5, 367–374.

Connolly, M. A., Gayer, M., Ryan, M. J., Salama, P., Spiegel, P., and Heymann. D. L. (2004). Communicable diseases in complex emergencies: impact and challenges. *The Lancet* 364, 1974–1983.

Das, P. (2004). Aid agencies facing health catastrophe in Darfur. *The Lancet Infectious Diseases* 4, 536.

Dick, M. H., Guillerm, M., Moussy, F., and Chaignat, C. L. (2012). Review of two decades of cholera diagnostics–how far have we really come? *PLoS Neglected Tropical Diseases* 6, e1845.

Estrada-Garcia, T. and Mintz, E. D. (1996). Cholera: Foodborne Transmission and Its Prevention. *European Journal of Epidemiology* 12: 461–469.

Fischer Walker, C. L., Perin, J., Aryee, M. J., Boschi-Pinto, C., and Black, R. E. (2012). Diarrhea incidence in low- and middle-income countries in 1990 and 2010: a systematic review. *BMC Public Health* 12, 220.

Goma Epidemiology Group. (1995). Public health impact of Rwandan refugee crisis: what happened in Goma, Zaire, in July, 1994? *The Lancet* 345, 339–344.

Griffith, D. C., Kelly-Hope, L. A., Miller, and M. A. (2006). Review of reported cholera outbreaks worldwide, 1995–2005. *American Journal of Tropical Medicine and Hygiene* 75, 973–977.

Guerin, P. J., Brasher, C., and Baron. E., et al. (2003). Shigella dysenteriae serotype 1 in west Africa: intervention strategy for an outbreak in Sierra Leone. *The Lancet* 362, 705–706.

Guerin, P. J., Brasher, C., and Baron, E., et al. (2004). Case management of a multidrug-resistant Shigella dysenteriae serotype 1 outbreak in a crisis context in Sierra Leone, 1999–2000. *Transactions of the Royal Society of Tropical Medicine & Hygiene* 98, 635–643.

Guevart, E., Solle, J., Noeske, J., Amougou, G., Mouangue, A., and Fouda, A. B. (2005). Mass antibiotic prophylaxis against cholera in the New Bell central prison in Douala during the 2004 epidemic. *Sante* 15: 225–227.

Gunnlaugsson, G., Einarsdottir, J., Angulo, F. J., Mentambanar, S. A., Passa, A., and Tauxe, R. V. (1998). Funerals during the 1994 cholera epidemic in Guinea-Bissau, West Africa: the need for disinfection of bodies of persons dying of cholera. *Epidemiology & Infection* 120, 7–15.

Imanishi, M., Kweza, P. F., and Slayton, R. B., et al. (2014). Household water treatment uptake during a public health response to a large typhoid fever outbreak in Harare, Zimbabwe. *American Journal of Tropical Medicine and Hygiene* 90, 945–954.

Jackson, B. R., Talkington, D. F., and Pruckler, J. M. et al. (2013). Seroepidemiologic survey of epidemic cholera in Haiti to assess spectrum of illness and risk factors for severe disease. *American Journal of Tropical Medicine and Hygiene* 89, 654–664.

Keddy, K. H., Sooka, A., Letsoalo, M. E., Hoyland, G., Chaignat, C. L., Morrissey, A. B., and Crump, J. A. (2011). Sensitivity and specificity of typhoid fever rapid antibody tests for laboratory diagnosis at two sub-Saharan African sites. *Bulletin of the World Health Organization* 89, 640–647.

Kerneis, S., Guerin, P. J., von Seidlein, L., Legros, D., and Grais, R. F. (2009). A look back at an ongoing problem: Shigella dysenteriae type 1 epidemics in refugee settings in Central Africa (1993–1995). *PLoS One* 4, e4494.

Kotloff, K. L., Nataro, J. P., and Blackwelder, W. C., et al. (2013). Burden and aetiology of diarrhoeal disease in infants and young children in developing countries (the Global Enteric Multicenter Study, GEMS): A prospective, case-control study. *The Lancet* 382, 209–222.

Lantagne, D. and Clasen, T. (2012). Point-of-use water treatment in emergency. *Waterlines* 31, 30–52.

Lantagne, D. S. (2008). Sodium hypochlorite dosage for household and emergency water treatment. *Journal of the American Water Works Association* **100**, 106–119.

Lantagne, D. S. (2008). CDC safe water system experience in developing countries during emergency situations. *Water Conditioning & Purification*.

Levine, M. M., Cohen, D., Green, M., Levine, O.S., and Mintz, E. D. (1999). Fly control and shigellosis. *Lancet* **353**, 1020.

Levine, M. M., Grados, O., Gilman, R. H., Woodward, W. E., Solis-Plaza, R., and Waldman, W. (1978). Diagnostic value of the Widal test in areas endemic for typhoid fever. *American Journal of Tropical Medicine and Hygiene* **27**, 795–800.

Liu, L., Johnson, H. L., Cousens, S., et al. (2012). Global, regional, and national causes of child mortality: an updated systematic analysis for 2010 with time trends since 2000. *The Lancet* **379**, 2151–2161.

Loharikar, A., Briere, E., Ope, M., et al. (2013). A national cholera epidemic with high case fatality rates–Kenya 2009. *Journal of Infectious Diseases* **208** Suppl 1, S69–77.

Luque Fernandez, M. A., Mason, P. R., Gray, H., Bauernfeind, A., Fesselet, J. F., and Maes, P. (2011). Descriptive spatial analysis of the cholera epidemic 2008–2009 in Harare, Zimbabwe: A secondary data analysis. *Transactions of the Royal Society of Tropical Medicine & Hygiene* **105**, 38–45.

Luquero, F. J., Banga, C. N., Remartinez, D., Palma, P. P., Baron, E., and Grais, R. F. (2011). Cholera epidemic in Guinea-Bissau (2008): the importance of "place". *PLoS One* **6**, e19005.

Luquero, F. J., Grout, L., Ciglenecki, I., et al. (2014). Use of Vibrio cholerae vaccine in an outbreak in Guinea. *New England Journal of Medicine* **370**, 2111–2120.

Lutterloh, E., Likaka, A., Sejvar, J., et al. (2012). Multidrug-resistant typhoid fever with neurologic findings on the Malawi-Mozambique border. *Clinical Infectious Diseases* **54**, 1100–1106.

Moore, P. S., Marfin, A. A., Quenemoen, L. E., et al. (1993). Mortality rates in displaced and resident populations of central Somalia during 1992 famine. *The Lancet* **341**, 935–938.

Morof, D., Cookson, S. T., Laver, S., et al. (2013). Community mortality from cholera: urban and rural districts in Zimbabwe. *American Journal of Tropical Medicine and Hygiene* **88**, 645–650.

MSF. (1997). *Refugee health: An approach to emergency situations*. Macmillan Education, Oxford, UK.

MSPP/CDC. (2010). *Haiti cholera training manual: A short course for healthcare providers*. Ministry of Public Health and Population Haiti/Centers for Disease Control and Prevention Atlanta, GA.

Naheed, A., Kalluri, P., Talukder, K. A., et al. (2004). Fluoroquinolone-resistant Shigella dysenteriae type 1 in northeastern Bangladesh. *Lancet Infectious Diseases* **4**, 607–608.

Neil, K. P., Sodha, S. V., Lukwago, L., et al. (2012). A large outbreak of typhoid fever associated with a high rate of intestinal perforation in Kasese District, Uganda, 2008–2009. *Clinical Infectious Diseases* **54**, 1091–1099.

Nelson, E. J., Nelson, D. S., Salam, M. A., and Sack, D. A. (2011). Antibiotics for both moderate and severe cholera. *New England Journal of Medicine* **364**, 5–7.

Oxfam. (2012). *Cholera outbreak guidelines: Preparedness, prevention and control*. Oxfam GB, Oxford, UK.

Page, A. L., Alberti, K. P., Mondonge, V., Rauzier, J., Quilici, M. L., and Guerin, P. J. (2012). Evaluation of a rapid test for the diagnosis of cholera in the absence of a gold standard. *PLoS One* **7**, e37360.

Parry, C. M., Hien, T. T., Dougan, G., White, N. J., and Farrar, J. J. (2002). Typhoid fever. *New England Journal of Medicine* **347**, 1770–1782.

Qadri, F., Khan, A. I., Faruque, A. S., et al. (2005). Enterotoxigenic Escherichia coli and Vibrio cholerae diarrhea, Bangladesh, 2004. *Emerging Infectious Diseases* **11**, 1104–1107.

Ries, A. A., Wells, J. G., Olivola, D., et al. (1994). Epidemic Shigella dysenteriae type 1 in Burundi: panresistance and implications for prevention. *Journal of Infectious Diseases* **169**, 1035–1041.

Robertson, R. C. and Pollitzer, R. (1939). Cholera in Central China During 1938 – Its Epidemiology and Control *Transactions of the Royal Society of Tropical Medicine & Hygiene* **XXXIII**, 213–232.

Rosborough, S. (2009). World update: cholera crisis in Zimbabwe. *Disaster Medicine & Public Health Preparedness* **3**, 11.

Schuller, M. and Levey, T. (2014). Kabrit ki gen twop met: Understanding gaps in WASH services in Haiti's IDP camps. *Disasters* **38** Suppl 1, S1–S24.

Sejvar, J., Lutterloh, E., Naiene, J., et al. (2012). Neurologic manifestations associated with an outbreak of typhoid fever, Malawi–Mozambique, 2009: an epidemiologic investigation. *PLoS One* **7**, e46099.

Shikanga, O. T., Mutonga, D., Abade, M., et al. (2009). High mortality in a cholera outbreak in western Kenya after post-election violence in 2008. *American Journal of Tropical Medicine and Hygiene* **81**, 1085–1090.

Shultz, A., Omollo, J. O., Burke, H., et al. (2009). Cholera outbreak in Kenyan refugee camp: risk factors for illness and importance of sanitation. *American Journal of Tropical Medicine & Hygiene* **80**, 640–645.

Sphere Project. (2004). *Humanitarian charter and minimum standards in disaster response.* The Sphere Project, Geneva, Switzerland.

Sumner, S. A., Turner, E. L., and Thielman, N. M. (2013). Association between earthquake events and cholera outbreaks: a cross-country 15-year longitudinal analysis. *Prehospital & Disaster Medicine* 28, 567–572.

Sutiono, A. B., Qiantori, A., Suwa, H., and Ohta, T. (2010). Characteristics and risk factors for typhoid fever after the tsunami, earthquake and under normal conditions in Indonesia. *BMC Research Notes* 3: 106.

Swerdlow, D. L., Malenga, G., Begkoyian, G., et al. (1997) Epidemic cholera among refugees in Malawi, Africa: treatment and transmission. *Epidemiology and Infection* 118, 207–214.

Swerdlow, D. L., Mintz, E. D., Rodriguez, M., et al. (1994). Severe life-threatening cholera associated with blood group O in Peru: implications for the Latin American epidemic. *Journal of Infectious Diseases* 170, 468–472.

UNICEF. (2013). UNICEF Cholera Toolkit UNICEF, New York, NY.

Ververs, M. and Narra, R. (2017). Treating cholera in severely malnourished children in the Horn of Africa and Yemen. *Lancet* 390, 1945–1946. http://dx.doi.org/10.1016/S0140-6736(17)32601-6.

World Health Organization. (1993). *Guidelines for cholera control.* World Health Organization: Geneva, Switzerland.

World Health Organization. (2003a). *Communicable disease toolkit: Case management of epidemic-prone diseases: Iraq.* World Health Organization: Geneva, Switzerland.

World Health Organization. (2003b). *Manual for the laboratory identification and antimicrobial susceptibility testing of bacterial pathogens of public health importance in the developing world.* World Health Organization: Geneva, Switzerland. Available at: http://apps.who.int/medicinedocs/documents/s16330e/s16330e.pdf.

World Health Organization. (2005a). *Guideline for the control of Shigellosis including epidemics due to Shigella dysenteriae type 1.* World Health Organization: Geneva, Switzerland.

World Health Organization. (2005b). *Diarrhoea treatment guidelines for clinic-based healthcare workers.* World Health Organization: Geneva, Switzerland.

World Health Organization. (2014). *Integrated management of childhood illness: Chart booklet.* World Health Organization: Geneva, Switzerland.

World Health Organization. (2016). Cholera, 2016. *Weekly Epidemiological Record* 92, 521–536.

World Health Organization. (2017). Meeting of the Strategic Advisory Group of Experts on immunization (April 2017) – conclusions and recommendations. *Weekly Epidemiological Record.* 92(22), 301–320.

Yee, E. L., Palacio, H., Atmar, R. L., et al. (2007). Widespread outbreak of norovirus gastroenteritis among evacuees of Hurricane Katrina residing in a large "megashelter" in Houston, Texas: Lessons learned for prevention. *Clinical Infectious Diseases* 44, 032–1039.

Yip, R. and Sharp, T. W. (1993). Acute malnutrition and high childhood mortality related to diarrhea. Lessons from the 1991 Kurdish refugee crisis. *The Journal of the American Medical Association* 270, 587–590.

Chapter 23

HIV

Kevin R. Clarke and Nathan Ford

Introduction

The human immunodeficiency virus (HIV) pandemic has seen significant changes over the last two decades. When HIV was first identified as the causative agent responsible for acquired immune deficiency syndrome (AIDS) in 1984, little was known about how to prevent and treat the disease (Barré-Sinoussi et al. 1983, Gallo, et al. 1984, Levy et al. 1984). HIV destroys the host immune system, leaving the infected individual susceptible to a host of infections and comorbidities that if untreated will lead to death. Early on in the pandemic, people developing symptoms, typically opportunistic infections such as tuberculosis (TB), cryptococcal meningitis or Kaposi sarcoma, would have less than one year to live.

From the late 1990s onwards, the availability of effective treatment, antiretroviral therapy (ART), and highly active antiretroviral therapy (HAART), completely changed the prognosis. The scaling up of antiretroviral therapy is estimated to have averted an estimated 4.2 million deaths in low- and middle-income countries between 2002 and 2012 (WHO 2013). People living with HIV today can, with good adherence to timely treatment, expect to live a near-normal life expectancy, in both high- and low-income settings. In South Africa, for example, life expectancy of HIV-infected adults receiving ART is about 80 percent of the normal life expectancy, provided people start treatment before advanced immunosuppression, defined as a CD4 count greater than 200 cells/μl (Johnson 2013).

Effective prevention methods are also available today that have helped reduce the global incidence of new infections. The number of people acquiring HIV infection globally declined by 20 per cent between 2001 and 2011 (WHO 2013).

Many of the early developments for treating HIV were developed in Western settings, using a highly-individualized approach that required specialized health staff and multiple laboratory investigations and therapeutic options. However, such an individualized approach was inappropriate to responding to the needs of the majority of people living with and dying from HIV who lived in resource-limited settings (Gilks et al. 2006).

In 2003, the World Health Organization (WHO) launched guidelines for scaling up ART in resource-limited settings (WHO 2004). These guidelines were framed within the context of a public health approach to HIV, and aimed to simplify and standardize the number of drugs and diagnostics needed to manage patients with HIV. Subsequent WHO guidelines have continued to promote ways to simplify care without compromising quality. Today the majority of HIV care can be delivered by nurses in the form of a single, daily treatment (WHO 2016).

The public health approach to managing HIV/AIDS is supportive of responding to the disease in the context of humanitarian emergencies. Initially however, interagency guidelines for response in humanitarian emergencies recommended against providing HIV treatment in emergency and postemergency settings (Griffiths and Ford 2013). Now it is recognized that providing HIV treatment should be part of the minimum package of care for people affected by crisis (UNHCR 2014).

Epidemiology, Risk Factors, and Transmission

Globally in 2016, 36.7 million people were estimated to be living with HIV. Prevalence is higher in low-income settings, and highest in southern Africa, where in some countries in the general adult population HIV prevalence exceeds 20 per cent. The high prevalence of TB in many of these countries further contributes to high excess mortality among people living with HIV as TB is a common coinfection among people living with HIV and remains a leading cause of hospitalization, illness, and death.

Disruption of health services in the context of humanitarian emergencies reduces access to treatment and care for people living with HIV. Recent examples include the armed conflict in the Democratic Republic of Congo (DRC), postelection violence in Kenya, flooding in Thailand, and the earthquake in Haiti. In this context, the nature of the emergency, as well as population and health system resiliency, may support continued treatment access despite adversity (Griffiths and Ford 2013, Bamrah et al. 2013).

HIV is transmitted through infected bodily fluids, notably blood and semen and, in the case of HIV-infected pregnant women, transmission to the fetus in utero or the infant during breastfeeding. As such, the main risk factors for HIV transmission include unprotected sexual intercourse, unsafe injection and blood transfusion, and lack of effective measures to prevent transmission from mother-to-child during pregnancy and breastfeeding. The efficiency of transmission varies significantly, from greater than 1 in 10 exposures for blood transfusion and mother-to-child transmission to near zero for unprotected oral sex (Patel et al. 2014). Each of these routes of transmission is amenable to prevention interventions that can significantly reduce or even eliminate the risk of onward infection.

Each of these risk factors may be exacerbated during humanitarian emergencies. During humanitarian emergencies, a safe blood supply may be limited. In addition, prevention programs may be disrupted, such as the provision of condoms, clean needles, and syringes, as well as HIV testing services. Further, access to antenatal and postnatal care for pregnant women may be restricted, including associated HIV testing and provision of ART to prevent mother-to-child transmission. Finally, widespread interruption of ART delivery conceivably would impair efforts to achieve population-epidemic control through the "treatment as prevention" strategy.

Particular attention needs to be paid to sexual assault, especially among women and children who are at higher risk during humanitarian emergencies. Specific interventions are needed to respond to the needs of these highly vulnerable groups, including appropriate violence-related wound care, immunization against tetanus, emergency contraception to prevent pregnancy, STI presumptive treatment, hepatitis B vaccination, and HIV postexposure prophylaxis. The collection of forensic specimens should be collected where facilities at the national level exist for analysis. Trauma counseling and referral for provision of legal assistance should also be offered.

While an individual's risk of sexual assault may be increased or access to HIV services may be impaired during humanitarian emergencies, especially those secondary to conflict, at a population level there has been insufficient data to support the hypothesis that conflict-related population movement and sexual violence increases HIV prevalence. A systemic review of published HIV prevalence surveys among conflict-related displaced and host populations in seven African countries did not identify increasing HIV prevalence trends associated with conflict (Spiegel et al. 2007). Of 12 refugee camps with available HIV prevalence data, only one had a higher prevalence than the surrounding host community (Spiegel et al. 2007). While individual vulnerability to HIV must be considered in HIV service delivery during humanitarian emergencies, the notion of conflict as a driver of population HIV prevalence is not supported by available evidence. As global gains are made in HIV prevention and treatment efforts, increasing attention is being paid to how the impact of humanitarian emergencies on HIV-epidemic control, with a growing number of people on lifelong ART, can be mitigated.

Prevention

Individual HIV prevention interventions are typically delivered in combination through a service delivery model called combination prevention. The UNAIDS Prevention Reference Group defines combination prevention programs as:

> Rights-based, evidence-informed, and community-owned programs that use a mix of biomedical, behavioral, and structural interventions, prioritized to meet the current HIV prevention needs of particular individuals and communities, so as to have the greatest sustained impact on reducing new infections. Well-designed combination prevention programs are carefully tailored to national and local needs and conditions; focus resources on the mix of programmatic and policy actions required to address both immediate risks and underlying vulnerability; and they are thoughtfully planned and managed to operate synergistically and consistently on multiple levels (e.g. individual, relationship, community, society) and over an adequate period of time (UNAIDS 2010).

HIV transmission can be prevented through a range of evidence-based behavioral, biomedical, and structural interventions. These are outlined in Figure 23.1.

Behavioral prevention interventions include HIV testing and risk reduction counseling, HIV education, peer counseling, and support groups. Biomedical interventions include the provision of antiretroviral drugs to either reducing HIV viral load to prevent onward transmission or preventing primary HIV infection. This includes postexposure prophylaxis, preexposure prophylaxis, and prevention of mother-to-child transmission (Baggaley et al. 2015).

Expanded ART for people living with HIV plays an important role in prevention strategy. The HIV Prevention Trials Network 052 Study enrolled 1,763 HIV-discordant couples across nine countries. The individual infected with HIV was randomized to either immediate ART or deferred ART initiation pending the onset of an AIDS-defining illness or a drop in CD4 count below 250 cells/μl. Early ART initiation reduced the risk of HIV transmission to the uninfected partner by 96 percent (Cohen et al. 2011). Biomedical prevention interventions also include needle exchange, opioid substitution therapy, male circumcision, blood safety interventions, and treatment of sexually transmitted infections.

Finally, structural prevention interventions address community or policy level issues that enable HIV transmission or serve as a barrier to access evidence-based prevention interventions. These may include community dialogue, policy reform, civil society advocacy, transportation issues, or housing for vulnerable populations.

HIV prevention interventions are often prioritized, adapted, and combined to target a population as well as the mode of transmission. Therefore, it is critical to understand factors influencing the epidemic to ensure that prevention interventions promoted are well adapted and likely to be impactful (UNAIDS 2016). Specifically, this means understanding national and local HIV epidemiology, populations most at risk, and how services may need to be adapted to reach the most vulnerable. Core HIV prevention interventions among displaced populations, particularly education and condoms, although critical, may be limited in impact by contextual factors, such as the desire to have children.

A community survey of 698 Sierra Leonean refugees living in Guinea assessed the common paradigm of whether increased knowledge and risk perception would lead to HIV avoidant behavior change. The analysis revealed no association between HIV knowledge and behavior change. Those with perceived HIV risk were less likely to report any avoidant behavior change. The study concluded that self-efficacy and autonomy required to translate risk perception into behavior change may not be present in some emergency-affected or vulnerable populations, such as women. For instance, in the survey the main reason reported for not using condoms was a desire to have children, which may or may not be an autonomous decision by the woman herself (Woodward et al. 2014).

Therefore, HIV prevention interventions aiming to improve knowledge or change risk perception may be inherently constrained, necessitating a better understanding of contextual factors through such methods as anthropologic interviews and community consultation. It is strongly advisable for humanitarian program managers to consult with available local and international HIV prevention stakeholders to ensure that basic and effective targeted HIV prevention interventions are provided.

While a comprehensive combination prevention program strategy is optimal, it may be necessary to prioritize HIV prevention activities during humanitarian emergencies. The Inter-Agency Standing Committee (IASC) guidelines highlight a number of core prevention activities to guide prioritization in emergency settings (IASC 2010). These include:

- HIV transmission prevention in healthcare settings
- Provision of good quality condoms
- Postexposure prophylaxis
- STI management
- Prevention of mother to child transmission
- Basic healthcare provision to key at-risk populations

Additional emergency response support to sectors such as protection, education, shelter, nutrition, and livelihood, as well as ready access to safe water, sanitation, and hygiene services, can reduce population vulnerability, thereby supporting broader HIV prevention efforts.

Specific minimum recommended interventions for each of these sectors in emergency settings are included in the IASC guidance for both the acute and expanded response. For instance, during the acute response protection efforts should include monitoring allegations of HIV-related human rights

Chapter 23: HIV

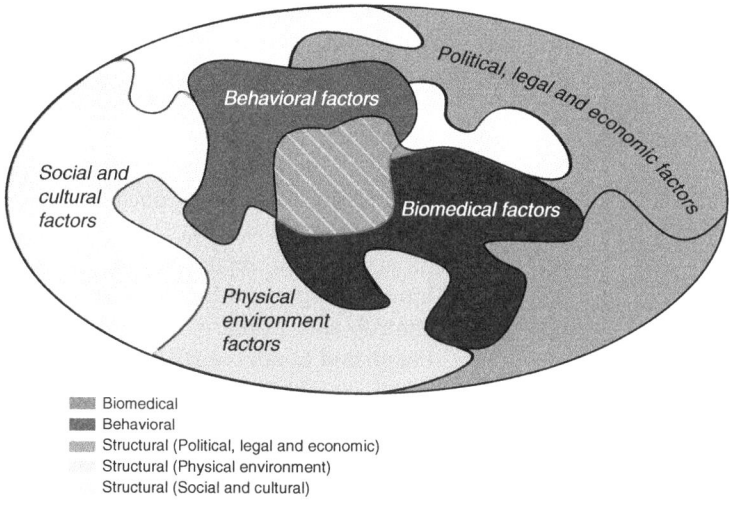

- Biomedical
- Behavioral
- Structural (Political, legal and economic)
- Structural (Physical environment)
- Structural (Social and cultural)

Biomedical intervention strategies to reduce exposure, transmission and/or infection
Male and female condom provision
Drug treatment including opioid substitution therapy, needle and syringe provision
Male circumcision
Biomedical prophylaxis – ARVs in PMTCT services, post exposure prophylaxis, etc.
ART initiation as soon as possible following a positive HIV diagnosis
Appropriate and accessible STI services
Blood safety, standard precautions in health care setting
etc.

Behavioural intervention strategies to promote individual risk reduction
HIV testing and risk reduction counseling
Behaviour change communication to promote partner reduction, condom use, uptake of HIV testing and counseling, etc.
HIV education
Interpersonal communication, including peer education and persuasion
Social marketing of prevention commodities
Cash incentives for individual risk avoidance
etc.

Social and cultural intervention strategies
Community dialog and mobilization, to demand services; for AIDS competence, etc.
Stigma reduction programmes
Advocacy and coalition building for social justice
Media and interpersonnal communication to clarify values, change harmful social norms
Education curriculum reform, expansion and quality control
Support youth leadership
etc.

Political, legal and economic strategies
Human rights programming
Prevention diplomacy with leaders at all levels
Community Microfinance/microcredit
Training/advocacy with police, judges, etc.
Policies re access to condoms (schools, prisons etc.)
Review and revise workplace policies
Stakeholder analysis & alliance building
Strategic advocacy for legal reform
Regulation/deregulation, taxes
etc.

Intervention strategies addressing physical environment:
Housing policy and standards
Enhance farming, other modes of subsistence, for food security
Infrastructure development – transportation, communications, etc.

Figure 23.1 HIV transmission prevention interventions
UNAIDS, 2010

violations while the expanded response should build local capacity to address human rights needs. Such guidance on activities for a cross-sectoral tiered response to HIV in emergency settings also offers a useful framework for humanitarian response evaluation.

Surveillance

HIV/AIDS is typically not included as a priority disease for EWARN surveillance during the acute phase of a humanitarian emergency. However, valuable public health information about the burden of HIV disease among host populations, refugees, or internally displaced persons should be collected through a review of existing epidemiology and prospective health information system data.

As mentioned earlier in the chapter, estimates of HIV disease burden are typically generated from national or subnational HIV seroprevalence surveys. These may be representative of the general population, subpopulations such as pregnant women, or approximated using statistical modeling such as Spectrum estimates used by UNAIDS (UNAIDS 2013). A review of existing population HIV/AIDS prevalence and HIV program service delivery data should be used to help estimate health service needs.

Valuable prospective health information system data related to HIV/AIDS service delivery can be collected during an emergency response. Selected HIV/AIDS service delivery indicators are incorporated into both the emergency and routine Health Information System (HIS) implemented by UNHCR (UNHCR 2010). Regular analysis of these data can provide valuable insight and feedback on HIV/AIDS service delivery uptake as compared to expected demand. Organizations providing HIV treatment services should document service delivery using national HIV program endorsed tools when feasible. HIV treatment data over time at a district or subnational level can be used to evaluate the resiliency of treatment services to emergency conditions, thereby directing contingency planning efforts.

Clinical Presentation

The clinical presentation and course of HIV infection from primary infection to AIDS has been well described. Recognition of clinical signs and symptoms of AIDS by humanitarian health workers, especially in high prevalence settings, and prompt linkage to HIV services may prove lifesaving. Following initial or primary infection with HIV, the virus infects a variety of cells within the body, prompting an initial immune response. Between 40 and 90 per cent of individuals with primary HIV infection develop an acute retroviral syndrome that typically manifests with flu-like symptoms, including fever, headache, sore throat and fatigue. This coincides with a period of active viral replication in the body until the immune response brings HIV replication under better control and primary infection symptoms subside (Sabin and Lundgren 2013).

In the absence of treatment, the period of time between primary HIV infection and the development of AIDS is highly variable. Age is a major contributing factor with vertically HIV-infected infants at particular risk of rapid disease progression. A pooled analysis of HIV-infected children in Africa prior to widespread ART availability observed that 52 per cent of children died by two years of age (Newell et al. 2004). By contrast, HIV disease progression in adults frequently occurs over many years with a very small but well-studied proportion of HIV-infected adults identified as long-term nonprogressors who may remain asymptomatic for seven years or longer (Sabin and Lundgren 2013). However, it is difficult to predict which patients will experience rapid versus slow progression; therefore, HIV treatment services rely on regular clinical and immunologic monitoring that increasingly favors early treatment as outlined in the treatment section below.

TB is a leading cause of morbidity and mortality among people living with HIV, with an estimated 360,000 deaths from HIV-associated TB in 2013. Persons living with HIV are 29 times more likely to progress to active TB disease than HIV uninfected individuals (WHO 2014). Therefore, diagnosis of either TB disease or HIV infection should prompt screening for the other infection. Colocation of TB and HIV diagnosis and treatment services is strongly recommended to simplify treatment access and monitor adherence. Tuberculosis is discussed in Chapter 29.

The advanced clinical manifestation of HIV infection is AIDS. AIDS is a life-threatening illness characterized by an immunocompromised state with illnesses that typically do not occur among individuals with a healthy immune system. If an HIV-infected individual has a CD4 lymphocyte count below the age-specific threshold or the presence of a WHO Stage 4 illness, they are considered to have AIDS (WHO 2007). While AIDS was once an inevitable outcome of HIV infection early in the epidemic, increasing global access to early testing and highly effective chronic treatment has reduced its occurrence. Nevertheless, the majority of patients starting treatment in low- and middle-income countries in 2016 did so with low CD4 counts (Anderegg & Kirk, 2016). Consequently, AIDS remains an important public health concern among underserved populations living with HIV and those with limited treatment options due to acquired viral resistance to available treatment.

In settings where protracted humanitarian emergencies have degraded or destroyed health infrastructure, improving population access to HIV services is challenging. In 2013, despite steady gains in HIV treatment coverage across sub-Saharan Africa, only 5 per cent of all estimated adults living with HIV in South Sudan were receiving treatment (UNAIDS 2014b). Treatment-experienced patients may present with AIDS after experiencing treatment interruptions, discontinuation, or prolonged periods of poor adherence. For example, this occurs in Southern Africa where economic migrants living with HIV struggle maintaining continued access to effective treatment options as they travel the region. Similarly, refugees and internally displaced persons on ART may be forced to live in settings with minimal or limited treatment options.

Diagnosis

Access to quality-assured HIV testing and counseling services is the critical first step identifying HIV infection and linking individuals to lifesaving treatment. HIV diagnostic services are increasingly integrated into routine health services, including during some humanitarian emergencies, to expand access and remove perceived barriers that HIV services require distinct service delivery models. Approaches to integrate HIV testing into primary or hospital care services are well described by WHO in opt-out or provider-initiated testing and counseling guidance. Relatively simple interventions to offer routine HIV testing at a refugee settlement clinic in Uganda resulted in a sixfold increase in the average number of HIV-infected cases identified each week (O'Laughlin et al. 2014).

Virological and Antibody Tests

HIV diagnostic tests either detect the virus itself, called virological tests, or detect antibodies produced by the body in response to HIV infection, called antibody tests.

In infants under 18 months of age, virological testing (where available), specifically HIV DNA PCR, is the standard of care internationally for diagnosing HIV infection. This is due to the persistence of vertically acquired maternal antibodies in infants that may lead to an incorrect diagnosis. Virological tests are more expensive, logistically complicated, and historically have been challenged by prolonged test result delivery timelines. However, they are critical for early infant diagnosis and early lifesaving treatment initiation. Current DNA PCR point-of-care and results delivery innovations being evaluated hold exciting potential for improved access to early infant diagnosis services.

In adults and children 18 months of age and older, point-of-care HIV antibody tests are the preferred method for diagnosis of HIV infection. These tests support rapid, same-day test result delivery, feasible integration into other health services, and the opportunity to provide counseling, prevention, and treatment referral support adapted to the results.

Repeat testing is required for both HIV diagnostic types if the individual has a negative result with a recent exposure.

The exact test kit and diagnostic algorithm to use is typically defined by existing national guidelines with additional global guidance provided by WHO. Multiple tests are required to confirm infection prior to the initiation of treatment. Many different models of HIV diagnosis service delivery models have been developed and evaluated. In addition to opt-out or provider-initiated testing and counseling models mentioned previously, HIV testing services may be provided through mobile outreach, community-based, target families of persons living with HIV, or be located at venues visited by key populations at high risk of HIV infection. The increasing availability of HIV self-testing kits offers the potential to develop new approaches to improving access to HIV testing in emergency settings. A comprehensive table of HIV testing service delivery models in both generalized epidemic settings and low or concentrated epidemic settings is available in the WHO guidance (WHO 2016).

Informed Consent

Informed consent is a fundamental aspect of HIV testing services, regardless of service delivery model chosen. HIV testing should never be coercive, should respect individual human rights, and autonomy, as well as the access needs of vulnerable populations. National guidelines typically establish informed consent and assent procedures when working with children, youth, and emancipated minors. IASC guidelines provide an action sheet for core activities to ensure HIV testing services are aligned with these principles (IASC 2010).

Quality Assurance

It is essential that all HIV diagnostic tests and counseling services undergo routine quality assurance measures to ensure accuracy. Diagnostic testing quality can be particularly compromised during humanitarian emergencies where poor test storage conditions, limited trained personnel, and competing priorities are common. A review identified various quality assurance intervention points for scaling-up HIV rapid testing in resource-limited settings which begins with prequalification prior to procurement and continues along the supply chain to include post-market surveillance of test kits. Importantly for emergency settings, early quality process decisions include HIV test kit selection with consideration for those that are ambient temperature stable and require relatively simple specimen collection, such as whole blood finger stick or oral fluid (Parekh et al. 2010). This quality assurance platform supported by WHO, the Global Fund, the President's Emergency Plan for AIDS Relief, and other stakeholders can be leveraged or adapted in humanitarian emergencies to ensure optimal products and protocols are implemented with a clear plan towards recovery once crisis subsides. Simple tools, such as a standardized HIV test log book, allow supervisors to monitor service delivery volume and enable early detection of HIV test kit performance concerns.

Treatment

International normative and evidence-based guidance strongly supports ART inclusion in the essential emergency health response. In 2006, an international expert panel representing WHO, UNHCR, UNAIDS, Médecins sans Frontières (MSF), and UNICEF issued a consensus statement highlighting historic disparities to HIV service access for populations affected by humanitarian emergencies and called for HIV service access to be implemented as an inalienable human right and public health necessity (WHO 2006). Soon thereafter, the IASC released guidance, recently updated, on HIV service delivery within a multisector humanitarian emergency response. The IASC guidance defines both the minimum initial response and expanded response elements for both the provision of care for HIV-related illnesses, as well as ART provision to those in need (IASC 2010).

The minimum HIV treatment response in humanitarian emergencies should include the identification of individuals in need of ART continuation and provision of ART to those newly diagnosed or previously on treatment. The minimum response should also include the provision of co-trimoxazole prophylaxis to all people living with HIV and HIV-exposed infants for opportunistic infection prevention.

The expanded response should include the continued expansion of care services, including prophylaxis and treatment services for opportunistic infections such as candidiasis, pneumonia, and cryptococcus, etc., as well as tuberculosis, malaria, catch-up vaccinations, and nutritional support. More detailed guidance on how to operationalize HIV treatment programs for migrant and crisis-affected populations in sub-Saharan Africa has been published to inform stakeholders beyond existing national and WHO HIV treatment guidance (UNHCR 2014).

Historically, the health response to humanitarian emergencies has excluded HIV treatment services, deferring to suspended or poorly supported routine HIV services provided through national HIV programs. These mutually exclusive choices can be dispelled in favor of increased emergency preparedness among national HIV programs alongside humanitarian multisectoral responses with integrated HIV service delivery. It is worth briefly understanding historic concerns with providing HIV treatment services to crisis-affected populations and comparing these to the expanded HIV treatment landscape today, to better appreciate the new paradigm of a public health approach to HIV service delivery. Some of these historic concerns and the current treatment paradigm are shown in Table 23.1.

Following landmark study results indicating improved health outcomes in adults when ART is

Table 23.1 Historic concerns and current HIV treatment paradigm for crisis-affected populations

Historic concerns with providing HIV treatment services to crisis-affected populations	Current HIV treatment paradigm for crisis-affected populations
• Adequate adherence too difficult and likely to result in poor patient outcomes	• Similar HIV treatment clinical and adherence outcomes have been achieved among conflict-affected and unaffected populations (Griffiths and Ford 2013) • Key service delivery preparedness and adaptation steps may contribute to this finding (Griffiths and Ford 2013) • Increasingly simple, even once daily, combination antiretroviral formulations • Increasingly standardized treatment regimens across national treatment programs • Treatment readiness and adherence counseling a constant feature of all HIV treatment services regardless of population • Increasing coverage of treatment means that displaced persons living with HIV may already be treatment experienced
• ART regimens too complex, especially for children	• Increasingly available heat-stable and fixed dose combination and pediatric combination antiretroviral formulations with continued advocacy for innovation • Family-based HIV treatment service delivery models and task sharing to expand pediatric HIV treatment access • Expanded treatment eligibility criteria for children offer streamlined assessment guidance
• Service delivery requirements are too intensive for emergency settings	• Point-of-care diagnostics and streamlined treatment guidance offer improved ability to integrate HIV treatment into emergency health delivery • Expanded HIV treatment availability through national treatment programs offers increasingly feasible referral options • Population displacement patterns are often predictable and can inform resource allocation
• HIV treatment is considered more appropriate for the postemergency recovery phase	• HIV is a chronic and treatable infectious disease that requires service delivery planning throughout the humanitarian emergency life cycle • Increased appreciation that, in addition to clinical benefits, HIV treatment helps to prevent new HIV infections

initiated early, when the CD4 count is above 500 cells/µl, the WHO's 2015 *Guideline on When to Start Antiretroviral Therapy and on Pre-Exposure Prophylaxis for HIV* represented a transformative shift and simplification in normative guidance for global HIV treatment (INSIGHT START Study Group et al. 2015, NIH 2015a, TEMPRANO ANRS 12136 Study Group et al. 2015). ART initiation is now recommended for all children, adolescents, and adults living with HIV irrespective of immune status (WHO 2016).

This increases the feasibility of HIV treatment integration into emergency health services. However, there remains an important role for trained clinical staff to diagnose and treat opportunistic infections. Laboratory diagnostics, such as CD4 count, are no longer required for ART initiation decisions, thus simplifying treatment requirements for emergency settings; however, CD4 cell count remains an important tool to identify people at an advanced stage of HIV disease. Point-of-care CD4 diagnostic platforms may provide a useful adjunct to HIV treatment services to assess disease risk.

ART for treatment purposes is always conducted using combination antiretroviral therapy. International HIV treatment programs have harmonized increasingly around an adult first-line treatment regimen containing tenofovir, lamivudine or emtricitabine, and efavirenz.

Table 23.2 Key clinic, program, and policy level innovations to support HIV treatment service delivery continuity during crisis

Clinic
- Three month or longer antiretroviral medication supplies to patients
- Expanded staff training on family-centered HIV service delivery, as well as acceptance of patient transfers without burdensome reevaluation as appropriate
- Patient-held HIV treatment cards to facilitate care and treatment transfer
- HIV diagnostic and medication buffer supply

Program
- Use of peer support groups to promote continued adherence and medication distribution
- Regular monitoring and coordination of HIV treatment service availability to inform patient referrals and supply distribution
- Integration of HIV service delivery within the emergency health package
- Mobile HIV treatment services

Policy
- Integration of emergency preparedness into national HIV guidance
- Task sharing, or the empowering of multiple different cadres in a health service delivery team, to provide family centered HIV service delivery
- HIV prevention and treatment service performance monitoring during humanitarian emergencies using IASC normative guidance as a reference standard
- Clear national formulary for antiretroviral medications with preference given to heat-stable fixed-dose combination formulations

This ART combination, recommended by the WHO, can be administered once daily in a single pill. By applying these guidelines, emergency health services in tandem with existing national HIV treatment programs can deliver treatment services at arguably less complexity than child malnutrition services, a service with historically strong commitment and implementation expertise among humanitarian emergency stakeholders. Newer antiretroviral drugs, notably dolutegravir, offer further potential for simplifing treatment through improved efficacy and safety, and since 2017 a number of countries began using dolutgravir as a preferred first-line antretroviral drug.

Program managers and healthcare workers responding to humanitarian emergencies may need to adapt and strengthen clinic protocols to ensure continued HIV treatment service delivery. Strategies to mitigate treatment interruption may require adapted service delivery models unique from nonemergency settings. MSF pioneered ART delivery in austere conflict-affected settings in 2003 and have developed a number of key best practices from experience in 22 ART delivery programs across West and Central Africa. These include program design strategies discussed further in the next section, as well as emphasis on patient adherence, emergency medication stock, and forced treatment interruption contingency planning, as well as medication stock security to ensure buffer stock access (O'Brien 2010). Key clinic, program, and policy-level innovations for implementation consideration to continue treatment during crisis, reported by MSF and elsewhere, are summarized in Table 23.2.

HIV Treatment Program Preparedness for Humanitarian Emergencies

By June 2014, 13.6 million people worldwide were receiving lifesaving antiretroviral therapy (UNAIDS 2014a). In 2013 an estimated $19.14 billion was available for HIV/AIDS response efforts. As these unprecedented global efforts to end AIDS increase the number of people receiving treatment services, there is a rising concomitant imperative to address the needs of this population also impacted by conflict, natural disaster, or economic crisis. Preparing for and addressing the needs of populations affected by humanitarian emergencies is crucial to preserve global public health gains and investment.

Emergency preparedness can be routinely integrated into national HIV/AIDS programs. Risk-informed programming, when applied to public health programs, utilizes known or anticipated hazard specific information to build program resilience to future shocks. For instance, repeated cycles of election violence involving subnational interethnic conflict may result in anticipated patterns of population displacement and HIV clinic closures. These risks can guide program preparedness by increasing HIV commodity buffer supplies to surrounding HIV clinics and preparing community support groups for the unique challenge of interethnic conflict.

For example, several studies evaluated the impact of 2010 postelection violence in Kenya on HIV care and treatment retention among adults and children. In a survey on chronic treatment for HIV or other diseases of 1,294 adult respondents residing in the three most heavily impacted provinces, fewer than 15 per cent of patients had more days of treatment interruption during the postelection violence compared to the month prior to violence onset. Key informant interviews supported an important role of increased medication supplies provided to patients in anticipation of the holidays and elections, as well as patient-held health cards in supporting continuity of care (Bamrah et al. 2013).

Similarly, a retrospective cohort analysis of children receiving HIV care and treatment services across 18 clinics in Rift Valley Province showed good retention despite the emergency. Of the 2,585 children living with HIV seen during the two months prior to postelection violence, only 7 percent failed to return to care during the four months after violence onset. Failure to return ranged from 1% to 24% comparing clinics, suggesting varying degrees of violence impact by locale. The clinic network utilized emergency task force coordination, engagement with humanitarian response actors, a nationwide patient telephone hotline, mass media communication messages on treatment access, and mobile outreach strategies. These likely played a critical role in maintaining patient retention (Vreeman et al. 2009). A thorough review of a region's hazard profile and adaptation of best practices can guide similar adaptive risk-informed programming decisions with the goal of building resilience for sustained treatment adherence.

Coordinated preparedness planning is needed not only to integrate emergency response into the national HIV/AIDS program, but to also engage donors and successfully interface with national disaster management authorities. Integrating clear preparedness guidance into national HIV/AIDS may identify anticipated gaps among donor funding streams that typically vary by the phase of emergency response (Hanson et al. 2008). Following postelection violence in Kenya in 2007, the government established a National Steering Committee for HIV Response in Emergency to bridge HIV/AIDS and disaster management units (USAID 2012).

Knowing the HIV epidemic at a subnational level prior to crisis is extremely useful to build resilient HIV treatment programs and effectively direct emergency support. Increasingly, HIV epidemiology surveys such as the Kenya AIDS Indicator Survey are being done at a subnational level and provide critical information on the burden of disease among populations of concern. Emergency humanitarian assistance frequently focuses on internally displaced persons or refugees in camp settings for good reason. However, in many crises there are far larger numbers of persons in need of HIV treatment who are still able to access preexisting treatment clinics, but the crisis has disrupted supply chains or human resources critical for sustained service delivery. Therefore, integration of HIV into coordinated emergency health sector support often requires an ongoing analysis of HIV epidemiology, treatment service utilization, and health commodity logistics.

Notes from the Field

Bukavu is a city of six hundred thousand in Eastern DRC. The region has experienced chronic conflict since the mid-1990s that in DRC is estimated to have resulted in around 4 million deaths between 1998 and 2004. HIV is a significant disease in the region, with an estimated adult prevalence of 4%–9% in Bukavu.

The international medical aid agency Médecins Sans Frontières (MSF) began providing HIV care in Bukavu in 2002, and by January 2006, 494 people had started ART. In 2004, armed forces invaded the city and the consequent conflict forced patients to be displaced and MSF expatriate staff running the HIV program to evacuate. Nevertheless, a number of contingencies were put in place to successfully minimize service disruption, including the establishment of communications networks between health staff and patients (e.g. via radio broadcasts, church groups, and posters); mapping and contact with other programs providing ART in neighboring regions; and the provision of patient personal identification cards listing antiretroviral medications and other important medical information such as comorbidities, medical allergies, and recent results of essential laboratory tests such as CD4 cell count (Culbert et al. 2007).

These contingencies helped maintain continuity of treatment despite service disruption and displacement of health staff and patients and have since been adopted by interagency guidelines.

References

Anderegg, N., and Kirk, O., for the IeDEA and COHERE Collaboration. Immunodeficiency at the start of combination antiretroviral therapy in low-, middle-, and high-income countries. 9th IAS Conference on HIV Science, Paris 23-26, 2017. Abstract MOAB0101.

Baggaley, R., Doherty, M., Ball, A., Ford, N., and Hirnschall, G. (2015). The strategic use of antiretrovirals to prevent HIV infection: A converging agenda. *Clin Infect Dis*, **60** (S3), S159–160.

Bamrah S., Mbithi, A., Mermin, J. H., Boo, T., Bunnell, R. E., Sharif, S., and Cookson, S. T. (2013). The impact of post-election violence on HIV and other clinical services and on mental health-Kenya, 2008. *Prehosp Disaster Med*, **28** (1), 43–51.

Barré-Sinoussi F., Chermann, J. C., Rey, F., et al. (1983). Isolation of a T-lymphotropic retrovirus from a patient at risk for acquired immune deficiency syndrome (AIDS). *Science*, **220** (4599), 868–871.

Cohen M., Chen Y., McCauley M., et al. (2011). Prevention of HIV-1 infection with early antiretroviral therapy. *NEJM* **365**, 493–505.

Culbert, H., Tu, D., O'Brien, D. P., Ellman, T., et al. (2007). HIV treatment in a conflict setting: Outcomes and experiences from Bukavu, Democratic Republic of the Congo. *PLoS Med*, **4** (5), e129.

Gallo, R. C., Salahuddin, S. Z., Popovic, M., Shearer, G. M., et al. (1984). Frequent detection and isolation of cytopathic retroviruses (HTLV-III) from patients with AIDS and risk for AIDS. *Science*, **224** (4648), 500–503.

Gilks, C. F., Crowley, S., Ekpini, R., Gove, S., et al. (2006). The WHO public health approach to antiretroviral treatment against HIV in resource-limited settings. *The Lancet*, **368** (9534), 505–510.

Griffiths, K. and Ford, N. (2013). Provision of antiretroviral care to displaced populations in humanitarian settings: A systematic review. *Med Confl Surviv*, **29** (3), 198–215.

Hanson, B. W., Wodak, A., Fiamma, A., and Coates, T. J. (2008). Refocusing and prioritizing HIV programmes in conflict and post-conflict settings: Funding recommendations. *AIDS*, **22** (S2), S95–S103.

Inter-Agency Standing Committee. (2010). Guidelines for addressing HIV in humanitarian settings (online). Available at: http://www.unaids.org/sites/default/files/media_asset/jc1767_iasc_doc_en_0.pdf (Accessed January 24, 2018).

INSIGHT START Study Group, et al. Initiation of Antiretroviral Therapy in Early Asymptomatic HIV Infection. N Engl J Med 2015; 373(9): 795-807.

Johnson, L. F., Mossong, J., Dorrington, R. E., Schomaker, M., et al. (2013). Life expectancies of South African adults starting antiretroviral treatment: Collaborative Analysis of cohort studies. *PLOS Med*, **10** (4), e1001418.

Levy, J. A., Hoffman, A. D., Kramer, S. M., Landis, J. A., et al. (1984). Isolation of lymphocytopathic retroviruses from San Francisco patients with AIDS. *Science*, **225** (4664), 840–842.

National Institutes of Health. (2015a). Guidelines for the use of antiretroviral agents in HIV-1 infected adults and Adolescents (online). Available at: https://aidsinfo.nih.gov/guidelines (Accessed January 24, 2018).

Newell, M., Coovadia, H., Cortina-Borja, M., Rollins, N., et al. (2004). Mortality of infected and uninfected infants born to HIV-infected mothers in Africa: a pooled analysis. *The Lancet*, **364** (9441), 1236–1243.

O'Brien, D. P., Venis, S., Greig J., et al. (2010). Provision of antiretroviral treatment in conflict settings: The experience of Medecins Sans Frontieres. *Conflict and Health*, **4** (12).

O'Laughlin, K. N., Kasozi, J., Walensky, R. P., Parker, R. A., et al. (2014). Clinic-based routine voluntary HIV testing in a refugee settlement in Uganda. *JAIDS*, **67** (4), 409–13.

Panel on Antiretroviral Guidelines for Adults and Adolescents. (2015). Guidelines for the use of antiretroviral agents in HIV-1-infected adults and adolescents. Department of Health and Human Services. Available at: www.aidsinfo.nih.gov/ContentFiles/AdultandAdolescentGL.pdf (Accessed June 5, 2015).

Parekh, B. S., Kalou, M. B., Alemnji, G., and Ou, C., et al. (2010). Scaling up HIV rapid testing in developing countries: comprehensive approach for implementing quality assurance. *American Journal of Clinical Pathology*, **134** (4), 573–584.

Patel, P., Borkowf, C. B., Brooks, J. T., Lasry, A., Lansky, A., and Mermin, J. (2014). Estimating per-act HIV transmission risk: A systematic review. *AIDS*, 28 (10), 1509–1519.

Sabin, C. A. and Lundgren, J. D. (2013). The natural history of HIV infection. *Curr Opin HIV AIDS*, 8 (4), 311–317.

Spiegel, P. B., Bennedsen, A. R., Claass, J., et al. (2007) Prevalence of HIV in conflict-affected and displaced people in seven sub-Saharan African countries: a systemic review. *Lancet*, **369** (9580), 2187–2195.

TEMPRANO ANRS 12136 Study Group, et al. A Trial of Early Antiretrovirals and Isoniazid Preventive Therapy in Africa. N Engl J Med 2015; 373(9): 808–22.

UNAIDS. (2010). *Combination HIV prevention: Tailoring and coordinating biomedical, behavioural and structural strategies to reduce new HIV infections*. UNAIDS: Geneva, Switzerland.

UNAIDS. (2013). Methodology – Understanding the HIV estimates (online). Available at: www.unaids.org/sites/default/files/en/media/unaids/contentassets/documents/epidemiology/2013/gr2013/20131118_Methodology.pdf (Accessed January 24, 2018).

UNAIDS. (2014a). *Fast track: Ending the AIDS epidemic by 2030*. UNAIDS: Geneva, Switzerland.

UNAIDS. (2014b). *The gap report*. UNAIDS: Geneva, Switzerland.

UNAIDS. (2016). Know your epidemic (online). Available at: www.unaids.org/en/dataanalysis/knowyourepidemic (Accessed July 16, 2017).

UNHCR. (2010). Health Information System (HIS) Reference Manual (online). Available at: www.unhcr.org/4a3114006.html (Accessed January 24, 2018).

UNHCR. (2014). *Guidelines for the delivery of antiretroviral therapy to migrants and crisis-affected persons in sub-Saharan Africa*. UNHCR: Geneva, Switzerland.

United States Agency for International Development. (2012). HIV treatment in complex emergencies (online). Available at: http://jsi.com/JSIInternet/Inc/Common/_download_pub.cfm?id=13042&lid=3 (Accessed January 24, 2018).

Vreeman, R. C., Nyandika, W. M., Sang, E., et al. (2009). Impact of the Kenya post-election crisis on clinic attendance and medication adherence for HIV-infected children in western Kenya. *Conflict and Health*, **3**(5).

Woodward, A., Howard, N., Kollie, S., Souare, Y., et al. (2014). HIV knowledge, risk perception and avoidant behaviour change among Sierra Leonean refugees in Guinea. *Int J STD AIDS*, 25c(11), 817–826.

World Health Organization. (2003). *Scaling up antiretroviral therapy in resource-limited settings: Treatment guidelines for a public health approach, 2003 revision*. WHO: Geneva, Switzerland.

World Health Organization. (2006). *Consensus statement, delivering antiretroviral drugs in emergencies: Neglected but feasible*. WHO: Geneva, Switzerland.

World Health Organization. (2007). *WHO case definitions of HIV for surveillance and revised clinical staging and immunologic classification of HIV-related disease in adults and children*. WHO: Geneva, Switzerland.

World Health Organization. (2013). *Global update on HIV Treatment 2013: Results, impact, and opportunities: WHO report in partnership with UNICEF and UNAIDS*. WHO: Geneva, Switzerland.

World Health Organization. (2014). *Global tuberculosis report 2014*. WHO: Geneva, Switzerland.

World Health Organization. (2016). *Consolidated guidelines on the use of antiretroviral drugs for treating and preventing HIV infection: Recommendations for a public health approach*, 2nd edition. WHO: Geneva, Switzerland.

Chapter 24

Malaria in Humanitarian Emergencies

Holly Williams, Marian Schilperoord, David A. Townes, and S. Patrick Kachur

Introduction

One of the earliest described diseases in human history, malaria remains a major global public health threat in the twenty-first century. Although disease surveillance and reporting remain incomplete in the majority of malaria endemic countries, the World Health Organization (WHO) tracks trends in morbidity and mortality through a combination of routine reporting systems and mathematical modeling. In 2013, there were 198 million clinical cases of malaria and 584,000 deaths, with an uncertainty interval of 124–283 million cases and 367,000–755,000 deaths, attributed to the disease worldwide (WHO 2014a). While still unacceptably high, these estimates have been declining consistently over the past decade and reflect profound progress in delivery of effective malaria prevention and control interventions to many endemic communities.

Malaria infection usually causes an illness with fever, chills, and generalized flu-like symptoms. Once ill, people with malaria can rapidly develop severe or complicated illness that may include confusion, convulsions, coma, respiratory distress, kidney failure, shock, bleeding problems, and other life threatening manifestations. Acute severe illness or repeated chronic infections are frequently fatal, but nearly all malaria illnesses and deaths are preventable. Even following recovery from severe or repeated infection, permanent disability and cognitive impairment from malaria are widespread (WHO 2014b).

Globally, more than 3.3 billion people are at risk of acquiring malaria. Transmission occurs in 99 countries, primarily in tropical and subtropical regions of Africa, South and Southeast Asia, the Middle East, and Central and South America. Isolated areas of transmission still persist in parts of Europe, Central Asia, North America, and the Caribbean (WHO 2014a). Approximation of the parts of the world where malaria transmission occurs is shown in Figure 24.1. The most intense malaria transmission is evident in sub-Saharan Africa and Southeast Asia.

In highly endemic parts of rural sub-Saharan Africa, people may be bitten by hundreds of infective mosquitoes throughout the year. In sub-Saharan Africa, malaria is a leading cause of morbidity and mortality (WHO 2014a). In these areas, malaria disproportionally afflicts young children, who have yet to develop partial protective immunity from repeated previous infections; pregnant women, especially those in their first and second pregnancies whose immunity to malaria is compromised during pregnancy; and other individuals from nonendemic or low transmission areas who lack protective immunity and migrate to or travel through regions of high transmission. In areas with less intense malaria transmission, such as Latin America and South and Southeast Asia, residents are likely to reach adult age without the frequent recurrent infections required to develop protective immunity and are therefore susceptible to severe and fatal illness at all ages.

In addition to the staggering public health impact, malaria impairs the economic productivity of individuals, families, communities, and whole nations where it occurs regularly. Malaria-endemic countries are among the most impoverished in the world, and malaria and poverty reinforce one another through a vicious circle. The global economic burden of malaria has been estimated at more than US$$12B per year (Sachs and Malaney, 2002).

Life Cycle and Transmission

Malaria is caused by protozoan parasites and transmitted by the bite of the female *Anopheles* mosquito. The malaria life cycle requires development in both human and mosquito hosts and is illustrated in Figure 24.2. Four species of malaria typically infect humans including *Plasmodium falciparum, Plasmodium vivax, Plasmodium ovale,* and *Plasmodium malariae.* The simian parasite species *Plasmodium knowlesi* has also been found to infect humans through natural, mosquito-borne transmission in isolated geographic

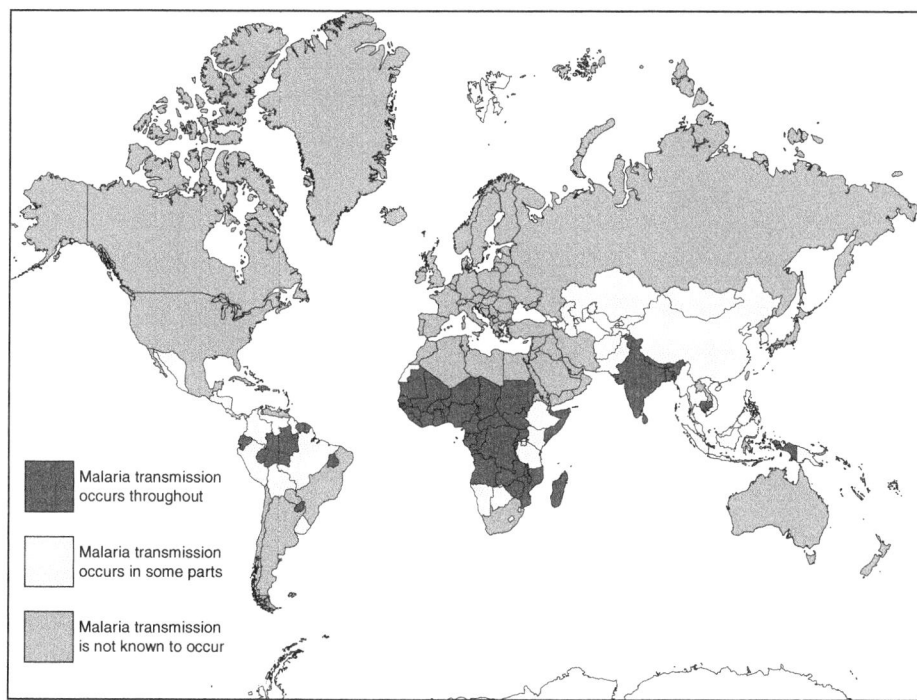

Figure 24.1 Approximation of the parts of the world where malaria transmission occurs
Courtesy of CDC, available at www.cdc.gov/malaria

settings in parts of Southeast Asia; however, this is rare and does not significantly contribute to the overall global burden of disease (Ennis et al. 2009).

Among the main four human malaria parasites, *P. falciparum* is most widely distributed and is most commonly associated with severe or fatal illness. It is prone to antimalarial drug resistance and remains the focus of many malaria control efforts worldwide. *P. vivax* is nearly as widespread and has become increasingly recognized for its potential to cause severe illness and extensive public health burden (Rogerson and Carter 2008, WHO 2015a). The other species of human malaria, *P. ovale* and *P. malariae*, exact a much smaller burden of human morbidity and mortality.

Malaria parasites, vector mosquitoes, and early hominids almost certainly evolved together over tens of millions of years. Based on genetic studies, falciparum malaria appears to have crossed over to humans from a related species of gorilla malaria more than 40 thousand years ago, most likely in central Africa. Human malaria greatly intensified with the advent of agriculture and expansion of human settlements over the past ten thousand years (Liu et al. 2010). It is likely that the Americas were free of human malaria until the arrival of European settlers in the sixteenth century. Each of the *Anopheles* mosquito species that transmit malaria around the world has a particular life span, ecological niche, and breeding and feeding behavior, to which the human malaria parasites have adapted. As a result, some vector species are more efficient at transmitting malaria than others. A particular mosquito's ecological niche, breeding and feeding habits, and other characteristics can present opportunities for interrupting the life cycle and preventing or reducing malaria transmission.

Burden of Disease

Although the ability to estimate the burden of malaria globally has improved, data on the malaria burden in humanitarian emergencies are much more limited. Of the 99 countries and territories that WHO considers malaria endemic, 91 (91.9%) of them host "persons of concern," defined by UNHCR to include populations of refugees, asylum-seekers, and internally displaced persons (IDPs) (UNHCR 2013c, RBM 2014). The number of persons of concern per host country varies greatly, ranging between two in Vanuatu and 4.7 million in Columbia.

Of the 99 endemic countries, 47.5 percent host more than 50 thousand persons of concern to

Section 3: Illness and Injury

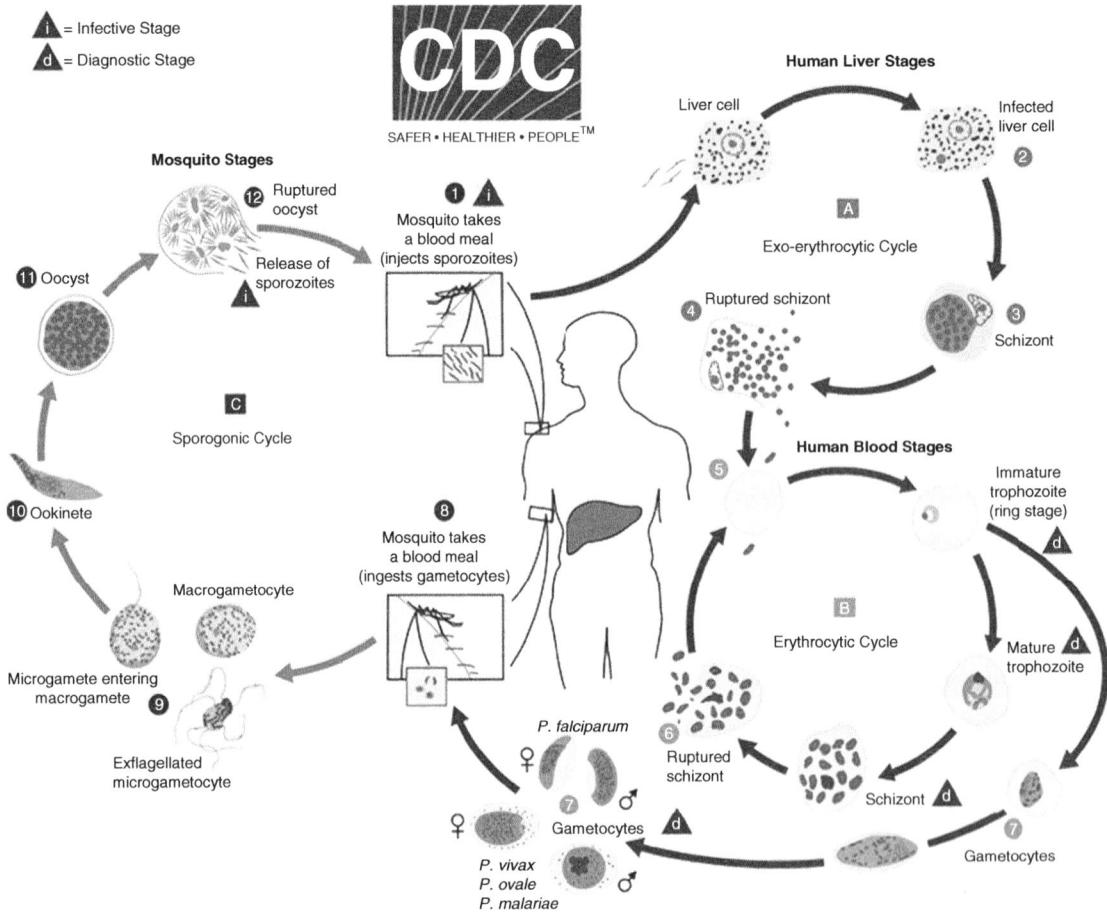

Figure 24.2 The malaria life cycle
The malaria parasite life cycle involves two hosts. During a blood meal, a malaria-infected female *Anopheles* mosquito inoculates sporozoites into the human host ❶. Sporozoites infect liver cells ❷ and mature into schizonts ❸, which rupture and release merozoites ❹. (Of note, in *P. vivax* and *P. ovale* a dormant stage [hypnozoites] can persist in the liver and cause relapses by invading the bloodstream, weeks or even years later.) After this initial replication in the liver (exo-erythrocytic schizogony Ⓐ), the parasites undergo asexual multiplication in the erythrocytes (erythrocytic schizogony Ⓑ). Merozoites infect red blood cells ❺. The ring stage trophozoites mature into schizonts, which rupture releasing merozoites ❻. Some parasites differentiate into sexual erythrocytic stages (gametocytes) ❼. Blood stage parasites are responsible for the clinical manifestations of the disease.
The gametocytes, male (microgametocytes) and female (macrogametocytes), are ingested by an *Anopheles* mosquito during a blood meal ❽. The parasites' multiplication in the mosquito is known as the sporogonic cycle Ⓒ. While in the mosquito's stomach, the microgametes penetrate the macrogametes generating zygotes ❾. The zygotes in turn become motile and elongated (ookinetes), ❿ which invade the midgut wall of the mosquito where they develop into oocysts ⓫. The oocysts grow, rupture, and release sporozoites ⓬, which make their way to the mosquito's salivary glands. Inoculation of the sporozoites into a new human host perpetuates the malaria life cycle ❶.
Courtesy of CDC, available at: www.cdc.gov/dpdx/malaria/index.html

UNHCR (UNHCR 2013a). Many of these host countries are low-to-middle-income countries that face serious health systems challenges, even without the presence of displaced populations. The World Bank characterizes 35 countries as "fragile situations" and 15 (42.9%) of these countries are malaria endemic (World Bank 2012). It has been estimated that up to 30 percent of malaria deaths in Africa occur in situations of war, local violence, or natural disasters (WHO 2000). Currently, there are numerous examples of malaria endemic countries facing situations of war and conflict including Nigeria, Somalia, Mali, Central African Republic, Democratic Republic of Congo, South Sudan, and Sudan (ACLED 2015, Council on Foreign Relations 2015). Two of these conflict-ridden countries, the Democratic Republic of Congo (DRC) and Nigeria, account for 33 percent of the global malaria cases (WHO 2014a).

Ninety percent of malaria deaths occur in the WHO African region, where the most vulnerable and poorest countries, including those mentioned above, suffer the greatest burden of malaria (WHO 2014a). In some settings, deaths from malaria may be higher than those resulting from conflicts (Chris et al. 2011). In spite of this, close to half of the African countries supporting populations of refugees and IDPs greater than ten thousand in size did not include this population in their malaria-related National Strategic Plan and Global Fund Proposals (Rounds 1–8) (Spiegel et al. 2010).

Much of the malaria data from humanitarian emergencies has been collected through the UNHCR Health Information System (HIS), which is utilized primarily in settled refugee camps and, more recently, in a few urban areas including Mafraz, Zarqa, and Erbid in Jordan, Nairobi, Kenya, and Douala and Yaounde in Cameroon. In 2014, as reported in the UNHCR HIS, malaria was the second leading cause of mortality and the third leading cause of morbidity in these settings (personal communication, Vincent Kahi, UNHCR, July 23, 2015). Much less is known about malaria among displaced persons who live in urban areas or in widely dispersed rural settings.

Malaria Control and Prevention

Implementing malaria control in the context of humanitarian emergencies presents many challenges. When establishing malaria control, understanding the broader sociocultural, political, economic, and environmental context of the emergency is critical. It is important to know the geographic origin of a displaced population, their route of travel, and where they settled, in order to understand their level of immunity and risks of transmission. For example, movement of nonimmune persons through or to an area of high transmission increases the risks of epidemics. Semi-immune populations may begin to lose their immunity if they reside in an area of low transmission for longer than a year, which increases their risk of infection if they return to an area of high transmission (Doolan et al. 2009). In addition, displacement of persons can weaken their immune system due to the arduous travel and emotional impact that results from fleeing conflict or natural disaster. Displaced individuals may be malnourished or have coinfections that may affect malaria-related morbidity and mortality, although the complex relationship between malnutrition and malaria morbidity is not well-understood (Fillol 2009). Malaria-related cell destruction, anorexia, and vomiting, may in turn, exacerbate malnutrition (Bloland and Williams 2003).

Initially, during a humanitarian emergency, there may be sparse or inadequate information to guide the establishment of malaria control interventions. Often, the size of the population at risk is not known. Further, there may be limited information on the efficacy of the anti-malarial medications and insecticides in use as levels of drug and/or vector resistance may be unknown.

Where displaced people settle and the type of shelter that is available may put them at added risk for malaria. There has been a shift in the last few years from refugees settling in camps to settling in urban areas. In 2013, only 35 percent of refugees lived in a planned/managed camp setting (UNHCR 2013b). For those who settle in dispersed rural areas or urban settings, planning coordinated malaria control is more of a challenge as it is more difficult to identify and reach these populations. Historically, displaced populations have not been included in national malaria control programming. Given the shift in settlement locations away from planned/managed camp settings, it becomes critically important that humanitarian actors and national malaria control programs collaborate to ensure that displaced, vulnerable populations can access malaria control programs, regardless of where they settle.

Depending on the humanitarian emergency, there may be overcrowding that increases the proximity and density of both susceptible and infected people (Bloland and Williams 2003). Generally, when displaced people initially settle, shelter is minimal, offering little protection from mosquitoes. These initial shelters often include teepee or lean-to type temporary shelter made from sticks, plastic sheeting, or pieces of cloth. More durable houses made of mud-daub walls that may ultimately replace these temporary shelters offer better (but far from adequate) protection from mosquitoes.

Displaced people often settle near water, particularly if they travel with animals, putting them at risk for malaria by living in close proximity to mosquito breeding sites. Livestock may also enhance the risk of transmission if the animals attract *Anopheles* mosquitoes.

Poor communication and collaboration among humanitarian actors can impede the provision of malaria control during humanitarian emergencies. This is more likely with large-scale humanitarian emergencies, when roles and responsibilities may be unclear, and it is difficult to know who is doing what in the emergency. Duplication of services can occur. For example, in the late 1990s, there was an outbreak of malaria in refugee camps along the western border of Tanzania. Upon closer investigation, it was found that there was a marked lack of coordination among nongovernmental organizations (NGOs) responsible for health care and malaria control. One NGO had the insecticide for indoor residual spraying (IRS) but no spray team, while another NGO had the spray team personnel but no insecticide. Improved malaria control occurred once all involved parties agreed to participating in a "task force" on malaria, which worked to ensure standardization across programs and better use of resources.

Finally, insecurity may result in displaced populations moving numerous times, which is disruptive to malaria control programs and causes difficulties in following up malaria cases. Lack of security also affects the ability of humanitarian actors to maintain malaria control, particularly if staff needs to be evacuated and/or if supply lines are disrupted leading to stockouts of key components of the malaria control program.

Health Services

During humanitarian emergencies, local health infrastructure may be absent or severely damaged, particularly in countries with limited resources prior to the humanitarian emergency. If health facilities are present, the sheer number of displaced persons requiring services may quickly overwhelm them. Early in the humanitarian emergency, there often is a lag until health services are established, funded, staffed, and supplied. Basic supplies such as diagnostic tests and antimalarial medications may be absent or in short supply. In addition, there may be a shortage of trained health personnel as trained health care professionals may leave the area due to the humanitarian emergency. Staff that does remain may suffer from shock and grief, as they are also victims. Further, referral services may not be available for cases of severe malaria, and if they are available, access may be impossible or impractical due to the security situation. Ongoing conflict can also limit access to health care facilities by vulnerable populations.

During the initial stages of a humanitarian emergency, the displaced population may not know where to find health services. In addition to the physiological vulnerabilities associated with malaria, such as pregnancy, it is important to understand vulnerability from a sociocultural or economic perspective in order to identify groups that are marginalized and hindered from accessing malaria care and treatment. Certain groups, such as the elderly, unaccompanied children, or the physically disabled, may have a more difficult time accessing health services and obtaining commodities, such as long-lasting insecticidal nets (LLINs), particularly in the chaos of the first few days of a humanitarian emergency.

Surveillance

Malaria surveillance is an essential public health function during humanitarian emergencies. An overview of surveillance is provided in Chapter 9.

In many humanitarian emergencies, collecting and analyzing malaria surveillance data often falls to clinical health care workers who may have little time for, interest in, or understanding of surveillance. Instead, surveillance may be viewed as an added burden to their already overworked clinical schedules. It is therefore critical when establishing a surveillance system that members of the health care staff are given explanations for *why* these data are collected and *how* to collect and interpret the data in order to improve malaria control. The surveillance system should be designed such that information flows in a timely manner, with practical interpretations of the data returned to the health care staff so programmatic decisions can be made and potential malaria outbreaks can be quickly identified and controlled.

A well-functioning malaria surveillance system can estimate the burden of malaria by age and sex and identify the most vulnerable populations. In addition, the system should be designed to identify the start and lifespan of an outbreak/epidemic, show disease trends over time, reflect changes in health care practices, and/or supplement other monitoring and evaluation activities to gauge the impact of malaria control interventions. For example, using surveillance data, one could see a trend in decreasing number of malaria cases in response to the introduction of a more efficacious antimalarial medication or, conversely, increasing number of malaria cases due to repeated stockouts of antimalarial medications. Data can be collected to determine changes in the malaria test positivity rate to better understand the proportion of suspected malaria cases that are confirmed (WHO 2014a). Knowing the demographic profile of the displaced population may help determine if there is a geographical distribution of sites where additional malaria control measures may be warranted, as the displaced population sleeps outdoors or conducts evening/night activities.

While drug efficacy and vector surveillance are important and are often a component of nonemergency malaria control, rarely is there time or resources to conduct such surveillance during a humanitarian emergency. Preemergency country data may be available to use as a baseline for programmatic decisions. However, if the humanitarian emergency becomes protracted, indicators that provide data on drug and insecticide efficacy, program effectiveness, prevention, case management, and treatment seeking behaviors become more important for monitoring and evaluating malaria control (WHO 2014a).

Case Definitions and Indicators

An essential component of an effective malaria surveillance system in a humanitarian emergency is that all partners implementing malaria control agree to a single, standardized case definition. During a humanitarian emergency, with multiple partners implementing malaria control, this may be exceedingly difficult, particularly in the early stages of the responses. For example, during the initial weeks following the Haiti earthquake in 2010, it took considerable time and effort to simply identify partners given constantly changing NGOs and other humanitarian actors, let alone gain consensus on a standardized case definition for surveillance purposes. This improved over time, but, as with other aspects of malaria control, clear, transparent, and frequent communication and willingness to collaborate are necessary and should be encouraged.

The WHO uses the following standardized case definitions for malaria that focus on diagnostic confirmation (WHO 2012a):

- **Confirmed malaria:** Suspected malaria case in which malaria parasites have been demonstrated in a patient's blood by microscopy or a rapid diagnostic test (RDT).
- **Presumed malaria:** Suspected malaria case without a diagnostic test to confirm malaria but nevertheless, treated presumptively as malaria.
- **Suspected malaria:** Patient illness suspected by a health worker to be due to malaria. The criteria usually include fever. All patients with suspected malaria should receive a diagnostic test for malaria, by microscopy or RDT.

The UNHCR's Health Information System (HIS) uses similar definitions and includes a weekly alert threshold (UNHCR 2010):

- **Confirmed malaria (uncomplicated or severe):** Any person with uncomplicated or severe malaria with laboratory confirmation of diagnosis by malaria blood film or other diagnostic test for malaria parasites.
- **To confirm a case:** Demonstration of malaria parasites in blood film by examining thick or thin smears, or by rapid diagnostic test kit for *Plasmodium falciparum*.
- **Weekly alert threshold:** 1.5 times the baseline. UNHCR also offers case definitions to differentiate between uncomplicated and severe malaria (UNHCR 2010).
- **Uncomplicated:** Any person with fever or history of fever within the past 48 hours (with or without other symptoms such as nausea, vomiting and diarrhea, headache, back pain, chills, myalgia) in whom other obvious causes of fever have been excluded.
- **Complicated (severe):** Any person with symptoms of uncomplicated malaria as well as drowsiness with extreme weakness and associated signs and symptoms related to organ failure such as disorientation, loss of consciousness, convulsions, severe anemia, jaundice, hemoglobinuria, spontaneous bleeding, pulmonary edema, and shock.
- **Case confirmation:** Demonstration of malaria parasites in blood film by examining thick or thin smears, or by RDT for *Plasmodium falciparum*.

There are standard indicators for malaria control that should be included in malaria surveillance in humanitarian emergencies. These include crude mortality, under five mortality, and malaria-specific mortality rates, proportional mortality, and morbidity due to malaria, malaria incidence, case-fatality rate for all confirmed malaria cases, case-fatality rate for all severe malaria cases, malaria test positivity rate, and proportion of population covered by malaria interventions (WHO 2013).

Limitations

There are limitations to malaria surveillance in humanitarian emergencies. Most surveillance systems reflect data from visits to health care facilities. It is estimated that in some settings less than 50 percent of patients with fever attend a health care facility even in the nonemergency context (WHO 2012b). The percentage of persons that attend health care facilities in a humanitarian emergency may vary widely depending on factors such as security, cultural acceptance of the health care provided, distance to and number of health care facilities, size of the displaced population, and availability of trained staff and antimalarial medications at the health care facilities. Surveillance data from patients attending health care facilities may not reflect the malaria burden in other parts of the displaced population who do not attend health care facilities (WHO 2012b).

In addition, there may be temporal and seasonal differences in health care facility attendance, particularly in the early stages of an emergency, as the size of the affected population may be too large or the damage to infrastructure too extensive, which may preclude access to health care facilities and diagnostic confirmation of malaria.

In recent years, the development and approval of rapid diagnostic test kits for detecting malaria infection has expanded greatly. Since 2010, WHO has recommended diagnostic testing prior to diagnosis and treatment of malaria illness for all age groups and in all malaria transmission zones (WHO 2011). The expansion of diagnostic testing for malaria presents an opportunity to revise reporting systems based on confirmed cases and could greatly improve the accuracy and reliability of malaria surveillance data.

Finally, data reporting from health care facilities may be incomplete and/or inaccurate. A multicountry evaluation of UNHCR HIS in 2008 identified a recurrent problem of lack of data cleaning, which affected the accuracy of the data.

Outbreak Response

In the context of a humanitarian emergency, malaria transmission can be heightened by population movement from hypoendemic to hyperendemic areas, inadequate shelter, environmental disruptions, seasonal changes in rain patterns or amounts, disrupted health care services, or lack of vector control measures (WHO 2013). In the setting of many humanitarian emergencies, historical data that might prove useful for baseline indicators are missing. During humanitarian emergencies, increasing numbers of confirmed malaria cases, changes in the malaria-specific case-fatality rate or increases in the malaria test positivity rate may be suggestive of a malaria outbreak/epidemic (WHO 2014a). Malaria outbreak detection and response may be included in a larger surveillance system, such as the early warning and response network (EWARN) that collects data for diseases with epidemic potential to identify outbreaks. EWARN requires diagnostic confirmation of malaria through microscopy or the use of RDTs (WHO 2012b). EWARN is discussed in Chapter 9.

The threshold or definition of a malaria outbreak will vary in different contexts. The Sphere Guidelines define a malaria outbreak as situation-specific: "An increase in the number of cases above what is expected for the time of year, among a defined population, in a defined area, may indicate an outbreak. Without historic data, warning signals include a considerable increase in the proportion of fever cases that are confirmed as malaria in the past two weeks and an increasing trend of case fatality rates over past weeks" (Sphere 2011). In one example, the alert threshold for confirmed malaria to be considered an outbreak may be "twice the average number of cases seen in the previous three weeks" (WHO 2012b).

In the context of a humanitarian emergency where the potential for an outbreak exists, it is critical to have a preparedness and outbreak/epidemic response plan in place, with full agreement and cooperation among all implementing partners, including the national malaria control program, if one exists, of the host country. Planning must consider budgetary constraints, availability and training needs of personnel, communication with the affected communities, supplies, and diagnostic capacities. Outbreak investigations should occur as quickly as possible in order to determine if scaling up of control activities is warranted (WHO 2014a).

Prevention

Prevention of malaria is essential in reducing the risk of infection and saving lives. It is an integral part of both malaria control programs and epidemic/outbreak response. Common malaria prevention approaches include vector control and personal protection against mosquito bites. In deciding the best approach, it is important to consider if malaria prevention will be useful and if so, what malaria prevention methods are most applicable and feasible given the context.

Long Lasting Insecticide Treated Nets (LLIN)

Long lasting insecticide treated nets (LLINs) are an effective means of preventing malaria infection. When used consistently and properly, LLINs are the most cost-effective method for malaria prevention, especially in rural areas of Africa, where the major malaria vector species bite indoors, late at night, and rest inside houses. Nets treated with an insecticide provide significant increased protection compared to untreated nets. If LLINs are part of the malaria prevention strategy during a humanitarian emergency, WHO Pesticide Evaluation Scheme (WHOPES) approved LLINs should be used (WHO 2010a). These nets are factory treated and last for two to three years.

During humanitarian emergencies, LLINs should be provided in sufficient numbers for universal coverage, which means providing coverage for everyone in the population exposed to transmission. Ideally, one LLIN should be distributed per two persons. Often, logistical, supply chain, and financial constraints prevent universal coverage.

In contexts where universal coverage cannot be achieved, populations at risk for significant morbidity and mortality from malaria should be prioritized including:

- Pregnant women
- Malnourished children of all ages
- Children under five years of age
- Individuals with chronic illnesses, including HIV

Additionally, all beds in hospitals, clinics, and stabilization centers should have LLINs.

The goal of LLIN campaigns in humanitarian emergencies is to have all members of the targeted population sleeping under an LLIN at nighttime. Mass distribution campaigns, often used at the beginning of a humanitarian emergency, can achieve rapid initial coverage; however, it is important that appropriate communication materials such as pictorial instructions on the correct use of the LLINs are provided. Distribution of LLINs alone without proper communication is not enough. Competing survival priorities, inadequate community engagement, and lack of education may lead to LLINs not being used correctly, not used consistently, not used at all, sold, or exchanged for other commodities.

Mass distributions should be combined with hanging up campaigns, properly planned door-to-door, involving a community-based workforce. Effective community promotion of campaigns is essential for successful malaria prevention. In addition to raising awareness of the use of LLINs, these campaigns encourage net acceptance, distribute nets, teach and support hanging of the nets, and monitor correct usage after the distribution.

As the situation permits, distributions may target more specific populations through distribution at antenatal clinics, during immunization programs, and at the primary health care facility. Monitoring and evaluation of bed net utilization is critical and should be assessed, ideally at one and six months post distribution.

One of the challenges in using LLINs in humanitarian emergencies is hanging LLINs in the temporary shelters that are often used by displaced persons. LLINs are not designed for use in these lean-to shelters made of plastic sheeting and often require additional resources to be used in this context.

Indoor Residual Spraying (IRS)

Indoor residual spraying (IRS) is used less often than LLINs in humanitarian emergencies as it requires substantial planning and resources and is not suitable for protecting individual households when people are spread over large distances or in temporary shelters. IRS is much more suitable where there are more permanent shelters in relative close proximity.

When used, the objectives of IRS are to reduce malaria transmission by reducing vector survivorship and density and thus human-vector contact. In the right context, IRS is a highly effective intervention to protect to entire communities through rapidly impacting vector populations (Pluess et al. 2010).

The effectiveness of IRS is highly dependent on the quality of the spraying operations. IRS is usually effective for three to six months and it is therefore critical that IRS be conducted at the appropriate time. To be an effective community control measure, IRS involves spraying an appropriate insecticide with coverage of at least 80 percent of dwellings to ensure that the majority of mosquitoes are exposed. Similar to LLINs, IRS is best suited to settings where most transmission involves a vector that bites and rests indoors.

The strategy for use of IRS has changed in recent years, taking into consideration the role of IRS in the context of universal LLIN coverage, the role of IRS in insecticide resistance management, and the reorientation of many national malaria control programs toward integrated vector management (IVM). In the setting of humanitarian emergencies, effective IRS programs should, where possible, be embedded into national malaria control programs. Preconditions for IRS spraying include:

- A population living in fixed dwellings with absorptive surfaces for the next three to six months
- Adequate information on local vectors, especially insecticide susceptibility and indoor versus outdoor feeding and resting behaviors
- Mosquitoes that enter and rest inside dwellings
- Commitment to, and social acceptance of, IRS by the population
- Households in close proximity of each other
- Sufficient program and system capacity to deliver good quality application of insecticide, ensuring that at least 80 percent of the dwellings are sprayed

IRS must be done in a manner that is safe for human health and not harmful to the environment. Only WHO-approved insecticides included on the WHOPES list should be used (WHO 2010a, WHO 2010b). Selection should be in consultation with the local WHO office and/or Ministry of Health. The use of the same insecticide for multiple successive IRS cycles is not recommended. It is preferable to have a rotation of a different insecticide class being used each year. If LLINs are being distributed, pyrethroids as insecticides should not be used in a spraying campaign. In addition to the insecticide, WHO provides specifications for compression sprayers, including how they must be maintained (WHO 2010c).

To monitor the quality of an IRS campaign, the following data should be collected immediately after the campaign:

- Percent of dwellings covered
- Amount of insecticide used per dwelling
- Percentage of households refusing spraying
- Percentage of spray pumps properly maintained and still working during and after the campaign

To monitor user acceptability of any IRS campaign postspraying, the following data should be collected one month after the campaign:

- Percentage of dwellings replastered, painted or washed
- Percentage of householders with complaints about IRS

Recently there has been interest in the use of insecticide-treated plastic sheeting (ITPS) in the construction of temporary shelters during humanitarian emergencies. There is still limited evidence for use of ITPS. LLINs and IRS remain the mainstays of malaria prevention in humanitarian emergencies.

Clinical Malaria

Overview

As discussed previously in the chapter, there are four important species of malaria, in terms of human infection, *P. falciparum, P. vivax, P. ovale* and *P. malariae*. Infection occurs following the bite of the female *Anopheles* mosquito, resulting in the malaria parasite within the salivary glands of the mosquito entering the human bloodstream. Malaria parasites initially infect the Kupffer cells of the liver. Parasites subsequently leave the liver to infect the red blood cells forming the asexual erythrocytic or blood stage of the parasite, resulting in the signs and symptoms of malaria. *P. falciparum* infection generally causes the most severe illness resulting in the greatest number of fatalities.

Depending on the species, the incubation period between the infective bite and the onset of signs and symptoms ranges from approximately 7 to 30 days. This is generally towards the shorter end of this range for *P. falciparum* and at the longer end for *P. malariae*. The usual incubation period for *P. falciparum* is between 7 and 14 days.

In *P. vivax* and *P. ovale* infections, some of the parasites remain dormant in liver cells as hypnozoites that may reactivate and infect red blood cells at a later time, resulting in an episode of malaria. These subsequent episodes, called malaria relapses, may occur months or even years after the initial episode of malaria. To prevent these relapses, treatment to eliminate the hypnozoite form of the parasite should be given after the initial episode of malaria in patients infected with these two species of parasites. This is detailed below.

Clinically, patients are categorized as having "uncomplicated" or "simple" malaria and "complicated" or "severe" malaria. As uncomplicated malaria may progress to complicated malaria, it requires timely and appropriate diagnosis and treatment. Complicated malaria is a life threatening medical emergency necessitating urgent and aggressive therapy (CDC 2010).

Uncomplicated (Simple) Malaria

Classically, malaria attacks last approximately 6–10 hours, including a cold stage with shivering and a sensation of cold, a hot stage with fever, headaches, vomiting, and seizures (in young children), and a sweating stage with sweats, return to normal temperature and fatigue. This pattern is actually uncommon and rarely observed. In addition, classically, there are tertian attacks that occur every second day in *P. falciparum, P. vivax,* and *P. ovale,* and quartan attacks that occur every third day in *P. malariae* including fever, chills, sweats, headaches, nausea and vomiting, and general malaise. While any or all of these symptoms may be present, this consistent periodicity is quite uncommon (CDC 2010).

Patients presenting with uncomplicated or simple malaria may demonstrate elevated temperature or fever, the most common finding, as well as perspiration, weakness, an enlarged spleen and/or liver, mild jaundice, and an increased respiratory rate.

Complicated (Severe) Malaria

Severe malaria occurs when infection results in organ failure or abnormalities in the blood or metabolism. In its most severe form, cerebral malaria, this includes abnormalities of the central nervous system including abnormal behavior, impairment of consciousness, seizures, and coma. Other manifestations include renal failure from hemolytic involvement in the kidneys, acute respiratory distress syndrome (ARDS) from an inflammatory reaction in the lungs often during treatment as a result of dying parasites, and low blood pressure from cardiovascular collapse. In addition, hemolysis may result in severe anemia and hemoglobinuria. Metabolic manifestations include metabolic acidosis, hypoglycemia, and abnormalities in coagulation. Finally, a parasitemia count of greater than 5 percent alone, with or without other findings, meets the definition of severe malaria (CDC 2010).

Diagnosis

The diagnosis of malaria is confirmed by identification of the malaria parasite in the blood of the patient.

Microscopy

The mainstay of malaria diagnosis is blood microscopy, including a thick and a thin blood smear. In a thick smear, a slide is prepared with many layers of cells. The cell membranes are then dissolved leaving intracellular contents, including any malaria parasites that may be then visualized under a microscope. The purpose of the thick smear is to concentrate the intracellular contents of thousands of cells so that malaria parasites will be visualized even if only a small percentage of cells are infected. In certain circumstances, a thick smear may be used to determine the parasitemia count and the malaria species. For example, the distinct gametocyte form of *P. falciparum* may be seen on a thick smear confirming the species. In general, however, a thick smear is used to simply confirm the diagnosis of malaria (CDC 2012, WHO 2010d).

In a thin smear, a slide is prepared so that a single layer of red blood cells is visualized under a microscope. Direct visualization of the intracellular malaria parasite confirms the diagnosis of malaria species. In addition, the parasitemia count may be calculated by determining the percentage of cells that are infected. This is one indicator of the severity of the disease. As previously mentioned, a parasitemia count of greater than 5 percent meets the definition of severe malaria. In addition, the species of malaria may be determined, as each of the four species that infect humans result in characteristic changes in the infected host red blood cells. A skilled microscopy technician may identify these changes in the infected red blood cells and determine the species of malaria. Thus, in the hands of a trained and experienced technician, a thin blood smear may confirm the diagnosis of malaria, determine the species, and indicate the general severity of the infection.

Rapid Diagnostic Tests (RDT)

Microscopy requires well-trained, highly skilled and experienced personnel and may not be practical in some settings, including humanitarian emergencies. Often in settings where adequate microscopy is unavailable or its capacity is exceeded, rapid diagnostic tests (RDT) are a reasonable alternative. Ideally, RDTs should be used with microscopy backup but in certain settings, including humanitarian emergencies, this is unrealistic. There are many different RDTs available and several different types utilizing different antigens for detection of the malaria parasites. Common antigens used for detection include histidine rich protein-2 (HRP-2) and plasmodium lactate dehydrogenase (pLDH).

Most RDTs report detection of *P. falciparum* specific antigens, answering the question, "Does this patient have *P. falciparum* malaria?" but give no indication of the severity of the infection. There are some multispecies RDTs that will detect different species of malaria; however, they should be used with caution, as the sensitivity and specificity may be inadequate. In addition, they need to be used in very specific and appropriate settings. Improper use may result in misleading results. For instance, in Haiti after the earthquake, several groups were using multispecies RDTs. *P. falciparum* is the only species of malaria endemic to Haiti yet there were several reports of "mixed infections" with *P. falciparum* and *P. vivax* based on these multispecies tests. It is likely that the *P. vivax* indicator line was responding to high-density *P. falciparum* infection resulting in a false positive for *P. vivax* infection (personal experience of Dr. David Townes).

At present, the Food and Drug Administration (FDA) has approved only one RDT for use in the United States. However, there are multiple tests that have been deemed acceptable by WHO for use in specific contexts outside the United States. The decision to utilize malaria RDTs and which RDT to choose should be made based on recommendations by WHO and in accordance to the national malaria control guidelines for the country in question (FIND 2015).

Clinical Diagnosis

For years, the mainstay of malaria diagnosis and the impetus for treatment was the presence of "fever" in a patient presenting in a malaria endemic country. The reliance on clinical diagnosis has likely resulted in overtreatment and may have contributed to the development of resistance to many antimalaria medications. Currently, this approach is generally considered inadequate. The diagnosis of malaria should be based on laboratory confirmation, ideally utilizing microscopy or RDTs with microscopy backup or in cases where microcopy is unavailable, RDTs alone.

There may be a role for clinical diagnosis in the setting of a malaria outbreak where the number of suspected cases would overwhelm diagnostic capacity; however, this is unusual especially since the advent of RDTs that are affordable and significantly less labor intensive than microscopy.

Treatment

The proper treatment for malaria will depend on the species or suspected species causing the infection, the severity of illness, and the national malaria treatment guidelines for that particular country. While not intended to provide specific clinical direction, some general principles include (WHO 2013):

- Infections with *P. falciparum* are the most dangerous in terms of morbidity and mortality. In endemic areas, malaria infections should be considered *P. falciparum* until the species is confirmed.
- In general, uncomplicated or simple malaria infections are treated with oral therapy; complicated or severe malaria requires intravenous or intramuscular therapy.
- The WHO recommendation for simple or uncomplicated malaria includes artemisinin combination therapy (ACT). Examples include artemether-lumefantrine (CoArtem®) and artesunate-amodiaquine (Coarsucam®) (WHO 2015b).
- Patients infected with *P. vivax* and *P. ovale* may require treatment not only for the acute infection, but in addition, for the hypnozoite form of the parasite. This treatment, commonly known as radical cure, often is done with a course of primaquine.
- Primaquine is currently the only drug available for the prevention of malaria relapse in cases of *P. vivax* and *P. oval* due to the hypnozoite form of the parasite that remain dormant in the liver after the initial infection. The standard primaquine course for the eradication of the hypnozoite form of the parasite may result in acute hemolysis in individuals with G6PD deficiency. It is generally recommended that individuals, especially those in high-risk populations, undergo G6PD testing prior to the administration of primaquine; however, this is not routinely done in CHEs.
- Guidelines for Treatment of Malaria in the United States may be found at: www.cdc.gov/malaria/resources/pdf/treatmenttable.pdf (CDC 2013).

Conclusion

Malaria remains a major public health concern in the setting of humanitarian emergencies. Displaced individuals may be at particularly high risk for malaria for a variety of reasons including inadequate shelter, proximity to mosquito breeding sites, relocation from hypoendemic regions through or to hyperendemic regions, and inadequate malaria prevention services. Once infected, displaced individuals may suffer significant morbidity and mortality from malaria due to malnutrition and inadequate or inaccessible health care services.

In the setting of a humanitarian emergency, malaria surveillance is critical to identify and respond to a malaria epidemic/outbreak. In addition, surveillance is useful in assessing the need for malaria control programs, as well as measuring the effectiveness of malaria control programs once they are in place. A key component of any malaria surveillance program is agreement on case definitions by all stakeholders.

The mainstay of malaria control in humanitarian emergencies is LLIN distribution. IRS may also be effective in the right context. It is important to include information, education, and communication about the proper use of bed nets in any distribution campaign, especially in the setting of a humanitarian emergency.

Malaria may be diagnosed by microscopy or rapid diagnostic test (RDT). Treatment depends on the local epidemiology (species transmitted, drug resistance potential), severity of the illness, and national guidelines of the country. Generally speaking, severe malaria is treated with intravenous or intramuscular medication and mild illness with oral medication. The WHO-recommended first line therapies for simple or uncomplicated malaria are ACTs.

Notes from the Field

Haiti (2010)

After the earthquake in Haiti in 2010, there was concern that there might be a malaria epidemic with over 1.2 million individuals displaced from their homes, many of whom were living outdoors, putting them at increased risk for malaria.

The decision was made that LLINs should be distributed to those displaced as part of a malaria control program. In addition, malaria was included in the surveillance system set up after the earthquake to follow trends and detect outbreaks of infectious diseases with epidemic potential.

There were several challenges in designing the proposed LLIN distribution. Given that Haiti is a low to medium transmission country, it was agreed that the goal should be universal coverage, as there was not a substantial level of immunity within the population. The first challenge was defining universal coverage.

In stable settings in sub-Saharan Africa, universal coverage may be determined by measuring the number of individuals or, more commonly, the number of sleeping spaces since multiple individuals may share a sleeping space, especially women and young children. To achieve universal coverage one should distribute one LLIN for each sleeping space.

However, in Haiti, it was impossible to calculate the number of individuals or sleeping spaces since the majority of displaced individuals were living in makeshift IDP camps in lean-to type shelters of plastic sheeting. The solution was to distribute one LLIN for small shelters and two LLINs for larger shelters.

The second challenge was hanging the LLINs in these makeshift shelters. LLINs are not designed to be hung in this type of temporary shelter and are not packaged with sufficient materials to hang them in this setting.

The third challenge was the lack of familiarity with LLINs, due to the low incidence of malaria. Thus, the distribution campaign needed to include a comprehensive educational component.

The combination of the second and third challenges resulted in a very resource- and labor-intensive LLIN distribution campaign. In the end, no malaria epidemic was detected. It was impossible to determine if the malaria control efforts made an impact.

References

ACLED – Armed Conflict Location and Event Data Project. (2015). Conflict Trends (No. 39). Real-time analysis of African political violence, July 2015. Available at: www.acleddata.com/wp-content/uploads/2015/08/ACLED_Conflict-Trends-Report-No.39-July-2015-pdf (Accessed August 31, 2015).

Bloland, P. and Williams, H. A. (2003). Malaria control during mass population movements and natural disasters, Roundtable on the Demography of forced migration. The National Academies Press: Washington, DC.

Centers for Disease Control and Prevention (CDC). (2010). Disease. Available at: www.cdc.gov/malaria/about/disease.html (Accessed June 10, 2014).

Centers for Disease Control and Prevention (CDC). (2012). Malaria diagnosis (U.S.) – microscopy. Available at: www.cdc.gov/malaria/diagnosis_treatment/microscopy.html (Accessed August 24, 2015).

Centers for Disease Control and Prevention (CDC). (2013). Guidelines for treatment of malaria in the United States. Available at: www.cdc.gov/malaria/resources/pdf/treattmenttable.pdf (Accessed June 10, 2014).

Chris, B., Singh S., and Sudarshi, D. (2011). Neglected tropical diseases, conflict, and the right to health. The causes and impacts of neglected tropical and zoonotic diseases: Opportunities for integrated intervention strategies.

Institute of Medicine (US) forum on microbial threats. National Academies Press (US): Washington, DC. A2.

Council on Foreign Relations. (2015). Global conflict tracker – Interactive guide to the world's conflict zones. Updated Aug 27, 2015. www.cfr.org/global/global-conflict-tracker/p32137#!/ (Accessed August 31, 2015).

Doolan, D. L., Dobaño, C., and Baird, J. K. (2009). Acquired immunity to malaria. *Clinical Microbiology Reviews*, **22**, 13–36. doi:10.1128/CMR.00025-08. Available at:www.ncbi.nlm.nih.gov/pmc/articles/PMC2620631/pdf/0025-08.pdf.

Ennis, J. G. et al. (2009). Simian malaria in a US traveler – New York, 2008. *MMWR*, **58**, 229–232.

Fillol, F. et al. (2009). Impact of child malnutrition on the specific anti-*Plasmodium falciparum* antibody response. *Malaria Journal*, **8**, 116.

Foundation for Innovative New Diagnostics (FIND). (2015). Available at: www.finddiagnostics.org/resource-centre/reports_brochures/malaria-diagnostic-test-report.html (Accessed May 29, 2015).

Liu, W. et al. (2010). Origin of the human malaria parasite *Plasmodium falciparum* in gorillas. *Nature*, **467**, 420–425.

Pluess, B. et al. (2010). Indoor residual spraying for preventing malaria. *Cochrane Database of Systematic Reviews*, **4**, CD006657. doi:10.1002/14651858.CD006657.pub2, Available at: http://onlinelibrary.wiley.com/doi/10.1002/14651858.CD006657.pub2/pdf/abstract

Rogerson, S. J. and Carter, R. (2008). Severe vivax malaria: Newly recognized or rediscovered? *PLOS Med*, 5, 3136.

Roll Back Malaria (RBM). Available at: www.rbm.who.int/endemiccountries.html (Accessed May 29, 2014).

Sachs, J. and Malaney, P. (2002). The economic and social burden of malaria. *Nature*, **415**:6872, 680–685.

Spiegel, P. et al. (2010). Conflict-affected displaced persons need to benefit more from HIV and malaria national strategic plans and Global Fund grants. *Conf Health*, **4**, 2.

The Sphere Project (2011). Humanitarian charter and minimum standards in humanitarian response. Practical Action Publishing: Rugby, UK.

United Nations High Commissioner for Refugees. (2010). Health Information System (HIS): Case definitions. Revised January 2010. Available at: www.unhcr.org/4614aa682.pdf, draft (Accessed July 17, 2015). United Nations High Commissioner for Refugees: Geneva, Switzerland.

United Nations High Commissioner for Refugees. (2013a). Mid-year trends, 2013. United Nations High Commissioner for Refugees: Geneva, Switzerland.

United Nations High Commissioner for Refugees. (2013b). UNHCR statistical yearbook, 2013, thirteenth edition. United Nations High Commissioner for Refugees: Geneva, Switzerland.

United Nations High Commissioner for Refugees. (2013c). UNHCR statistical online populations database: Sources, methods and data considerations. Available at: www.unhcr.org/en-us/statistics/country/45c06c662/unhcr-statistical-online-population-database-sources-methods-data-considerations.html.

World Bank. (2012). Fragile and conflict affected situations. The World Bank: Washington, DC.

World Health Organization. (2000). Press release WHO/46. World Health Organization: Geneva, Switzerland. Available at: http://reliefweb.int/report/sierra-leone/third-african-malaria-deaths-due-conflict-or-natural-disaster (Accessed July 17, 2015).

World Health Organization. (2010a). WHO Pesticide Evaluation Scheme (WHOPES). World Health Organization: Geneva, Switzerland. Available at: www.who.int/whopes/en (Accessed May 29, 2014).

World Health Organization. (2010b). WHO recommended insecticides for indoor residual spraying against malaria vectors. World Health Organization: Geneva, Switzerland. Available at: www.who.int/whopes/Insecticides_IRS_Malaria_09.pdf (Accessed May 29, 2014).

World Health Organization. (2010c). WHO Pesticide Evaluation Scheme (WHOPES). World Health Organization: Geneva, Switzerland. Available at: www.who.int/whopes/equipment/en/ (Accessed May 29, 2014).

World Health Organization. (2010d). Basic malaria microscopy. Part I. Learner's guide, 2nd edition. World Health Organization: Geneva, Switzerland.

World Health Organization. (2011). Universal access to malaria diagnostic testing: An operational manual. World Health Organization; Geneva, Switzerland. Available at: http://apps.who.int/iris/bitstream/10665/44657/1/9789241502092_eng.pdf

World Health Organization. (2012a). Disease surveillance for malaria control: An operational manual. World Health Organization; Geneva, Switzerland. Available at: www.who.int/malaria/areas/surveillance/operationalmanuals/en/ (Accessed Aug 20, 2015).

World Health Organization. (2012b). Outbreak surveillance and response in humanitarian emergencies. WHO Guidelines for EWARN implementation. World Health Organization: Geneva, Switzerland. Available at: http://apps.who.int/iris/bitstream/10665/70812/1/WHO_HSE_GAR_DCE_2012_1_eng.pdf (Accessed July 17, 2015).

World Health Organization. (2013). Malaria control in humanitarian emergencies: An inter-agency handbook. 2nd edition. World Health Organization: Geneva, Switzerland.

World Health Organization. (2014a). World malaria report, 2014. World Health Organization: Geneva, Switzerland.

World Health Organization. (2014b). Severe malaria. World Health Organization: Geneva, Switzerland.

Available at: www.who.int/malaria/publications/atoz/who-severe-malaria-tmih-supplement-2014.pdf

World Health Organization. (2015a). Control and elimination of *Plasmodium vivax* malaria: a technical brief. World Health Organization: Geneva, Switzerland. Available at: www.who.int/malaria/publications/atoz/9789241509244/en/

World Health Organization. (2015b). Guidelines for the treatment of malaria. 3rd edition. World Health Organization: Geneva, Switzerland.

Chapter 25
Acute Malnutrition

Carlos Navarro-Colorado, Eva Leidman, and Maureen L. Gallagher

Introduction

Acute malnutrition and micronutrient deficiencies are often the consequences of food insecurity and disease that result from long standing poverty, humanitarian emergencies, or a superposition of both. Malnutrition is directly associated with a higher mortality risk (Toole et al. 1992; Golden 1996). It also increases the frequency and case-fatality of many communicable diseases, such as measles (HTP 2011a). The identification and treatment of malnourished individuals is an important component of the response to humanitarian emergencies.

The diagnosis and treatment of acute malnutrition continues to be a very active area of research and innovation. Protocols and strategies have evolved at a great pace in the last decades (HTP 2011a). Protocols recommending high protein diets in nutrition rehabilitation centers were replaced with specialized foods and medical treatment in inpatient treatment centers, and then by community based treatment using ready to use foods with medical treatment in coordination with the scale-up of programs to integrate nutrition into health systems in emergency and nonemergency settings (Golden 2010, Ahmed et al. 1999). New protocols and approaches continue to be tested and translated into international recommendations and national protocols (Golden 2010, Ahmed, et al. 1999, Golden 1982).

This chapter provides an overview of current practice for diagnosis and treatment of acute malnutrition and micronutrient deficiencies. A strategic shift in the focus of current treatment programs, which puts more emphasis on health system strengthening and integration of treatment into primary health and community based programs, is also discussed.

Acute Malnutrition

Two distinct clinical and physiological conditions are included in the term acute malnutrition: wasting, or marasmus, and edematous malnutrition, or kwashiorkor. Each has a complex etiology, pathogenesis and clinical presentation. In both wasting and edematous malnutrition, acute malnutrition reflects recent changes in dietary intake and acute infection.

Wasting/Marasmus

Wasting, or marasmus, is characterized by extreme thinness. It represents the result of a process of reductive adaptation, whereby the body utilizes peripheral body tissue to fuel and maintain essential body functions in an effort to preserve energy and body nutrients. This complex process results in visible tissue reduction affecting mostly fat and muscle.

Wasting progresses through a continuum encompassing mild, moderate, and severe acute malnutrition. If untreated, the condition may become complicated by infection and other nutrient and physiological imbalance resulting in complicated severe acute malnutrition. At this stage, the functional capacity of the heart, kidneys, liver, and gut is progressively reduced. This results in greatly increased vulnerability of each of these systems to further complications. The most common causes of death include hypoglycemia, dehydration, cardiovascular decompensation with pulmonary edema, and infections (Ashworth 2001). The characteristics of the patient with complicated severe acute malnutrition are such that the clinician has little margin for error during treatment (Golden 1996).

Edematous Malnutrition/Kwashiorkor

Edematous malnutrition, or kwashiorkor, is characterized by bilateral pitting edema of the limbs. Fluid usually accumulates first in feet and legs, but severe cases may present with edema of the hands, arms, and face as well. Bilateral pitting edema in feet and legs, in the epidemiological context of a nutritionally challenged population, is usually considered as diagnostic of edematous malnutrition. When affecting children, this is also known as kwashiorkor. Edematous malnutrition in adults requires a differential diagnosis to exclude liver, kidney, or heart disease, as well as careful consideration of specific signs and symptoms of other conditions and of malnutrition.

It is not fully understood why some cases progress towards wasting while others develop Kwashiorkor, often in the same setting. Despite the usual finding of low protein in blood, the edema of Kwashiorkor is not thought to be of osmotic origin. Rather, it is the result of loss of permeability of the cell membrane, possibly due to free radical damage resulting from excessive production of free radicals in response to external factors such as measles infection, aflatoxin, etc., or a lack of specific antioxidant nutrients in the diet (Golden 1982). The key role of intestinal flora in this process has recently been suggested, but needs further investigation (Blanton et al. 2016).

The hypotheses that marasmus was caused by low energy intake and kwashiorkor by a low-protein diet was presented in the nineteenth century and held into the 1980s. This theory has since been disproven by a large body of metabolic research; alternative hypotheses have been proposed (Golden 2002).

Complicated Severe Acute Malnutrition (SAM)

Complicated Severe Acute Malnutrition (SAM), whether derived from acute wasting or severe kwashiorkor, is characterized by an overall nutrition failure involving profound physiologic and metabolic changes that can affect all organs, systems, and cells in the body, with an increased risk of death. Complicated SAM is usually diagnosed by the addition of specific clinical complications. The most important of these complications used to identify complicated SAM is anorexia.

Acute malnutrition increases the risk of acquiring other acute and chronic conditions such as measles or tuberculosis and increases the risk of complications and death from such conditions. SAM may also alter the presentation of certain conditions and complications, making them more difficult to diagnose and treat.

The medical and nutritional treatment of wasting and edematous malnutrition follow the same principles and protocols (with small differences) and are usually organized as part of the same therapeutic programs.

Diagnosis and Classification

Diagnosis of acute malnutrition is done through proxy measurements:

- Wasting is diagnosed using anthropometry, the measurement of the human body. The specific anthropometric indicators used for diagnosis are different for each age group.
- In all age groups, edematous malnutrition is assessed by clinical observation of bilateral pitting edema in feet and legs. Clinical assessment is also used to identify complications and adapt treatment accordingly.

The metabolic changes present in severe wasting and edematous malnutrition are not specific and cannot be used for diagnostic purposes. Laboratory changes are often difficult to interpret due to changes in body composition, hemodilution, and the presence of complications. Use of laboratory testing in the management of acute malnutrition is often limited to diagnosis of infection and some specific associated conditions but does not play a role in the diagnosis of complicated acute malnutrition itself.

While individuals of any age can develop acute malnutrition, children between the ages of 6 and 59 months are generally the most nutritionally vulnerable individuals in a population and are therefore the focus of most emergency nutrition programs.

Children 6–59 Months

As discussed in Chapter 12, for children 6–59 months, two key anthropometric indicators are used for diagnosing wasting: weight-for-height and Middle Upper Arm Circumference (MUAC).

Weight-for-Height

Weight-for-height is a metric that compares the weight of a child to that of a standard reference population of children of the same sex and height or length. The most commonly used reference population is the WHO Growth Standard (WHO GS) population, a multi-country sample of children developed by WHO in 2006 (WHO 2009). The distance from the patient's value to the expected or median value in the standard population is measured in a continuous scale in Z-scores. This is a statistical unit equivalent to one standard deviation from the reference population median. For example, a zero Z-score value means that a child has the expected weight for their height and sex. A weight below the expected value will

Table 25.1 Classification of acute malnutrition in children 6–59 months

Nutrition Indicator	Moderate Acute Malnutrition (MAM)	Severe Acute Malnutrition (SAM)
Weight-for-height	≥-3 SD and <-2 SD	<-3 SD
MUAC	≥115 mm and <125 mm	<115 mm
Bilateral edema	No	Yes

produce a negative Z-score. A cutoff of −2 Z-scores for weight-for-height defines moderate acute malnutrition (MAM) and −3 Z-scores defines severe acute malnutrition (SAM). The WHO GS is both a reference in that it is a common measure allowing comparisons across populations and a standard in that it is a norm indicating the ideal way children are expected to grow. Other nonnormative references, such as the NCHS reference, have been progressively abandoned in recent years (de Onis et al. 2006).

MUAC

MUAC is a measure of lean body mass on the upper left arm. The MUAC value can be compared to a reference population as is done for weight-for-height; however, the absolute value is more commonly used by practitioners for diagnosis. It is possible for a child to be classified as malnourished by one indicator but not the other (Grellety and Golden 2016).

Children 6–59 months are considered severely malnourished if they present with bilateral edema, have a weight-for-height Z-score less than −3 SDs below the reference population median, and/or have a MUAC measurement below 115 mm. They are considered moderately malnourished when determined to have a weight-for-height Z-score between −2 and −3 SDs below the reference median or have a MUAC measurement ≥115 and <125 mm. This is shown in Table 25. 1.

Older Children and Adolescents

Acute malnutrition in older children and adolescents is particularly difficult to identify through anthropometry due to the fast changes in body shape and size during puberty. Malnutrition may itself affect the age at which puberty occurs, further complicating its assessment (Kulin et al. 1982).

For children and adolescents 5–19 years of age, WHO recommends the use of Body Mass Index (BMI), calculated as the weight (kg) over the square of the height (m^2), adjusted for age. This is often impractical in the field and identifies acute malnutrition with less precision than weight-for-height does in children. As with weight-for-height, Z-scores for BMI-for-age are derived from the WHO Growth Standards (WHO 2007c). A Z-score between −2 and −3 SDs identifies moderate acute malnutrition and a Z-score below −3 is considered severe acute malnutrition. There is no expert agreement on MUAC cutoffs for adolescents.

Adults

In some humanitarian emergencies, other age groups may develop malnutrition in large numbers. This may be secondary to disease such as HIV, TB or other related to food shortages. Dependent adults, the disabled, and the elderly are often at higher risk of malnutrition in these situations and may go unnoticed in emergency nutrition assessments if they are not actively assessed.

Malnutrition in adults and nonpregnant women is often identified using BMI. A BMI below 16 is considered severe thinness (WHO 1995b). The term thinness or "Chronic Energy Deficiency" is generally used when describing adults with low BMI, rather than wasting, as it may represent a chronic condition rather than an acute one (WHO 1995b).

MUAC is also used for the diagnosis of malnutrition in adults; however, there are no recommended standard cutoffs. Research on appropriate cutoffs is ongoing (Tang, 2017).

In all cases, a single measure of BMI or MUAC is thought to be of limited use for assessing an individual's risk of illness or benefit from treatment (WHO 1995a). These measures should be used in combination with the assessment of clinical signs and symptoms to improve diagnostic specificity. Common signs used for diagnosis include recent weight loss (a 10% weight loss in the last month reported by the patient or documented by the clinician) and physical weakness (e.g., grip strength) for which there is no other clinical explanation (Navarro-Colorado 2006). Inability to stand is sometimes used as a late marker of acute malnutrition. These signs and symptoms are taken as an indication of malnutrition if they cannot be explained as the consequence of another known condition and are present in the context of poor access to sufficient nutritious foods.

At the population level, a rapid increase on the number of adults presenting with moderate or severe thinness indicates that they are most likely suffering from acute malnutrition. Stable rates of moderate and severe thinness in the population are common in deprived populations and may represent a mix of cases of chronic malnutrition and acute malnutrition.

If untreated, severe acute malnutrition in adults and elderly people very often evolves to edematous malnutrition, with fluid retention in the pericardium, lungs, and intestinal space. This is uncommon in children with nutritional edema. Edematous malnutrition in adults requires a differential diagnosis to exclude liver, kidney, or heart disease.

Pregnant and Lactating Women

BMI and other indices based on a single weight measurement cannot be used in pregnant women due to the body weight that is consequence of the growth of the fetus as well as the placenta, gland and adipose tissue. MUAC is the preferred anthropometric index for pregnant women, as it is not expected to be affected by pregnancy and therefore does not require knowledge about gestational age. The average increase in MUAC during pregnancy is generally less than 0.5 cm (PAHO 1991). Additionally, low MUAC is associated with adverse birth outcomes including low birthweight as well as higher maternal mortality during the first year postpartum (WHO 1995a, Christian, 2008). While pregnant and lactating women can develop edematous malnutrition, particularly during later stages of pregnancy, most pregnant women develop some degree of edema in the legs during a normal pregnancy (WHO, 1995a).

WHO recommends the use of low MUAC to identify SAM in pregnant women (WHO, 2013). However, there is no global consensus on an appropriate threshold. A conservative cut-off of <23 cm has been recommended for emergency contexts (Ververs, 2013). If the weight of the mother before the pregnancy or during the first trimester is known, this can be used to monitor the evolution of the pregnancy but not to evaluate the nutritional status of the woman.

Infants

Management of severe acute malnutrition in infants is given separate consideration given important physiological differences from older children. For example, thermoregulation and gastrointestinal functions are relatively immature. Severe acute malnutrition in infants less than 6 months old is assessed as a weight-for-length <-3 Z-scores or presence of bilateral pitting edema, according to current WHO recommendations (WHO, 2013). No single MUAC criteria for identifying acute malnutrition in infants under 6 months of age currently exists (Kerac et al. 2015). The need for inpatient care is assessed through clinical signs. These include one or more of the following: any serious clinical or medical complication; visible wasting (recent weight loss or failure to gain weight); ineffective attachment, positioning or suckling; or pitting edema (WHO, 2013). Infants may also be admitted to nutrition programs when there is presence of significant risk factors such as absence of the mother or the child has a disability. Current research regarding identification of malnutrition using anthropometric indexes in this age group is limited; research is ongoing.

Treatment

The treatment of acute malnutrition cannot be limited to replenishment of the patient's energy and nutrient needs. Instead, the treatment requires the provision of specific nutrients in balanced amounts, together with specific medical interventions for stabilization of the metabolism and treatment of infection and other complications when present. The treatment protocols for associated conditions and complications that may be appropriate in a well-nourished child could be inefficient, or even dangerous, in a child with complicated SAM. Therefore, it is always advised that doctors and nurses treating patients with SAM are specifically trained to do so.

The medical and nutritional treatment of acute malnutrition, whether wasting or edematous malnutrition, is usually organized as part of a single therapeutic program. Treatment for both conditions follows the same principles and protocols with minor differences.

Community-Based Management of Acute Malnutrition (CMAM)

Community-based management of acute malnutrition (CMAM) has been endorsed by major nutrition agencies (e.g., WHO, WFP, UNICEF, and the UN Standing Committee on Nutrition) as the standard of care for management of acute malnutrition in both emergency and development contexts (WHO 2007a).

Today, with effective treatment following current protocols, recovery rates of over 75 percent are expected (Sphere 2011). The treatment of acute malnutrition continues to be an area of active research and innovation.

CMAM relies on the application of well-known community based strategies, previously developed in community health programs, to the treatment of malnutrition. It became feasible in the late nineties with the development of ready-to-use-therapeutic-foods (RUTF) which are easily administered at home by a family member. With current protocols and an optimum program setup, only children with complicated SAM should be treated as inpatients.

Components of CMAM

- Community mobilization and outreach, including activities aimed at early case finding and sensitizing the community to the management of malnutrition
- Targeted Supplementary Feeding Program (tSFP), including clinical management of cases of moderate acute malnutrition (MAM) aimed at both treating identified cases and decreasing the incidence of SAM
- Outpatient Therapeutic Care, including clinical management of individuals with SAM with no medical complications through outpatient facilities involving regular (weekly or biweekly) provision of medical services and treatment and the distribution of specialized foods to be consumed at home
- Inpatient Stabilization Center, including inpatient clinical management of individuals with SAM who have medical complications through treatment at inpatient centers until their recovery allows continuation of treatment as outpatients or full discharge

The four components are part of one comprehensive program for addressing acute malnutrition. Cases identified by active case finding and community mobilization are triaged to either a supplemental feeding program (SFP) or an outpatient therapeutic program (OTP). If found to have complications, patients are referred from the OTP to a stabilization center (SC). Ideally, the four components of CMAM should be managed by a single organization as part of the national health services of the country. In practice, different components of CMAM may be managed by different organizations, as part of the national health service or as independent facilities. Since the treatment of each child often requires passage through different components of CMAM, in these situations interagency coordination becomes of paramount importance to ensure the integrity of treatment and efficient implementation of protocols to prevent and treat malnutrition.

Community Mobilization and Outreach

Community outreach is an integral part of the CMAM package aimed at ensuring both early detection and referral of cases of acute malnutrition to the appropriate CMAM component. As with other public health interventions, community participation can make activities more adapted, relevant, efficient, and effective (Burtsher 2013). When effective, community mobilization increases demand for treatment services, thus improving coverage of the programs. Mobilization entails increasing awareness of CMAM among all members of the community about the CMAM program, including information on the rationale for treatment activities, what treatment entails, who is eligible for what services, and where treatment services are located. Community mobilization activities depend on the context but may include community dialogues related to the causes of malnutrition, meetings with key community members and organizations, training of community members to help in case finding and referral, as well as nutrition education.

Children whose malnutrition is identified in the earlier stages and who are referred to treatment early are less likely to incur complications, and therefore will recover faster, sustain lower mortality and consume fewer program resources. Early detection is promoted with screenings to measure MUAC and identify edema. CMAM includes the use of both active and passive methods of identifying children that are acutely malnourished but not yet in treatment. Active case finding generally involves trained individuals visiting all households in the community to measure all children. Alternatively, caregivers may be called to bring their children to a central location, such as a school or religious center, for a community mass screening. When case finding is integrated into routine health services, as part of pediatric consultations or routine growth monitoring, this is considered passive screening. Mobilization can also encourage self-referral,

Table 25.2 Common community-level barriers to early detection and referral to CMAM programs

Common Barrier	Summary	Suggested Actions
Lack of awareness of malnutrition and services	Caregivers who are not aware of signs and symptoms of malnutrition or who recognize the condition, but do not know that treatment is available.	Improving the content, frequency, and method of disseminating information. A successful strategy includes integrating messages into other health campaigns (e.g., maternal and child health weeks).
High (opportunity) costs	Visiting a site for treatment can involve both direct and indirect costs, such as cost of transport or loss of income. The (opportunity) costs may change by season.	Reducing the frequency of visits (e.g., from weekly to biweekly), conducting home visits where community based health workers are active (task shifting), providing compensation/incentives for attendance (e.g., vouchers or food supplements), opening new treatment sites closer to the target population.
Distance to the site	Caregivers may have to travel long distances to visit a site for treatment. Travel may be expensive, require a long time in transit, and can be risky in the context of a conflict setting. Distant sites may become inaccessible in rainy season.	Opening additional treatment sites, increasing the number of health facilities providing services, conducting home visits (task shifting), and/or providing vouchers for transport.
Previous rejection	Children who are screened in communities and referred to treatment, but sent back home without treatment because they were found to not be malnourished. Children who are turned away from treatment because a site is full.	Standardizing the criteria for screening and admission. Working to ensure health facilities and treatment centers are not overcrowded through increasing treatment days, task shifting, or opening more centers. Improving communication between health workers and caregivers.
Staff/beneficiary interactions	Service provider communication and way of treating the caregiver/beneficiary is not positive.	Improving communication between health workers and caregivers and improving quality of services.
Stockout of therapeutic foods (RUTF)	Malnourished children are sent back home without treatment when therapeutic foods (RUTF) are not available, resulting in loss of trust in the program/treatment.	Ensuring appropriate supplies are in place to prevent stock outs including systems for tracking stock and reporting stock outs. Establish systems to communicate stock outs to caregivers with children in treatment.

Source: Puett et al. 2013 and Rogers and Guerrero 2014

where a caregiver brings a child to a treatment center independent of a referral based on their own assessment of the child's nutritional or health status.

In addition to case finding, community mobilizers play a key role in the program by following up patients that are enrolled in treatment but skip a scheduled visit. In these cases, the community worker visits the patient's home to determine the reason why the patient was absent and, if appropriate, encourage the patient to return for treatment. Community mobilizers may also work with nutritionists or health workers to evaluate the feeding practices of children who are not responding to care.

During humanitarian emergencies, there often exist considerable barriers to early detection, referral, and effective treatment. Table 25.2 outlines common community-level barriers, and suggested actions that can be integrated into community mobilization strategies to help overcome them.

Section 3: Illness and Injury

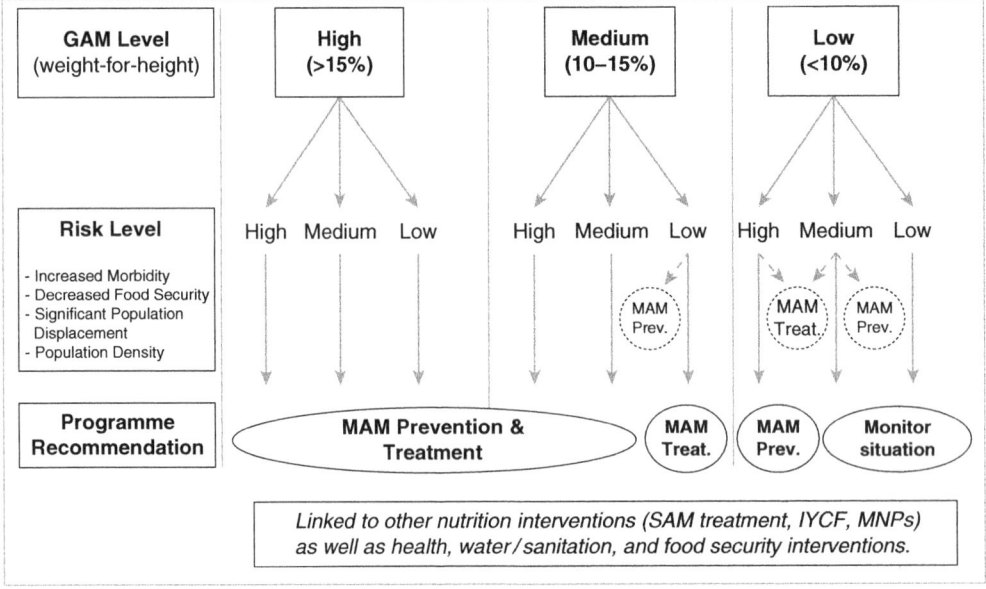

Figure 25.1 Management of moderate acute malnutrition program objective decision tool
Source: MAM Task Force 2014 courtesy of the Global Nutrition Cluster

Targeted Supplementary Feeding Programs

Targeted supplementary feeding programs aim to rehabilitate the nutritional status of individuals with MAM and to prevent individuals with MAM from deteriorating and developing SAM. By improving the nutritional status of patients with MAM, tSFPs also reduce morbidity and mortality risk from other conditions.

Current guidance recommends that the decision to start a tSFP be based on both an analysis of the current situation plus the risk of deterioration. Prevalence of GAM, as assessed by weight-for-height, is the key indicator of the current situation at the population level. Risk of deterioration is based on four factors: 1. increased risk of morbidity and likelihood of an infectious disease outbreak; 2. decreased food security due to disrupted food availability, access, or utilization; 3. significant population displacement; and 4. high population density. Programs for treatment of MAM are recommended where there are large numbers of children with MAM currently (GAM >10%) or where prevalence is lower but the situation is expected to deteriorate (risk level is assessed as high or medium) (MAM Task Force 2014). This approach is shown in Figure 25-1.

In establishing a tSFP, the program operation, the target group, nutrition products, duration of the program, and mechanism of delivery need to be considered (MAM Task Force 2014). In humanitarian emergencies, tSFPs focus on children 6–59 months, pregnant and lactating women 6 months postpartum (PLW), and people living with chronic illness such as HIV or TB. In some contexts, the mothers of severely malnourished infants less than 6 months may be admitted into tSFP. Infants under 6 months with malnutrition are not admitted into supplemental feeding, but are instead referred for inpatient care. If assessments identify other population subgroups that are nutritionally vulnerable, the group may also be considered eligible for treatment.

The program delivery mechanism should be adapted to the local context to ensure the greatest coverage for tSFP activities. tSFP programs are often provided in the same location as OTP services, and/or associated with a health center, but can be organized separately. Supplementary feeding centers may be implemented as fixed sites, where services are provided at one set location, or by mobile teams. In a mobile setup, the team providing SFP services changes locations daily in a planned schedule, so that one team can cover up to five or six feeding sites on different days of the week. Mobile strategies can enable programs to provide service to rural population closer to their residences.

There are many other local factors that need to be considered in designing the program during an emergency response. For example, in a response where general food rations are insufficient, nutritional products distributed through tSFPs intended for the malnourished child may be shared among family members. It therefore may be appropriate to increase distributions to account for this inevitability. Additionally, in most settings tSFP distribute foods as dry rations to be prepared at home. In some situations, beneficiaries are unable to prepare the dry rations, such as besieged populations, institutionalized patients, or when cooking facilities and firewood are not available. Ready-to-use supplementary foods (RUSF) are often used in these settings. Alternatively, the tSFP can be implemented as on-site feeding where patients visit the center daily and receive prepared meals made from fortified blended foods twice a day. Wet feeding is discouraged because of the high risk of cross infection among individuals; it has been less frequently used since the advent of RUSF.

Individuals are admitted into tSFPs when they are identified as moderately malnourished. Once admitted, patients regularly visit the tSFP site until rehabilitated. Patients are asked to revisit the tSFP on a regular interval, usually every two weeks. Weekly schedules for treatment may be necessary in some emergencies. During each visit, the patients receive a clinical examination. Their anthropometric status is measured to assess evolution of treatment and help make a decision about continuation of treatment. Supplementary foods for nutritional rehabilitation are then provided. Medical treatment is provided at each visit following a predefined schedule. In addition, the patients and their caretakers may receive health education and participate in cooking demonstrations.

Patients are discharged once they recover their nutritional status. Discharge criteria remains an area of ongoing research (WHO 2010). The establishment of a discharge policy for a specific program is a decision based on the assessment of the patient evolution and programmatic considerations (i.e., resources available, integration with other programs, etc.). They are specific to each response. Current guidance recommends discharging based on the criteria for which the patient was admitted. For example, patients admitted based on a low MUAC value should be discharged once they have a MUAC of 125 mm or greater for two consecutive visits. A patient admitted based on low weight-for-height Z-score should be discharged when this indicator reaches −1.5 Z-scores or higher for two consecutive visits. Most national guidelines also recommend that patients should not be discharged less than 2–3 months after admission to ensure nutritional replenishment.

Supplementary foods provided at tSFP programs must be energy-dense and rich in micronutrients. The nutrient content of the supplementary food for children 6–59 months is designed to support a weight gain of 5 g/kg/day (WSHO 2012a). Programs generally provide 1,000–1,200 kcal per person per day with 20 to 45 grams of protein per 1,000 kcal. These amounts assume that these are *supplemental* rations (i.e., they do not cover all needs) and that the patient's basic diet consists primarily of cereals, pulses, and variable amounts of breast milk (WHO 2012a). When this is not the case, the supplemental ration should be adapted to increase or decrease its amount and vary its composition so as to supplement the local diet appropriately. Other groups, such as pregnant women or the elderly, will need different amounts of supplementation based on their nutritional status and the baseline diet.

Supplements are generally provided as either:
- Fortified Blended Foods (FBFs) – usually distributed in the form of dry rations or premixes with vegetable oil. They require additional preparation at home, by mixing with warmed water. or
- Ready to Use Supplementary Foods (RUSFs) – energy-dense fortified foods that are presented as ready to eat and require no additional preparation.

FBFs are generally made with a base of corn, soy, and/or wheat flour. The blends are made with dried skimmed milk powder for children 6–24 months of age and without milk powder for children above 24 months and adults (UNICEF, 2016). The majority of RUSFs are lipid-based products made with peanuts or chickpeas. Ready to Use Foods (RUFs) designed for treatment of moderate acute malnutrition are commonly referred to as RUSF to differentiate them from those for treatment of severe acute malnutrition (RUTF).

Macro and micronutrients specifications for food products used in the treatment of MAM are described in a 2012 WHO Technical Note (WHO 2012a). While similar and compliant with the WHO guidance and *Codex Alimentarius*, the nutritional content of the FBFs and the RUFs available on the market are not identical in terms of mineral and vitamin composition, given adjustments in the formulation to account for factors such as preparation (WHO 2012a). A large number of studies have aimed at assessing the advantages of RUFs over FBFs in terms of efficacy and cost-effectiveness. Current evidence suggests that treatment with RUSF may result in somewhat greater weight gain and higher recovery rates (Nackers et al. 2010, Patel et al. 2005, Ndekha et al. 2009, Perez-Exposito and Klein 2009, and Karakochuk et al. 2012).

Medical Treatment

There is no universally-ratified consensus on routine medical treatment for management of MAM (Annan et al. 2014). However, the following medical treatment is a common regimen provided as part of routine care in tSFPs (UNHCR and WFP 2011):

- Presumptive treatment of worm infections for children 12–59 months of age with an anthelmintic such as albendazole or mebendazole
- Iron and folic acid supplementation for children, pregnant and lactating women with anemia
- Vitamin A supplementation for children aged 6–59 months of age
- Measles vaccination for all children aged 9 months to 15 years of age

Exact recommendations should be adjusted according to national protocols, or in their absence, international recommendations.

The SFP may also be used as a point of care to administer other ongoing programs such as expanded program on immunization (EPI), health education, breastfeeding promotion, or distributions of nonfood items.

Outpatient Therapeutic Care

The main objective of therapeutic care is to save the lives of individuals with severe acute malnutrition (SAM). This is achieved through the provision of specific nutrients in balanced amounts, together with treatment of complications when they occur. Treatment entails more than the replenishment of the patient's energy and nutrient needs. As stated previously, treatment protocols for associated conditions and complications that may be appropriate in a well-nourished child could be inefficient, or even dangerous, for a child with complicated SAM. With effective management of severe cases, programs can achieve recovery rates as high as 90 percent (Collins and Sadler 2002).

For the purpose of treatment, cases of SAM are classified as either complicated or uncomplicated. Patients with SAM with no medical complications are treated in outpatient facilities (OTPs), whereas those with complications are treated at inpatient facilities, special units in hospitals, or stabilization centers (SCs).

Patients are classified as complicated and requiring of inpatient care if they present with (HTP 2011b, Collins and Yates 2003):

- Anorexia (lack of appetite) as demonstrated by an appetite test, or
- Severe bilateral pitting edema, or
- Marasmus with any level of bilateral pitting edema, or
- The presence of other medical complications including intractable vomiting, convulsions, lethargy, decreased consciousness, unconsciousness, lower respiratory tract infection, high fever, severe dehydration, severe anemia, hypoglycemia, or hypothermia.

Infants less than 6 months are frequently admitted into inpatient care as they lack the reflexes to swallow the solid foods used in outpatient care. Ongoing research is exploring the possibility to treat these patients at the community level as well.

Patients are classified based on a medical examination following the same procedures recommended for any sick patient, including medical history and physical examination. An appetite test is also performed, as a lack of appetite is sometimes the only sign of medical complication for an acutely malnourished individual (HTP 2011a).

In the context of a humanitarian emergency, establishment of OTPs and SCs is justified when the number of severely malnourished individuals exceeds the number that can be treated at existing hospitals and clinics and where trained professionals are available to staff the centers. In practice, this means that therapeutic feeding programs are a component of nearly every emergency response. Outpatient therapeutic feeding activities are reintegrated into the primary health system when the number of patients drops back to preexisting capacity (UNHCR and WFP 1999).

Inpatient Stabilization Center

Treatment of severe acute malnutrition is organized into three phases:

- Stabilization phase focused on the treatment of medical complications such as hypoglycemia,

dehydration and infections and stabilization of physiologic function.
- Transition phase that starts after appetite has returned, medical complications are under control, and edema has started decreasing.
- Rehabilitation phase that focuses on catchup growth. The rehabilitation phase is now managed through outpatient care for most patients.

The decision to transfer a patient from inpatient to outpatient care is determined by clinical assessment, not anthropometric measurement (WHO 2013). Complicated SAM cases are generally stabilized and referred to outpatient care within 7 to 10 days of admission (HTP 2011a).

During the stabilization phase, nutritional treatment in inpatient units is achieved by feeding an exclusive diet of F75 reconstituted milk. The term F75 refers to the number of kcals (75 kcal or 31 kJ/100 mL) in the formulation. Patients receive frequent, small doses calculated according to their weight. Frequency of feeding, usually 6 to 12 feeds per day, depends on the number of days in treatment. However, when staff capacity is scarce, use of standard six feedings per day is recommended. Children 6–59 months receive 100 kcal/kg/day during stabilization. Feeding during stabilization is not aimed at gaining weight. The patient should not receive any other foods during this phase of treatment. Force feeding is strictly avoided (HTP 2011a).

During the transition phase, as the patient prepares for outpatient care, RUTF is introduced gradually. Treatment with F75 or F100 reconstituted milks (100 kcal or 420 KJ/100 mL) is continued until appetite fully returns. The milk formulas are similar; however, F100 contains higher doses of protein (2.9 gr/100 ml) than F75 (0.9 gr/100 ml) and higher sodium, among other differences.

Patient's weight, degree of edema, body temperature, clinical signs, and outcome of each feeding (e.g., refusal, vomiting) should be monitored and recorded at least daily. Warning signs of deterioration include increased edema, signs of fluid retention, and significant refeeding diarrhea. During the stabilization phase, recovery of appetite and improvement of complications are the main signs that the metabolism of the patient has been stabilized. This generally takes between two and four days. Once stabilized and able to consume RUTF, the patient may be transferred to an outpatient facility to complete treatment. On some occasions, the patient may need to stay longer in the inpatient facility to complete treatment of an associated condition, or may stay due to a lack of OTP services near their home, absence of a caregiver to take charge of the treatment at home, or other exceptional situations.

Running an inpatient facility is labor intensive given the complexity of treatment and the frequency of feedings. Inpatient care facilities are usually staffed with nurses and physicians, feeding assistance (one per ten patients), cleaners, kitchen staff, and a dedicated supervisor. All these health workers need to be trained specifically in the treatment of complicated SAM. In particular, physicians and nurses making decisions over individual treatment of patients with complicated SAM need to be trained explicitly on the treatment of malnutrition.

In humanitarian emergencies, this standard inpatient care may be provided at a standalone structure or integrated in an existing hospital or care center. Ideally, a dedicated room or rooms should be established for this purpose, to minimize cross infection with other patients in the pediatric ward.

Nutritional Treatment at Outpatient Therapeutic Programs

Outpatient centers provide therapeutic care to patients with uncomplicated SAM and patients who have recovered from complicated SAM in inpatient care. OTPs aim to rehabilitate cases and support catchup growth. The nutritional treatment in OTPs is based on the distribution of RUTFs in doses of 150–220 kcal/kg/day for children 6–59 months (WHO 2013).

The nutritional composition of RUTF is based on extensive metabolic and clinical research. It is similar in composition to that of F100 with several key differences. First, a lipid (usually a peanut paste) replaces some of the dried skim milk. Second, as it lacks water, RUTF is more than five times as energy dense as F100 (543 kcal/100 g compared to 100 kcal/100 g in F100). Additionally, RUTF contains a low dose of iron not contained in F100 (HTP 2011a). RUTF is most commonly distributed in sachets containing about 500 kcals (92 g). RUTF biscuits (e.g., BP100), with a similar micronutrient profile, can also be used for children over 24 months and eaten directly. It is important to offer clean drinking water along with the RUTF in order to improve its absorption.

Education of the patient or the caregiver is an important part of OTP programs. Educational messages should emphasize the need to offer safe water, proper hygiene and storage, and the feeding schedule. Messages should describe RUTF as a food and medicine not to be shared with other children. Although RUTF covers all the nutrient and caloric needs for recovery from malnutrition, patients may want to eat family meals. This is acceptable provided the RUTF is taken first. In addition, for children under 24 months, mothers should be encouraged to continue or reinitiate breastfeeding.

As with SCs and SFPs, OTPs in emergencies can be standalone structures or be associated to a health center. OTPs and SFPs are often run out of the same facilities. The centers are open for admissions daily. Once admitted, patients visit the centers once a week or once every two weeks. These centers are usually run by frontline health workers.

Medical Treatment in Therapeutic Care

Routine medical treatment is an important part of the treatment of SAM both in inpatient and outpatient care. Routine medical treatment of SAM includes:

- Antibiotics such as amoxicillin, started at admission.
- Antimalarial medications if malaria is prevalent and the patient has a positive malaria test or clinical symptoms. This should follow national protocols.
- Anthelmintic medications such as albendazole or mebendazole, for children at least 1 year of age, administered as a single dose during the second week of treatment in OTP, and after recovery of appetite in inpatient care.
- Vitamin A administered as a single dose at first visit, unless vitamin A is part of other daily supplements (such as F-75, F-100, or RUTF) as these already contain sufficient vitamin A. Vitamin A is contraindicated for cases of kwashiorkor.
- Measles vaccination, often given on admission to children older than 9 months and repeated at discharge or after four weeks.

Routine use of antibiotics aims to address the high rate of infection in patients with SAM. However, routine use in the treatment of uncomplicated SAM is an area of debate given concerns about efficacy in less severe patients. Current guidelines suggest the use of antibiotics for uncomplicated SAM, but not for those with MAM. Randomized, double-blind, placebo controlled trails have had inconsistent findings with respect to the effect of antibiotics on mortality rates and recovery (Isanaka 2016, Manary et al. 2012).

Specific treatment for associated conditions and complications may be added by the trained clinician. At the OTP, this consists of treatment of minor illnesses or transfer to inpatient care or a medical facility.

Inpatient care may involve additional or alternative treatment, such as the use of second-line antibiotics, which require specialized knowledge of SAM's metabolism and treatment protocols. In particular, the use of IV lines for treatment of complications, including dehydration, is strictly avoided except in case of septic shock or septicemia, as a result of the high risk of fluid overload and pulmonary edema during the first days of recovery from SAM. For patients with severe dehydration that are not in shock, slow rehydration either orally or by nasogastric tube is preferred. Use of half-strength standard WHO low-osmolality oral rehydration solution or ReSoMal (rehydration solution for severely malnourished children) is recommended unless the child has cholera (WHO 2013).

Emotional and Physical Stimulation

Emotional and physical stimulation is considered an integral part of recovery from SAM in order to prevent developmental delays, mental disorders, and other sequelae. Special programs and protocols for emotional and physical stimulation have been developed and adapted to the work in inpatient and outpatient care and should be implemented in all programs (Kerac et al. 2012).

Discharging Patients

As with programs for MAM, current recommendation for discharging patients from therapeutic care is that the indicator used to confirm SAM and enroll the patient should be used to assess nutritional recovery. When a tSFP program is functional, the children may be moved from the OTP to the SFP when they reach criteria of moderate malnutrition to complete recovery there. If such a program is unavailable, the children should be kept in the OTP until complete recovery. Weight gain should be monitored but not used as a criterion for discharge.

Management of Acute Malnutrition in Infants

For malnourished infants below 6 months of age, treatment prioritizes continued breastfeeding or reestablishment of breastfeeding, when appropriate. Reinstatement of breastfeeding for the mother or another female caregiver is achieved by a method called supplementary suckling technique, where the infant is fed an overdiluted preparation of F100 through a tube attached to the mother's nipple, thereby stimulating milk production, and at the same time, feeding the infant (WHO 2013). Infants cannot be provided standard F100 given the risk of hypernatremia with dehydration. The mother is also stimulated to breastfeed, and once she starts producing milk, the amount of therapeutic milk given is reduced until the child is gaining weight on breastmilk alone. Wet nursing is encouraged when relactation is not a viable option.

Medical treatment guidelines suggest that inpatients receive parenteral antibiotics and appropriate treatment for any medical complications (WHO 2013). Broad-spectrum oral antibiotics such as amoxicillin are recommended for outpatient infants in weight-adjusted doses. Folic acid is routinely given at admission. Iron can be added to F100 once a child is suckling well and begins to gain weight.

Infants can be referred to outpatient care when they are free of medical complication, are clinically well and have an appetite, demonstrate sufficient weight gain in response to breastfeeding or replacement feeding, and are up to date on vaccinations. They can be discharged as recovered when they demonstrate adequate weight gain and a weight-for-length of ≥ -2 Z-scores (WHO 2013).

Management of Acute Malnutrition in Persons Infected with HIV

HIV infected malnourished patients can recover their nutritional status with the same therapeutic feeding approaches as children who are not HIV infected. The protocols require only minor modifications to the antibiotic regimen. In addition, HIV infected patients who qualify should receive antiretroviral drug treatment. To prevent toxicity, antiretroviral drugs are started only when nutritional status starts improving and any metabolic disturbances have been corrected.

Management of Acute Malnutrition in Adolescents, Adults, and Older People

Treatment of adolescents and adults follow similar protocols as children 6–59 months with fewer calories per kilogram, as the energy requirements of adults are considerably less than for children (Collins et al. 1998). The amount of therapeutic food required is inversely related with age. For example, the energy requirement for treatment of malnutrition at 10 years old (75 kcal/kg) is nearly double that for a 70-year-old (40 kcal/kg) (WHO 1999a). Treatment with antibiotics is recommended, as is the provision of vitamin A, except for pregnant women (WHO 1999a).

Malnourished adults are generally initially admitted for inpatient care. There is some limited evidence, however, to support outpatient management for adult patients with an appetite. Patients are discharged when they have regained appetite, are gaining weight, and have no remaining clinical conditions, including edema. A weight gain of 15 percent is often recommended (HTP 2011a).

Monitoring and Evaluation

Efficacy of CMAM programs is assessed both as the efficacy of the program to recover the children that are admitted to the program (performance statistics) and the ability of the program at recruiting malnourished children into the program (program coverage). The following sections provide an overview of methods for measuring both performance statistics and coverage.

Performance Statistics

Patients attending a supplementary or therapeutic feeding program are recorded in a dedicated registration book. They are often given an individual patient card summarizing their status and evolution. For outpatient care, the patient nutritional and health status are assessed at each visit. In inpatient facilities, the patient is assessed daily. In either case, a decision on the continuation or interruption of treatment is made and recorded in both the registration book and patient card. Performance indicators are then calculated based on collated discharge data from each treatment center.

There are key indicators monitored for any given period of time, typically a month:

Recovery Rate

Recovery rate is a measure of successful treatment and includes in the numerator the number of beneficiaries who are discharged after meeting the discharge criteria for the center. For OTP, this includes patients that are discharged to a tSFP or patients successfully treated in OTP where there is no tSFP. The denominator must include all children discharged from the program, regardless of the reason for discharge.

$$\left(\frac{Number\ successfully\ discharged\ as\ recovered}{Total\ discharges}\right) \times 100$$

Mortality Rate

Mortality rate includes in the numerator the number of beneficiaries that died from any cause while registered in the program. Deaths rarely occur at the program site in community-based programs. For this reason, active investigation of the status of patients that stop attending the center needs to be done in order to estimate the mortality rate of the program. The denominator must include all children discharged from the program, regardless of the reason for discharge.

$$\left(\frac{Number\ died\ while\ in\ the\ program}{Total\ discharges}\right) \times 100$$

Defaulter Rate

Defaulter rate includes both confirmed defaulters (those known to be alive as verified during a home visit) and unconfirmed defaulter (those absent for unknown reason but who could in fact be unrecorded deaths and therefore misclassified.) Defaulting is defined as missing two consecutive scheduled visits. The denominator must include all children discharged from the program regardless of the reason for discharge. Defaulter rate is interpreted as an indicator of accessibility and acceptability.

$$\left(\frac{Number\ defaulters\ nonconfirmed + Number\ defaulters\ confirmed}{Total\ discharges}\right) \times 100$$

Nonrecovery Rate

Nonrecovery rate includes beneficiaries that have care discontinued due to medical referral and transfer to a health facility as well as beneficiaries considered nonresponders, those that do not meet the discharge criteria after a predefined length of treatment, generally 3–4 months. For tSFP programs, nonrecovery rate also includes beneficiaries transferred to a therapeutic program such as a stabilization center or outpatient therapeutic care center.

Total discharges do not include patients that move to another equivalent facility but remain under treatment in the program. Additional indicators, such as the average length of stay or percentage of relapses, can be calculated using available administrative data.

Sphere key minimum standard for supplementary feeding programs specify that at least 75 percent of all discharged beneficiaries should recover, less than 3 percent die, and less than 15 percent default (Sphere 2011). For therapeutic programs (SCs and OTPs), Sphere specifies a less than 10 percent death rate as a minimum standard; however, other guidelines suggest that a standard of less than 3 percent can also be acheived at therapeutic programs (Sphere 2011, Navarro-Colorado, et al. 2012).

The above indicators should be calculated for each treatment facility, as well as collated at the program level, to understand program performance and provide remedial action when and where needed. In each program, these indicators should always be treated as flags for further investigation. If a treatment site or the whole program are underperforming, it's important to understand why, including what are the specific barriers hindering recovery. Understanding the specific challenges can help target interventions, improve quality, and obtain better outcomes. For example, if there are barriers to patients accessing care in a specific site or the overall program, a program may reconsider the locations of treatment sites or decentralizing feeding centers. If defaulter rates are high because stockouts are common, improving reporting of commodity stocks and employing defaulter tracking may be a more relevant intervention.

Performance statistics need to be calculated separately for each age and treatment group, since the expected performance may not be the same for children and pregnant and lactating women. In SFP, it is important to separate the performance statistics of children that have been admitted directly to the program with MAM from those that were referred after being cured in OTP, often referred as "TFP follow up" since the discharge criteria for this group is based in time in the program rather than in nutritional evolution.

Trends in the number of admissions are also monitored. However, this information is interpreted with caution, as an increase may indicate an increase in

$$\left(\frac{Number\ medical\ referrals + Number\ of\ non-response + Number\ of\ transfers\ to\ therapeutic\ care}{Total\ discharges}\right) \times 100$$

prevalence of malnutrition in a community, improvements in coverage, or an increase in the catchment population resulting from immigration to an area. Information on total admissions is essential for planning logistics and tracking commodity needs such as nutrition products, medication, and staff. Significant increases can also suggest a need to open additional treatment centers.

Coverage

Coverage is a measure of the number of patients that are receiving treatment for acute malnutrition in a specific area as a proportion of all patients with acute malnutrition in that area. Coverage is a critical indicator of program efficacy. A high-quality program with excellent recovery rates (90%) yet low coverage (30%) will meet the need of a lower proportion of children in need than programs of average quality with relatively low recovery rates (50%) and high coverage (70%), in which case met need is higher. As with other performance indicators, coverage may change rapidly due to changes in the quality of the program (i.e., stockouts, rumors) and the context in which the program operates (e.g., rainy season, which limits access, violence, population displacement). Hence, continuous monitoring of coverage would be a better measure of program efficacy than one-off measurements.

Coverage can be thought of as a composite indicator that flags barriers at all steps of a CMAM program. For example, coverage will be poor if there are failures in community mobilization (e.g., lack of awareness of malnutrition or the CMAM program, stigma, poor coverage of CHWs, and screenings), failures in provision of care (e.g., stockouts of commodities, long wait times, absent staff), barriers in accessing services (far distances, high opportunity costs) and other nonprogram barriers (insecurity, heavy rains, displacement). The Sphere Standards recommend specific coverage indicators for nutrition interventions in rural (50%), urban (70%), and camp environments (90%) (Sphere 2011).

Measuring coverage is an area of particular interest, given recent evidence that coverage in many contexts is low, often 40 percent or lower, even when community-based programs are operating with good support (Young, et al. 2004, Rogers and Guerrero 2014). Assessing coverage of treatment of SAM is complicated from a methodological point of view. As SAM is a relatively rare condition (generally less than 5 percent of children 6–59 months of age even in nutrition emergencies), identifying large enough sample sizes to achieve interpretable precision using population representative methods of sampling is challenging. Alternative methods, such as those that involve active case finding, often referred to as *active and adaptive methods,* including snowball sampling and chain-referral sampling, may introduce selection bias particularly in IDP, refugee, or urban settings where population movement is significant (Myatt et al. 2012). Additionally, survey methods estimate point coverage, which is coverage at a particular period in time. While this provides a useful snapshot, it gives no indication of how coverage is changing over time. A dynamic coverage indicator is thought to be more useful for program monitoring as it helps interpret changes in admission.

Work is ongoing to improve the methods by which we monitor and evaluate coverage achieved by CMAM programs. This includes improved analysis of routine program data, rapid community assessments to identify and address barriers to service access and uptake, as well as methods of estimating coverage. Given these difficulties in measuring coverage, and the complexity of interpreting coverage estimates, programs often also monitor geographic coverage. Geographic coverage is interpreted as the maximum coverage that a program can achieve (UNICEF 2015). Geographic coverage considers the number and location of treatment centers. Sphere guidelines recommend that nearly all (90%) of patients should be within one-day return walk to a treatment site or within one-hour walk if the program involves wet rations (on-site feeding). Geographic coverage is generally assessed as a mapping exercise, where the location of treatment centers and the location of patients are mapped to identify areas where geography may be a barrier. The proportion of health facilities offering CMAM services is also sometimes considered (UNICEF 2015).

Micronutrient Malnutrition

Micronutrient malnutrition encompasses several types of undernutrition that are the result of inadequate intake, absorption, or utilization of specific micronutrients. Micronutrient deficiency diseases (MDD) are the clinical diseases that occur because of lack of specific micronutrients.

Populations affected by emergencies are often at greater risk for MDD for many reasons. First, displaced populations are often dependent on external sources for food. Despite increased awareness among international organizations and considerable efforts to improve the micronutrient content of food rations, refugee populations dependent upon external food aid continue to be at high risk for micronutrient deficiency, particularly in contexts with insufficient food supply as a result of problems with access, importation, or limited funding (Dye 2007). Limited research suggests that micronutrient deficiencies may be greater among camp-based refugees than those living among the host population (Bilukha et al. 2014). Additionally, populations affected by humanitarian emergencies may also experience higher prevalence of diarrheal disease and infectious diseases, such as malaria or helminth infections, which can affect absorption and result in deficiencies (HTP 2011a).

Vitamin A, iodine, and iron deficiencies are the most prevalent MDDs globally, with an estimated two million people at risk (Bhutta et al. 2013). Some deficiencies are rarely seen in populations not affected by a humanitarian emergency. The following section discusses some key micronutrient conditions of public health importance in refugee and displaced populations.

Vitamin Deficiencies

Vitamin A

Vitamin A deficiency is considered a problem of public health significance in nearly all low-income countries, affecting nearly a third of preschool-age children (190 million) and 19 million pregnant women (WHO 2009).

Vitamin A deficiency causes a range of eye conditions including xerophthalmia, night blindness, corneal scars, and permanent blindness. Vitamin A deficiency is the leading cause of preventable pediatric blindness. Deficiencies in vitamin A have also been shown to cause weakened resistance, which can increase the severity of infectious diseases and risk of death (WHO 2009). Higher mortality rates from measles and diarrhea have been well documented in vitamin A deficient populations (Stevens et al. 2015). Individuals with clinical signs of xerophthalmia can be treated with an oral dose of vitamin A. In most cases, individuals will spontaneously recover without sequelae. Vitamin A deficiency is defined as serum retinol levels less than 0.70 μmol/L (Sommer and Davidson 2002).

Periodic supplementation is recommended in settings where vitamin A deficiency is a public health problem. Vitamin A supplementation has been added to the Expanded Program for Immunization (EPI) list and is commonly combined with polio eradication campaigns. Twice annual supplements containing 200,000 IU of vitamin A for children 1–5 years of age, with half doses for infants 6–11 months of age, are routine in many countries. In many high-risk countries, supplementation of mothers within six weeks of delivery is also recommended; however, coverage of this intervention remains low (WHO 2009).

In emergency contexts, vitamin A is recommended to be distributed to children aged 6 months to 15 years in tandem with measles immunization campaigns (UNICEF 2004; MSF 1997). Vitamin A supplementation may also be given to specific at risk groups including cases of measles, cases of severe and moderate malnutrition, and women at delivery. Supplementation is not recommended for infants under six months of age or pregnant women, given the risk of teratogenic effect on the fetus.

Efforts are also made to ensure vitamin A rich rations. Many foods are naturally rich in vitamin A, including fresh fruits (e.g., mangoes, cantaloupe), vegetables (e.g., sweet potatoes, carrots, dark leafy greens), fish, liver, and red palm oil. Vitamin A is also included in many fortified blended foods as well as vegetable oil.

Vitamin B1 (Thiamin)

In contrast to vitamin A deficiency, deficiencies in B vitamins, including deficiencies in niacin, riboflavin, and thiamin, are rarely seen outside emergency contexts. One of the most common vitamin B deficiencies is vitamin B1 (thiamin). Deficiencies in thiamin can result in beriberi. Beriberi occurs among populations where there is a diet high in carbohydrates and low in thiamin. This classically occurs among populations dependent on rations based on polished, nonparboiled rice. However, outbreaks among non-rice-eating populations do occur, such as in 2000 in North Eastern Kenya among pastoralists who primarily consumed maize (Stevens et al. 2001). Beriberi may also occur with alcoholism or with the consumption of foods containing antithiamin enzymes such as raw fish and some teas. As beriberi generally occurs among populations where energy intake is good and energy expenditure high, beriberi is not the consequence of starvation (Golden 1997).

There are three main types of beriberi:
- Dry beriberi presents as general dysfunction of the nervous system, loss of sensation in the feet, and weakness of the muscles.
- Wet beriberi is characterized by heart failure with signs of edema and hyperdynamic circulation.
- Infantile beriberi is associated with irritability, slight edema, and loss of crying voice.

Outbreaks of beriberi can be challenging to diagnose as the clinical features can be difficult to differentiate from other conditions in the absence of laboratory diagnostics.

Moderate beriberi can be treated with oral thiamin. Severe cases may require intravenous doses. After careful examination, patients can be given a flooding dose, as thiamin is not toxic in large quantities. In wet and infantile beriberi, response to treatment is rapid. Dry beriberi is often less responsive to treatment. At a population level, prevention measures should be in place to assure thiamin content in the general ration is sufficient. This can be done through diversification of the diet, ensuring adequate amounts of beans and ground nuts, or though fortification of blended foods. In the context of an outbreak, weekly mass drug supplementation may be advisable; however, ensuring access to fortified foods may be more feasible.

Vitamin B2 (Riboflavin)

Deficiencies in vitamin B2 (riboflavin) can result in ariboflavinosis or angular stomatitis, affecting the corners of the mouth. Inflammation of the tongue (glossitis), crackling of the lips (cheilosis), and conjunctivitis may also occur.

Riboflavin is understood to play a role in the absorption of other micronutrients, principally zinc and iron, such that poor riboflavin status contributes to anemia when iron intakes are low (Agte et al. 1998, Powers 2003).

Populations at highest risk are those dependent primarily on unfortified cereal flours or rice. Riboflavin deficiency is also often endemic in populations whose diets do not contain dairy products and meat (Powers 2003). Biochemical signs of depletion arise within only a few days of dietary deprivation (Powers 2003).

Treatment with vitamin B complex is recommended for cases with riboflavin deficiency. Long term, rations should be updated to contain sufficient riboflavin, 1.35–1.8 mg/d for adolescents (Blanck et al. 2002). Fortification of cereal flour or provision of fortified blended foods is often most feasible.

Vitamin B3/PP (Niacin)

Vitamin B3 (niacin) deficiency is known as pellagra, which presents as the three Ds: *dermatitis*, followed by *diarrhea* and *dementia*. Dermatitis appears on parts of the body exposed to sunlight, often around the nose and eyes, in a distinctive butterfly sign and around the neck, sometimes termed Casal's necklace after Gasper Casal who first described the condition (HTP 2011b).

Outbreaks of pellagra have been documented where niacin rich foods such as ground nuts, dried fish, and meats have not been provided in emergency rations. The 1990 outbreak of pellagra in Malawi among Mozambican refugees involving nearly 20 thousand cases is considered the most extensive reported since World War II and largely attributed to the absence of groundnuts and limited niacin in the food rations for a prolonged period (MMWR 1991). Subsequent outbreaks have been reported, including in Angola in 2001 (Young et al. 2004). Attack rates are generally higher among adult women (Malfait et al. 1993).

In the immediate term, weekly mass drug supplementation of niacin as well as vitamin B complex to the entire population is recommended once the outbreak is confirmed. Long-term supplementation is not recommended. Rather, rations should contain sufficient niacin, at least 6.6 mg per 1,000 kcal (MMWR, 1991).

Vitamin C (Scurvy)

Deficiencies in vitamin C present as scurvy. Cases of scurvy can be identified by characteristic bleeding gums, as well as petechiae, perifollicular hemorrhages, and painful joints. These symptoms are proceeded by weakness and irritability, dull aching pains, and weight loss (WHO 1999b). In children, vitamin C deficiency is called Moeller-Barlow disease, generally observed in nonbreastfed infants around 5–6 months of age (WHO 1999b). Vitamin C deficiency also increases risk of anemia.

Scurvy is most prevalent in semidesert areas, cold climates, and drought-affected areas that have limited provisions of fresh fruit, vegetables, and animal products such as milk. Scurvy is endemic in drought-affected regions of Afghanistan (Leborgne et al. 2002). Outbreaks have been identified in Ethiopian refugees in Somalia (1982), Somalia refugees in Hartisheik, Ethiopia (1989), Ethiopian refugees in Kassala, Sudan (1991), and among drought-affected pastoralists in Wajir, Kenya (1994) (WHO 1999b, Young et al. 2004).

The recommended dose of vitamin C remains debated; however, cases are often observed when intake of vitamin C is below 10–15 mg per day (MSF 1997, WHO 1999b). Cases can be managed with oral doses of vitamin C. Left untreated, scurvy can be fatal. Where the risk of outbreak is high, food fortification, food diversification, and drug supplementation to vulnerable groups (women, children, and the elderly) are recommended. However, vitamin C is not very stable and is destroyed quickly by heat and air, making fortification more challenging with vitamin C than other micronutrients.

Mineral Deficiencies

Iron Deficiency Anemia

Iron deficiency anemia is believed to be the most prevalent form of micronutrient malnutrition. The WHO estimates that 2 billion people are anemic, mostly due to iron deficiency (Camaschella 2015). In their review of anemia prevention strategies, UNHCR reported that anemia was a problem of serious public health importance, defined by WHO as greater than 40 percent prevalence among refugees in more than half of the sites assessed (UNHCR 2008).

Iron deficiency is responsible for more than half of nutritional anemia cases globally. Nutritional anemia includes anemia due to deficiencies in iron, folate, iron B12, and vitamin A. Malaria, hookworm, and schistosomiasis are other major causes of anemia. Iron deficiency is characterized by abnormally low blood hemoglobin concentrations, <110 g/L in children 6–59 months of age and pregnant women, <115 g/L in children 5–11 years of age, <120 g/L in children 11–14 years of age and nonpregnant women, and <130 g/L in men (WHO 2011). Adjustments to these thresholds should be made for individuals who reside at significant elevations above sea level or are smokers, conditions known to increase hemoglobin concentrations. Rapid testing of hemoglobin levels to diagnose anemia is now widely used in the field; however, differential diagnosis of the cause of anemia is rarely possible (MSF 1997).

Iron deficiency anemia is often identified among populations that do not eat meat. Iron is best absorbed from heme iron sources such as liver, beef, or lamb. However, iron is better regulated from nonheme plant sources, including dark leafy greens such as spinach, beans, and whole grains. Iron absorption can be increased by also increasing consumption of vitamin C. Many cereals, tea, and coffee inhibit absorption.

Pregnant and lactating women, as well as children aged 6 to 36 months, have higher iron needs and therefore are at higher risk for iron deficiency anemia. In all contexts, regardless of prevalence, iron or folic acid and iron supplements are recommended for pregnant women (Sazawal 2006). Maternal supplementation can also protect against deficiency in newborns. As noted previously, severely malnourished children should not receive iron supplements during the first two weeks of treatment.

Following a technical consultation on anemia in refugees in 2008, UNHCR guidelines have been revised to include the blanket use of micronutrient powders (MNP) at the household level and lipid-based nutrient supplements (LNS) for children aged 6–23 months in contexts where prevalence of anemia is high (UNHCR 2008).

Generally, iron deficiency anemia can be treated with oral supplementation. Concurrent supplements of vitamin C can help iron absorption. If present, parasitic infections should also be treated. Where anemia is the result of malaria, antimalarial drugs should be administered, but iron is not recommended unless associated iron deficiency is confirmed, as iron supplementation has been shown to increase severity and mortality from malaria in children (WHO 2012b).

Iodine

Iodine is essential to the synthesis of thyroid hormones. Deficiency in iodine is a primary cause of impaired cognitive development and mental disorders. The spectrum of conditions linked to iodine deficiency, known collectively as iodine deficiency disorders (IDD), include goiter and cretinism. Deficiency in pregnant women can also result in stillbirth and miscarriages.

Universal salt iodization was endorsed as the main strategy for elimination of IDD in 1993 (WHO 2014). More than 120 countries now implement salt iodization programs (WHO 1994). Deficiencies in iodine remain a public health problem primarily in areas where salt is not fortified with iodine and where iodine content in soil is low. Unlike other micronutrient deficiencies, dietary diversification generally will not reduce prevalence of IDD in endemic areas where food is grown in soil with low iodine levels. Inclusion of iodized salt in general food distributions is generally sufficient to prevent IDD. Recent literature has even demonstrated excess dietary iodine intake among long-term refugees dependent on rations (Seal et al. 2006). Goiter can be treated with oral doses of iodine. Cretinism cannot be treated, but can be prevented with prophylactic doses of iodine for pregnant women.

Zinc

Zinc is found in all cells, and consequently, deficiencies in zinc have broad physiologic implications, effecting protein synthesis, cell growth and differentiation, and immune function. Supplementation with zinc has been shown to reduce the duration, severity, and incidence of diarrheal episodes (Bhutta et al. 2000). Zinc supplementation along with provision of oral rehydration salts (ORS) is recommended treatment for diarrhea (Khan and Selen 2011). Given that diarrheal episodes are a primary cause of weight loss among children, particularly in humanitarian emergency settings, zinc supplementation is considered a key nutrition intervention. Zinc supplementation may also reduce incidence of acute lower respiratory infections, such as pneumonia, as well as malaria (Bhutta et al. 1999, Sazawal et al. 1998).

Zinc is widely present in foods, with the highest concentrations found in meat, fish, shellfish, nuts, seeds, legumes, and wholegrain cereals. However, zinc from wholegrain cereals and legumes is absorbed less efficiently than from animal products, as absorption is inhibited by fiber and phytates (Shah et al. 2016). Therefore, zinc deficiencies are more common in populations primarily dependent on these sources.

Zinc supplements come in a variety of forms. Supplementation can be achieved with tablets, pills, powders, or syrups of common zinc salts. WHO recommends a supplemental dose of 20 mg per day for 10–14 days to treat diarrhea in children aged 6 to 59 months (WHO 2016). There are no standard recommendations for dose or frequency of preventive supplementation with zinc (Mayo-Wilson et al. 2014).

Prevention and Treatment

Recognizing that multiple micronutrient deficiencies are often present among populations dependent on diets with limited diversity, the current strategy of emergency programs is toward prevention of micronutrient deficiencies with fortified and blended foods, as well as promotion of dietary diversity where feasible. The policy of most major food aid donors is that all blended foods, oils, and salts should be fortified with one or multiple micronutrients. For example, cereal flours may be fortified with B vitamins, oil is usually fortified with vitamin A, and salt is usually fortified with iodine.

Blended foods such as corn soy blend (CSB) are also routinely distributed in general ration distributions as an alternative to maize or flour in humanitarian emergencies. CSB Plus and similar products contain a premix containing vitamin A, vitamin D3, vitamin E, vitamin K, B vitamins, vitamin C, biotin, niacin, folic acid, iodine, iron, zinc, potassium, calcium, and phosphorus (USAID 2016). Micronutrient powders (MNP) and lipid-based nutrient supplements (LNS), which both contain a mix of micronutrients, have been endorsed for use in prevention of micronutrient deficiencies among refugees (UNHCR 2011). LNS are fortified pastes that contains vitamins and minerals in addition to providing energy. MNPs provide only vitamins and minerals, not energy.

In addition to the provision of these products, a variety of other prevention strategies may be considered, depending on the context. An effective prevention strategy with long-term impact is likely to use a combination of different approaches. The relevance of each will depend on the primary source of food (whether general food rations or otherwise), access to local markets, and availability of land for cultivation. These strategies include:

- Inclusion of nutrient-rich commodities in food aid rations. For example, ground nuts (peanuts) are a good source of *niacin* (vitamin B3). Including fresh food items can help address micronutrient deficiencies. However, large scale provision of fresh fruits and vegetables can be a challenge.
- Promotion of home gardening and agricultural development. The distribution of seeds, tools, and other agricultural inputs may allow populations to grow vegetables and fruit or livestock for home consumption or sale. However, access to land may be a major constraint, particularly in refugee

camps or in areas which are insecure. Access to adequate water may also be a limiting factor.
- Increasing income generation or distribution of cash and/or vouchers. Increasing household income can help to improve the dietary intake of micronutrients by increasing diet diversity. This strategy assumes the displaced population has access to markets where they can spend cash or vouchers.
- Promotion of recommended infant and young child feeding practices. Promotion of exclusive breastfeeding and appropriate complementary feeding practices are critical public health interventions that also contribute to maintaining micronutrient status. Exclusive breastfeeding up to six months of age, followed by the introduction of age-appropriate, nutritionally adequate and safe complementary foods with continued breastfeeding, are very important for the nutritional status and health of children.
- Ensuring adequate health care and a healthy environment. Good health is very important in maintaining good nutrition and micronutrient status. Examples of public health interventions that may contribute to preventing micronutrient deficiencies include: measles vaccination, provision of good sanitation, hygiene promotion including hand washing, and programs to control malaria.
- Ensuring access to adequate nonfood items. If households are lacking nonfood items such as cooking pots, soap, or assets such as tools, they may choose to use available food stocks or assets to buy these rather than to improve the quantity or quality of their diet.
- Increasing the size of the general food ration. This can facilitate diet diversification by exchange or trade. This approach may be particularly useful when there are inadequate supplies of micronutrient-rich food aid commodities, and the beneficiaries have access to markets where micronutrient-rich foods are available.

Integrating Management of Acute Malnutrition into National Health Systems

Treatment of acute malnutrition has traditionally been understood as an emergency intervention, whereby treatment programs for acute malnutrition are scaled-up in response to a humanitarian emergency and scaled back down once the situation has stabilized. This approach presumes that acute malnutrition is a temporary phenomenon, like an outbreak of measles, with a clear start and end (Hailey and Tewoldeberha 2010). In fact, the prevalence of acute malnutrition in nonemergency contexts is not zero. Millions of children suffer from acute malnutrition in nonhumanitarian emergency settings (UNICEF 2015). The traditional model also presumes that cases of acute malnutrition during nonemergency times can be treated by the existing health system. This is often inaccurate, unless a specific program has been established at the national level to support treatment of malnutrition at the health system. While CMAM programs can be very effective in the context of a humanitarian emergency with the supplemental resources and qualified staff from international donors and humanitarian agencies, the treatment of malnutrition as described is often not feasible in post-emergency and developing contexts. This is particularly true in contexts with limited health care budgets and only a handful of clinicians for every one hundred thousand people (Park et al. 2012). When a humanitarian emergency begins, there is always a time lag between the rise in prevalence of acute malnutrition and the detection and response with additional resources. This is especially problematic if these additional cases cannot be treated within the existing health system.

In response to this situation, humanitarian agencies have proposed to address these limitations by focusing on building the capacity of the existing health system to manage acute malnutrition as part of the emergency response. The aim of this approach is to support Ministries of Health (MoH) to provide treatment for acute malnutrition according to standard protocols during times of nonemergency, as well as scale-up care during the lag time between the observed rise in prevalence of GAM and the international response during a humanitarian emergency.

For the success and scale-up of these services, it is important that health staff at all levels take responsibility for the screening, diagnosis, and management of acute malnutrition. This health system–based approach implies that international stakeholders shift their role in management of acute malnutrition from that of implementer to facilitator in support of health ministries in the management of acute malnutrition (Israel and Gallagher 2013). Acting as

Table 25.3 WHO pillars of health system strengthening in the context of treatment of acute malnutrition

Pillar	Definition	Examples of support linked to malnutrition
Leadership/ governance	Strategic policies, oversight of the system and regulation; bringing together public, private and volunteer sectors	Support in development of policies and guidelines for CMAM, IYCF, micronutrient supplementation
Health care financing	Health financing policies; tools and information on health spending; cost projections	Lobbying for funding for nutrition activities; including costs for nutrition programs commodities (e.g., RUTFs) in the national budget
Health workforce	Developing and sustaining the qualified human resource structure to meet health needs	Including treatment of acute malnutrition in training curriculums; on the job training for current health care providers
Essential medicines/ technology	Timely and regular availability of medicines and equipment	Supporting the supply chain by directly transporting or joint planning; review of supply systems
Information and research	Data to monitor the health system's performance, influence policy and decision making	Technical support of Health Information System and integration of nutrition indicators; support to strengthening data management systems; use of mobiles and other electronic devices
Service delivery	Diagnosis and treatment of disease; promotion of best practices for health	On the job coaching with health workforce on CMAM and other nutrition specific interventions.

a facilitator may include several roles. Stakeholders may complement programs with the MoH by working with clinicians in the health system to jointly provide services, they may serve as field support to the MOH providing on the job training, and they may work in an advisory role to the MoH seconded to help draft guidance and protocols.

Strengthening the whole health system means focusing on the pillars of leadership and governance, health care financing, health workforce, medical products and technology, information and research, and service delivery. Table 25.3 outlines how these six pillars for health system strengthening can be understood in the context of treatment of acute malnutrition (WHO 2007b).

References

Agte, V. V., Paknikar, K. M., and Chiplonkar, S. A. (1998). Effect of riboflavin supplementation on zinc and iron absorption and growth performance in mice. *Biological trace element research*, 65(2), 109–115.

Ahmed, T., Ali, M., Ullah, M. M., Choudhury, I. A., Haque, M. E., Salam, M. A., Rabbani, G. H., Suskind, R. M., and Fuchs, G. J. (1999). Mortality in severely malnourished children with diarrhoea and use of a standardised management protocol. *Lancet*, 353(9168), 1919–1922.

Annan, R. A., Webb, P., and Brown, R. (2014). *Management of moderate acute malnutrition (MAM): Current knowledge and practice.* CMAM forum (online). Available at: www.cmamforum.org/Pool/Resources/MAM-management-CMAM-Forum-Technical-Brief-Sept-2014.pdf.

Ashworth, A. (2001). Treatment of severe malnutrition. *J Pediatr Gastroenterol Nutr*, 32(5), 516–518.

Bhutta, Z. A., Bird, S. M., Black, R. E., et al. (2000). Therapeutic effects of oral zinc in acute and persistent diarrhea in children in developing countries: pooled analysis of randomized controlled trials. *Am J Clin Nutr*, 72(6), 1516–1522.

Bhutta, Z. A., Black, R. E., Brown, K. H., et al. (1999). Prevention of diarrhea and pneumonia by zinc supplementation in children in developing countries: pooled analysis of randomized controlled trials. Zinc Investigators' Collaborative Group. *J Pediatr*, 135(6), 689–697.

Bhutta, Z. A., Salam, R. A., and Das, J. K. (2013). Meeting the challenges of micronutrient malnutrition in the developing world. *Br Med Bull*, 106, 7–17.

Bilukha, O. O., Jayasekaran, D., Burton, A., et al. (2014). Nutritional status of women and child refugees from Syria-Jordan, April-May 2014. *MMWR Morb Mortal Wkly Rep*, 63(29), 638–639.

Blanck, H. M., Bowman, B. A., Serdula, M. K., et al. (2002). Angular stomatitis and riboflavin status among adolescent Bhutanese refugees living in southeastern Nepal. *Am J Clin Nutr*, 76(2), 430–435.

Blanton, L. V., Charbonneau, M. R., Salih, T., et al. (2016). Gut bacteria that prevent growth impairments transmitted by microbiota from malnourished children. *Science*, 351(6275).

Burtsher, D. (2013). *Involving communities: Guidance document for approaching and cooperating with communities* (online). Available at: https://evaluation.msf.org/sites/eva luation/files/involving_communities_0.pdf (Accessed on July 6, 2017).

Camaschella, C. (2015). Iron-deficiency anemia. *N Engl J Med*, 373(5), 485–486.

Christian P, Katz J, Wu L. Risk factors for pregnancy-related mortality: a prospective study in rural Nepal. Public Health. 2008 Feb;122(2):161–72. Epub 2007 Sep 10.

Collins, S., Myatt, M., and Golden, B. (1998). Dietary treatment of severe malnutrition in adults. *Am J Clin Nutr*, 68(1), 193–199.

Collins, S. and Sadler, K. (2002). Outpatient care for severely malnourished children in emergency relief programmes: a retrospective cohort study. *Lancet*, 360(9348), 1824–1830.

Collins, S. and Yates, R. (2003). The need to update the classification of acute malnutrition. *Lancet*, 362(9379), 249.

de Onis M., Onyango, A.W., Borghi, E., et al. (2006). Comparison of the World Health Organization (WHO) child growth standards and the National Center for Health Statistics/WHO international growth reference: implications for child health programmes. *Public Health Nutr*, 9(7),942–947.

Dye, T. D. (2007). Contemporary prevalence and prevention of micronutrient deficiencies in refugee settings worldwide. *Journal of Refugee Studies*, 20(1), 108–119.

Golden, M. H. (1982). Protein deficiency, energy deficiency, and the oedema of malnutrition. *Lancet*, 1(8284), 1261–1265.

Golden, M. H. (1996). Severe malnutrition, in D. J., Weatherall, J. G. G. Ledington, and D. A. Warrell, eds. *Oxford Textbook of Medicine*, 3rd edition. Oxford: Oxford University Press, pp. 1278–1296.

Golden, M. H. (1997). Diagnosing beriberi in emergency situations. *Field Exchange*, (1), 17.

Golden, M. H. (2002). The development of concepts of malnutrition. *J Nutr*, 132(7), 2117s–2122s.

Golden, M. H. (2010). Evolution of nutritional management of acute malnutrition. *Indian Pediatr*, 47(8), 667–678.

Grellety, E. and Golden, M. H. (2016). Weight-for-height and mid-upper-arm circumference should be used independently to diagnose acute malnutrition: policy implications. *BMC Nutrition*, 2(1), 1–17.

Hailey, P. and Tewoldeberha, D. (2010). Suggested new design framework for CMAM Programming. *Field Exchange*, (39), 41.

Harmonized Training Package. (2011a). *Module 4: Micronutrient malnutrition*. Oxford: Emergency Nutrition Network (ENN).

Harmonized Training Package. (2011b) *Module 13: Management of severe acute malnutrition*. Oxford: Emergency Nutrition Network (ENN).

Isanaka, S., Langendorf, C., Berthe, F., et al. (2016). Routine amoxicillin for uncomplicated severe acute malnutrition in children. *N Engl J Med*, 374(5), 444–453.

Israel, A. D. and Gallagher, M. (2013). From vertical to horizontal: Experiences & recommendation in integrating SAM treatment to the health system, abstract for conference presentation, in International SAM Conference, London.

Karakochuk, C., van den Briel, T., Stephens, D., et al. (2012). Treatment of moderate acute malnutrition with ready-to-use supplementary food results in higher overall recovery rates compared with a corn-soya blend in children in southern Ethiopia: an operations research trial. *Am J Clin Nutr*, 96(4), 911–916.

Kerac, M., McGrath, M., Grijalva-Eternod, C., et al. (2012). Psychosocial aspects of malnutrition management in *Management of Acute Malnutrition in Infants (MAMI) Project*. Available at: https://scholar.google.com/scholar?q=Management+of+Acute+Malnutrition+in+Infants+(MAMI)+Project+2012&hl=en&as_sdt=0&as_vis=1&oi=scholart&sa=X&ved=0ahUKEwic2_Gro_vXAhUW6WMKHSCYBSwQgQMIJTAA. (Accessed December 1, 2017).

Kerac, M., Mwangome, M., McGrath, M., et al. (2015). Management of acute malnutrition in infants aged under 6 months (MAMI): current issues and future directions in policy and research. *Food Nutr Bull*, 36(1 Suppl), S30–S34.

Khan, W. U. and D.W., S. (2011). *Zinc supplementation in the management of diarrhoea*: e-Library of Evidence for Nutrition Actions (eLENA) (online). Available at: www.who.int/elena/titles/bbc/zinc_diarrhoea/en/ (Accessed July 6, 2017).

Kulin, H. E., Bwibo, N., Mutie, D., et al. (1982). The effect of chronic childhood malnutrition on pubertal growth and development. *Am J Clin Nutr*, 36(3), 527–536.

Leborgne, P., Wilkinson, C., Montembaut, S., and Ververs, M. T. (2002). Scurvy outbreak in Afghanistan: an investigation by Action Contre la Faim (ACF) and WHO. *Field Exchange*, (17) 27.

Malfait, P., Moren, A., Dillon, J. C., et al. (1993). An outbreak of pellagra related to changes in dietary niacin among Mozambican refugees in Malawi. *Int J Epidemiol*, **22**(3), 504–511.

MAM Task Force. (2014). *Moderate acute malnutrition: A decision tool for emergencies*: Geneva, Switzerland: Global Nutrition Cluster.

Manary, M. J., Maleta, K. and Trehan, I. (2012). *Randomized, double-blind, placebo-controlled trial evaluating the need for routine antibiotics as part of the outpatient management of severe acute malnutrition.* Washington, DC: FHI 360/FANTA-2 Bridge (online). Available at: www.fantaproject.org/sites/default/files/resources/FANTA-CMAM-Antibiotic-Study-2).Mar2012.pdf (Accessed on July 9, 2017).

Mayo-Wilson, E., Junior, J., Imdad, A., et al. (2014). Zinc supplementation for preventing mortality, morbidity, and growth failure in children aged 6 months to 12 years of age (Review). *Cochrane Database of Systematic Reviews*, **15**(5), CD009384.

Médecins Sans Frontières (MSF). (1997). Refugee Health: An approach to emergency situations. G. Hanquet, general editor.

Myatt, M., Guevarra, E., Fieschi, L., et al. (2012). *Semi-Quantitative Evaluation of Access and Coverage (SQUEAC)/Simplified Lot Quality Assurance Sampling Evaluation of Access and Coverage (SLEAC) technical reference.* Washington, DC: FHI 360/FANTA (online). Available at: www.fantaproject.org/sites/default/files/resources/SQUEAC-SLEAC-Technical-Reference-Oct2012_0.pdf (Accessed on July 9, 2017).

Nackers, F., Broillet, F., Oumarou, D., et al. (2010). Effectiveness of ready-to-use therapeutic food compared to a corn/soy-blend-based pre-mix for the treatment of childhood moderate acute malnutrition in Niger. *J Trop Pediatr*, **56**(6), 407–413.

Navarro-Colorado, C., Andert, C., Mates, E., et al. (2012). *Minimum reporting package for emergency supplementary and therapeutic feeding programmes* (online). Available at: www.cmamforum.org/Pool/Resources/MRP-UserGuidelinesFINAL-2012.pdf (Accessed on July 9, 2017).

Navarro-Colorado, C. (2006). *Adult malnutrition in emergencies: An overview of diagnosis and treatment.*

Ndekha, M., van Oosterhout, J. J., Saloojee, H., et al. (2009). Nutritional status of Malawian adults on antiretroviral therapy 1 year after supplementary feeding in the first 3 months of therapy. *Trop Med Int Health*, **14**(9), 1059–1063.

Outbreak of pellagra among Mozambican refugees–Malawi, 1990. (1991). *MMWR Morb Mortal Wkly Rep*, **40**(13), 209–213.

PAHO. (1991). *Maternal nutrition and pregnancy outcomes. Anthropometric Assessment, Scientific Publication No 529.* Washington, DC: Pan American Health Organization.

Park, S. E., Kim, S., Ouma, C., et al. (2012). Community management of acute malnutrition in the developing world. *Pediatr Gastroenterol Hepatol Nutr*, **15**(4), 210–219.

Patel, M. P., Sandige, H. L., Ndekha, M. J., et al. (2005). Supplemental feeding with ready-to-use therapeutic food in Malawian children at risk of malnutrition. *J Health Popul Nutr*, **23**(4), 351–357.

Perez-Exposito, A. B., and Klein, B. P. (2009). Impact of fortified blended food aid products on nutritional status of infants and young children in developing countries. *Nutr Rev*, **67**(12), 706–718.

Powers, H. J. (2003). Riboflavin (vitamin B-2) and health. *Am J Clin Nutr*, **77**(6), 1352–60.

Puett, C., Swan, S. H., and Guerrero, S. (2013). *Access for all, Volume 2: What factors influence access to community-based treatment of severe acute malnutrition?* London: Coverage Monitoring Network.

Rogers, E., and Guerrero, S. (2014). *Access for all: What can community-based SAM treatment learn from other public health interventions to improve access and coverage?* London: Coverage Monitoring Network (online). Available at: www.cmamforum.org/Pool/Resources/Access-for-All-(Vol-3)-CMAM-learning-from-other-PH-interventions-CMN-2014.pdf (Accessed on July 9, 2017).

Sazawal, S., Black, R. E., Jalla, S., et al. (1998). Zinc supplementation reduces the incidence of acute lower respiratory infections in infants and preschool children: a double-blind, controlled trial. *Pediatrics*, **102**(1 Pt 1), 1–5.

Sazawal, S., Black, R. E., Ramsan, M., et al. (2006). Effects of routine prophylactic supplementation with iron and folic acid on admission to hospital and mortality in preschool children in a high malaria transmission setting: community-based, randomised, placebo-controlled trial. *Lancet*, **367**(9505), 133–143.

Seal, A. J., Creeke, P. I., Gnat, D., et al. (2006). Excess dietary iodine intake in long term African refugees. *Public Health Nutr*, **9**(1), 35–39.

Shah, D., Sachdev, H. S., Gera, T., et al. (2016). Fortification of staple foods with zinc for improving zinc status and other health outcomes in the general population (Review). *Cochrane Database of Systematic Reviews*, (6), CD010697.

Sommer, A., and Davidson, F.R. (2002). Assessment and control of vitamin A deficiency: the Annecy Accords. *J Nutr*, **132**(9 Suppl), 2845s–2850s.

Stevens, D., Araru, P., and Dragudi, B. (2001). Outbreak of micronutrient deficiency disease: did we respond appropriately? *Field Exchange*, 12–14.

Stevens, G. A., Bennett, J. E., Hennocq, Q., et al. (2015). Trends and mortality effects of vitamin A deficiency in children in 138 low-income and middle-income countries between 1991 and 2013: a pooled analysis of population-based surveys. *Lancet Glob Health*, **3**(9), e528–536.

The Sphere Project. (2015). Humanitarian charter and minimum standards in humanitarian response. P. Greaney, S. Pfiffner, and D. Wilson, eds. Practical Action Publishing: Rugby: United Kingdom.

Tang A, Chung M, Dong K, et al. Determining a Global Mid-Upper Arm Circumference Cutoff to Assess Underweight in Adults (Men and Nonpregnant Women). Washington, DC: FHI 360/FANTA.

Toole, M. J., Malkki, R. M., Blake, P. A., et al. (1992) Famine-affected, refugee, and displaced populations: Recommendations for public health issues. *MMWR Recomm Rep*, **41**(Rr-13), 1–76.

United Nations Children Fund. (2016). Management of severe acute malnutrition in children: Working towards results at scale (online). Available at: www.unicef.org/eapro/UNICEF_program_guidance_on_manangement_of_SAM_2015.pdf (Accessed on July 9, 2017).

United Nations Children Fund. Technical bulletin No 16. Supercereal products (online). Available at: www.unicef.org/supply/files/Supercereal_Products_(CSB).pdf (Accessed on July 9, 2017).

United Nations Children Fund, World Health Organization. (2004). WHO/UNICEF joint statement: Reducing measles mortality in emergencies (online). Available at: www.who.int/immunization/diseases/WHO_UNICEF_Measles_Emergencies.pdf (Accessed on July 9, 2017).

United Nations Children Fund, World Health Organization, World Bank Group. (2015). Joint child malnutrition estimates – Levels and trends (2015 edition) (online). Available at: www.who.int/nutgrowthdb/estimates2014/en/ (Accessed on July 9, 2017).

United Nations High Commissioner for Refugees. (2008). UNHCR strategic plan for anaemia prevention, control and reduction. Reducing the global burden of anaemia in refugee populations (online). Available at: www.unhcr.org/4b8e854d9.pdf (Accessed on July 9, 2017).

United Nations High Commissioner for Refugees. (2011). UNHCR operational guidance on the use of special nutritional products to reduce micronutrient deficiencies and malnutrition in refugee populations. UNHCR: Geneva (online). Available at: www.unhcr.org/4f1fc3de9.pdf (Accessed on July 9, 2017).

United Nations High Commissioner for Refugees, World Food Program. (1999). Selective Feeding Programmes in Emergency Situations, 1999 (online). Available at: www.who.int/nutrition/publications/en/selective_feeding_emergencies.pdf (Accessed July 9, 2017).

United Nations High Commissioner for Refugees, World Food Program. (2011). Guidelines for selective feeding: The management of malnutrition in emergencies. Geneva (online). Available at: www.unhcr.org/4b7421fd20.html (Accessed on July 9, 2017).

United States Agency for International Development. (2016). Corn Soy Blend Plus commodity factsheet (online). Available at: www.usaid.gov/what-we-do/agriculture-and-food-security/food-assistance/resources/implementation-tools/corn-soy (Accessed July 9, 2017).

Ververs M, Antierens A, Sackl A et al. Which Anthropometric Indicators Identify a Pregnant Woman as Acutely Malnourished and Predict Adverse Birth Outcomes in the Humanitarian Context? PLoS Curr. 2013 June 7; 5.

World Health Organization. (1994). Iodine and health: Eliminating iodine deficiency disorder safely through salt iodization. WHO: Geneva (online). Available at: http://apps.who.int/iris/bitstream/10665/58693/1/WHO_NUT_94.4.pdf?ua=1 (Accessed July 9, 2017).

World Health Organization. (1995a). Physical status: The use and interpretation of anthropometry. Report of a WHO expert committee. Technical Report Series No. 854. World Health Organization: Geneva.

World Health Organization. (1995b). Maternal anthropometry and pregnancy outcomes. A WHO Collaborative Study: Introduction. *Bull World Health Organ*, 73 suppl, 1–6.

World Health Organization. (1999a). Management of severe malnutrition: A manual for physicians and other senior health workers.

World Health Organization. (1999b). Scurvy and its prevention and control in major emergencies (online). Available at: www.unhcr.org/4cbef0599.pdf (Accessed July 9, 2017).

World Health Organization. (2007b). Everybody's business: Strengthening the health system to improve health outcomes. WHO: Geneva (online). Available at: www.who.int/healthsystems/strategy/en/ (Accessed July 9, 2017).

World Health Organization. (2007c). Growth reference 5–19 years (online). Available at: www.who.int/growthref/en (Accessed July 9, 2017).

World Health Organization. (2009). Global prevalence of vitamin A deficiency in populations at risk 1995–2005. WHO global database on vitamin A deficiency. Geneva: WHO, 2009 (online). Available at: http://apps.who.int/iris/bitstream/10665/44110/1/9789241598019_eng.pdf. (Accessed July 9, 2017).

World Health Organization. (2010). Consultation on the Programmatic Aspects of the Management of Moderate Acute Malnutrition in Children under five years of age. WHO: Geneva (online). Available at: www.who.int/nutrition/topics/moderatemalnutrition_consultation_programmaticaspects_MM_report.pdf (Accessed July 9, 2017).

World Health Organization. (2011). Haemoglobin concentrations for the diagnosis of anaemia and assessment of severity, Vitamin and Mineral Nutrition Information System, Editor. WHO: Geneva (online). Available at: www

.who.int/vmnis/indicators/haemoglobin.pdf (Accessed July 9, 2017).

World Health Organization. (2012a). Technical note: Supplementary foods for the management of moderate acute malnutrition in infants and children 6–59 months of age. World Health Organization: Geneva (online). Available at: www.who.int/nutrition/publications/moderate_malnutrition/9789241504423/en/ (Accessed July 9, 2017).

World Health Organization. (2012b). Daily iron and folic acid supplementation in pregnant women: Guideline. WHO: Geneva (online). Available at: www.who.int/nutrition/publications/micronutrients/guidelines/daily_ifa_supp_pregnant_women/en/ (Accessed July 9, 2017).

World Health Organization. (2013). Guideline: Updates on the management of severe acute malnutrition in infants and children. World Health Organization: Geneva.

World Health Organization. (2014). Guideline: Fortification of food-grade salt with iodine for the prevention and control of iodine deficiency disorders. 2014, WHO: Geneva (online). Available at: http://apps.who.int/iris/bitstream/10665/136908/1/9789241507929_eng.pdf?ua=1 (Accessed July 9, 2017).

World Health Organization. (2016). Zinc supplementation in the management of diarrhoea: e-Library of Evidence for Nutrition Actions (eLENA) (online). Available at: www.who.int/elena/titles/zinc_diarrhoea/en/ (Accessed July 9, 2017).

World Health Organization, United Nations Children's Fund. (2009). WHO child growth standards and the identification of severe acute malnutrition in infants and children: A Joint Statement by the World Health Organization and the United Nations Children's Fund. WHO and UNICEF: Geneva.

World Health Organization, World Food Programme, United Nations System Standing Committee on Nutrition. (2007a). Community Based Management of Severe Acute Malnutrition (online). Available at: www.who.int/nutrition/topics/Statement_community_based_man_sev_acute_mal_eng.pdf (Accessed July 9, 2017).

Young, H., Borrel, A., Holland, D., et al. (2004). Public nutrition in complex emergencies. *Lancet*, **364**(9448), 1899–1909.

Chapter 26

Measles

Eugene Lam, Allen Gidraf Kahindo Maina, Lisandro Torre, Muireann Brennan, and James L. Goodson

Introduction

Measles is a highly infectious acute viral disease and major cause of childhood morbidity and mortality worldwide including during humanitarian emergencies (Toole and Waldman 1990, Lam et al. 2015a, Liu et al. 2015, Strebel et al. 2016). Humans are the only host for the measles virus which is spread by transmission of aerosolized respiratory droplets from person to person. Despite the availability of a safe and effective vaccine, measles is one of the leading causes of death among young children globally, responsible for 114,900 deaths in 2014 (Perry et al. 2015, WHO 2015b). Measles infection is associated with serious complications, including an increased susceptibility to other infectious agents because of measles-induced immunosuppression and exacerbation of vitamin A deficiency, both especially critical during humanitarian emergencies (WHO 2005a). Infants and children under five years of age are at heightened risk for contracting measles and developing complications (WHO 2005b).

Before widespread use of measles vaccines, measles was estimated to cause 5–8 million deaths annually (WHO 2009). Since the introduction of the first measles vaccine in the early 1960s, there have been dramatic reductions in measles infections and deaths. Increased use of measles-containing vaccine (MCV) in routine vaccination programs and mass vaccination campaigns, also called supplementary immunization activities (SIAs), has resulted in remarkable progress in reducing measles incidence and mortality worldwide, particularly in the Americas where there is no longer endemic transmission of the measles virus.

Eradication

In July 2010, an expert advisory panel convened by the World Health Organization (WHO) concluded that measles can and should be eradicated. These conclusions have since been endorsed by the WHO Strategic Advisory Group of Experts (SAGE) and the World Health Assembly (WHA) (WHO 2010a). In 2012, the WHA endorsed the Global Vaccine Action Plan (GVAP) with a major objective to eliminate measles in five WHO regions by 2020. In addition, the Measles & Rubella Initiative launched the 2012–2020 Global Measles and Rubella Strategic Plan with goals aligned to the GVAP (WHO 2012a).

Since 2013, all six WHO regions have adopted goals to eliminate measles by 2020 (WHO 2012a). However, major challenges to global measles eradication have been identified, including difficulties in achieving high vaccination coverage in settings with high population density, natural disasters, war, and civil unrest, which cause interruptions in vaccination activities and population displacement, and the increasing frequency of international travel and forced displacement that facilitate measles virus importations and transmission (Strebel et al. 2016). Implementation of effective prevention strategies as well as outbreak preparedness and response among displaced populations in the setting of complex humanitarian emergencies is critical because movement of susceptible populations increases the risk of virus introduction and large outbreaks and has the potential to challenge progress toward measles elimination globally.

Outbreaks

Humanitarian emergencies in the setting of natural disasters, famine, war, large-scale population movements, and outbreaks of emerging pathogens can cause disruptions in immunization services and create persistent reservoirs for vaccine-preventable diseases (VPDs) and for the measles virus, in particular. Protracted armed conflict, especially in the absence of a centralized government, can cripple efforts to provide basic public health services to local civilian populations, including the delivery of vaccinations to children. Prevention of VPD outbreaks should be a high priority in these settings. Measles outbreaks, when they occur, can quickly overwhelm already marginalized health systems and cause significant morbidity and mortality. Measles SIA planning and implementation during humanitarian emergencies should engage local leaders in microplanning and social mobilization, focusing on hard-to-reach areas, improving training, and conducting house-to-house canvassing during the SIA.

To prevent large measles outbreaks and reach elimination goals, vaccination efforts must achieve and maintain high 2-dose MCV coverage to reach the population immunity threshold required for herd immunity. In refugee settings, Sphere minimum standards for humanitarian response include providing two doses of MCV to every child, monitoring 2-dose MCV coverage, including informal settlements and host communities in vaccination plans, and conducting periodic measles risk assessments, accounting for the likely population immunity based on the situation of the displaced population's country of origin (Sphere Project 2011). Outbreak preparedness activities should include high-quality surveillance for measles cases, appropriate case management, and maintaining a capacity for rapid outbreak response. To reach susceptible populations, outbreak response immunization (ORI) strategies should be based on epidemiological analyses of measles surveillance data, particularly the age distribution of reported cases and results of measles risk assessments.

During the emergency phase of a humanitarian emergency and at the beginning of any mass displacement event, measles vaccination is considered one of the top priorities by humanitarian workers because of the high prevalence of risk factors such as malnutrition, overcrowding, insufficient sanitation, and lack of access to healthcare services, that increase the severity of measles morbidity and mortality (WHO 2012c). To achieve and maintain ≥95% two-dose vaccination coverage, it is paramount to have a strong infrastructure in operations, cold chain capacity, surveillance, and outbreak response. The health infrastructure often deteriorates quickly during a crisis, resulting in undervaccination of large birth cohorts. During a humanitarian emergency, pools of measles-susceptible populations can accumulate quickly due to the interruption of routine vaccination programs. Recently, a growing number of security issues related to access to health services in conflict areas, as seen in the Syrian conflict, have resulted in additional operational challenges and a need to develop new programmatic strategies in delivering vaccines to vulnerable populations. In such settings, full implementation of measles elimination strategies should be a priority to achieve the WHO recommended high vaccination coverage with two MCV doses. Working with local authorities, and negotiating "days of tranquility" or humanitarian cease-fires has proven to be a successful strategy in the Global Polio Eradication Initiative (WHO 2016). Measles elimination efforts have proven that identification of susceptible subpopulations and mapping and reaching all communities with immunizations is necessary for eliminating chains of transmission from all reservoirs. Due to its highly infectious nature, measles is most often the first VPD that one encounters in areas of low immunization coverage; as such, measles is an important indicator for guiding targeted public health action.

Clinical Presentation

Measles virus is an enveloped ribonucleic acid (RNA) virus, a member of the *Morbillivirus* genus in the paramyxoviridae family, and occurs naturally only in humans (WHO 2009). The measure of the transmissibility of an infectious agent is its basic reproduction number (R_0), which is defined as the average number of secondary cases generated by a primary case in a completely susceptible population. Measles has an R_0 of 12–18, making it the most infectious communicable disease known (Durrheim et al. 2014). Measles is transmitted from an infected person to a susceptible person via aerosolized respiratory droplets, usually through coughing and sneezing (Kouadio et al. 2010). Measles infection begins with cell entry of the virus in the lungs. The virus then spreads via the lymphoid tissues and immune cells throughout the body causing an acute viremia and a systemic infection (WHO 2015a, Strebel et al. 2016). The incubation period is approximately 7–21 days (Zenner and Nacul 2012).

The prodromal phase starts approximately four days prior to rash onset, and is characterized by fever greater than 38°C (100.4°F), cough, coryza (runny nose), and/or conjunctivitis (red eyes with discharge). During the prodromal phase, generally 1–2 days before the onset of rash, multiple small bluish-white plaques known as Koplik spots may appear on the surface of the buccal mucosa, occurring in ~70 percent of patients with measles (Xavier and Forgie 2015, PAHO 2005).

Koplik spots are pathognomic for measles. Since they first appear before rash onset, they can be an important clinical finding for early case detection and initiation of treatment, isolation procedures, and outbreak response, particularly in refugee settings without access to confirmatory laboratory testing. The measles rash that occurs 3–4 days after the onset of fever is maculopapular rather than vesicular and typically starts on the face and spreads to the core and extremities (Pickering et al. 2012). The rash generally lasts 3–7 days and fades in the same pattern as it appeared (PAHO 2005). Persons with measles are considered infectious from four days before until four days after onset of rash.

Since measles is an acute systemic viral infection that spreads to the organs throughout the body and leads to immunosuppression, it can cause severe illness and death, particularly in persons with malnutrition and comorbidities and when treatment is delayed or suboptimal. Measles infection depletes immune cells and causes a transient immunosuppression that lasts for at least 1–2 months, and longer in some cases. Common complications of measles include acute otitis media, diarrhea, and pneumonia (WHO 2005a). Acute encephalitis occurs in <1% of measles infections, occurs more frequently in adults, and can lead to permanent brain damage (Pickering et al. 2012). The risk of serious measles complications and death is highest among children <5 years of age and adults >20 years. Pneumonia causes approximately 60 percent of measles deaths and is more common in young patients. Persons with malnutrition, particularly vitamin A deficiency, are especially vulnerable to severe measles infection and complications (WHO 2005a). In these cases, measles infection can further deplete vitamin A levels, ultimately leading to blindness, and in some cases, death (Heymann 2008). In humanitarian emergencies, the combination of measles infection and acute malnutrition can be lethal. Vitamin A supplementation has been shown to significantly reduce measles mortality; therefore, it is a critical part of case management and mass measles vaccination campaigns.

Epidemiology

Natural infection with measles provides lifelong immunity. Introduction of measles vaccination into routine immunization programs and increasing measles vaccination coverage changes measles epidemiology (Goodson et al. 2011). Prior to the widespread use of measles vaccine starting in the early 1960s, epidemic cycles of measles occurred every two to three years, and virtually everyone experienced measles infection during childhood. In the pre-vaccine era, 90 percent of individuals were infected by age 10. Generally, the introduction of measles vaccination leads to decreasing measles incidence, longer interepidemic periods and a shift in the age distribution of remaining cases toward older children and young adults. In settings with prolonged periods of low measles incidence and without high 2-dose MCV coverage, measles-susceptibility accumulates across a wide age range. When measles outbreaks occur in these settings, the age distribution of cases is wide, and it can be challenging to determine the target age groups for ORI strategies. During humanitarian emergencies, it is important to consider the historical vaccination coverage and epidemiology of measles in the target population group to determine the age groups at risk for measles. Of course, if routine vaccination services were interrupted due to a crisis or if there were marginalized populations that had poor access to vaccination, then large numbers of unimmunized infants and young children would have accumulated and would be at risk for measles. While some common measles risk factors, such as nonvaccination, are universal, others will vary by setting, and efforts should be made in each crisis to identify key risk factors for measles in that particular population.

Risk Factors

Displaced populations, including refugees, are at risk for contracting measles, which contributes to all-cause mortality in emergencies (Kouadio et al. 2010). A survey conducted in the Tuareg refugee camps of Mauritania in 1992 showed that 40 percent of all childhood deaths were due to measles (MSF 1997, Paquet 1992). Measles is of particular and immediate concern during a humanitarian emergency or mass displacement event because the conditions created by a humanitarian emergency facilitate the rapid spread of measles. In humanitarian emergencies, poor living conditions and crowding tend to occur during the first phase of population displacement. A crowded camp environment, with insufficient water and sanitation, and poor nutrition status and low immunization coverage of the camp population, increase the likelihood of an infectious disease outbreak and higher morbidity and mortality if an outbreak should occur (Kouadio et al. 2010). In addition, health infrastructure may be overwhelmed by additional and urgent workload, and routine immunization programs may be disrupted. In this situation, measles outbreaks are more probable and deadlier, and rapid measles transmission may result in an outbreak beyond the capacity of the host government to manage. For all these reasons, preventive measles vaccination campaigns are a priority during humanitarian emergencies.

Measles outbreaks among displaced populations have been documented in the published literature, including outbreaks in Tanzania, Ivory Coast, Darfur, Ethiopia, Somalia and Kenya (WHO 2004, Kamugisha et al. 2003, Kouadio et al. 2009, Navarro-Colorado et al. 2014). In 2011, an outbreak of measles occurred among Somali refugee populations in Ethiopia and Kenya who had migrated to refugee camps because of famine, drought, and conflict. The arduous journey of the Somali refugees from their homes in the areas of armed conflict to the camps sometimes took weeks without access to food and health services and took a large toll on their health. By the time the refugees arrived in the camps, they were generally in poor health and many were malnourished (Navarro-Colorado et al. 2014). A facility-based assessment of risk factors for measles mortality among cases during this outbreak found gastrointestinal and respiratory complications were common, and malnutrition and neurologic complications were associated with increased measles mortality (Mahamud et al. 2013). The physical environment of the camps with high population density and over crowding put them at higher risk of contracting measles, and their malnutrition from the long journey increased the risk of severe measles complications.

Population movement between camps and host communities and large influxes of new refugees into camps can contribute to measles outbreaks (Kamugisha et al. 2003, Kouadio et al. 2009, Navarro-Colorado et al. 2014, Guerrier et al. 2009). For example, a large influx of undervaccinated refugees from Burundi to refugee camps in Tanzania resulted in a severe measles outbreak during 2000–2001 (Kamugisha et al. 2003). In 2003 and 2004, in Cote d'Ivoire, a measles outbreak occurred in transit camps for Liberian refugees; transmission was documented among refugees and the Ivorian host community (Kouadio et al. 2010). These findings highlight the need to coordinate vaccination activities between refugee populations and host communities to prevent and respond to outbreaks.

Case Fatality

The measles case fatality rate (CFR) varies by setting and access to care and is typically less than 1 percent in developed countries, but it can range from 3%–6% in developing countries. Among vulnerable populations in humanitarian emergencies, measles can be especially devastating, with CFRs often higher than those observed in stable populations (Connolly et al. 2004, Kouadio et al. 2010, Mahamud et al. 2013).

Identified factors associated with an increased risk of death due to measles include younger median age of cases, increased intensity of measles virus exposure, increased likelihood of secondary infections, malnutrition (especially vitamin A deficiency), low educational level, poverty, crowded living conditions, and large household size. Many of the factors that lead to high measles CFRs are common in humanitarian emergencies. Displaced populations often have acute malnutrition, interrupted health services, or poor access to healthcare and preventive services. In emergency settings, measles CFRs among children and infants have been reported as high as 30%–40% (PAHO 2005) and 10%–30% in other displaced populations (Heymann 2008, WHO 2005a). During a measles outbreak in 1985 among Ethiopian refugees in Wad Kowli camps in Sudan, the CFR was 32 percent (Shears et al. 1987). During an outbreak among Turkmen and Uzbek refugees in Afghanistan in 2000–2001, the CFR was 15 percent (Bosnan et al. 2002).

Risk Assessment

It is important to take into account local epidemiologic factors when assessing the risk for a measles outbreak. The WHO SAGE Working Group on Vaccination in Humanitarian Emergencies published a framework for decision-making as well as a qualitative epidemiological risk assessment specific for VPDs in acute emergencies (WHO 2012c). This risk assessment should be carried out quickly within the first few days of the emergency, continued as long as necessary, and consists of three steps. The first step is a consideration of general risk factors that are cross-cutting for infectious diseases in emergencies, including high burden of malnutrition, overcrowding, and a lack of water, sanitation, and hygiene. Each general

Table 26.1 Epidemiological risk assessment classification for vaccination interventions in an acute emergency (WHO 2012c)

		Level of risk due to general factors		
		High	Medium	Low
Level of risk due to factors specific to the VPD	High	Definitely consider	Definitely consider	Possibly consider
	Medium	Definitely consider	Possibly consider	Do not consider
	Low	Do not consider	Do not consider	Do not consider

risk factor is assigned a rating of high, medium, or low based on expert opinion. The second step is a consideration of risk factors specific to an infectious disease or VPD such as measles. Each risk factor specific to the VPD is assigned a rating of high, medium, or low, based on a variety of factors including population immunity, geography, climate, seasonality, and burden of disease within the population. Finally, those conducting the assessment must determine the overall risk of a measles or other VPD outbreak, based on the cross-tabulation of risks to guide and prioritize vaccination interventions as shown in Table 26.1. Along with the overall classification, the timing, epidemic potential, and age groups most affected should also be considered when prioritizing the need for vaccination efforts in an acute emergency (WHO 2012c).

More recently, a quantitative risk assessment tool specific to measles was developed by WHO (Lam et al. 2015b, Harris et al. 2016, Ducusin et al. 2015, Kriss et al. 2016). If feasible, use of the measles risk assessment tool is recommended to assess district-level risk in the displaced population's country of origin as well as in the host country. In an emergency setting, it is recommended that the risk assessment be carried out separately for different populations. An adapted version of the measles risk assessment tool is being developed for emergency settings to assess the level of integration and immunization coverage among both displaced and host populations.

Outbreak Preparedness and Response

Measles Vaccine

The measles vaccine is a safe, effective, and inexpensive live attenuated vaccine. It can be administered concurrently with inactivated vaccines as well as with some other live attenuated vaccines including mumps and rubella (Heymann 2008, WHO 2009, Strebel et al. 2016). Measles vaccine is highly effective at conferring immunity to recipients, reaching 95 percent effectiveness with a single dose given at ≥12 months of age. The vaccine must be stored in a cold chain (2°–8°C) (Heymann 2008). Before reconstitution, the vaccine can be stored for up to one year prior to the expiry date from the manufacturer. The lyophilized vaccine must be reconstituted with the specific sterile water diluent from the manufacturer by trained medical staff. Human error during reconstitution and lack of adherence to vaccine storage and handling requirements have caused avoidable adverse events and deaths. Once reconstituted, the vaccine must be kept in cold chain and discarded after six hours because of the loss of potency and the risk of bacterial contamination from exposure to light and temperatures greater than 8°C (Heymann 2008). Vaccine vial monitoring (VVM) is an effective way of determining if there have been problems with refrigerators or freezers used to store the vaccine, or if there has been a break in the cold chain during emergencies (WHO 2005b).

To reach the requisite herd immunity and achieve measles elimination, WHO recommends providing two doses of MCV (WHO 2009). A second dose increases the likelihood that each person seroconverts and acquires immunity, therefore reducing the number of measles-susceptible persons in the population. Epidemiological and biological factors are considered when deciding the timing for the first dose. Infants born to immune mothers passively acquire IgG antibodies from their mothers that protect them from measles for the first few months of life. The same antibody that protects the infant early in life can also prevent seroconversion following vaccination if the vaccine is given too early (Durrheim et al. 2014). These maternal antibodies are usually no longer present in infants aged six to nine months, which is why WHO has set six months as the lower age limit when planning a vaccination campaign (WHO 2009). Although this is a live vaccine, children with asymptomatic human immunodeficiency virus (HIV) infection should also receive vaccination, as they are at a greater risk of becoming severe measles cases (WHO 2009, Polonsky et al. 2015).

Measles Vaccination Strategies

WHO recommends that the first MCV dose be given to children 9 to 11 months in a nonoutbreak setting and a second dose delivered either through routine immunization services or supplementary immunization activities (SIAs) (WHO 2009). Children aged six to eight months who receive vaccination during an outbreak should be revaccinated at nine months of age for their first dose of measles vaccination as part of the EPI schedule. Measles vaccination campaigns should also incorporate vitamin A distribution to children aged 6 months to 5 years during emergencies. During an outbreak in an emergency, the target age group for vaccination is expanded to 6 months to 14 years, with a minimum target age range of 6 to 59 months (Kamugisha et al. 2003). However, the target age group should be determined by examination of the epidemiology of cases and the historical vaccine coverage in the country of origin of the affected population (Salama et al. 2004).

The available literature for the WHO African Region reports various target age-groups for measles vaccination campaigns among displaced populations. For example, a series of mass measles vaccination campaigns were conducted in the internally displaced persons (IDP) camps in Gulu district of Northern Uganda from 1997 to 2001, targeting children under five years of age (Mupere 2005). In contrast, a regional measles vaccination campaign conducted in 2004 targeted children aged 9 months to 15 years in IDP camps and surrounding communities in West and North Darfur (CDC 2004). The different age groups targeted within each outbreak response reflect the evolution of recommendations and guidance provided during the past 15 years. There is an increasing consideration of the importance of examining the local epidemiology and context of measles virus transmission in various settings in order to determine target age groups in outbreak response (Kaiser 2014).

While target age groups typically include those between 6 months and 14 years, it is important to consider the immunization status of older refugees because of the possible long interruption in vaccination programs due to conflict. Outbreaks of measles can affect refugees older than 15 years of age because they have never been exposed to wild virus or the vaccine (Navarro-Colorado 2014). For example, in the 2011 measles outbreak among Somali refugees residing in Kenya and Ethiopia, ORI campaigns initially targeted children aged 6 months to 14 years (Kaiser 2014, Navarro-Colorado 2014). However, cases continued to rise despite vaccination efforts. Upon review of epidemiological data, it was recognized that most cases occurred in persons aged 15 years or older, and the upper age limit for the campaign was expanded to include persons up to 30 years of age. Expanding routine vaccination programs to include older refugees is an emerging topic in humanitarian response.

Because of unplanned periodic influxes of new susceptible populations during humanitarian emergencies, unique vaccination strategies are needed to address the specific needs of refugee and IDP populations. Emphasis should be placed on the importance of early vaccination of displaced persons upon arrival at camps according to existing guidelines (Sphere Project 2011). Establishment of vaccination posts or health screening desks that are integrated with registration desks at reception centers in camps and with transit centers at crossing points might also ensure timely screening of those with measles and help provide appropriate case management during mass population movement (Mahamud 2013). In settings where refugees or IDPs are situated both in camp and noncamp settings and integrated into host communities, there will be a need for coordination of vaccination efforts among camp settings, host communities, and possibly the refugee country of origin.

Measles Vaccination Campaigns

Emergency preventive measles vaccination is a public health priority among displaced populations and should be initiated as soon as possible (Connolly et al. 2004, WHO 2005a, Heymann 2008, Toole and Waldman 1990). Even in settings where displaced populations have come from areas of relatively high immunization coverage, there is still the potential for an outbreak due to the highly contagious nature of the disease (WHO 2005a). The control of measles in humanitarian emergencies has focused on the mass vaccination of refugees at transit centers or upon arrival in camps and during measles outbreak response.

Vaccination programs during emergencies are complicated by the nature of the emergency. Planning and organization of a vaccination campaign are discussed further in Chapter 16. During the acute phase of an emergency, if there is high population movement, the risk for measles infection depends on a host of factors including the immunization coverage of both the moving population and the host population. Once a population is established in a camp, seldom is the population stable. Often, refugees move in and out of the camps and their movement is difficult to track, making surveillance and the results of coverage surveys potentially biased. For instance, in the measles outbreak in transit camps within urban Abidjan, Ivory Coast, that was precipitated by close interactions between Liberian refugees and Ivorian host communities, both the displaced and host communities had apparent immunity gaps for VPDs (Kouadio et al. 2010). In such a situation, it is recommended to vaccinate both groups of susceptible persons. Mass measles vaccination campaigns were conducted for both refugee and nondisplaced populations in Abidjan (Kouadio et al. 2009). Additionally, the humanitarian community had to adapt to new circumstances as it is becoming common for refugees to live outside camps within the host communities in more urban environments (Grais et al. 2011). This presents challenges when setting up vaccination programs and surveillance systems.

Another consideration for vaccination programs during humanitarian emergencies is the location of the vaccination sites. As mentioned earlier, some populations may be relatively stable within a camp, while others have high movement between camps and host communities. Campaigns can choose to utilize fixed vaccination sites at health facilities, mobile teams that move around the camp or migrant areas to reach populations, or a combination of both (WHO 2012c). These considerations vary based on the situation and must be evaluated by the immunization team.

In humanitarian emergencies, logistical issues are a big challenge. Displaced populations are rarely located near the best-served areas in a country. Refugee camps are often located in areas chosen by host governments and often put in rural areas far from urban centers. Usually, routine immunization programs reach rural border areas slowly, so refugees may find themselves in a host population with lower vaccination coverage and where measles virus may be circulating. In 2004, a measles campaign was launched in South Darfur and West Darfur. The campaign was impeded by challenges in West Darfur due to the security situation, and access to both areas was limited because of the start of the rainy season (CDC 2004). Vaccinators must determine the needs in terms of transportation, storage and cold-chain capacity, and the safety and security of vaccination teams (WHO 2012c). A 2002 measles campaign in Vietnam targeted rural communes where there was little cold-chain capacity and thus relied heavily on vaccine vial monitors (VVM) to ensure administration of safely stored vaccines (WHO 2002, WHO 2005b). These logistical issues can impede the speed and coverage of immunization campaigns.

Additional logistical concerns such as the cost and availability of vaccines should also be considered during the planning of vaccination campaigns. It is not always possible to vaccinate the entire target population and difficult opportunity-cost choices need to be made when planning. Some of the difficulties of including older age groups in a campaign are logistical, including a lack of sufficient numbers of trained vaccinators and the cost of additional vaccine and supplies to reach a larger target population (Grais et al. 2011).

Finally, social mobilization and informed consent are also concerns in setting up a vaccination campaign. Social mobilization is essential in spreading the word about the campaign. Clear messages about the campaign must be developed beforehand and campaigns should mobilize local leaders including religious and community leaders to help publicize it (WHO 2012c). The extent and medium of the communication will depend on the situation and urgency of the campaign. Informed consent is also a critical ethical factor of planning a campaign. The amount of information and way that it is communicated needs to take into consideration the health-literacy status and perceived understanding of the risks and benefits of the vaccine among the population (WHO 2012c). Campaigns have devised various ways to tackle this issue, including group education before vaccination in the waiting room and use of visual aids (WHO 2012c)

Because of these challenges, collaboration with key agency and community partners is crucial in outbreak response vaccination strategies. In 2004, grassroots community organizations and mass media were engaged to inform and mobilize persons in IDP camps in West and North Darfur for a measles vaccination campaign targeting those aged 9 months to 15 years (WHO 2004). Given the insecurity in Western Darfur and limited access because of the rainy season, this large-scale vaccination campaign was made possible through stakeholder cooperation, including negotiations with opposition forces to allow vaccinations to take place in hard-to-reach areas (CDC 2004, WHO 2004).

Treatment

Management of severe measles and its complications during humanitarian emergencies can be extremely difficult. Therefore, every effort should be made to achieve ≥95% 2-dose measles vaccination coverage to prevent outbreaks as an effective alternative (Mahamud et al. 2013). It is critical to maintain preparedness for a measles outbreak response, including managing and treating measles patients. Hospital admission criteria should be clearly defined. Whenever possible, outpatient case management is preferred over hospitalization, to avoid nosocomial transmission. Isolation procedures at triage, outpatient, and inpatient facilities should be clear and strictly followed, particularly once a measles outbreak is confirmed. No specific antiviral treatment exists for the treatment of measles infection.

Appropriate case management, consisting of prevention and treatment of symptoms and complications from measles infection, is needed to reduce morbidity and mortality. Supportive management of measles usually involves managing fluids, nutritional therapy, and a full regimen of vitamin A supplementation. WHO recommends giving vitamin A supplementation to children to reduce the severity of the infection and decrease mortality. Table 26.2 shows the recommended doses of vitamin A according to target age groups and various types of immunization contacts (WHO 2015c).

Depending on the numbers affected, it may be necessary to create a small unit for children with measles and their mothers to support their care (WHO 2005a). Other recommendations include enrollment of patients in feeding programs if necessary, but only after they have passed the infectious phase (WHO 2005a). Oral rehydration and antibacterial treatment may also be needed to manage the illness and its complications (Grais et al. 2011, Kouadio et al. 2010).

Measles Surveillance

In refugee settings and humanitarian emergencies, disease surveillance is a high priority, and several complementary surveillance systems might be needed. New arrivals of refugees or IDPs may introduce measles virus into a setting, so priority should be placed on rapidly establishing disease surveillance covering the population, particularly in areas with the newest refugee arrivals (Mahamud et al. 2013). For example, in concurrent measles outbreaks in the Dollo Ado refugee camp in Ethiopia and the Dadaab refugee camp in Kenya during 2010–2011, the initial cases occurred among new arrivals from Somalia, a country that was experiencing an ongoing measles outbreak (CDC 2012, Navarro-Colorado 2014). Additionally, a measles outbreak during 2000–01 in four established Burundi refugee camps in Tanzania was an extension of an outbreak in Burundi and precipitated by a large influx of new arrivals who were

Table 26.2 Potential target groups and immunization contacts for prevention of vitamin A deficiency (VAD) in countries with VAD

Target population for vitamin A supplementation	Immunization contact	Vitamin A does
Infants 6 to 11 months	- Routine EPI contacts from 6 months onwards (e.g., DTP3 if given at 6 months) - Measles / yellow fever at 9 months - EPI campaigns (polio, NIDs, measles, SIAs, etc.)	100,000 IU
Children 12 to 59 months	- Delayed primary immunization contacts - Routine EPI booster contacts >12 months (e.g., DTP booster, measles second dose) - EPI campaigns	200,000 IU

Source: WHO 2015c

inadequately vaccinated (Kamugisha et al. 2003). It is crucial that surveillance data from all available sources for the population in humanitarian emergencies be monitored and analyzed for rapid case detection and outbreak response. The following describes the various sources of measles surveillance used during emergencies and highlights the need to hold frequent meetings to communicate and cross check data among surveillance systems within refugee camp settings, the refugee country of origin, and the host government.

Case-based Surveillance

Effective measles surveillance includes case-based surveillance with individual case investigation and blood specimen collection for laboratory testing to confirm measles.

A suspected measles case is defined as:

- An acute illness characterized by fever and rash and either cough, coryza, or conjunctivitis (WHO 2013).

A suspected case can also be identified by a clinician who suspects an illness is caused by the measles virus infection (WHO 2013). Suspected measles cases are confirmed on the basis of laboratory findings or an epidemiologic linkage.

An epidemiologically linked confirmed measles case is defined as:

- A clinical case of measles that has not been confirmed by a laboratory but is geographically and temporally related (with dates of rash onset occurring between 7 and 21 days apart) to a laboratory-confirmed case or (in the event of an outbreak) to another epidemiologically confirmed measles case (WHO 2010b).

The most common methods of laboratory confirmation include detection of measles-specific IgM antibodies in serum samples using enzyme-linked immunosorbent assay (ELISA) or identification of the measles virus RNA in nasopharyngeal swabs, oral fluid, or urine through reverse transcription polymerase chain reaction (RT-PCR) (Kutty et al. 2014). During outbreaks, nasopharyngeal swab specimens are collected to identify measles virus genotypes. Suspected cases are also confirmed by epidemiologic linkage to laboratory-confirmed cases or other epidemiologically linked cases. In 2014, 187 (96%) countries used case-based surveillance, and 191 (98%) had access to standardized quality-controlled testing through the WHO Global Measles and Rubella Laboratory Network (GMRLN) (Perry et al. 2015).

Global Measles and Rubella Laboratory Network (GMRLN)

The Global Measles and Rubella Laboratory Network (GMRLN) was established in 2000 and includes more than seven hundred laboratories in all six WHO regions to provide standard procedures for measles case confirmation, virus identification and characterization, and monitoring global distribution of genotypes. The WHO recognizes 24 genotypes of measles virus and has established a set of reference genetic sequences for each. Following global vaccination activities and elimination efforts, circulating wild-type measles virus genotypes have decreased from the original 24 recognized genotypes to only 13 that were detected and reported during 2005–2014 (WHO 2015d). Of note, measles virus genotypes or strains do not vary in their transmissibility or virulence, and the immune response generated by vaccination protects against all genotypes. It is important to collect specimens for genotyping from all measles outbreaks to track virus transmission pathways, identify surveillance gaps, and to conduct molecular epidemiological studies of measles virus transmission (Plotkin 2013).

Early Warning and Response Network (EWARN)

The most common surveillance systems in humanitarian emergencies are the WHO Early Warning and Response Network (EWARN) and the United Nations High Commission for Refugees (UNHCR) Health Information System (HIS). The EWARN was developed by the WHO to meet surveillance needs and provide high quality data during an emergency (WHO 2012b). It is comprised of two main elements including immediate reporting, which triggers an alert during the early stages of an outbreak, and weekly reporting (WHO 2012b). These two elements complement each other to identify outbreaks and monitor morbidity and mortality. The EWARN is most useful at the start of an emergency (the acute phase) when surveillance systems have been disrupted, underperforming, or, in some cases, non-existent. The EWARN is meant to serve as a stopgap measure while routine systems recover or more permanent systems are installed. Since measles is a disease with epidemic potential, it is included as a priority disease in the EWARN.

The EWARN is easy for clinicians and field workers in emergencies to implement with simple case definitions and alert statuses (Morof et al. 2013). To provide flexibility and to be as sensitive as possible, the EWARN relies on syndromic case definitions. A suspected case of measles is any person with fever, a generalized maculopapular (nonvesicular) rash and one or more of the following: cough, coryza, or conjunctivitis. Additionally, any person in whom a clinician suspects measles is considered a suspected case. Any suspected case should generate an outbreak signal, which then results in investigation and verification to determine if there is an outbreak (WHO 2012b).

The EWARN epidemic alert threshold for measles is one suspected case. Although the EWARN does not require laboratory confirmation, it is still important to seek laboratory confirmation at a regional or international reference laboratory when an outbreak is suspected. Once the emergency has concluded, the EWARN should be reintegrated into normal surveillance activities. A more in-depth description of the EWARN is found in Chapter 9.

Health Information System (HIS)

The UNHCR Health Information System (HIS) was developed in 2002 with the goal of introducing standardized data collection reporting tools to refugee camps (Haskew et al. 2010). While the EWARN is established during the acute phase of an emergency, the HIS is created for routine reporting of key health indicators in camp settings. The system uses standard indicators and internationally recognized benchmarks. It is not as robust as a national surveillance system, but it is a useful tool for refugees and provides data that can assess the health situation in a camp and steer programing and resources towards activities where they are most needed.

For measles, the HIS provides a system for reporting coverage of measles vaccination and vitamin A among infants less than one year. The system also collects information on the vaccine wastage rate, which is the proportion of doses of the measles vaccine that is supplied but not administered. The morbidity section of the HIS collects information on the weekly number of measles cases tallied at the facility level, with the threshold for an outbreak being one reported measles case. The HIS uses the same measles case definition as the WHO (UNHCR 2010). The weekly reporting allows for monitoring for trends; however, the HIS is facility-based and does not detect cases not seeking care or referred.

Community-based Surveillance

Community-based surveillance is an active surveillance system that can help find cases before they arrive at a health facility; it is an important component of surveillance in humanitarian emergencies. Rapid measles case detection, early treatment, and case management reduces measles morbidity and mortality, particularly in refugee settings. Community-based surveillance relies on trained community volunteers who are based in the community and interact directly with households to recognize suspect cases of measles based on a broad case definition and refer them to a health facility for further evaluation (Johns Hopkins 2008). Like the EWARN, it uses the same syndromic case definition for measles. Community volunteers refer any suspect case to a health facility.

It is critical that staff working on the various surveillance systems communicate on a regular basis, frequently, to share findings and coordinate efforts. This will ensure early case detection, confirmation, and appropriate outbreak response.

Notes from the Field

Horn of Africa (2010)

Devastating measles outbreaks occurred in the Horn of Africa in 2010–11 during a humanitarian emergency caused by severe drought, famine, war, large-scale population movements, and overcrowded refugee camps. In Somalia, measles is endemic, and massive influxes of nearly six hundred thousand refugees moved into camps in Kenya and Ethiopia (CDC 2012). During 2010–11, a total of 16,135 measles cases were reported in Somalia, the majority of which (78%) occurred among children aged <5 years; 9,756 and 2,566 measles cases were reported in Ethiopia and Kenya, respectively, with wide age distributions among cases. In the outbreaks in Kenya and Ethiopia, unimmunized adults likely contributed to sustained measles virus transmission and experienced significant measles morbidity and mortality. In Dadaab, 15 (47%) of 32 reported measles deaths were among unvaccinated women aged ≥15 years; of those, seven were aged ≥30 years.

In the Dadaab refugee camps in Kenya, an outbreak began in July 2011, coinciding with a large influx of refugees from Somalia where a measles outbreak was ongoing; the majority of cases (59%) were among refugees aged ≥15 years. Between March and September 2011, a series of outbreak response immunizations (ORIs) were conducted, targeting several age groups: children aged 9 months to 14 years during the March–April ORI; children aged 6 months to 5 years during the August ORI; and adults aged 15 to 29 years during the September ORI. In addition, in August 2011, measles vaccination was provided to new arrivals aged 6 months to 29 years, all hospitalized pediatric patients, and unvaccinated household contacts of measles cases aged 6 months to 14 years. Beginning in October 2011, reported cases decreased as the numbers of newly arriving refugees decreased. Similarly, a measles outbreak occurred in the Dollo Ado refugee camps in Ethiopia during July–October 2011, with 436 cases (44% aged ≥15 years). As a result of the age distribution of cases, routine measles vaccination was expanded in September 2011 to include new arrivals aged 6 months to 29 years, followed by a decrease in the number of new arrivals and reported cases.

Despite a series of ORI activities, the outbreaks continued in part because of narrow age ranges for the populations targeted for vaccination and periodic influxes of new arrivals. In retrospect, restricting vaccination upon arrival to camps and in routine immunization clinics to children aged 6–59 months (Ethiopia) and 9–59 months (Kenya) was too narrow a response. In Dadaab, Kenya, a measles vaccination campaign was conducted for children aged 9 months to 14 years during March–April 2011. However, the outbreaks continued in both settings; eventually, vaccination campaigns with expanded target age groups up to 29 years of age were conducted in camps in both countries (Navarro-Colorado et al. 2014).

This experience demonstrated the need for measles outbreak response strategies to be adjusted to changing measles epidemiology, including measles-susceptibility in older age groups in emergency settings (Kaiser 2014). ORI strategies should be designed based on a rapid measles risk assessment accounting for the historical vaccination coverage and measles epidemiology of the population using data from the districts of origin, as well as the refugee setting and host country. Measles outbreak preparedness and response plans should be established that include policies for using expanded target age groups for vaccination activities and contingency plans for vaccine supply to avoid delays in procurements and shortages. Also, in refugee settings, strategies should be implemented to achieve and maintain high (≥95%) routine two-dose MCV coverage, rather than the previous approach of implementing a routine one-dose measles vaccination strategy.

Conclusion

During humanitarian emergencies, displaced populations are at increased risk of measles transmission. The landscape of measles continues to evolve as epidemiological data suggest that it is no longer only a childhood disease. This has implications for measles prevention and control in humanitarian emergency settings, specifically, the need for wider target age group for ORI and preventive vaccination campaigns. Risk assessments are needed in each specific humanitarian emergency setting and should include an assessment of the country of origin to determine risk in the specific districts from which the displaced population is coming. An adapted measles risk assessment tool specific for displaced populations would be useful to assess the unique risk factors, including population movement, crowded living conditions, and nutritional deficiencies, often encountered in humanitarian emergency settings. In addition, high quality surveillance is needed to ensure early case detection and to mount a rapid effective response and reduce morbidity and mortality.

Measles infection can lead to serious complications and death, particularly among displaced populations. Outbreak preparedness and response must be maintained in emergency settings, including appropriate case management and isolation procedures. While there is no specific antiviral treatment for measles, case management with supportive symptomatic treatment and vitamin A supplementation is recommended.

In conclusion, measles is one of the most infectious diseases known and is responsible for significant morbidity and mortality during humanitarian emergencies. A highly effective measles vaccine is available and can prevent outbreaks in emergencies if high two-dose vaccination coverage is achieved.

Population displacement can threaten global measles elimination efforts. The trend of increasing numbers of humanitarian emergencies globally, with growing insecurity and destruction of cold chain and infrastructure for transportation, poses new and emerging challenges in providing lifesaving measles vaccines, especially in conflict settings. Coordination of vaccination activities between camp settings and the surrounding communities in the host country is therefore critical.

Acknowledgement

We would like to thank Anyie Li and Jennifer Head for their editorial assistance and help in review of the current literature. We also thank Jim Alexander for his comments.

References

Bosnan, A., Dil, S., Kakar, F., et al. (2002). Measles mortality among Afghan refugees' children. *Pakistan Journal of Medical Research*, 41, 123–125.

Centers for Disease Control and Prevention. (2004). Emergency measles control activities–Darfur, Sudan, 2004. *Morbidity and Mortality Weekly Report*, 53, 897–899.

Centers for Disease Control and Prevention. (2008). Manual for the surveillance of vaccine-preventable diseases (online). Available at: www.cdc.gov/vaccines/pubs/surv-manual/index.html (Accessed Nov 5, 2015).

Centers for Disease Control and Prevention. (2012). Measles–Horn of Africa, 2010–2011. *Morbidity and Mortality Weekly Report*, 61, 678–684.

Cohn, J. (2014) The challenge of vaccinating in emergency settings: policy and advocacy implications. *International Journal of Infectious Diseases*, 21S, 51.

Connolly, M. A., Gayer, M., Ryan, M. J., et al. (2004). Communicable diseases in complex emergencies: impact and challenges. *Lancet*, 364, 1974–1983.

Davidkin, I., Jokinen, S., Broman, M., et al. (2008). Persistence of measles, mumps, and rubella antibodies in an MMR-vaccinated cohort: a 20-year follow-up. *The Journal of Infectious Diseases*, 197, 950–956.

De Serres, G., Boulianne, N., Meyer, F., et al. (1995). Measles vaccine efficacy during an outbreak in a highly-vaccinated population: incremental increase in protection with age at vaccination up to 18 months. *Epidemiology and Infection*, 115, 315–323.

Ducusin, M. J., de Quiroz-Castro, M., Roesel, S., et al. (2015). Using the World Health Organization Measles Programmatic Risk Assessment Tool for monitoring of supplemental immunization activities in the Philippines. *Risk Analysis*, May 7. doi:10.1111/risa.12404.

Durrheim, D. N., Crowcroft, N. S., and Strebel, P. M. (2014). Measles – The Epidemiology of Elimination. *Vaccine*, 32, 6880–6883.

Goodson, J. L., Masresha, B. G., Wannemuehler, K., et al. (2011). Changing epidemiology of measles in Africa. *Journal of Infectious Diseases*, 204 Suppl 1, S205–S214.

Grais, R. F. and Juan-Giner, A. (2014). Vaccination in humanitarian crises: satisficing should no longer suffice. *International Health*, 6, 160–161.

Grais, R. F., Strebel, P., Mala, P., et al. (2011). Measles vaccination in humanitarian emergencies: A review of recent practice. *Conflict and Health*, 5, 211.

Guerrier, G., Zounoun, M., Delarosa, O., et al. (2009). Malnutrition and mortality patterns among internally displaced and non-displaced population living in a camp, a village or a town in Eastern Chad. *PLoS One*, 4, e8077.

Harris, J. B., Badiane, O., Lam, E., et al. (2016). Application of the World Health Organization Programmatic Assessment Tool for risk of measles virus transmission-Lessons learned from a measles outbreak in Senegal. *Risk Analysis*, 36, 1708–1717.

Haskew, C., Spiegel, P., and Tomczyk, B. (2010). A standardized health information system for refugee settings: rationale, challenges and the way forward. *Bulletin of the World Health Organization*, 88, 792–794.

Heymann, D. L. (2008). *Control of communicable diseases manual*, 19th edition, Washington, DC: American Public Health Association.

Johns Hopkins Bloomberg School of Public Health & International Federation of Red Cross and Red Crescent Societies. (2008). Public health guide in emergencies (online). Available at: http://reliefweb.int/sites/reliefweb.int/files/resources/Forward.pdf?wb48617274=62F43829 (Accessed July 7, 2017).

Kaiser, R. (2014). Emergency settings: be prepared to vaccinate persons aged 15 and over against measles. *The Journal of Infectious Diseases*, 210, 1857–1859.

Kamugisha, C., Cairns, K. L. and Akim, C. (2003). An outbreak of measles in Tanzanian refugee camps. *The Journal of Infectious Diseases*, 187, S58–S62.

Kouadio, I. K., Kamigaki, T. and Oshitani, H. (2010). Measles outbreaks in displaced populations: a review of transmission, morbidity and mortality associated factors. *BMC International Health and Human Rights*, 10, 5.

Kouadio, I. K., Koffi, A. K., Attoh-Toure, H., et al. (2009). Outbreak of measles and rubella in refugee transit camps. *Epidemiology and Infection*, 137, 1593–1596.

Kriss, J. L., De Wee, R. J., Lam, E., et al. (2016). Development of the World Health Organization Measles Programmatic Risk Assessment Tool using experience from the 2009 measles outbreak in Namibia. *Risk Analysis*, Feb 19. doi:10.1111/risa.12544

Kutty, P., Rota, J., Bellini, W., et al. (2014). *VPD Surveillance Manual*. 6th ed. Atlanta, GA: CDC (online). Available at: www.cdc.gov/vaccines/pubs/surv-manual/chpt07-measles.pdf (Accessed Nov 8, 2015).

Lam, E., McCarthy, A., and Brennan, M. (2015a). Vaccine-preventable diseases in humanitarian emergencies among refugee and internally-displaced populations. *Human Vaccines & Immunotherapeutics*, **11**, 2627–2636. doi:10.1080/21645515.2015.1096457.

Lam, E., Schluter, W. W., Masresha, B. G., et al. (2015b). Development of a district-level programmatic assessment tool for risk of measles virus transmission. *Risk Analysis*, May 15. doi:10.1111/risa.12409.

Lebaron, C. W., Beeler, J., Sullivan, B. J., et al. (2007). Persistence of measles antibodies after 2 doses of measles vaccine in a postelimination environment. *Archives of Pediatrics and Adolescent Medicine*, **161**, 294–301.

Liu, L., Oza, S., Hogan, D., et al. (2015). Global, regional, and national causes of child mortality in 2000–13, with projections to inform post-2015 priorities: an updated systematic analysis. *Lancet*, **385**, 430–440.

Mahamud, A., Burton, A., Hassan, M., et al. (2013). Risk factors for measles mortality among hospitalized Somali refugees displaced by famine, Kenya, 2011. *Clinical Infectious Diseases*, **57**, e160–e166.

Markowitz, L. E., Albrecht, P., Orenstein, W. A., et al. (1992). Persistence of measles antibody after revaccination. *The Journal of Infectious Diseases*, **166**, 205–208.

Médecins Sans Frontières (1997). *Refugee health: An approach to emergency situations*. London, UK: Pan Macmillan.

Morof, D. F., Abou-Zeid, A., and Brennan, M. (2013). An Evaluation of an Early Warning Alert and Response Network (EWARN) in Darfur, Sudan. *The Medical Journal of Cairo University*, **81**, 209–217.

Mupere, E., Onek, P., and Babikako, H. M. (2005). Impact of emergency mass immunisations on measles control in displaced populations in Gulu district, northern Uganda. *East African Medical Journal*, **82**, 403–408.

Navarro-Colorado, C., Mahamud, A., Burton, A., et al. (2014). Measles outbreak response among adolescent and adult Somali refugees displaced by famine in Kenya and Ethiopia, 2011. *The Journal of Infectious Diseases*, **210**, 1863–1870.

Pan American Health Organization. (2005). Measles Elimination Field Guide, 2nd edition (online). Available at: www.paho.org/immunization/toolkit/resources/paho-publication/field-guides/Measles-Elimination-2nd-edition.pdf?ua=1 (Accessed November 8, 2015).

Paquet, C. (1992). Rèfugiès Touaregs dans le sud-est de la Mauritanie. Paris: Epicentre.

Perry, R. T., Murray, J. S., Gacic-Dobo, M., et al. (2015). Progress toward regional measles elimination – worldwide, 2000–2014. *Morbidity and Mortality Weekly Report*, **64**, 1246–1251.

Pickering, L. K., Baker, C. J., and Kimberlin, D. W. (2012). Red Book: Report of the Committee on Infectious Diseases, 29th edition, Elk Grove Village, IL: American Academy of Pediatrics.

Plotkin, S. A., Orenstein, W. A., and Offit, P. A. (2013). Vaccines, 6th edition, Atlanta: Elsevier Inc.

Polonsky, J. A., Singh, B., Masiku, C., et al. (2015) Exploring HIV infection and susceptibility to measles among older children and adults in Malawi: A facility-based study. *Int J Infect Dis,* **31**, 61–67.

Salama, P., Spiegel, P., Talley, L., et al. (2004). Lessons learned from complex emergencies over past decade. *Lancet*, **364**, 1801–1813.

Shears, P., Berry, A. M., Murphy, R., et al. (1987). Epidemiological assessment of the health and nutrition of Ethiopian refugees in emergency camps in Sudan, 1985. *British Medical Journal (Clinical Research Edition)*, **295**, 314–318.

The Sphere Project. (2011). Essential health services SPHERE Handbook: Humanitarian Charter and Minimum Standards in Humanitarian Response (online). Available at: www.spherehandbook.org/ (Accessed Nov 5, 2015).

Strebel, P. M., Papania, M. J., Gastañaduy, P. A., et al. (2016). Measles vaccine, in: S. A., Offit, W. A., Plotkin, and P. A. Orenstein (eds.), *Vaccines*, 7th Edition, Philadelphia, PA: Elsevier Inc., pp. 579–618.

Toole, M. J. and Waldman, R. J. (1990). Prevention of excess mortality in refugee and displaced populations in developing countries. *JAMA*, **263**, 3296–3302.

United Nations High Commissioner for Refugees. (2010). Health Information System (HIS): Case Definitions (online). Available at: www.unhcr.org/4614aa682.pdf (Accessed Nov 5, 2015).

World Health Organization. (2002). Technical review of vaccine vial monitor implementation (online). Available at: www.who.int/immunization_standards/vaccine_quality/vvm_technical_review_report.pdf (Accessed Nov 8, 2015).

World Health Organization. (2004). Prevention of measles deaths in Darfur, Sudan. *Weekly Epidemiological Record*, **79**, 344–8.

World Health Organization. (2005a). Communicable disease control in emergencies (online). Available at: http://whqlibdoc.who.int/publications/2005/9241546166_eng.pdf?ua=1. (Accessed Nov 5, 2015).

World Health Organization. (2005b). Monitoring vaccine wastage at country level (online). Available at: http://apps.who.int/iris/bitstream/10665/68463/1/WHO_VB_03.18.Rev.1_eng.pdf. (Accessed January 29, 2018).

World Health Organization. (2009). Vaccine position papers: Measles (online). Available: www.who.int/wer/2009/wer8435.pdf (Accessed March 30, 2015).

World Health Organization. (2010a). Global eradication of measles: report by the Secretariat (online). Available at http://apps.who.int/gb/ebwha/pdf_files/wha63/a63_18-en.pdf (Accessed Nov 5, 2015).

World Health Organization. (2010b). Monitoring progress towards measles elimination. *Weekly Epidemiological Record*. **85**, 490–494 (online). Available at www.who.int/wer/2010/wer8549.pdf?ua=1 (Accessed March 10, 2016)

World Health Organization. (2012a). World Health Organization. Global measles and rubella strategic plan: 2012–2020 (online). Available at www.who.int/immunization/newsroom/Measles_Rubella_StrategicPlan_2012_2020.pdf. (Accessed Nov 5, 2015).

World Health Organization. (2012b). Outbreak surveillance and response in humanitarian emergencies (online). Available at: www.who.int/diseasecontrol_emergencies/publications/who_hse_epr_dce_2012.1/en/.(Accessed Nov 5, 2015).

World Health Organization. (2012c). SAGE Working Group on Vaccination in Humanitarian Emergencies, Vaccination in Acute Emergencies: a Framework for Decision Making (online). Available at: www.who.int/immunization/sage/meetings/2012/november/FinalFraft_FrmwrkDocument_SWGVHE_23OctFullWEBVERSION.pdf (Accessed Nov 5, 2015).

World Health Organization. (2013). Measles elimination field guide (online). Available at: www.wpro.who.int/immunization/documents/measles_elimination_field_guide_2013.pdf?ua=1. (Accessed Nov 5, 2015).

World Health Organization. (2015a). *Disease outbreak news* (online). Available: www.who.int/csr/don/en/ (Accessed Nov 5, 2015).

World Health Organization. (2015b). *Measles* (online). Available: www.who.int/mediacentre/factsheets/fs286/en/ (Accessed Nov 5, 2015).

World Health Organization. (2015c). Vitamin A supplementation (online). Available: www.who.int/immunization/programmes_systems/interventions/vitamin_A/en/index1.html / (Accessed Nov 5, 2015).

World Health Organization. (2015d). Genetic diversity of wild-type measles viruses and the global measles nucleotide surveillance database (MeaNS). *Weekly Epidemiological Record*, **90**, 373–380.

World Health Organization. (2016). Health as a Bridge for Peace – HUMANITARIAN CEASE-FIRES PROJECT (HCFP) (online). Available: www.who.int/hac/techguidance/hbp/cease_fires/en/ (Accessed February 23, 2016).

Xavier, S. and Forgie, S. E. D. (2015). Koplik spots revisited. *Canadian Medical Association Journal*, **187**(8), 600.

Zenner, D. and Nacul, L. (2012). Predictive power of Koplik's spots for the diagnosis of measles. *The Journal of Infection in Developing Countries*, **6**, 271–275.

Chapter 27

Meningococcal Disease

Sarah Mbaeyi, Amanda Cohn, and Matthew Coldiron

Introduction

Meningococcal disease is an acute and potentially life-threatening infection due to the bacterium *Neisseria meningitidis*. A leading cause of bacterial meningitis, *N. meningitidis* is notable for its ability to cause large-scale epidemics, making it a potential concern in humanitarian emergencies. Other causes of bacterial meningitis include *Streptococcus pneumoniae* and *Haemophilus influenzae*.

Neisseria meningitidis is a gram-negative diplococcus. Meningococci are classified into serogroups based on the composition of their capsular polysaccharide. Twelve serogroups of meningococcus have been identified, although six (A, B, C, W, X, Y) account for nearly all human disease.

Epidemiology

Meningitis Belt

Meningococcal disease is found worldwide, with rates of disease varying by region (Halperin et al. 2012). The highest incidence of disease is observed in the meningitis belt of sub-Saharan Africa, a region stretching from Senegal to Ethiopia and home to over four hundred million people as shown in Figure 27.1. Meningococcal disease is hyper-endemic in this region, with major epidemics every 8 to 12 years when incidence rates may reach 1,000 cases per 100,000 population (Greenwood 1999). Epidemics occur during the dry season from December to June, characteristically ending once the rainy season begins. Serogroup A has accounted historically for 90% of meningococcal meningitis cases in this region and can lead to widespread epidemics (Campagne et al. 1999). In recent years, large serogroup C epidemics have been reported in Nigeria and Niger (Sidikou, et al. 2016; Funk, et al. 2014; Chow, et al. 2016). Serogroups W and X have also caused outbreaks.

The epidemiology of meningococcal disease in regions of Africa outside the meningitis belt as well as in Asia and the Middle East is generally characterized by low endemic rates with occasional outbreaks. North America, South America, Europe, and Australia experience low annual rates of meningococcal disease of 0.3–2 cases/100,000 population, primarily due to sporadic cases of serogroups B, C, and Y (Halperin et al. 2012).

In meningitis belt countries, rates of disease are highest in persons younger than 30 years, particularly among children aged 5–14 years (Campagne et al. 1999). Outside the meningitis belt, the highest rates of disease are observed in infants under the age of 1 year, with increased rates also observed in adolescents (Cohn et al. 2010).

Several outbreaks of meningococcal meningitis in refugee camps have been reported in the literature, primarily due to serogroup A disease, in Thailand (1980), Sudan (1985, 1989, 1999, 2007), Ethiopia (1989, 1993), Guinea (1993), Uganda (1994), and the Democratic Republic of the Congo (1994) (Haelterman et al. 1996; Moore et al. 1990b; Santaniello-Newton and Hunter, 2000; Benca et al. 2007). While outbreaks may be localized to refugee camps, they often occur in the context of a larger epidemic in the surrounding area.

With widespread introduction of the serogroup A conjugate meningococcal conjugate vaccine, MenAfriVac™, described later in the chapter, substantial declines in the number of confirmed serogroup A and suspected meningitis cases have been observed in the meningitis belt (Lingani et al. 2015; Trotter et al. 2017). However, with the continued introduction and use of this vaccine, along with the emergence of large-scale serogroup C epidemics in recent years, the prevention, surveillance, and control of meningococcal disease in this region remains essential.

Chapter 27: Meningococcal Disease

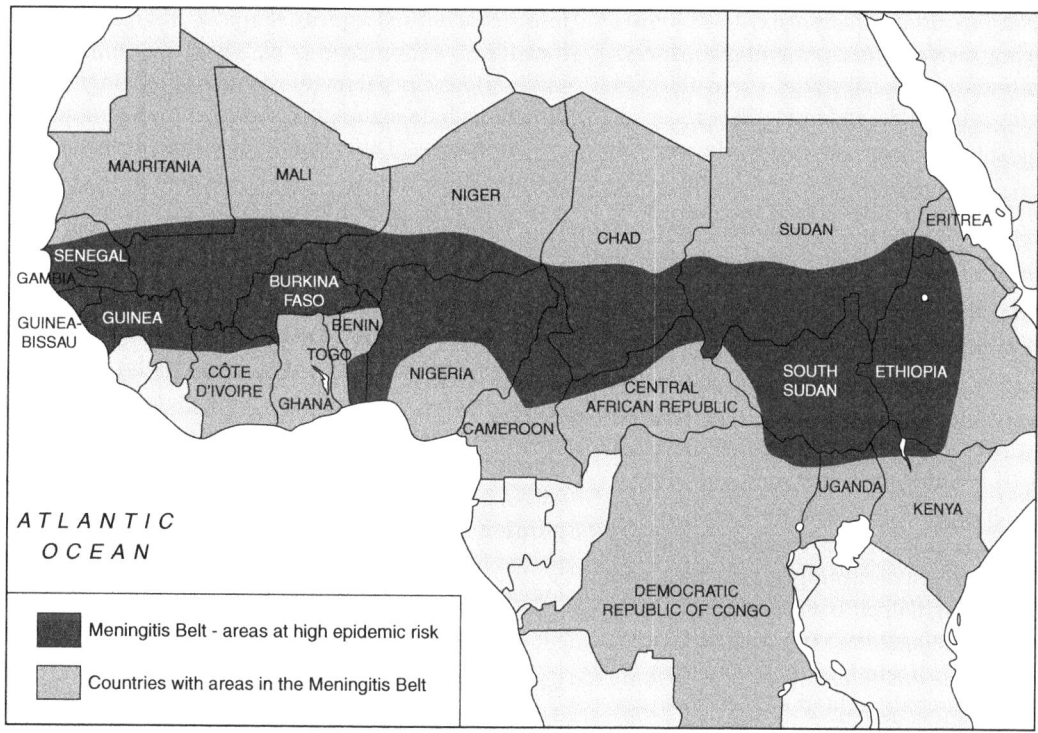

Figure 27.1 The sub-Saharan African meningitis belt
Source: CDC Yellowbook, 2016. Available at: wwwnc.cdc.gov/travel/yellowbook/2016/infectious-diseases-related-to-travel/meningococcal-disease.

Risk Factors

Humans are the only natural reservoir for *Neisseria meningitidis*. Approximately 10% of persons carry the organism asymptomatically in the nasopharynx at any given time (Caugant et al. 1994). Rates of meningococcal carriage are highest in adolescents and young adults (Yazdankhah and Caugant, 2004). Transmission occurs from human-to-human through respiratory droplets or secretions. In most persons, carriage is innocuous and serves as an immunizing process whereby protective antibodies against disease are developed (Kremastinou et al. 1999). In a small proportion of carriers, the bacteria penetrate the mucosa and enter the bloodstream, resulting in systemic disease.

Risk factors for meningococcal disease include organism, host, and environmental factors. Crowded living conditions, such as university dormitories and military barracks, can facilitate transmission of the organism (Bruce et al. 2001; Baker et al. 2000). Smoking and exposure to second-hand smoke may damage the nasopharynx mucosa, thereby increasing the risk of developing meningococcal disease (Fischer et al. 1997; Kriz et al. 2000). Preceding upper respiratory infections have likewise been demonstrated to increase risk of infection (Moore et al. 1990a). In addition, asplenia, such as in persons with sickle-cell disease, is a risk factor for disease (Fijen et al. 1999). Risk of disease is particularly elevated among household and childcare contacts of a meningococcal case (De Wals et al. 1981; Munford et al. 1974). This risk among close contacts is highest in the first few days after symptom onset (Munford et al. 1974).

Environmental and climate conditions are thought to predispose the meningitis belt to recurrent epidemics. Harmattan winds from the Sahara Desert create a hot, dry, dusty environment particularly during the months December through March. Environmental factors such as low humidity, high temperatures, and high levels of mineral dust are thought to play a role in the location and seasonality of meningococcal epidemics (Garcia-Pando et al. 2014). These environmental factors are thought to predispose to nasopharyngeal irritation and breakdown in mucosal integrity, thus facilitating invasive disease acquisition.

Persons living in refugee camps may be at higher risk of acquiring meningococcal meningitis due to crowding and poor nutritional status, particularly in areas where the disease is endemic (Moore et al. 1990a). In addition, the high rates of acute respiratory infections in refugee camps may be an additional risk factor for meningococcal meningitis in these settings.

Prevention

Several vaccines are available for the prevention of meningococcal meningitis. The monovalent serogroup C conjugate vaccine and the quadrivalent serogroup A, C, W, Y conjugate vaccine are available in industrialized countries and are routinely recommended for targeted age groups (CDC 2013). However, these vaccines are not routinely available for use for the prevention of meningococcal disease in hyperendemic meningitis belt countries. Since 2010, a new serogroup A conjugate vaccine, MenAfriVac™, has been rolled out in meningitis belt countries via mass vaccination campaigns in the 1–29 year age group followed by introduction of the vaccine into the routine immunization programs in at-risk countries (Marc LaForce, et al. 2009). Recombinant protein-based serogroup B vaccines are also available and recommended for certain populations in some industrialized countries; however, given the low burden of serogroup B in meningitis belt countries, serogroup B vaccines are not recommended.

In industrialized countries, where most cases are sporadic or part of outbreaks that occur infrequently and are of lower magnitude than those seen in hyperendemic countries, chemoprophylaxis of close contacts of meningitis cases is recommended to prevent further spread (Cohn et al. 2013). However, in meningitis belt countries, chemoprophylaxis of household contacts is recommended only during non-epidemic settings (WHO 2014). Chemoprophylaxis is not currently recommended during epidemics in the meningitis belt, as the benefits are unclear and the logistical and financial constraints imposed by mass chemoprophylaxis may divert scarce resources away from vaccination efforts and case management.

Clinical Presentation and Course

Meningococcal disease often initially presents similarly to common, less serious illnesses such as viral infections, but subsequently rapidly progresses to serious illness (Thompson et al. 2006). The most common serious clinical manifestations of meningococcal disease include meningitis, sepsis, and pneumonia.

Symptoms of meningitis in children and adults include sudden onset of fever, headache, neck stiffness, vomiting, photophobia, lethargy, altered mental status, and seizures. In children less than 2 years of age, meningitis may present with non-specific features such as a gradual onset of fever, poor feeding, irritability, and in infants, a bulging fontanel (Ragunathan et al. 2000; Wong et al. 1999).

N. meningitidis can also cause meningococcemia (meningococcal infection of the bloodstream) with or without meningitis. Meningococcemia often presents with a petechial or purpuric rash and can progress to purpura fulminans and septic shock. The incubation period for meningococcal disease is usually less than four days, but ranges from one to ten days after exposure.

Suspected meningococcal disease is a medical emergency as it can rapidly progress to fulminant disease, multi-organ failure, and death within hours. Persons with suspected meningococcal disease should be evaluated and treated at a healthcare facility as soon as possible. Without treatment, the case fatality ratio for meningococcal disease is 75–80%. Even with antimicrobial treatment, approximately 10 percent of patients die. Among survivors, 10–20% develop permanent neurologic sequelae, including sensorineural hearing loss, cognitive deficits, seizures, and limb loss (Edward and Baker 1981).

Diagnosis

While the diagnosis of bacterial meningitis may be inferred based on clinical presentation, laboratory confirmation is important for individual case management as well as for effective outbreak response in order to select the appropriate vaccine to be used for a mass vaccination campaign.

Diagnosis of meningitis is made by collection of cerebrospinal fluid (CSF) through a lumbar puncture (LP) often performed by a physician or, in some countries, a nurse or other qualified healthcare worker. This procedure consists of inserting a needle into the lower back between the fourth and fifth lumbar vertebrae (L4–L5), whereby fluid is collected from the thecal sac surrounding the spinal cord. CSF is normally a clear, colorless fluid. In a patient with bacterial meningitis, CSF is often cloudy or purulent, but may be clear or bloody.

CSF of suspected meningitis cases should be analyzed in a laboratory to determine the causative organism. In developing countries, the most commonly available tests for the diagnosis of bacterial meningitis include culture, Gram stain, latex agglutination, and polymerase chain reaction (PCR) (WHO 2011). Isolation of *N. meningitidis* through culture is the diagnostic gold standard. PCR testing detects meningococcal DNA, which can be useful when the organism cannot be isolated by culture, such as in the event that the patient is treated with antibiotics prior to CSF collection or in the setting of suboptimal specimen storage and transport conditions. In most developing countries, PCR tests are available only at a reference laboratory. Gram stain can identify the likely causative organism, with identification of intracellular gram negative diplococci indicative of *N. meningitidis*. However, Gram stain is not confirmatory and cannot distinguish among meningococcal serogroups.

Latex agglutination or immunochromatographic tests can also be used for rapid identification of the meningococcal capsular polysaccharides, although readings of results are subjective and may lack sensitivity.

Treatment

Given the high rates of morbidity and mortality from meningococcal disease, effective antimicrobial treatment should be initiated as soon a diagnosis of meningitis is suspected. Ideally, collection of the diagnostic CSF specimen should be performed prior to antibiotic treatment when possible and when the patient's clinical condition permits, in order to identify the causative organism. Antimicrobial treatment prior to collection of the specimen may lead to a false negative result. Treatment however, should not be delayed until the diagnostic results are available. Further, the inability to perform a lumbar puncture should not preclude prompt treatment.

Several antimicrobial choices are available for the treatment of meningitis, and when available, clinicians should adhere to national meningitis treatment protocols or guidelines. During meningitis outbreaks in the meningitis belt, WHO guidelines recommend a seven-day course of ceftriaxone for children aged under two months, and a five-day course of ceftriaxone for adults and children greater than age two months (WHO 2014). A single dose of ceftriaxone is no longer recommended for the treatment of meningitis. While effective against meningococcal infections, single-dose therapy is not effective against the other causes of bacterial meningitis (*S. pneumoniae*, *H. influenzae*), which are likely to constitute a higher proportion of meningitis cases following MenAfriVac™ introduction.

In addition to antimicrobial therapy, supportive therapy including hydration, adequate nutrition, antipyretics, anticonvulsive therapy, and pain management should be provided as needed. Given the seriousness of the illness and the requirement for intravenous or intramuscular antimicrobials and supportive care, persons with suspected meningitis require close observation.

Surveillance and Outbreak Detection

Surveillance of meningococcal disease is critical in order to rapidly identify, confirm, and respond to outbreaks. In addition, understanding the local epidemiology of disease over time allows for the planning of effective preventive measures and allocation of resources for case management and future outbreak response. Given that meningococcal meningitis presents similarly to other forms of bacterial and viral meningitis, surveillance is generally conducted on the basis of suspected meningitis conforming to a standard case definition.

In stable settings, routine reporting of cases should be performed through the national reporting systems according to guidelines set forth by that country. Routine surveillance should be conducted year-round and intensified in meningitis belt countries during the epidemic season, December to June. Health facility staff should be trained on the standardized case definition, CSF collection, meningitis case management, and case reporting. In sub-Saharan Africa, where the vast majority of meningococcal meningitis epidemics occur, national meningitis surveillance is conducted through the Integrated Disease Surveillance and Response (IDSR) system, and in many countries, through WHO enhanced meningitis or case-based surveillance systems (WHO 2009, WHO 2010).

The meningitis case definition found in the WHO guidance for meningitis outbreaks is shown in Table 27.1 All cases responding to the standard case definition are reported weekly as aggregate case and death counts. In addition, case-level data, such as age, sex, residence, immunization status, and onset date

Table 27.1 WHO Meningitis Case Definition

Suspected Meningitis Case	Confirmed Meningitis Case
Any person with a sudden onset of fever (>38.5°C rectal or 38.0°C axillary) and one of the following signs - neck stiffness, flaccid neck, bulging fontanelle, convulsion, or other meningeal sign	Isolation or identification of the causal pathogen (*Neisseria meningitidis, Streptococcus pneumoniae, Haemophilus influenzae* type b) from the CSF of a suspected or probable case by culture, PCR, or agglutination test

Source: WHO 2014

Table 27.2 Epidemiological Thresholds for Suspected Meningitis in the Meningitis Belt

Population	Alert Threshold	Epidemic Threshold
30,000–100,000 persons	3 cases/100,000 population in 1 week	10 cases/100,000 population in 1 week
< 30,000 persons	2 cases in one week or higher incidence than in non-epidemic year	5 cases in one week or a doubling of incidence in a 3-week period
Special situations involving groups of people such as refugees or displaced persons, closed institutions, mass gatherings	N/A	Immediate response when 2 cases of meningococcal disease are confirmed in 1 week

Source: WHO 2014.

should be collected in order to appropriately target outbreak response activities. Alert and epidemic thresholds have been defined based on population size as shown in Table 27.2. It is important to note that these thresholds were developed for countries in sub-Saharan Africa at greatest risk for epidemics and are not appropriate for other regions for which a threshold should be based on the local epidemiology of meningitis.

In the meningitis belt, when the population is over 30,000 persons, attack rates are calculated to monitor disease incidence over time. When the population is below 30,000, thresholds are defined based on the number of cases in a week and comparisons to the number of cases in previous years. To calculate the weekly attack rate:

$$\text{Attack rate} = \frac{\text{Number of suspected meningitis cases in a district during 1 week}}{\text{Population}} \times 100,000$$

During a humanitarian emergency, large numbers of persons may be displaced and population figures may be unavailable, unreliable, or rapidly changing. Thus, the calculation of an accurate attack rate may not be possible. In these settings, the number of suspected meningitis cases should be monitored closely. Doubling of meningitis cases in a short period of time should alert clinicians and public health authorities of a potential epidemic. Two confirmed cases of meningococcal meningitis in a week in a refugee camp is an indication for mass vaccination (WHO 2014). The epidemiologic situation in non-displaced persons in the communities surrounding the refugee camps should also be a factor in determining whether the reported number of cases constitutes an outbreak.

In the setting of a humanitarian emergency, existing national surveillance systems may be overwhelmed and unable to provide timely data necessary for decision-making and response. In these settings, implementation of an early warning alert and response network (EWARN) may be necessary to quickly identify and respond to meningococcal and other disease outbreaks. In the WHO EWARN system, a single case of suspected meningitis in a crowded camp setting triggers the alert threshold (WHO 2012). In order for reactive mass vaccination campaigns to be effective, they must be instituted early in the course of the outbreak, and thus the alert threshold should trigger a set of immediate and rapid preparations in case the epidemic threshold is crossed (Varaine et al. 1997). The epidemic threshold signifies the need for prompt response, including mass vaccination and strengthening of resources for case management. Due to the high case burden during a suspected outbreak, it may not be feasible to collect CSF specimens on each suspected meningitis case. Ideally, specimens should be collected on at least the first ten cases. After the causative agent of the outbreak is confirmed, regular collection of specimens should be maintained, as increases due to other meningococcal serogroups as well as sporadic cases of *S. pneumonaie* and *H. influenzae* can occur.

Outbreak Response

During an outbreak, meningococcal vaccines are used for prevention of additional cases through reactive immunization campaigns. Once the epidemic threshold has been crossed, it is recommended to conduct a mass immunization campaign as soon as possible, and within four weeks. Such campaigns should target the entire population at risk using the appropriate vaccine for the causative serogroup. In outbreaks during a humanitarian emergency, refugees as well as non-refugees in an affected area should be targeted in the reactive vaccination campaign.

When available, conjugate monovalent or quadrivalent vaccine should be used for outbreak response. For serogroup A outbreaks in sub-Saharan Africa, the conjugate serogroup A meningococcal vaccine should be used. For outbreaks due to other meningococcal serogroups in meningitis belt countries, if conjugate vaccines are not available, polysaccharide vaccines (AC, ACW, ACWY) should be used according to the causative serogroup (WHO 2011).

Due to suboptimal immune responses in young children, the minimal impact of the vaccine on nasopharyngeal carriage, and the short duration of protection, polysaccharide vaccines are not preferred for prevention outside the outbreak setting (Granoff et al. 2013). Currently no vaccine against serogroup X is available.

Notes from the Field

Central Africa Republic (2013)

The violent events of 2013 and 2014 in the Central African Republic (CAR) produced a massive movement of the population to neighboring countries, including Chad, where nearly 100,000 displaced persons, some refugees, some Chadian returnees, had arrived by the end of 2014.

Following the 2013 Strategic Advisory Group of Experts (SAGE) guidelines for vaccination in humanitarian emergencies based on the evaluation of epidemiologic risks, Médecins Sans Frontières (MSF) and the Ministry of Health decided to offer a package of three vaccines for arriving refugees: measles for children 6 months to 15 years, oral polio for children aged under five years and the MenA conjugate vaccine for persons aged 1–29 years. These decisions were taken because of poor vaccination coverage in CAR for polio and measles, recent polio outbreaks in Chad, and Chad's location in the meningitis belt. While Chad had recently completed the introduction of MenAfriVac™, the refugees arriving from the CAR had not yet been vaccinated.

In three separate camps, a total of 43,955 persons received MenAfriVac™, representing 60%–85% of the total target population, depending on the camp. In most sites, coverage among children under 15, around 90 percent, was much higher than for those aged 15–29. Host communities were also targeted by the vaccination campaigns. While MenAfriVac™ can be used in a controlled temperature chain, during these campaigns, since other vaccines required storage in a cold chain, the MenAfriVac™ was stored in the traditional manner.

Several important lessons were learned about the use of MenAfriVac™ in this context. First, planning and logistic preparation can be quite complex in the acute phase of humanitarian emergencies. As the target group for MenAfriVac™ includes persons older than the target groups for "traditional" vaccination, social mobilization should be tailored, specifically towards older age groups, reminding them of the importance of vaccination, as they may consider themselves too old for routine vaccination or may not see the urgency in vaccination outside an epidemic period.

Given the multifaceted intervention, it was also important to design a flow around the vaccination site that ensured all necessary vaccines were administered properly, including one team per antigen, and that crowds and beneficiary flow could be controlled. For example, MenAfriVac™ was the first injectable vaccine administered, and those not eligible for the measles vaccination then left the patient circuit.

References

Baker, M. et al. (2000). Household crowding a major risk factor for epidemic meningococcal disease in Auckland children. *Pediatr Infect Dis J.*, **19**(10), 983–990.

Benca, J. et al. (2007). Meningococcal meningitis among displaced and refugee camps in southern Sudan. *Neuro Endocrinol Lett*, **28** Suppl 2, 44.

Bruce, M. G. et al. (2001). Risk factors for meningococcal disease in college students. *JAMA*, **286**(6), 688–693.

Campagne, G. et al. (1999). 77(6), 499–508.

Caugant, D. A. et al. (1994). Asymptomatic carriage of Neisseria meningitidis in a randomly sampled population. *J Clin Microbiol*, **32**(2), 323–330.

CDC. (2013). Prevention and Control of Meningococcal Disease: Recommendations of the Advisory Committee on Immunization Practices. *Morbidity and Mortality Weekly Report*, **62**, 1–22.

Chow et al. (2016). Invasive meningococcal meningitis serogroup C outbreak in northwest Nigeria, 2015 – third consecutive outbreak of a new strain. Plos Currents. July 7, 2016.

Cohn, A. C. et al. (2010). Changes in Neisseria meningitidis disease epidemiology in the United States, 1998–2007: Implications for prevention of meningococcal disease. *Clin Infect Dis*, **50**(2), 184–191.

Cohn, A. C. et al. (2013). Prevention and control of meningococcal disease: recommendations of the Advisory Committee on Immunization Practices (ACIP). *MMWR Recomm Rep*, **62**(RR-2), 1–28.

De Wals, P. et al. (1981). Meningococcal disease in Belgium. Secondary attack rate among household, day-care nursery and pre-elementary school contacts. *J Infect*, **3**(1 Suppl), 53–61.

Edwards, M. S. and C. J. Baker. (1981). Complications and sequelae of meningococcal infections in children. *J Pediatr*, **99**(4), 540–545.

Fijen, C. A. et al. (1999). Assessment of complement deficiency in patients with meningococcal disease in The Netherlands. *Clin Infect Dis*, **28**(1), 98–105.

Fischer, M., Hedberg, K., Cardosi, P., Plikaytis, B. D., Hoesly, F. C., Steingart, K. R., Bell, T. A., Fleming, D. W., Wenger, J. D., and Perkins, B. A. (1997). Tobacco smoke as a risk factor for meningococcal disease. *The Pediatric Infectious Diseases Journal*, **16**(10), 979–983.

Funk et al. (2014). Sequential outbreaks due to a new strain of *Neisseria meningitidis* in northern Nigeria, 2013–2014. PLoS Currents. December 2014.

Garcia-Pando, C. P. et al. (2014). Meningitis and climate: From science to practice. *Earth Perspectives*, **1**(14).

Granoff, D. M., Pelton, S., and Harrison, L. H. (2013). Meningococcal Vaccines, in S. Plotkin and P. Offit, eds., *Vaccines* (6th edition), Edinburgh, Scotland: Elsevier/Saunders, 388–414.

Greenwood, B. (1999). Manson Lecture: Meningococcal meningitis in Africa. *Trans R Soc Trop Med Hyg*, **93**(4), 341–353.

Haelterman, E. et al. (1996). Impact of a mass vaccination campaign against a meningitis epidemic in a refugee camp. *Trop Med Int Health*, **1**(3), 385–392.

Halperin, S. A. et al. (2012). The changing and dynamic epidemiology of meningococcal disease. *Vaccine*, **30** Suppl 2, B26–B36.

Hellenbrand, W. et al. (2011). What is the evidence for giving chemoprophylaxis to children or students attending the same preschool, school or college as a case of meningococcal disease? *Epidemiol Infect*, **139**(11), 1645–1655.

Kremastinou, J. et al. (1999). Detection of IgG and IgM to meningococcal outer membrane proteins in relation to carriage of Neisseria meningitidis or Neisseria lactamica. *FEMS Immunol Med Microbiol*, **24**(1), 73–78.

Kriz, P., Bobak, M., and Kriz, B. (2000). Parental smoking, socioeconomic factors, and risk of invasive meningococcal disease in children: a population based case-control study. *Arch Dis Child*, **83**(2), 117–21.

LaForce, F. Marc et al. (2009). Epidemic meningitis due to Group A Neisseria meningitidis in the African meningitis belt: a persistent problem with an imminent solution. *Vaccine*, **27** Suppl 2, B13–B19.

Lingani et al. (2015). Meningococcal meningitis surveillance, 2004–2013. Clinical Infectious Diseases. **61**(5): S410-415.

Moore, P. S. et al. (1990a). Respiratory viruses and mycoplasma as cofactors for epidemic group A meningococcal meningitis. *JAMA*, **264**(10), 1271–1275.

Moore, P. S. et al. (1990b). Surveillance and control of meningococcal meningitis epidemics in refugee populations. *Bull World Health Organ*, **68**(5), 587–596.

Munford, R. S. et al. (1974). Spread of meningococcal infection within households. *Lancet*, **1**(7869), 1275–1278.

Preblud S. R., Horan, J. M., and Davis, C. E. (1979). Meningococcal disease among Khmer refugees in Thailand,. In D. Allegra, P. Nieburg, and M. Grabe, eds., *Emergency refugee health care – A chronicle of the Khmer refugee assistance operation*, 1979–1980. CDC, 65–69.

Ragunathan, L. et al. (2000). Clinical features, laboratory findings and management of meningococcal meningitis in England and Wales: report of a 1997 survey. Meningococcal meningitis: 1997 survey report. *J Infect*, **40**(1), 74–79.

Santaniello-Newton, A. and Hunter, P. R. (2000). Management of an outbreak of meningococcal meningitis in a Sudanese refugee camp in Northern Uganda. *Epidemiol Infect*, **124**(1), 75–81.

Sidikou et al. (2016). Emergence of epidemic *Neisseria meningitidis* in Niger, 2015: An analysis of national surveillance data. Lancet Infectious Diseases. **16**(11):1288–1294.

Thompson, M. J. et al. (2006). Clinical recognition of meningococcal disease in children and adolescents. *Lancet*, **367**(9508), 397–403.

Trotter et al. (2017). Impact of MenAfriVac in nine countries of the African meningitis belt, 2010-2015: an analysis of surveillance data. Lancet Infectious Diseases. **17**(8):867–872. http://apps.who.int/iris/bitstream/10665/144727/1/WHO_HSE_PED_CED_14.5_eng.pdf?ua=1&ua=1

Varaine, F. et al. (1997). Meningitis outbreaks and vaccination strategy. *Trans R Soc Trop Med Hyg*, **91**(1), 3–7.

Wong, V. K., Hitchcock, W., and Mason, W. H. (1989). Meningococcal infections in children: a review of 100 cases. *Pediatr Infect Dis J*, **8**(4), 224–227.

World Health Organization. (2009). Standard operating procedures for enhanced meningitis surveillance in Africa.

World Health Organization. (2010). Technical guidelines for integrated disease surveillance and response in the African region.

World Health Organization. (2011a). Laboratory methods for the diagnosis of meningitis caused by Neisseria meningitidis, Streptococcus pneumoniae, and Haemophilus influenzae. Geneva: WHO Press.

World Health Organization. (2011b). Meningococcal vaccines: WHO position paper, 2011. *Weekly epidemiologic record*, **47**(86), 521–540.

World Health Organization. (2012). Outbreak surveillance and response in humanitarian emergencies: WHO guidelines for EWARN implementation.

World Health Organization. (2013). Meningococcal disease in countries of the African meningitis belt, 2012 – emerging needs and future perspectives. *Weekly Epidemiological Report*, **88**(12), 129–136.

World Health Organization. (2014). Revised guidance on meningitis outbreak response in sub-Saharan Africa. *Wkly Epidemiol Rec*, **89**, 580–586. http://apps.who.int/iris/bitstream/10665/144727/1/WHO_HSE_PED_CED_14.5_eng.pdf?ua=1&ua=1

Yazdankhah, S. P. and Caugant, D. A. (2004). Neisseria meningitidis: an overview of the carriage state. *J Med Microbiol*, **53**(Pt 9), 821–32.

Mental Health

Barbara Lopes Cardozo and Richard Francis Mollica

Introduction

Worldwide, there is a considerable burden of morbidity, mortality and disability associated with mental illnesses. The Global Burden of Disease Study indicated depression as the fourth leading disease burden in 1990 and is predicted to move to second place by 2020 (Murray and Lopez 1996). Further, five of the ten leading causes of disability globally were due to psychiatric conditions. Mental health is a core public health issue in emergency settings including during humanitarian emergencies. In these settings, the need for a mental health approach is critical. Although the Global Burden of Disease report did not concentrate on emergencies, the burden of mental illness is likely much greater among traumatized and displaced populations. Despite the challenges of assessing the prevalence of mental illness in emergency settings, studies reveal the serious impact of conflict and natural disasters on mental health (Mollica, et al. 2004). The need to address mental health issues in humanitarian emergencies has become evident in recent years.

Not only manmade or natural disasters have major mental health consequences – the psychological consequences and effects on mental health on individuals and populations in the event of epidemics, such as severe acute respiratory syndrome (SARS) (Tam 2004), H1N1 (Goodwin 2009), HIV/AIDS, Ebola (De Roo 1998), and other infectious diseases, are enormous.

Suicide, which is closely related to mental illness, is another concern in humanitarian emergencies. It is the main contributor to mortality associated with mental illness. More than 90 percent of people who die from suicide have a mental disorder. Suicide is among the top 20 leading causes of death globally for all ages. Every year nearly one million people die from suicide (WHO 2011b). Mental illness, primarily depression, alcohol-use disorders and abuse, violence, loss, cultural and religious beliefs (e.g., belief that suicide is a noble resolution of a personal dilemma), local epidemics of suicide, isolation, a feeling of being cut off from other people, and barriers to accessing mental health treatment represent major risk factors for suicide (CDC 2013). Most importantly, suicide risk may be higher in countries affected by war and conflict and especially among refugees.

Unfortunately, few studies have been conducted to detect the risk of suicide among refugees resettled to third countries. Additionally, there is no research assessing suicide risk in refugee camps. One study however showed that Bhutanese refugees who were resettled to the US were at a higher risk for suicide compared with the general US population or the estimated annual global suicide rate for all persons (Cochran 2013). Another study found suicidal ideation was associated with posttraumatic stress disorder (PTSD) in postwar Kosovo (Wenzel et al. 2009).

Focus on the interconnectedness of physical and mental health cannot be ignored in humanitarian emergencies. The Surgeon General's landmark report on mental health in 1999 raised awareness about the interconnectedness of the mind and the body with physical and mental health (Office of the Surgeon General 1999). Physical health cannot be adequately addressed without also addressing mental health. The Surgeon General's Report highlighted the potential impact of mental illness on a person's ability to understand and practice health promotion and disease prevention.

Three decades ago little was known about the importance of identifying and caring for the mental health impact of manmade and natural disasters. This is no longer the case. Not only have the links between mental health and physical health been firmly established in humanitarian emergencies, but also effective culturally valid clinical and preventative strategies efforts have emerged (Mollica 2011).

Burden of Disease

Until 1988, no mental health surveys had been conducted among refugee or war-affected populations.

Chapter 28: Mental Health

In 1988, the first on-site mental health survey was conducted among the Cambodian refugees staying in Site 2, a Thai refugee camp on the Cambodian border. This survey showed a 37 percent prevalence of PSTD and 68 percent depression (Mollica 1993). A cross-sectional survey conducted in 1996 of Bosnian refugee adults living in a camp established by the Croatian government near the city of Varazdin showed that 39 percent and 26 percent of reported symptoms met Diagnostic Statistical Manual (DSM) criteria for depression and PTSD, respectively (Mollica et al. 1999). A mental health survey in Kosovo, conducted shortly after the end of the war in 1999, showed that 17 percent of the people had symptoms of PTSD (Lopes Cardozo et al. 2000). In a follow-up survey in 2000, this number increased to 25 percent (Lopes Cardozo et al. 2003). A 2002 nationwide mental health survey in Afghanistan revealed that the prevalence within the population for symptoms of depression was 68 percent; 72 percent of the population had symptoms of anxiety. The prevalence of the Afghan people with symptoms of PTSD was 41 percent (Lopes Cardozo et al. 2004).

In comparison, in a given year, major depressive disorder affects approximately 6.7 percent of the U.S. population age 18 and older, and about 3.5 percent of people in this age group have PTSD (NIMH 2011, Kessler et al. 2005). An overview of mental health surveys in populations affected by war and conflict that conducted from 1993 until the present is shown in Table 28.1. Compared with prevalences for depression and PTSD in the US population, people in war-torn countries have much higher levels of symptoms of PTSD and depression. The prevalence of serious mental disorders such as PTSD among refugees resettled to Western countries has been estimated to be ten times higher than the age-matched general population (Fazel et al. 2005).

Risk and Mitigating Factors

Individual

Mental health surveys have identified a number of risk factors associated with poorer mental health outcomes. Exposure to traumatic experiences is a major risk factor linked to the development of not only PTSD, but also depression and poorer social functioning (Lopes Cardozo et al. 2000). In several surveys, women were shown to be at higher risk than men for developing mental health problems. Specific risk patterns were identified for different countries, which included a history of psychiatric illness or physical illness, torture, and separation or death of family members (de Jong et al. 2001). In a study among Guatemalan refugees in Chiapas, Mexico, respondents who had witnessed a massacre were at risk for elevated anxiety symptom scores (Sabin et al. 2003).

Community

At the community level, poor quality of camp conditions was associated with higher risk of developing PTSD in a number of countries (de Jong et al. 2001). In a refugee camp in Thailand, economic activity was significantly associated with decreased likelihood of depression (Mollica et al. 2002). Another study in Thailand among Karenni refugees in the Thai-Burmese border camps identified several psychosocial risk factors, some of which could be modified by changes in refugee policy in the Karenni camps (Lopes Cardozo et al. 2004). In particular, the policy to forbid movement, employment, and cultivation of land outside the camps appeared to negatively affect the social functioning and mental health of the Karenni refugees. The psychosocial well-being of refugees would probably improve by amending refugee policy to allow for income generation and movement outside camps.

Identifying Mental Health and Psychosocial (MHPS) Needs

In a humanitarian emergency, it is important to identify the specific mental health and psychosocial needs of the affected community. As early as possible, a rapid Mental Health and Psychosocial (MAPS) assessment should be conducted. A guideline on assessing MHPS needs and resources in humanitarian emergencies can be found at:

- www.who.int/mental_health/resources/toolkit_mh_emergencies/en/

As soon as feasible during a humanitarian emergency a comprehensive MHPS survey should be conducted. Survey methodology is discussed in detail in Chapter 8. The main difference between conducting MHPS surveys compared with surveys in other public health fields lies for the most part in the types of questions and instruments being used. In most cases, to perform a MHPS survey it will be necessary to adapt standard instruments according to the context and culture. Qualitative methods using key

Table 28.1 Mental health surveys in populations affected by war and conflict that conducted from 1993 until the present

Study Group	Prevalence of PTSD (%)	Prevalence of Depression (%)	Nonspecific mental health morbidity (%)	Screening method	Reference
Cambodian refugees in Thailand	37.2	67.9		HTQ HSCL-25	Mollica et al. (1993)
Bosnian refugees in Croatia	26	39		HTQ HSCL-25	Mollica et al. (1999)
Kosovar Albanians in Kosovo	17.1	N/A	43 (11 mean score)	HTQ GHQ-28	Lopes Cardozo et al. (2000)
Rwandan Refugees in Tanzania	N/A	N/A	50 (14 mean score)	GHQ-28	De Jong et al. (2000)
Afghan population	42.1	67.7			Lopes Cardozo et al. (2004)
Karenni (Burmese) refugees in Thailand	4.6	41.8		GHQ-28 HSCL-25 HTQ	Lopes Cardozo et al. (2004)
Sri Lanka internally displaced persons in Jaffna	7.0	30.7		HSCL-25 HTQ	Husain et al., 2011
Cambodia (Siem Reap)	20.6	49.5		HSCL-25 HTQ	Mollica et al. 2013
Algeria	Lifetime: 37.4			LESHQ CIDI	De Jong JT et al. (2001)
Ethiopia	Lifetime: 15.8			LESHQ CIDI	De Jong JT et al. (2001)
Gaza	Lifetime: 17.8			LESHQ CIDI	De Jong JT et al. (2001)
U.S. Population	12-month: 3.5	12-month: 6.7		CIDI	Kessler, Chiu, et al. (2005)
	Lifetime: 6.8	Lifetime: 16.6		(modified)	Kessler, Berglund, et al. (2005)

informants and, if necessary, focus group discussions should be used to identify specific traumatic events and stressors, coping mechanisms and support systems, the way symptoms of mental illness are expressed in the culture, terminology, and functioning. According to the findings of this qualitative assessment, the questions of the instruments for a quantitative MPHS survey can be adapted or formulated.

A key to valid cross-cultural assessment lies in establishing equivalence with regard to language, concepts, and scales within and between cultures and ethnic groups. Because of a general lack of cross-culturally validated mental health instruments, it is difficult to compare populations in different countries and different cultural contexts. The best possible solution at this time for measuring the mental health status of populations in humanitarian emergencies is to use instruments that have at least been validated and field-tested in a number of countries. In an emergency setting, the specific instrument should be culturally validated for the specific country and context

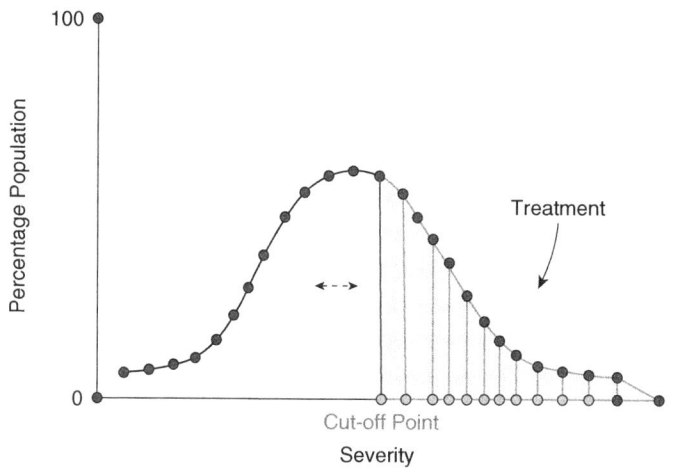

Figure 28.1 Establishing a cut-off point for mental health screening and treatment

where they will be used. Resources, however, are often not available to do so.

Instruments that have been used in many MHPS surveys in humanitarian emergencies are the Hopkins Symptom Checklist (HSCL) measuring symptoms of anxiety and depression, and the Harvard Trauma Questionnaire (HTQ) measuring trauma events and PTSD symptoms as defined in the DSM-IV. Another instrument developed by the World Health Organization (WHO) is the Self-Reporting Questionnaire (SRQ-20) that measures general psychological distress. SRQ-20 has good validity and reliability for adults (≥15 years) and can be used both as a self- or interviewer-administered questionnaire. It consists of 20 closed questions covering expression of distress, the total score corresponding to the sum of positive responses. It has been validated in several countries including Rwanda, India, Vietnam, and Brazil.

PTSD, depression, anxiety, and other mental health disorders common in humanitarian emergencies need to be identified, but this could be a challenge since they can manifest in a variety of ways in different populations and cultures. Culture influences the clinical presentation and distribution of mental illnesses. However, the more severe the psychopathology, the more likely a diagnosis is applicable across cultures – for example, schizophrenia. The Harvard Program in Refugee Trauma (HPRT) has developed a screening manual that addresses all of the major issues in the development and use of culturally valid screening instruments to identify those traumatized and in need of care (Mollica 2004). This includes the role of preliminary needs assessments and the establishment of resource-based cut-off points based upon the psychometric properties of known instruments such as the HSCL and HTQ. The method of establishing a cut-off point for mental health screening and treatment is shown in Figure 28.1.

In humanitarian emergencies, mental health problems may go undiagnosed and untreated because symptoms of mental illness may be expressed differently than in Western societies. In many cultures, for example, psychological problems are expressed as physical symptoms (e.g., headache, bodily pains, stomach aches, etc.).

The Diagnostic Statistical Manual-5 (DSM-5) has introduced a new terminology called "cultural concept of distress" (CCD). The concept refers to different ways groups of people in a particular culture may experience, understand, and express distress (DSM-5). It has been suggested that inclusion of CCD in epidemiological studies can improve detection of psychological distress that may otherwise be missed using conventional instruments (Kohrt et al. 2013).

Overall, those assigned to determining the mental health impact of humanitarian emergencies must decide how to identify and screen for traumatized persons at high risk for mental health problems, psychiatric morbidity, and health-related physical illness. This is not an easy task, especially in resource-poor environments, in light of the reality that almost all affected persons will exhibit some forms of emotional distress. The aims and goals of mental health screening must be clearly defined and acknowledged at the outset of a disaster. Resources must be linked to the capacity to provide culturally effective care.

Best Practices

Emergency Risk Communication

During a humanitarian emergency, especially from sudden onset disasters such as an earthquake, other natural disasters, technological disasters, or outbreak of a disease, risk and crisis communication is very important. The stress of uncertainty and anxiety about the events may make some people physically ill. They may experience stress-related symptoms such as headaches, upset stomach, and pain (Reynolds and Seeger 2012). It may be a problem when the worried-well burden a healthcare system that may already be overloaded during a humanitarian emergency. Early and good communication with the public may help avoid unnecessary use of resources. As an example, after a volcano eruption in Colombia, when an entire village was buried under the mud, many people were demanding vaccinations against tetanus, even those who were far removed from the disaster site and were not injured at all (personal communication, Lopes Cardozo).

Six principles of good crisis risk communication to persons affected by a humanitarian catastrophe are (Reynolds and Seeger 2012):

- Be first
- Be right
- Be credible
- Express empathy early
- Promote action
- Show respect

It is important for the communicator to understand that in crisis, people often manifest psychological reactions that may become psychological barriers if they are not handled well. In an emergency, these include individuals experiencing fear, anxiety, confusion, and even dread. Contrary to popular myths, it is actually quite uncommon for people to panic (Reynolds and Seeger 2012). Most people are able to act rationally even when faced with extreme stress. It is not the role of mental health professionals and spokespersons to make these feelings go away; rather it is helpful to acknowledge these feelings in an empathetic way. If feelings of fear go unchecked, feelings of hopelessness and helplessness and eventually withdrawal, if the person becomes overwhelmed by fear, may set in (Reynolds and Seeger 2012). To avoid this, it is helpful to set the community or the individual on a course of action, including encouraging people to take action and asking them to do things that are constructive and helpful in the given crisis. Anxiety is reduced by action and gives a sense of control (Reynolds and Seeger 2012). The WHO established in an important historic declaration the context and overall aim of clear crisis communication (Petevi 2000).

Two additional principles of clear communication are (Reynolds and Seeger 2012):

- Do no harm
- Establish a dialogue

Guidelines

For many years, mental health interventions were not routinely included in humanitarian emergency response. Lack of knowledge about the burden of mental illness and uncertainty about the right approach for mental health and psychosocial programs in humanitarian emergencies made it difficult for humanitarian agencies to implement mental healthcare. The Interagency Standing Committee (IASC) Guidelines on Mental Health and Psychosocial Support (MHPS) in Emergency Settings were created in 2007 to address the latter. In the IASC Guidelines, the composite term mental health and psychosocial support (MHPSS) was used to describe "any type of local or outside support that aims to protect or promote psychosocial well-being and/or prevent or treat mental disorder."

These guidelines were based on a consensus approach among many agencies, that were implementing or considering implementing MHPSS programs. Although the guidelines were based on a best practices approach and not backed up by outcome evaluations and other scientific evidence (Lopes Cardozo 2008), these guidelines proved to be a major step forward in the MHPS field. Furthermore, mental health has now also been included in the SPHERE Standards (2011) as an essential health service.

The IASC Guidelines describe the concept of an intervention pyramid that outlines the type of services from basic to specialized, at each stage of the pyramid, from larger to fewer numbers of people needing different levels of care. This is shown in Figure 28.2.

Chapter 28: Mental Health

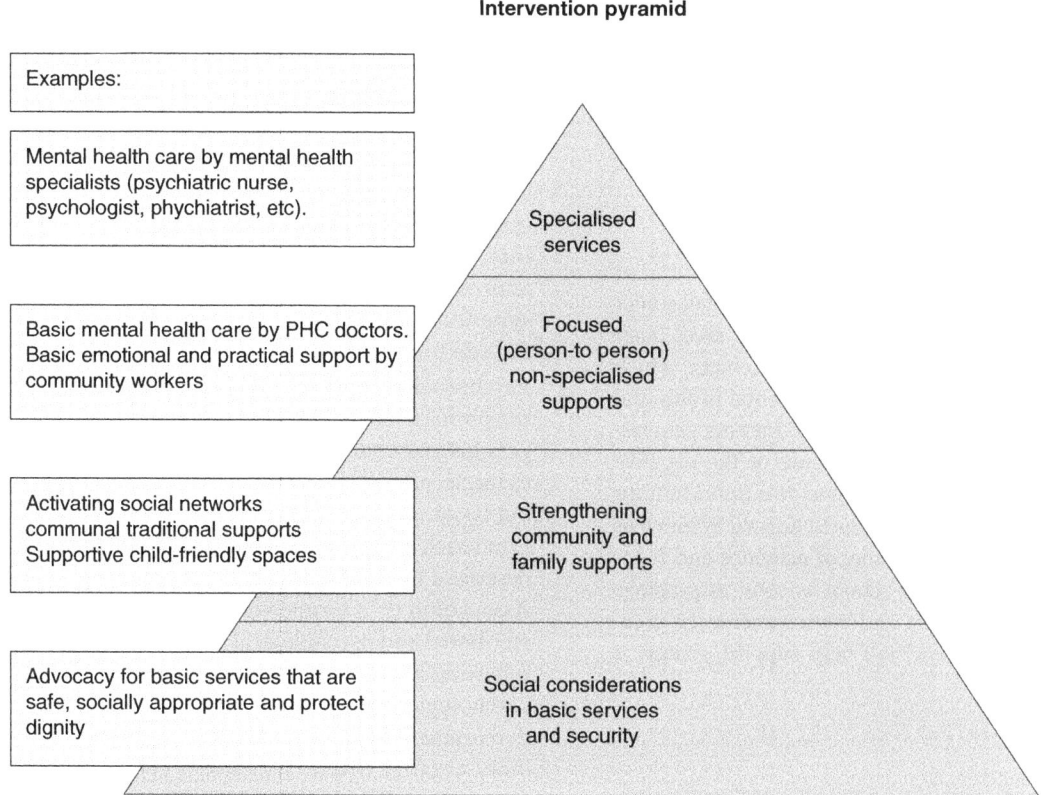

Figure 28.2 Intervention pyramid outlining the type of services from basic to specialized
Source: Interagency Steering Committee Reference Group on Mental Health and Psychosocial Support, 2010

Generally, intervention at the base of the pyramid tends to be more focused on the social aspects of psychosocial interventions. Those at the top level of the pyramid are focused towards people who suffer from serious mental illness and/or have substantial impairment in daily functioning because of emotional problems. The assistance directed at this segment of the population should include psychological or psychiatric support for people with severe mental disorders. Such problems require either referral to specialized services, if they exist, or initiation of longer term training and supervision of primary healthcare providers in psychiatric skills. While these specialized services are needed for only a small percentage of the population, in most large emergencies this group amounts to thousands of individuals (IASC 2007).

During the emergency phase, the IASC Guidelines recommend establishing services through the primary healthcare system to address urgent psychiatric problems and ensuring availability of essential psychotropic medications at health facilities. In the post emergency or reconsolidation phase of an emergency, the IASC Guidelines recommend training and supervision of primary healthcare workers in basic mental health knowledge and skills. Education of humanitarian aid workers and community leaders in basic psychological skills is also recommended. Medication for psychiatric patients should be made readily available in the reconsolidation phase. Finally, collaboration with traditional healers is encouraged (IASC 2007).

Treatment Approaches

Integrating Mental Healthcare

According to WHO, around 75 percent of people with psychiatric, neurological, and substance use disorders in developing countries do not have access to proper care and treatment. WHO also reports that the resources available for mental health are insufficient, inequitably distributed, and are inefficiently used. The WHO Mental Health Gap Action Programme (mhGAP) aims to scale up mental health services for psychiatric, neurological, and substance use disorders especially for low- and middle-income countries (WHO 2012b). The WHO focus is on utilizing primary healthcare providers to provide basic mental healthcare. This emphasis on primary healthcare applies to humanitarian emergencies as well.

Community Approach

Certain types of mental health interventions fall under the spectrum of the term psychosocial. In most post-emergency situations, poverty is a big problem, which may have a substantial effect on the mental health and well-being of the affected population. Income generating projects can help overcome some of the negative effects of poverty and lack of income. It is important for children that the situation returns to normal as much as possible by facilitating recreational activities and helping children to go back to school as soon as possible. Depending on the culture and environment, the creation of community-based self-help support groups is useful.

Counseling

There is a gap in scientific knowledge of the effectiveness of treatment approaches in humanitarian emergencies, postconflict environments, and in low-resource countries. During and after humanitarian emergencies, a variety of treatment approaches have been used by international humanitarian organizations, mental health institutions, and mental health professionals. The more commonly implemented mental health practices are counseling, nonpharmacological management of mental disorders by general healthcare providers, and training of nonspecialized personnel such as community workers and teachers (Tol et al. 2011). A systematic review of the literature focusing on acute humanitarian emergencies revealed a small number of treatment evaluation studies (N = 16) of which only about a third used randomized controlled trial methodology. Because of the heterogeneity of these studies, it is not possible to provide strong recommendations for MHPS intervention in humanitarian emergencies (de Jong et al. 2014). At this time, the following recommendations are made until further research is conducted:

- **Counseling** is a commonly used method of treatment but can mean different things to different people. Sometimes, it is understood as a form of psychotherapy, other times as a basic supportive intervention. A review of the scientific literature revealed that culturally adapted counseling interventions were more likely to result in an effective intervention than generic counseling approaches. Trained, clinically supervised, lay counselors implemented most of the reviewed interventions. Nonculturally adapted counseling approaches did not affect anxiety and depression symptoms; those that were culturally adapted did (de Jong et al. 2014).

- **Psychosocial Debriefing** was originally thought as the pinnacle of care for highly traumatized persons and communities and widely used, for example, after the 9/11 Twin Tower catastrophe, but has dramatically fallen out of favor (Van Emmerick et al. 2002). Psychosocial Debriefing as described by the American Psychological Association is "a formal version of providing emotional and psychological support immediately following a traumatic event; the goal of psychological debriefing is to prevent the development of post-traumatic stress disorder and other negative effects" (American Psychological Association, Division 12, 2008). The timing of debriefing and the professional level of support have varied considerably. The cultural appropriateness of asking persons to state openly, and often to a stranger from an outside community, the precise details of their traumatic experiences has been challenged as highly questionable and may even increase the individual's emotional distress, including the symptoms of PTSD (Rose et al. 2001).

- **Psychological First Aid (PFA)** is listed as the best practice in humanitarian emergency environments and increasingly practiced by humanitarian workers. The 2011 SPHERE Standards mentions Psychological First Aid as one of the major interventions in emergencies. The SPHERE Handbook describes Psychological First Aid as a "humane, supportive response to a fellow human being who is suffering and who may need support. It entails basic, non-intrusive pragmatic care with a focus on listening but not forcing talk, assessing needs and concerns, ensuring that basic needs are met, encouraging social support from significant others and protecting from further harm."

- PFA has become increasingly popular and is being applied extensively in humanitarian emergencies, especially since debriefing has fallen out of favor. Yet there is an absence of quantitative data containing evidence to support PFA following traumatic events. However, it is apparent scientifically that certain risk factors, such as traumatic dissociation and lack of support, are associated with higher rates of emotional distress, and quite possibly lead to PTSD and depression (Bisson and Lewis 2009).
- Clearly, crisis intervention needs to address these factors. There is also a widespread belief in the humanitarian aid community that a sense of safety, hope, connectedness, and caring by the international community and humanitarian aid workers be promoted actively. The cultural and interpersonal sensitivity of the affected communities and families, however, must guide PFA with a major enforcement and buy-in by the local community and its leadership (National Child Traumatic Stress Network and National Center for PTSD 2006).

Treatment of DSM Mental Health Disorders

The Diagnostic and Statistical Manual of Mental Disorders (DSM), published by the American Psychiatric Association, contains common language and standard criteria for the classification of mental disorders.

The most common DSM psychiatric disorders occurring during humanitarian emergencies are depression, anxiety, complex grief, and posttraumatic stress disorder (PTSD). People with preexisting mental disorders (e.g., bipolar illness, schizophrenia, and substance abuse) may experience an exacerbation in their symptoms due to increased stress, lack of medication, and the collapse of the mental health treatment system. The management and the treatment of the latter chronic mental illnesses are beyond the scope of this chapter.

Depression and Anxiety

Depression in the aftermath of humanitarian emergencies is common and the majority of patients respond well to treatment. Treatments that have been shown to be effective are antidepressant medications and psychotherapy or a combination of both. Older types of antidepressants such as tricyclic antidepressants (TCAs) (e.g., amitriptyline) are effective but usually have more side effects than newer antidepressants such as selective serotonin reuptake inhibitors (SSRIs) (e.g., fluoxetine, paroxetine) or the atypical antidepressants (e.g., bupropion). Benzodiazepines are not recommended for the treatment of depression. Nevertheless, they are often overprescribed in the context of humanitarian emergencies due to lack of knowledge and training of healthcare providers and sometimes lack of availability of other psychotropic medications. Additionally, a meta-analysis showed that different psychotherapeutic interventions are effective with more robust evidence for cognitive-behavioral therapy, interpersonal therapy, and problem-solving therapy (Barth et al. 2013). However, few of these studies have been in emergency or low-resource settings. One study in rural Uganda showed that group interpersonal psychotherapy was highly effective for the treatment of major depression and dysfunction (Bolton et al. 2003). It is important to keep in mind that it may take several weeks before antidepressant medications take effect and that it is necessary to continue treatment for at least six months to a year and much longer in some patients. Continued treatment and follow-up may be a problem in emergency settings.

Anxiety disorders are also common during humanitarian emergencies. In Western countries with a lot of resources, treatments that have been shown to be effective are cognitive behavioral therapy (CBT) and medication in particular benzodiazepines (e.g., diazepam, clonazepam, alprazolam) and for some patients' SSRI antidepressants. However, CBT is often not a form of psychotherapy that is being practiced or taught to psychotherapists in humanitarian emergency settings. Acute anxiety after exposure to extreme stressors such as traumatic events in an emergency is initially best managed following the principles of PFA. If this approach is not sufficient, primary care providers could consider prescribing a benzodiazepine for a short period of time (Jones 2011). For a diagnosis of major depression, related disorders and generalized anxiety need to be addressed; the basic symptom criteria in the new DSM-5 have not significantly changed (APA 2013).

Posttraumatic Stress Disorder (PTSD) and Acute Stress Disorder (ASD)

PTSD may occur if people are exposed to traumatic or stressful events, serious injury, or sexual violence.

Effective treatment includes psychotherapy, especially CBT. Exposure therapy is a specific form of CBT that is considered the gold standard, first-line intervention for PTSD in Veterans (Eftekhari et al. 2013). Eye movement desensitization and reprocessing (EMDR) is another type of cognitive behavioral therapy for PTSD. The goal of all forms of CBT is ultimately to change how patients react to trauma memories. Other types of psychotherapy may also be helpful, such as group therapy, or psychodynamic psychotherapy, but the evidence of their effectiveness from clinical trials and more rigorous studies is limited. SSRIs have also been shown to be effective in many cases. Venlafaxine, a serotonin-norepinephrine reuptake inhibitor (SNRI), has also shown efficacy in the treatment of PTSD (Jeffreys 2014).

The evidence for efficacy of these treatments for PTSD during humanitarian emergencies and in its aftermath is scarce. However, a literature review focusing on CBT versus other PTSD psychotherapies as treatment for women victims of war-related violence revealed that various forms of CBT, including cognitive processing therapy (CPT), culturally adapted CPT, and narrative exposure therapy (NET) contribute to the reduction of PTSD and depression severity among these women (Dossa and Hatem 2012). In one study in the Democratic Republic of Congo, a conflict-affected country, group psychotherapy reduced PTSD symptoms and combined symptoms of depression and anxiety, and improved functioning among women survivors of sexual violence (Bass et al. 2013). A few studies have also been conducted among traumatized refugees who were resettled in the US (Hinton 2004). CPT was effective in decreasing PTSD symptoms among refugees who had arrived from Afghanistan and Bosnia (Schulz et al. 2006). However, there were some limitations to this study, including lack of a control group.

There is some evidence that early intervention with modified prolonged exposure therapy may prevent the development of PTSD (Rothbaum et al. 2012). To date, however, no PTSD prevention studies have been conducted in humanitarian emergencies.

Acute Stress Disorder (ASD) follows the same symptoms as PTSD in the Diagnostic and Statistical Manual of Mental Disorders (DSM-5). The difference is that these symptoms occur in the first 30 days after the trauma exposure. If the symptoms last for longer than 30 days after the traumatic event, a diagnosis of PTSD needs to be considered. The new trauma- and stressor-related disorders category in the DSM 5 are helpful for identifying and treating ASD and PTSD, which are relatively common in humanitarian emergencies. In the DSM-5, the diagnostic criteria have been clarified and clearly link the occurrence of severe traumatic or stressful events to the potential for the development of ASD or PTSD if the symptoms persist for more than 30 days. With a clearer diagnostic category, clinicians will be more likely to choose the correct treatment options.

Grief Reactions

Although most individuals are highly resilient to loss, the unnatural death and loss of a loved one (spouse, child, relative and friends) can lead to grief reactions so severe that the bereaved becomes emotionally and physically ill. All cultures have traditional and cultural ceremonies and prescribed rituals associated with grief and mourning. However, studies have demonstrated that those who have had a child murdered, suffer an unnatural death, or disappear in an emergency are especially prone to complex grief reactions that last longer than the cultural norm and are associated with major depression. The DSM-IV allowed for an "exclusion criteria" for depression associated with grief so that a normal grief reaction would not be misdiagnosed as a mental illness and associated with possible stigma and use of medication. These exclusion criteria have been removed in the DSM-5. Some mental health professionals believe this may lead to a medicalization of the grief reaction. Others say it will lead to proper treatment of depression affecting the bereaved. A new disorder in the DSM-5 called Persistent Complex Bereavement Disorder has also been proposed. This disorder describes grief reactions with persistent and severe sadness, feelings of being stuck on the loss, and invasive images and yearning for the deceased person. These symptoms continuing six months after the loss, need to be identified because they can be severe and debilitating.

Grief reactions are so common in humanitarian emergencies that it is necessary that the relief workers:

- Know the cultural expression and the traditional support of grief
- Be able to identify those who are developing a major grief-related physical and mental illness and provide the proper care

While cultural and religious ceremonies, counseling, and medication are often effective in caring for grief reactions, those with Persistent Complex Bereavement Disorder are often refractory to these treatments and will need specialized care (Shear et al. 2011).

Mental Health and Chronic Disease

There is emerging evidence that refugees, persons who have experienced natural disasters, and those impacted by conflict and war have increased levels of long term chronic disease attributable to their traumatic experiences and high levels of distress (Kinzie et al. 2008, Spiegel et al. 2010, Roberts et al. 2012). Specific traumatic events, such as torture, rape, disappearance of a loved one, unnatural death of a family member, and a history of child abuse, have the potential for negatively affecting a person's health and mental health status. While traumatic events can lead to negative health outcomes directly, mental health outcomes such as PTSD and depression can be mediators of poor health and physical disease. In a recent study in the Siem Reap province, it was found that traumatic experiences 25 years earlier impacted directly on functional and perceived health, whereas with more recent traumatic experiences the effect on mental health was directly related to PTSD and depression (Mollica et al. 2014). Other authors have further confirmed the relationship between trauma, PTSD, and health outcomes (Sledjeski et al. 2008, Spitzer et al. 2009).

Key work in mainstream populations in this area was initiated by Felitti and his colleagues. Their initial research called The Adverse Childhood Experiences Study (ACE study) (Anda et al. 2006) demonstrated the impact of adverse childhood trauma on the physical health of fifteen thousand middle-class American patients. This research is now being expanded to include highly traumatized populations who have experienced extreme violence, such as refugees, displaced persons, and those affected by natural disasters and humanitarian crises. Those working with highly traumatized patients and communities in the emergency phase must lay the groundwork for the prevention of chronic illness such as diabetes, hypertension, and heart disease that will have a major impact on trauma survivors within the immediate or more long-term future. Those who experience trauma are more likely to die at a younger age, develop serious physical illnesses, exhibit poor mental health, smoke more, use drugs and alcohol more, exercise less, and have poor eating habits (Anda et al. 2006). The direct and indirect impact of trauma-related mental health disorders such as PTSD and depression are now clearly linked to increased mortality and morbidity. Research has set the stage for the humanitarian community to advance the prevention and care of chronic medical disorders as a top priority that needs to be grounded in early interventions during the emergency phase. Mollica and his colleagues have built on this new approach to elaborate a new H^5 model (human rights, humiliation, healing, health promotion, housing/habitat) for the care of displaced populations and other highly traumatized populations (Mollica et al. 2014).

Gender-based Violence and Women's Health

Over the past quarter century, a major revelation has occurred within the international community concerning populations affected by mass violence and natural disaster: the major abuse of women in humanitarian emergencies is sexual violence (Goldfeld et al. 1988). The physical and emotional abuse of women can occur at epidemic proportions as witnessed in Haiti after the recent earthquake (Gage and Gutchinson 2006, Kolbe and Hutson 2006, Small et al. 2008). Gender-based violence not only includes rape but all forms of sexual abuse including trafficking, enslavement, and domestic violence. It can affect males and children as well as females. Gender-based violence is highly associated with emotional distress and psychiatric disorders (e.g., PTSD and depression), drug and alcohol abuse, and similar behavior. The experience of rape and sexual abuse is associated with numerous medical problems including sexually transmitted infections (STIs), HIV-AIDS, hepatitis C, infertility, and a plethora of other women's health illnesses and symptoms.

Disasters create an environment for gender-based violence due to the disruption of normal social life and social structures, dislocation, death, loss of family members, a chaotic living environment (poor housing, homelessness, lack of electricity), and a living environment without lights (WHO 2002, Chew and Ramdas 2005). All of the latter factors can facilitate the physical and emotional abuse of the traumatized populations, especially women, children, and the elderly. A history of widespread domestic violence and other forms of gender-based violence prior to the disaster almost guarantees that it will occur and even be enhanced during the new crisis and emergency phase. Therefore, humanitarian aid during the emergency phase of the humanitarian crisis must be prepared to prevent and treat gender-based violence, such as arresting and prosecuting those who prey on survivors of a catastrophe when they are most vulnerable and susceptible to victimization.

In addition to gender-based violence, the overall vulnerability of women during and after disasters can be extreme (Carballo et al. 2005). Women are at a much greater risk of death, impact on pregnant women can be extreme, contraception and family planning breaks down, and poverty and care giving roles are expanded. Social taboos, for example, for women and girls in Bangladesh after the 1998 floods revealed increased rashes and urinary tract infections because the women were not able to wash out menstruation rags properly in private and had no access to clean water for washing. Women's health issues can be associated with major mental health problems and emotional distress. Yet, little is still known about women's health and mental health in complex emergencies (American College of Obstetricians 2010).

Humanitarian Aid Workers

Humanitarian work is demanding and stressful (Lopes Cardozo et al. 2004, Ursano et al. 2006). A typical deployment may include uncertainty over deployment time, travel to an unfamiliar location with uncertain living accommodations or work responsibilities, exposure to victims or destruction, personal risk of injury, worries over family or work back home, political sensitivities and reentry into work or home life (Eriksson et al. 2001, Lopes Cardozo et al. 2005). Humanitarian work in complex emergencies is increasingly dangerous. One review noted deaths among international humanitarian workers working for nongovernmental organizations have increased since 1985 (Sheik et al. 2000, Lancet 2006). Much in the same way that organizations attempt to reduce individual risks associated with other occupational work exposures such as work-space injuries or exposure to biological or toxic agents, organizations that employ aid workers or responders are identifying the need for policy and programs that address the psychological consequences of such work (Antares Foundation, 2012). Several studies and surveys have been conducted describing the consequences of stress among international humanitarian aid workers (Lopes Cardozo et al. 2005, Holtz et al. 2002, Lopes Cardozo et al. 2012) and local staff working in humanitarian emergencies (Eriksson et al. 2012, Ager et al. 2012, Lopes Cardozo et al. 2013). In a survey among expatriate humanitarian aid workers in Kosovo, symptoms of depression were common, but symptoms of PTSD were not, although there was substantial exposure to trauma. Aid workers who were on their first assignment were at higher risk for developing mental problems than those who had been deployed several times. However, aid workers who had been on five or more assignments were again at higher risk to develop mental problems. Organizational support was an important mitigating factor.

The IASC guidelines on mental health and psychosocial support in emergency settings provide guidance to prevent and manage mental health problems and psychosocial well-being among staff and volunteers (IASC 2007, action sheet 4.4, pages 87–92). Many of the same principles of staff care have also been described in the Antares guidelines (Antares Foundation 2012), and in agency-specific guidance for staff mental health and psychosocial support (Welton-Mitchell 2013). These guidelines recommend that humanitarian agencies have written policy in place, screen and assess staff before every assignment, provide training and prepare staff for an assignment, monitor staff, and provide ongoing support during the assignment. In case a crisis occurs (i.e., hostage taking, medical illness, shooting, attack on the compound, etc.), the agency should be prepared to provide specific interventions as needed. Immediately after the assignment is over, the agency needs to actively assist with the reentry process of the staff member. The agency should keep in contact with the staff member even after the end of the assignment and offer any additional support if necessary.

International Humanitarian Aid Workers

Based on the result of a longitudinal study among international humanitarian aid workers (Lopes Cardozo et al. 2012), organizations deploying aid workers should consider the following policy recommendations for maximizing staff wellness:

Prior to Deployment
- Screen aid workers for history of mental illness and family risk factors

- Provide stress awareness and stress management training

During Deployment
- Providing the best possible living accommodations, workspace, and reliable transportation
- Having an organizational policy and management structure in place to ensure a reasonable workload, adequate management, and recognition for achievements

During and After Deployment
- Stimulate support networks which have shown to be very important mitigating factors
- Connect with family and friends back home (expatriate aid workers)

  The organization should encourage:
- Involvement in social support
- Facilitate peer support networks by helping to organize them
- Institute liberal telephone and Internet use policies, paid for by the organization, which will help increase social support networks of deployed staff

National Humanitarian Aid Workers

Few studies have explored the consequences of the stress of humanitarian aid work among national staff (employees who are drawn from the local population). Even though national staff far outnumber expatriates/international staff and make up the majority of the workforce in many humanitarian organizations, entitlements to services, including basic healthcare, psychological support, medical evaluation, salaries and other benefits, organizational support structures, and security policies for national staff are generally less comprehensive than for expatriate staff (McCall and Salama 1999). In addition, national staff have often personally suffered traumatic experiences and extreme stress related to the humanitarian emergencies in their countries (Lopes Cardozo et al. 2005, Lopes Cardozo and Salama 2001).

In a series of three cross-sectional surveys, the mental health of local staff was examined in Uganda, Jordan, and Sri Lanka, (Ager et al. 2013, Eriksson et al. 2012, Lopes Cardozo et al. 2013). In these studies, local staff reported high levels of exposure to chronic stressors related to both setting and work environment.

Of the workers in

Uganda	Jordan	Sri Lanka
50%	25%	51%

experienced five or more categories of traumatic events

| 68% | 55% | 58% |

high levels of symptoms of depression, anxiety, and PTSD

| 53% | 50% | 53% |

diagnosis of anxiety

| 26% | 19% | 19% |

diagnosis of depression diagnosis of PTSD

From the results of the field surveys in these three countries, the following generic recommendations to national humanitarian organizations for their workers have been extracted. These recommendations are relevant to organizations that employ national staff in humanitarian emergencies in other countries. The recommendations include:

- Teach stress-management techniques as a regular part of staff training
- Fortify social support mechanisms, including peer support networks
- Avoid excessive hours spent at work and provide adequate down time
- Practice good management principles, offer specialized training to managers to increase the skills necessary for their work: project planning, time management, motivating staff, and assessing and providing corrective feedback on performance
- Provide continuing education on mental health issues, while raising awareness that the issues can apply to everyone, including staff
- Create access to psychological support for all staff
- Decrease chronic stressors related to the workplace
- Provide psychosocial skills training and a sustainable support system to aid the staff in their work with beneficiary populations
- Address the high levels of depression and anxiety symptoms in these workers

Conclusion

Mental health in humanitarian emergencies is a significant issue that needs to be addressed. Currently, most mental health interventions in humanitarian emergencies are based on best practices and empirical evidence rather than evidence-based research. More research is needed to improve the standard of care. Humanitarian organizations must include mental healthcare of their staff in standard organizational policies.

Notes from the Field

Kosovo (1999)

After a decade of violent conflict in Kosovo, there were many anecdotal reports about mass rape of women by Serbian troops. An international NGO decided to send a psychiatrist from a European country to assist the rape victims with any mental health problems. The program consisted mainly of counseling of rape victims. This seemed to make sense because there was a lack of mental health professionals in Kosovo at the time. However, the international psychiatrist did not speak Kosovar Albanian. Even though this was a well-intentioned effort, several things went wrong including:

- There was no communication with the mental health professionals in Kosovo who were starting up a training program at that time, so the whole approach lacked sustainability. After the international psychiatrist left, there was no follow-up care in place for the women
- Since the international psychiatrist did not speak the local language, the use of an interpreter was necessary, and it was difficult to communicate with the women
- Because the counseling took place in a building that was clearly marked for survivors of rape, other people in the community knew who was being treated there and for what reason, which stigmatized the women in a country where victims of rape can become outcasts in their family
- An opportunity was missed to build capacity of local staff
- The effectiveness of a counseling program for women who have become victims of mass rape has never been evaluated.

From this experience, there were several lessons learned:

- First do no harm – identification of women who have been raped could place them at risk in some cultures

- Integrate mental health services from international organizations during an emergency into existing services or train local (mental) health professionals.

Acknowledgements: Nicholas DiStefano, Ha Young Lee, Cole Youngner, Julia Smith, and Justin Williams

References

Ager, A., Pasha, E., Yu, G., et al. (2012). Stress, mental health, and burnout in national humanitarian aid workers in Gulu, northern Uganda. *Journal of Traumatic Stress*, **25**, 713–720.

American College of Obstetricians. (2010). Preparing for disasters: Perspectives on women. American College Obstetricians and Gynecologists Committee Opinion Number 457 Available at: www.acog.org/Resources-And-Publications/Committee-Opinions/Committee-on-Health-Care-for-Underserved-Women/Preparing-for-Disasters-Perspectives-on-Women (Accessed 8 July 2017).

American Psychiatric Association. (2013). Diagnostic and Statistical Manual of Mental Disorders, 5th Edition: DSM-5. American Psychiatric Association.

Anda, R. F., Felitti, V. J., Bremner, J. D., et al. (2006). The enduring effects of abuse and related adverse experiences in childhood – A convergence of evidence from neurobiology and epidemiology. *European Archives of Psychiatry and Clinical Neuroscience*, **256**(3) 174–186.

Antares Foundation. (2012). Managing stress in humanitarian workers: Guidelines for good practice. Third edition. Available at: www.antaresfoundation.org/ (Accessed 8 July 2017).

Barth, J., Munder, T., Gerger, H., et al. (2013). Comparative efficacy of seven psychotherapeutic interventions for patients with depression: A network meta-analysis. *PLoS Med* **10**(5), 1–17, doi: 10.1371/journal.pmed.1001454.

Bass, J. K., Annan, J., McIvor Murray, S., et al. (2013). Controlled trial of psychotherapy for Congolese survivors of sexual violence. *New England Journal of Medicine*, **368**(23), 2182–2191.

Bisson, J. I., and Lewis, C. (2009). Systematic review of psychological first aid. July 31. Available at: http://mhpss.net/?get=178/1350270188-PFASystematicReviewBissonCatrin.pdf (Accessed 8 July 2017).

Bolton, P., Bass, J., Neugebauer, R., et al. (2003). Group interpersonal psychotherapy for depression in rural Uganda: A randomized controlled trial. *Journal of the American Medical Association*, **289**(23), 3117–3124.

Carballo, M., Hernandez, M., Schneider, K., et al. (2005). Impact of the Tsunami on reproductive health. *Journal of the Royal Society of Medicine*. **98** (9), 400–403.

Centers for Disease Control and Prevention (CDC). (2013). National Center for Injury Prevention and Control. Page last updated August 15-2016. Available at: www.cdc.gov/violenceprevention/suicide/riskprotectivefactors.html (Accessed 8 July 2017).

Chew, L., Ramdas, K. N. (2005). Caught in the storm: The impact of natural disasters on women. The Global Fund for Women. Available at: www.globalfundforwomen.org/wp-content/uploads/2006/11/disaster-report.pdf (Accessed July 8 2017).

Cochran, J., Geltman, P., Ellis, H., et al. (2013). Suicide and suicidal ideation among Bhutanese refugees – United States, 2009-2012. *Morbidity and Mortality Weekly Report*, **62**(26), 533-536.

De Roo, A., Ado, B., Rose, B., et al. (1998). Survey among survivors of the 1995 Ebola epidemic in Kikwit, Democratic Republic of Congo: Their feelings and experiences. *Tropical Medicine and International Health*, 3(11), 883-885.

Dossa, N. I., and Hatem, M. (2012). Cognitive-behavioral therapy versus other PTSD psychotherapies as treatment for women victims of war-related violence: A systematic review. *The Scientific World Journal*, **2012**, 1-19, doi:10.1100/2012/181847.

Eftekhari, A., Ruzek, J. I., Crowley, J. J., et al. (2013). Effectiveness of national implementation of prolonged exposure therapy in Veterans Affairs care. *JAMA Psychiatry*, 70(9), 949-955, doi: 10.1001/jamapsychiatry.2013.36.

Eriksson, C. B., Cardozo, B. L., Foy, D. W., et al. (2012). Pre-deployment mental health and trauma exposure of expatriate humanitarian aid workers: Risk and resilience factors. *Traumatology*, 19(1) 41-48, doi:10.1177/1534765612441978.

Eriksson, C. B., Kemp, H. V., Gorsuch, R., et al. (2001). Trauma exposure and PTSD symptoms in international relief and development personnel. *Journal of Traumatic Stress*, **14**(1), 205-212.

Fazel, M., Wheeler, J., and Danesh, J. (2005). Prevalence of serious mental disorder in 7000 refugees resettled in western countries: a systematic review. *Lancet*, 365, 1309-1314.

Gage, A. J., and Gutchinson, P. L. (2006). Power, control, and intimate partner sexual violence in Haiti. *Archives of Sexual Behavior*, 35 (1), 11-24.

Goldfeld, A., E., Mollica, R., F., Pesavento, B., H., et al. (1988). The Physical and Psychological Sequelae of Torture Symptomatology and Diagnosis. *JAMA*, **259**(18), 2725-2729.

Goodwin, R., Haque, S., Neto, F., et al. (2009). Initial psychological responses to Influenza A, H1N1 ("Swine flu"). *BMC Infectious Diseases*, 9(166), 1-6.

Hinton, D. E., Pham, T., Tran, M., et al. (2004). CPT for Vietnamese refugees with treatment-resistant PTSD and panic attacks: A pilot study. *Journal of Traumatic Stress*, 17, 429-433.

Hobfoll, S. E., Bell, C. C., et al. (2007). Five essential elements of immediate and mid-term mass trauma intervention: Empirical evidence. *Psychiatry*, **70**, 283-315.

Holtz, T. H., Salama, P., Cardozo, B. L., et al. (2002). Mental health status of human rights workers, Kosovo, June 2000. *Journal of Traumatic Stress*, **15**(5), 389-395.

Husain, F., Anderson, M., Lopes Cardozo, B., et al. (2011). Mental health and displacement in postwar Jaffna District, Sri Lanka. *Journal of the American Medical Association*, **306** (5), 522-531.

IASC Reference Group for Mental Health and Psychosocial Support in Emergency Settings. (2010). Mental health and psychosocial support in humanitarian emergencies: What Should humanitarian health actors know? Geneva. Available at: www.who.int/mental_health/emergencies/what_humanitarian_health_actors_should_know.pdf (Accessed 8 July 2017).

Inter-Agency Standing Committee. (2007). IASC Guidelines on Mental Health and Psychosocial Support in Emergency Settings. Available at: www.who.int/mental_health/emergencies/guidelines_iasc_mental_health_psychosocial_june_2007.pdf (Accessed 8 July 2017).

International Medical Corps. (2013). Approach to Mental Health and Psychosocial Support(MHPSS) Case Management. Available at: http://mhpss.net/?get=208/1382622139-MCsapproachtoMHPSSCaseManagementOct2012.pdf (Accessed 3 June 2014).

Jeffreys, M. (2014). Clinician's guide to medications for PTSD. PTSD: National Center for PTSD. Available at: www.ptsd.va.gov/professional/treatment/overview/cliniciansguide-to-medications-for-ptsd.asp (Accessed 8 July 2017).

Jones, K. (2011). "Psychopharmacology: Acute phase" in Disaster psychiatry: Readiness, evaluation, and treatment, in F. J. Stoddard, A. Pandya, and C.L. Katz, eds., *American Psychiatric Publishing, Inc*, Arlington, VA, pp. 241-260.

de Jong, J. P., Scholte, W. F., Koeter, M. W., et al. (2000). The prevalence of mental health problems in Rwandan and Burundese refugee camps. *Acta Psychiatric Scandinavica*, **102**(3), 171-177.

de Jong, K. (2011). Psychosocial and mental health interventions in areas of mass violence. A community-based approach. Médecins Sans Frontières – Operational Centre Amsterdam. 2nd edition. Available at: www.msf.org/sites/msf.org/files/old-cms/source/mentalhealth/guidelines/MSF_mentalhealthguidelines.pdf (Accessed 8 July 2017).

de Jong, K., Knipscheer, J. W., Ford, N., et al. (2014). The efficacy of psychosocial interventions for adults in contexts of ongoing man-made violence—A systematic review. *Health*, **6**, 504-516.

de Jong, J. T., Komproe, I. H., Van Ommeren, M., et al. (2001). Lifetime events and posttraumatic stress disorder in 4 postconflict settings. *Journal of the American Medical Association*, **286**(5), 555-562.

Kessler, R. C., Berglund, P., Delmer, O., et al. (2005). Lifetime prevalence and age-of-onset distributions of DSM-IV disorders in the National Comorbidity Survey Replication. *Archives of General Psychiatry*, **62**(6), 593–602.

Kessler, R. C., Chiu, W. T., Demler, O., et al. (2005). Prevalence, severity, and comorbidity of 12-month DSM-IV disorders in the National Comorbidity Survey Replication. *Archives of General Psychiatry*, **62**, 617–627.

Kinzie, J. D., Riley, C., McFarland, B., et al. (2008). High prevalence of diabetes and hypertension among refugee psychiatric patients. *The Journal of Nervous and Mental Disease*, **196**, 108–112.

Kohrt, B., Rasmussen, A., Kaiser, B., et al. (2013). Cultural concepts of distress and psychiatric disorders: Literature review and research recommendations for global mental health epidemiology. *International Journal of Epidemiology*, **42**(2), 365–406.

Kolbe, A. R. and Hutson, R. A. (2006). Human rights abuse and other criminal violations in Port-au-Prince, Haiti: a random survey of households. *Lancet*, **368**, 864–873.

Lancet. (2006). A tribute to aid workers, editorial, 368, 620.

Lopes Cardozo, B. (2008). IASC guidelines need a more evidence-based approach: a commentary on the guidelines on mental health and psychosocial support in emergency settings. *Intervention: The International Journal of Mental Health, Psychosocial Work and Counselling in Areas of Armed Conflict*, **6**, (3/4), 252–254.

Lopes Cardozo, B., Bilukha, O., Gotway, C., et al. (2004). Mental health, social functioning and disability in postwar Afghanistan. *Journal of the American Medical Association*, **292**, 575–584.

Lopes Cardozo, B., Gotway, C., Eriksson, C., et al. (2012). Psychological distress, depression, anxiety, and burnout among international humanitarian aid workers: A longitudinal study. *PLoS ONE*, 7(9), 1–13, doi:10.1371/journal.pone.0044948.

Lopes Cardozo, B., Holtz, T., Kaiser, R., et al. (2005). The mental health of expatriate and Kosovar Albanian humanitarian aid workers. *Disasters*, **29**(2), 152–170.

Lopes Cardozo, B., Kaiser, R., Gotway, C. A., et al. (2003). Mental health, social functioning and feelings of hatred and revenge of Kosovar Albanians one year after the war in Kosovo. *Journal of Traumatic Stress*, **16**(4), 351–360.

Lopes Cardozo, B. and Salama, P. (2001). Mental health of humanitarian aid workers in complex emergencies, in Y. Danieli, ed. Sharing the front line and the back hills: International protectors and providers: Peacekeepers, humanitarian aid workers and the media in the midst of crisis. Amityville, NY: Baywood Publishing, pp. 242–255.

Lopes Cardozo, B., Sivilli, T. I., Crawford, C., et al. (2013). Factors affecting mental health of local staff working in the Vanni region, Sri Lanka. *Psychological Trauma: Theory, Research, Practice, and Policy*, **5**(6), 581–590. doi:10.1037/a0030969.

Lopes Cardozo, B., Talley, L., Burton, A., et al. (2004). Karenni refugees living in Thai-Burmese border camps: traumatic experiences, mental health outcomes, and social functioning. *Social Science and Medicine*, **58**, 2637–2644.

Lopes Cardozo, B., Vergara, A., Agani, F., et al. (2000). Mental health, social functioning and attitudes of Kosovar Albanians following the war in Kosovo. *Journal of the American Medical Association*, **284**(5), 569–577.

McCall, M. and Salama, P. (1999). Selection, training, and support of relief workers: an occupational health issue. *British Medical Journal*, **318**(7176), 113–116.

Mollica, R. F., (2004). Measuring trauma, measuring torture. Harvard Program in Refugee Trauma, Cambridge.

Mollica, R. F., ed. (2011). Textbook of global mental health: Trauma and recovery: A companion guide for field and clinical care of traumatized people worldwide. Harvard Program in Refugee Trauma, Cambridge.

Mollica, R. F., Brooks, R., Tor, S., et al. (2014). The enduring mental health impact of mass violence: a community comparison study of Cambodian civilians living in Cambodia and Thailand. *International Journal of Social Psychiatry*, 60(1), 6–20, doi: 10.1177/0020764012471597.

Mollica, R. F., Cui, X., McInnes, K., et al. (2002). Science-based policy for psychosocial interventions in refugee camps. *Journal of Nervous and Mental Disease*, **190**, 158–166.

Mollica, R. F., Donelan, K., Tor, S., et al. (1993). The effect of trauma and confinement on functional health and mental health status of Cambodians living in Thailand-Cambodia border camps. *Journal of the American Medical Association*, **270**(5), 581–586.

Mollica, R. F., Lopes Cardozo, B., Osofsky, H. J., et al. (2004). Mental health in complex emergencies. *Lancet*, **364**, 2058–2067.

Mollica, R. F., McInnes, K., Sarajlić, N., et al. (1999). Disability associated with psychiatric comorbidity and health status in Bosnian refugees living in Croatia. *Journal of the American Medical Association*, **282**(5), 433–439.

Mollica, R. F., et al. (2015). Lindert, J., Levav, I., (eds.) Violence and mental health: Its manifold faces. *The New H5 Model of Refugee Trauma and Recovery*. Springer, New York, pp. 341–378.

Murray, C. J. and Lopez, A. D. (1996). Evidence-based health policy–Lessons from the global burden of disease study. *Science*, **274**(5288), 740–743.

National Child Traumatic Stress Network and National Center for PTSD, (2006), Psychological first aid: Field operations guide, 2nd edition.

National Institutes of Mental Health (NIMH). (2011). Post-traumatic stress disorder among adults. Available at: www.nimh.nih.gov/health/statistics/prevalence/post-traumatic-stress-disorder-among-adults.shtml (Accessed 8 July 2017).

Office of the Surgeon General. (1999). Center for Mental Health Services. Mental health: A report of the Surgeon General. National Institute of Mental Health. Available at: http://profiles.nlm.nih.gov/ps/access/NNBBHS.pdf. (Accessed 8 July 2017).

Patel, V. (2003). Where there is no psychiatrist: A mental health care manual. The Royal College of Psychiatrists.

Petevi, M., ed. (2000). WHO Declaration of Cooperation: Mental health of refugees, displaced peoples, and other populations affected by conflict and post-conflict situations. Geneva: WHO.

Prince, M., Patel, V., Saxena, S., et al. (2007). Global mental health 1. No health without mental health. *Lancet*, **370**, 859–77, doi:10.1016/S0140-6736(07)61238-0.

Reynolds, B. and Seeger, M. (2012). Crisis and emergency risk communication. Atlanta: Centers for Disease Control and Prevention. Available at: https://emergency.cdc.gov/cerc/manual/index.asp (Accessed 8 July 2017).

Roberts B., Patel P., and McKee M. (2012). Non-communicable diseases and post-conflict countries. *Bulletin World Health Organization*. **90**: 2-2A.

Rose, S., Bisson, J., Churchill, R., et al. (2001). Psychological debriefing for preventing post-traumatic stress disorder (PTSD). The Cochrane Data Base of Systematic Reviews, Issue 3.

Rothbaum, B. O., Kearns, M. C., Price, M., et al. (2012). Early intervention may prevent the development of posttraumatic stress disorder: a randomized pilot civilian study with modified prolonged exposure. *Biological Psychiatry*, **72**(11), 957–963, doi: 10.1016/j.biopsych.2012.06.002.

Sabin, M., Lopes Cardozo, B., Nackerud, L., et al. (2003). Factors associated with poor mental health among Guatemalan refugees living in Mexico 20 years after civil conflict. *Journal of the American Medical Association*, **290** (5), 635–42.

Schulz, P. M., Resick, P. A, Huber, L. C., and Griffin, M.G. (2006). The effectiveness of cognitive processing therapy for PTSD with refugees in a community setting. *Cognitive and Behavioral Practice*, **13**, 322–331.

Shear, M. K., et al. (2011). Complicated grief and related bereavement issues for DSM-V. *Depression Anxiety*, **28**, 103–117.

Sheik, M., Gutierrez, M. I., Bolton, P., et al. (2000). Deaths among humanitarian workers. *British Medical Journal*, **321** (7254), 166–168.

Sledjeski, E. M., Speisman, B., and Dierker, L. C. (2008). Does number of lifetime traumas explain the relationships between PTSD and chronic medical conditions? Answers from National Comorbidity Survey-Replication (NCS-R). *Journal of Behavioral Medicine*. **31**, 341–349.

Small, M. J., Gupta, J., Frederic, R., Joseph, G., Theodore, M., and Kershaw, T. (2008). Intimate partner and non partner violence against pregnant women in rural Haiti. *International Journal of Gynecology and Obstetrics*, **102**, 226–233.

The Sphere Project. (2011). Sphere Handbook: Humanitarian Charter and Minimum Standards in Humanitarian Response, Chapter 2.5. Essential health services – mental health. Available at: www.sphereproject.org/resources/download-publications/?search=1%26keywords=%26language=English%26category=22 (Accessed 8 July 2017).

Spiegel, P. B., Checchi, F., Colombo, S., and Paik, E. (2010). Health-care needs of people affected by conflict: future trends and changing frameworks. *Lancet*, **375**, 341–345.

Spitzer, C., Barnow, S., Volzke, H., et al. (2009). Trauma, posttraumatic stress disorder, and physical illness: Findings from the general population. *Psychomatic Medicine*, **71**, 1021–1027.

Tam, C. W. C., Pang, E. P. F., Lam, L. C., et al. (2004). Severe acute respiratory syndrome (SARS) in Hong Kong in 2003: Stress and psychological impact among frontline healthcare workers. *Psychological Medicine*, **34**, 1197–1204, doi: 10.1017/S0033291704002247.

Tol, W. A., Barbui, C., Galappatti, A., et al. (2011). Mental health and psychosocial support in humanitarian settings: Linking practice and research. *Lancet*, **378** (9802), 1581–1591, doi: 10.1016/S0140-6736(11)61094-5.

UNHCR. (2013). Operational Guidance Mental Health & Psychosocial Support Programming for Refugee Operations. Available at: www.unhcr.org/525f94479.html (Accessed 8 July 2017).

Ursano, R. J., Cerise, F. P., Demartino, R., et al. (2006). The impact of disasters and their aftermath on mental health. *Primary Care Companion to the Journal of Clinical Psychiatry*, **8**(1), 4–11.

Van Emmerik, A. R. P., Kamphuis, J. H., Hulsbosch, et al. (2002). Single session debriefing after psychological trauma: A meta-analysis. *Lancet*, **360**, 766–771.

van Ommeren, M., Saxena, S., and Saraceno, B. (2005). Mental and social health during and after acute emergencies: emerging consensus? *Bulletin of the World Health Organization*, **83**, 71–76.

Welton-Mitchell, C. E. (2013). UNHCR'S mental health and psychosocial support for staff. Available at: www.unhcr.org/51f67bdc9.html (Accessed 8 July 2017).

Wenzel, T., Rushiti, F., Aghani, F., Diaconu, G., Maxhuni, B., Zitterl, W. (2009). Suicidal ideation, post-traumatic stress and suicide statistics in Kosovo.

An analysis five years after the war. Suicidal ideation in Kosovo. *Torture*, **19**(3), 238–247.

World Health Organization. (2002). Gender and Health in Disasters.

World Health Organization. (2011a). The Interagency Emergency Health Kit. Available at: www.who.int/medicines/publications/emergencyhealthkit2011/en/ (Accessed 8 July 2017).

World Health Organization. (2011b). Psychological first aid: Guide for field workers. Available at: http://whqlibdoc.who.int/publications/2011/9789241548205_eng.pdf (Accessed 8 July 2017).

World Health Organization. (2012a). mhGAP intervention guide for mental, neurological and substance use disorders in non-specialized health settings: Mental Health Gap Action Programme (mhGAP). Available at: www.who.int/mental_health/publications/mhGAP_intervention_guide/en/ (Accessed 8 July 2017).

World Health Organization. Mental Health Gap Action Programme (mhGAP). (2012b). 4th meeting of the mhGAP forum. Hosted by WHO in Geneva on 10 October 2012 Summary Report of the Meeting. Available at: www.who.int/mental_health/mhgap/mhGAP_forum_2012.pdf?ua=1 (Accessed 8 July 2017).

Chapter 29

Tuberculosis

Michelle Gayer and Susan Temporado Cookson

Introduction

This chapter outlines the epidemiology of tuberculosis (TB) among populations affected by humanitarian emergencies, including factors that lead to the increased vulnerability of these populations and TB control programs within this context. In the acute phase of a humanitarian emergency, TB is not one of the primary infectious diseases killers and as such, is rarely a priority. Despite the fact that it is the number one infectious disease killer, it is often left to the recovery phase (Martins et al. 2006). However, TB, if neglected, can quickly result in increased morbidity and mortality. Specific guidance for treating TB is not covered to any extent in this chapter and is deferred to the standards promulgated by ministries of health in host countries, international aid agencies, and the World Health Organization (WHO).

Epidemiology

Global

In 1993, WHO declared tuberculosis as a global public health emergency. Today, TB ranks as the leading global killer from a single infectious agent but is a curable disease. In 2015, an estimated 1.8 million people died from TB (of whom 0.4 million also are human immunodeficiency virus [HIV]-infected), and there were 10.4 million new TB cases (WHO 2016a). Of note in the same year, HIV infection killed 1.1 million and is no longer among the top 10 causes of death (WHO 2017a). The disease burden among women and children is high. Over one-third of the TB deaths and new cases (34% each) occurred among women and 10% of new cases occurred among children.

The majority of new TB cases occur in the African and South-East Asian WHO regions. These two WHO regions have 21 (70%) of the 30 high TB burden countries (WHO 2016a). For 2015, these 30 high TB burden countries have an estimated TB incidence of 195 per 100,000 population compared with an estimated global TB incidence of 142 per 100,000 population (95% uncertainty interval 119–166 per 100,000) or an almost 30% greater incidence (WHO 2016a). The TB incidence by WHO region for 2015 is shown in Table 29-1.

Table 29.1 TB incidence by WHO region, 2015

Region	Incidence per 100,000 population (lower limit, upper limit) Rate	Number (thousands) (lower limit, upper limit)
African	275 (239–314)	2,720 (2,360–3,110)
Americas	27 (25–29)	268 (250–287)
Eastern Mediterranean	116 (86–149)	749 (561–965)
European	36 (33–38)	323 (299–349)
South-East Asian	246 (167–339)	4,740 (3,230–6,540)
Western Pacific	86 (78–94)	1,590 (1,440–1,740)

Source: World Health Organization. Global Tuberculosis Report, 2016. Statistical limits derived from the modeling exercise.

Emergency Affected Populations

Sudden changes in TB incidence can result from rapid influx of persons from countries with a high burden of TB. This may occur in a humanitarian emergency, such as during a time of conflict, or during a natural disaster, such as a drought or flood. Until the advent of the Arab Spring in 2010, these humanitarian emergencies and natural disasters mainly occurred in the same two WHO regions as the majority of new TB cases, the high TB burden countries of Africa, and South-East Asia. Arab Spring has affected persons from countries with lower TB burden; however, the TB epidemic and the migration of persons from environmental deterioration or state disruption overlap geographically. In 2015 among the 30 high TB burden countries, all but two (Lesotho and the Philippines) were either the country of origin or the country of asylum for one thousand refugees or more. Of these 28 countries with available numbers, an average of 97,853 refugees originated from the countries and 195,856 asked for asylum within the countries. In 2015, of the 16.1 million refugees or persons in refugee-like situations, almost 20 percent originated from and 30 percent took asylum in a high TB burden country (UNHCR 2016). This is shown in Table 29.2. Furthermore, for 2015, among the internally displaced persons, 15 percent resided in six of the 30 high TB burden countries (UNHCR 2016). High rates of TB prevalence or incidence have been observed among internally displaced persons (IDPs) across a diversity of countries after times of war. For example, this has been found among IDPs following the 1980–1992 civil war in El Salvador, during the 1992–93 military conflict subsequent to independence

Table 29.2 Refugee and refugee-like numbers by origin or asylum high TB burden countries, 2015

High TB Burden Countries by Region	Origin Number		Asylum Number	
African Region				
Angola	11,869		15,555	
Cen. African Rep.	471,104		7,330	
Congo	14,781		44,955	
Dem. Rep. of Congo	541,499		383,095	
Ethiopia	85,834		736,086	
Kenya	7,905		553,912	
Lesotho	17		31	
Liberia	9,994		36,505	
Mozambique	57		5,622	
Namibia	1,476		1,737	
Nigeria	167,988		1,395	
Sierra Leone	4,895		760	
South Africa	449		121,645	
Tanzania	6,221		211,845	
Zambia	344		26,447	
Zimbabwe	21,344		6,950	
Subtotal, n (%)	1,345,777	(49.1)	2,153,870	(44.0)
Americas Region				
Brazil, **n (%)**	895	(0.03)	8,707	(0.18)
Eastern Mediterranean Region				
Pakistan, **n (%)**	297,835	(10.9)	1,561,162	(31.9)

Table 29.2 (cont.)

High TB Burden Countries by Region	Origin Number		Asylum Number	
European Region				
Russian Federation, n (%)	67,050	(2.4)	314,506	(6.4)
South-East Asia Region				
Bangladesh	12,173		231,958	
Dem. People's Rep. Korea	1,103		-*	
India	9,881		201,381	
Myanmar	451,807		-	
Thailand	222		108,261	
Subtotal, n (%)	475,186	(17.3)	541,600	(11.1)
Western Pacific Region				
Cambodia	12,803		76	
China	212,911		301,052	
Indonesia	13,956		5,957	
Papua New Guinea	339		9,510	
Philippines	593		269	
Vietnam	313,156		-	
Subtotal, n (%)	553,758	(20.2)	316,864	(6.5)
Total Refugee Number in High Burden Countries	2,740,501		4,896,709	
Percentage of Total Refugees (N = 16,121,427)	17.0%		30.4%	

* A dash (-) indicates that the value is zero or not available. Source: United Nations High Commissioner for Refugees. Global trends, Forced displacement in 2015, 2016.

from the Soviet Union in Georgia, and following the 1997–99 war in the Republic of the Congo (Barr and Menzies 1994, Weinstock et al. 2001, M'Boussa et al. 2002). In the Congo and El Salvador studies, the rate of TB increased two and three times, respectively, compared with prewar estimates (M'Boussa et al. 2002, Barr and Menzies 1994). During the early 1990s, in Bosnia and Herzegovina, TB cases increased 50 percent compared with the wartime period (Ljubic and Hrabac 1998).

Similar high TB rates have been observed among Tibetan refugees in India, Kosovar refugees in Norway, Syrian refugees in Jordan, and among refugee populations resettled in the United States and elsewhere (Bhatia et al. 2002, Rysstad and Gallefoss 2003, Cookson et al. 2015, Hadzibegovic et al. 2005). A systematic review of crisis-affected populations (those experiencing displacement, armed conflict, or natural disasters), largely found elevated rates of TB notification and of TB prevalence (Kimbrough et al. 2012). Some of these higher prevalence rates may be because of increased detection. During humanitarian emergencies, nongovernmental organizations (NGOs) may be involved in the response, resulting in more active case detection. In the United States, resettled refugees are offered free initial domestic health assessments in contrast to immigrants. This more active system may lead to the higher TB prevalence seen among refugees compared with other foreign-born persons.

Besides high rates of TB among displaced populations, studies demonstrate high rates of TB-associated mortality and high rates of drug-resistant TB. In Guinea-Bissau, TB patients affected by the 1998 civil war compared with prewar TB patients had a mortality rate ratio, adjusted for age, sex, HIV-status, residence and length of treatment, of 3.3 and 2.3 for the intensive (first 2 months of treatment) and continuation (subsequent 4 to 6 months of treatment) phases, respectively (Gustafson et al. 2001).

Studies have also identified drug-resistant TB among resettling refugees in such countries as the United Kingdom, Sweden and the United States (Callister et al. 2002, Brudey et al. 2004, Oeltmann et al. 2008). In northeastern Kenya, comparing camp refugee with nonrefugee patients showed 3.7 greater odds of having drug-resistant TB (Githui et al. 2000). More recently, large numbers of Somali refugees have been found to have multidrug resistant (MDR) TB (Cain et al. 2015). A cluster of MDR-TB cases also has been identified in Europe among 29 persons fleeing hardship in the Horn of Africa (Walker et al. 2018).

Contributing Factors

Although large proportions of refugees and IDPs originate from or currently reside in one of the 30 high TB burden countries, additional factors may lead to their progression to TB disease. With migration, because of deteriorating environmental or governmental conditions, whether within one's country or across international borders, there might be a drop in caloric intake because of destroyed crops or markets, disruption of shelter or basic services with exposure to the elements, and unsafe drinking water or poor hygiene and sanitation practices. These factors can lead to depression of the immune system and increased susceptibility to water- and foodborne infectious diseases. All these factors might result in greater risk of progression to active TB disease among those with latent *Mycobacterium tuberculosis* infection (LTBI). In addition, during humanitarian emergencies, the diminution of medical services has led to an increase in patients lost to follow up for their treatment (M'Boussa et al. 2002) or the healthcare system no longer being able to provide treatment because of lack of medications or staff, or destroyed facilities. Another risk for drug-resistant TB with probably greater prevalence among displaced populations is that patients may have a greater tendency to seek care from nonregulated providers or pharmacies as seen in Somalia (Turpie 2008). These providers may use nonstandardized treatment regimens and the medication may be of poor quality. Therefore, lack of compliance with standardized treatment can be seen among the patients, providers, and pharmacies.

Clinical Course

Stigma

In addition to previously discussed factors, stigma can impact any TB patient, whether displaced or living in his or her home. TB has received many names through the years, such as white plague, referring to the pallor caused by the anemia of chronic disease, or consumption, referring to the cachexia of TB patients. These names have stigma attached. In the current era of HIV, the stigma of TB has the additional fears of coinfection with HIV for many living in Africa and elsewhere (Kipp et al. 2011a).

Studies have found TB patients expressing feelings of shame and having fears of isolation and rejection by their spouses, families, community, employers, or even the healthcare system itself (Kipp et al. 2011a, Zachariah et al. 2012). In addition, these feelings have been associated with delays in seeking care and nonadherence with treatment (Murray et al. 2013, Kipp et al. 2011b), the former potentially leading to increased transmission of TB and the latter to increased risk of developing drug-resistant TB.

Displaced persons are isolated by either a disaster and/or destruction of their home and community. In humanitarian emergencies, fear abounds with the breakdown of authority and increased levels of insecurity. In addition to delaying their seeking of care, these persons have been found to have self-treatment behaviors. These behaviors of delayed treatment and increased self-treatment have been described among Ethiopian TB patients living in a conflict zone (Gele and Bjune 2010). Both of these behaviors can have a negative impact of the clinical course of TB patients.

Infection vs. Disease

Displaced persons have high rates of LTBI, as seen in El Salvador during the 1980–92 civil war (Barr and Menzies 1994). Additionally, the travel conditions of their journey itself can be a factor for increased risk of LTBI as seen among asylum seekers (Sarivalasis et al. 2012, Cookson and Maloney 2017). In addition, overcrowding, as can occur in spontaneous settlements or refugee camps, has been associated with TB transmission (Lönnroth et al. 2009). WHO estimates that of the nearly one-quarter global population with LTBI, 10 percent will develop active disease over their lifetime. Malnutrition increases the incidence of active TB among those with LTBI (Cegielski and McMurray 2013). Therefore, displaced persons living in overcrowded conditions have increased risk factors for LTBI and suffering from food insecurity and malnutrition have increased risk factors for active TB disease, if LTBI is present.

Signs and Symptoms

Signs and symptoms of TB disease depend on the site of the disease. TB can travel outside the lungs (the usual port of entry) or disseminate to any part of the body, such as the meninges, and cause disease, such as TB meningitis. Young children (mainly those less than 5 years of age) and HIV-infected persons have a greater risk for this disseminated or extrapulmonary TB. Systematic symptoms of TB include night sweats, fever, weight loss, pallor, and fatigue. For pulmonary TB, cough of two weeks duration or longer, hemoptysis, and chest pain while breathing or coughing are common. Young children may have no symptoms, except failure to gain weight or weight loss. HIV-infected persons and young children may have little or no findings on chest X-ray or just mediastinal adenopathy.

Diagnosis and Treatment

The International Standards of Tuberculosis Care (ISTC) has defined 13 standards for diagnosis and treatment of TB disease (TB CARE I 2014):

1. Ensure early diagnosis by having providers (i) be aware of TB risk factors and (ii) perform prompt evaluation and diagnostic tests for TB suspects
2. Evaluate all patients, including children, with unexplained (i) cough of two weeks or longer or (ii) chest X-ray findings suggestive of TB
3. Have all patients, including children, capable of producing sputum, submit samples (i) two sputum specimens for microscopy or (ii) one for GeneXpert® MTB/RIF[1] (Cepheid®, Sunnyvale, CA)
4. Perform microbiological testing of appropriate specimens of all patients, including children, from sites suspected to be involved with extrapulmonary TB
5. Start anti-TB treatment for patients with suspected pulmonary TB, even if initial testing is negative, while awaiting further testing
6. Examine respiratory specimens in all children with suspected intrathoracic TB, whenever possible
7. Have provider (i) prescribe appropriate treatment regimen, (ii) monitor adherence, and (iii) address, when needed, factors leading to interruption or discontinuation of treatment
8. Use quality-assured drugs for all patients on WHO recommended first-line treatment
9. Use patient-centered approach to treatment, based on patient's needs and mutual respect
10. Monitor response to anti-TB treatment with follow-up sputum smear microscopy at completion of initial phase (two months)
11. Assess likelihood of drug-resistant TB
12. Treat patients with or highly likely to have drug-resistant TB with specialized regimens with quality-assured second-line anti-TB treatment
13. Maintain records of (i) all medication, (ii) bacteriologic response, (iii) outcomes, and (iv) adverse reactions for all patients

Since these standards for diagnosis, WHO has studied and found that the Xpert MTB/RIF Ultra assay is noninferior to the Xpert MTB/RIF assay (WHO 2017b). Diagnostic testing can be difficult to perform in emergency and postdisaster settings. At best, smear microscopy has been performed in the past. However, there is increased experience with GeneXpert® (see Notes in the Field). GeneXpert (Cepheid®, Sunnyvale, CA) is a cartridge-based, fully automated machine those cartridge reagents can rapidly identify the deoxyribonucleic acid (DNA) of *M. tuberculosis* and determine rifampin resistance for over 90 percent of strains using nucleic acid amplification tests (NAAT). The International Organization for Migration (IOM) has been using the GeneXpert® for several years among migrant, refugee, and host communities in Cambodian, Ethiopia, Nepal, Thailand and elsewhere (Gagnidze 2012). They have found it user-friendly and easy to perform with generally simple installation and training.

There are well-established criteria for establishing TB control programs in emergency situations (WHO 2007). When displacement is prolonged, as seen among refugees in such places as Kenya and the Thai-Burmese border or among internally displaced persons in such protracted conflicts in Afghanistan and Somalia, delay in treatment until the emergency is over may no longer be appropriate (Coninx 2010). Consequently and recently, TB control has been included in "international responses to relieve suffering in many major humanitarian crises"; however, control during emergencies needs sufficient evaluation and documentation of its feasibility and benefit (WHO, Eastern Mediterranean Region, 2015).

Different public-private partnerships in conflict-affected areas have had success in providing quality TB care and treatment, with Médecins Sans Frontières reporting the most on their experience (Heldal et al. 2007, Ndongosieme et al. 2007, Keus et al. 2003, Hehenkamp and Hargreaves 2003, Liddle et al. 2013). Strategies that have been tried include establishing the Manyatta regimen for patients to remain onsite in a home-type setting during treatment in such different countries as East Timor and southern Sudan (Keus et al. 2003, Heldal et al. 2007); developing a 3-tier protocol for evacuation of (i) international staff alone, (ii) with warning, for staff and community, and (iii) without warning, for all; and "runaway bags" with anti-TB medication (Hehenkamp and Hargreaves, 2003). This idea of "runaway" or "go" bags has also been used for preparation for natural disasters. Because of lessons learned from Hurricane Katrina by the Louisiana and Texas TB programs, they each gave their patients, in advance of Hurricane Rita, a two- to four-week supply of anti-TB medication in case directly observed therapy was interrupted (CDC 2006a). Other TB program preparation included:

- Creating line lists of patients in parishes and counties that might be affected
- Ensuring the patient had a list of phone numbers to reestablish contact with other TB programs, if displaced
- Obtaining contact information for patients' relatives and friends in other parts of the country
- Ensuring backup copies of patients' records were available for potential sharing with new TB programs, if patients displaced
- Moving essential TB supplies and medication stock to safer inland locations

Although these preparations were undertaken by United States TB programs for an ensuing large-scale natural disaster, many of these preparations are potential good practices for TB control programs in conflict-prone areas.

Challenges still exist with public-private partnership for TB control, such as lack of institutional development, difficult and prolonged transitions to national programs, difficulty ensuring compliance with national and WHO treatment guidelines, expatriate provider turnover, and sustainability (Heldal et al. 2007, Ndongosieme et al. 2007). Many of these issues have been seen in East Timor and the Democratic Republic of the Congo, leading to the national authority delaying their ability to take over this vital control activity of public health.

The chapter is not intended to be a guide for the care and treatment of patients with suspected TB. The reader is referred to ISTC (TB CARE I, 2014), WHO (WHO 2010a, WHO 2011, WHO 2014a), specific nongovernmental organization (NGO), such as Médecins Sans Frontières (MSF and Partners in Health, 2014), or country-specific guidance for appropriate treatment of TB patients, both first- and second-line anti-TB regimens. Additional guidance is available through the Curry International Tuberculosis Center (Curry International Tuberculosis Center 2016).

Prevention

The central principles for preventing transmission of and progression to TB are the same in the setting of humanitarian emergencies as in more stable settings.

Individual

The most important prevention measure an individual with TB disease can do is to adhere with prescribed anti-TB treatment. As mentioned above, in areas prone to unrest and conflicts, mechanisms can exist, such as "go" or "runaway" bags, to ensure continuation of therapy. In addition, issues associated with the stigma of having TB disease need to be addressed with use of patient-centered approach to treatment to further ensure adherence.

The TB patient, until noninfectious, or a person suspected of having TB disease, should:

- Stay away from other persons as much as possible
- Stay in well-ventilated areas, such as outside, and away from others
- Cover his or her mouth for any cough, sneeze, or laughter, with a tissue or rag if possible and discard the dirty tissue or rag in a safe manner

Infant

WHO recommends BCG (Bacille Calmette-Guérin) vaccine as an important tool in the global fight against

TB, until new vaccines are available, for infants born or living in parts of the world where the disease is common. BCG is fairly effective in protecting young children from severe TB complications; however, it does have less protection against pulmonary TB for older children and adults (Colditz et al. 1994, Rodrigues and Smith 1990). Regardless of the receipt of BCG vaccination, providers need to educate their patients of the need to come to the health facility if they develop TB symptoms. All children and HIV-infected family members of patients with TB diagnosed, regardless of prior BCG vaccination, need to be assessed for active TB disease.

Healthcare Setting

Hospitalized patients with suspected TB should be provided with sputum pots or mugs. These should have a cover and contain a disinfectant.

In 2008, WHO launched the public health strategy for resource-limited countries called Three I's to reduce the impact of TB among HIV-infected persons, these are:

1. **ICF**: Intensive case finding of TB cases
2. **IPT**: Isoniazid preventive therapy for persons with LTBI or living in areas with >30% LTBI prevalence
3. **IC**: Infection control measures for vulnerable patients, health care workers, the community, and those living in congregate settings.

Active case finding, part of intensive case finding (ICF), should begin as soon as possible, usually after the acute phase of the emergency or crisis. After assessment to exclude active TB, isoniazid prevention therapy (IPT) should not only be begun as soon as possible for HIV-infected persons but also for young children (less than five years of age) of sputum smear-positive mothers. In addition, if the child is breastfed, this needs to be continued (WHO 2010a). Family members, especially young children and those infected with HIV, have the greatest risk of developing active TB, if infected. A prophylactic dose of isoniazid (adults: isoniazid 5 mg/kg or 300 mg daily; children: isoniazid 10 mg/kg daily, or maximum 300 mg daily) should be given for at least six months, once active TB disease is ruled out.

Infection control (IC) should be in place for any displaced populations (WHO 2008). The measures do not require sophisticated infrastructure but basically include:

- Prompt detection of infectious patients
- Airborne precautions, and
- Treatment of people who have suspected or confirmed TB disease

For healthcare facilities there is a three-level hierarchy of infection control measures and include:

1. Administrative measures
2. Environmental controls
3. Use of respiratory protective equipment (Cookson and Jarvis 1997)

The first level, administrative measures, is the most important and impacts the largest number of people. It is, again, prompt identification of patients with presumptive TB disease to reduce the risk of uninfected people developing LTBI or TB disease in a healthcare facility. Patients suspected or diagnosed as having TB disease must be separated from other patients, especially young children and HIV-infected patients. The second level of the hierarchy, environmental controls, means ensuring good ventilation and reducing crowding in healthcare facilities, including their waiting rooms, to reduce the amount of bacteria in the air. If the patient with TB or presumptive TB is hospitalized, the facility needs to have good infection control, which means good ventilation and as much sunlight exposure as possible. Good ventilation can be as simple as ensuring that all the doors and windows are open and that air flow is from the patient to the outside, without anyone between the patient and the window or door. Administrative measures and environmental control minimize the number of areas in the healthcare facilities where exposure to TB may occur and therefore must be initiated before the provision of respirators.

Control

In nonemergency settings, the objectives of any TB program were to detect at least 70 percent of new smear-positive TB cases existing in the population and to cure at least 85 percent of those case. Identifying and curing smear-positive pulmonary TB patients should be a priority. The 2016–2020 Stop TB Strategy has updated these objectives to reaching 90% of all people who need TB treatment, including 90 percent of people in key populations, and achieving at least 90 percent treatment success (Stop TB Partnership, 2015). The basis of any effective TB program was first outlined in The Stop TB Strategy 2006–15 and since updated for after 2015 (WHO 2006, WHO 2016b, WHO 2016c).

The six components of this strategy are:

1. Pursue high-quality directly observed therapy-short course (DOTS) expansion and enhancement

2. Address TB-HIV, MDR-TB, and the needs of poor and vulnerable populations
3. Contribute to health system strengthening based on primary health care
4. Engage all care providers
5. Empower people with TB and communities through partnership
6. Enable and promote research

There are guidelines and tools available on-line to facilitate all components of The Stop TB Strategy (WHO 2006). The first component of the strategy is critical in all settings, although the approach and operationalization may be adapted in emergencies. This entails having an effective drug supply and management system, electronic recording and reporting systems, TB surveillance, treatment and program management guidelines, TB recording and reporting formats, laboratory and diagnostic strengthening, and legislation and management (including planning, human resources, training, and supervision). The updated strategy has been adapted to meet the needs of displaced populations or migrants to include such innovations as mobile clinics and family-supported treatment to improve diagnosis and treatment (Dhavan et al. 2017).

A TB control program that is poorly implemented can potentially do more harm than good. Such a program can potentially contribute to the development and subsequent spread of multiple drug-resistant bacilli. Therefore, certain criteria have been developed for implementing a TB control program in emergency settings (WHO 2007).

Identification of Need

The following criteria should be used to decide whether a TB program in emergency settings is needed (WHO 2007):

- Epidemiological data indicate that TB is an important health problem among the population concerned
- The acute emergency phase is over (in some settings where death rates are <1 per 10000 per day or usually when basic survival needs of of the population are being met as defined by SPHERE standards).
- Essential clinical services are available to treat priority/common conditions
- Basic package of health services is accessible to a large part of the population so that persons with presumptive TB suspects can be found and appropriate investigation or referral arranged

Criteria for Implementation

The first and main component of the Stop TB Strategy is to pursue high-quality DOTS expansion and enhancement. For this, the five key criteria which need to be in place, and what these require, are outlined below (WHO 2006):

1. Political commitment with sustained financing. This includes a legal and regulatory framework, financing for staffing, laboratory, drugs, and operations.
2. Case detection through quality-assured bacteriology. This requires community awareness and information, laboratory services including trained staff, infrastructure, equipment, supplies, and maintenance.
3. Standardized treatment with supervision and patient support. This requires functioning primary and referral health services, including trained staff at community level and health care facilities to allow appropriate patient care and compliance, and contact management, as per ISTC and WHO Tuberculosis Treatment Guidelines (TB CARE I 2014, WHO 2010a).
4. An effective drug supply and management system. This entails efficient procurement, warehousing, distribution, avoiding shortages and expiry, prepositioning, and drug quality control.
5. Monitoring and evaluation system, and impact measurement. This includes program planning and management, an effective health information system, and regular supervision.

Steps in Implementation

In order to move forward after fulfilling the criteria for implementation, several key concrete steps need to be taken, including:

- Mobilizing political support for measures to ensure treatment compliance
- Limiting TB drugs from being disseminated outside the program
- Establishing coordination mechanisms with local authorities and implementing partners
- Assessing program implementation capacities (treatment sites, staffing, supply chain, laboratory, logistics, funding)
- Developing a budget and obtaining necessary funds and elaborating a work plan
- Developing a local protocol for implementation

A local protocol is not just about treatment, but entails writing memoranda of understanding (MoU) between potential NGO program coordinators and the lead agency, which whenever possible should be the in-country national TB program (NTP). This should outline steps in patient management including diagnosis, treatment categories and regimens, and follow-up as per ISTC, WHO, MSF/Partners in Health, or country-specific guidance or treatment guidelines. In addition, it should describe establishing a recording and reporting system, supervision to assure proper monitoring and evaluation, managing drugs procurement, storage, distribution and supply chain, and contingency planning for potential interruptions to the program implementation in coordination with the NTP.

The key steps in implementation of a TB program in emergency settings described above are outlined in Figure 29.1, adapted from World Health Organization, 2007.

Disruptions to Ongoing Programs

Whether in a stable or emergency setting, disruptions to ongoing programs can occur for various reasons. For example, a natural disaster, conflict, or civil unrest can cause sudden population displacement and/or destruction of facilities, records, or supplies, forcing a cessation in normal activities. Some events that cause disruption to the program can be anticipated, and contingency planning should take place to mitigate the effects.

The objective of any intervention when TB programming is initially disrupted is the continuity of treatment of those already on treatment to avoid the development drug resistance and to enhance the chance of cure. This was outlined in the document from WHO, Eastern Mediterranean Regional Office (2015) to occur in the acute phase of the emergency.

Detection of new cases is not a priority until treatment continuation is restored and the initial emergency phase of lifesaving and essential services can be broadened to more comprehensive care with stability of services, patient load, and staffing. However, in the postacute recovery phase of the emergency, health authorities need to ensure funds are secured for TB control by inclusion in donor proposals (WHO, Eastern Mediterranean Region 2015).

Thus, the priority is to locate the people already on treatment and restore their treatment as soon as possible.

Key actions include:
- Address the cause of disruption, if possible
- Provide wide health education and mobilize the community to trace patients already on treatment
- List health facilities, NGOs or private providers that can continue TB drug distribution
- Ensure appropriate supply and storage of TB drugs
- Ensure TB drug distribution to listed facilities
- Establish referral system from community to facilities
- Ensure treatment guidelines distributed
- Map any laboratory facilities remaining and link to facilities
- Ensure laboratories supplied with basic microscopy and at least one for culture or GeneXpert
- Put into place a monitoring and supervision system

Patients may have lost their TB treatment cards, so it will be important to locate treatment regimens at facilities or ensure that trained clinicians get the best possible understanding of the diagnosis and treatment regimen for that individual.

Specific protocols must be followed as per WHO treatment guidelines based on duration of treatment to date plus or minus sputum results (WHO 2010a):

- For treatment interruptions of less than one month, treatment can be continued with compensation for missing doses
- Treatment interruptions for one to two months will require repeat sputum testing and treatment options based on both the length of the initial therapy prior to disruption and sputum results
- Interruption of treatment of two or more months classifies the patient as lost to follow up and requires repeat sputum testing and treatment options based only on the sputum results
- In the event that patient records are not available and regimen is unknown, protocols as per WHO treatment guidelines should be followed after determining the duration the treatment and performing two sputum smears on all patients

The anti-TB drugs supply chain needs to be maintained to ensure continuity of treatment and prevent future disruptions.

Contingency Planning

Contingency planning is an essential element of any TB program and should consider all potential types of

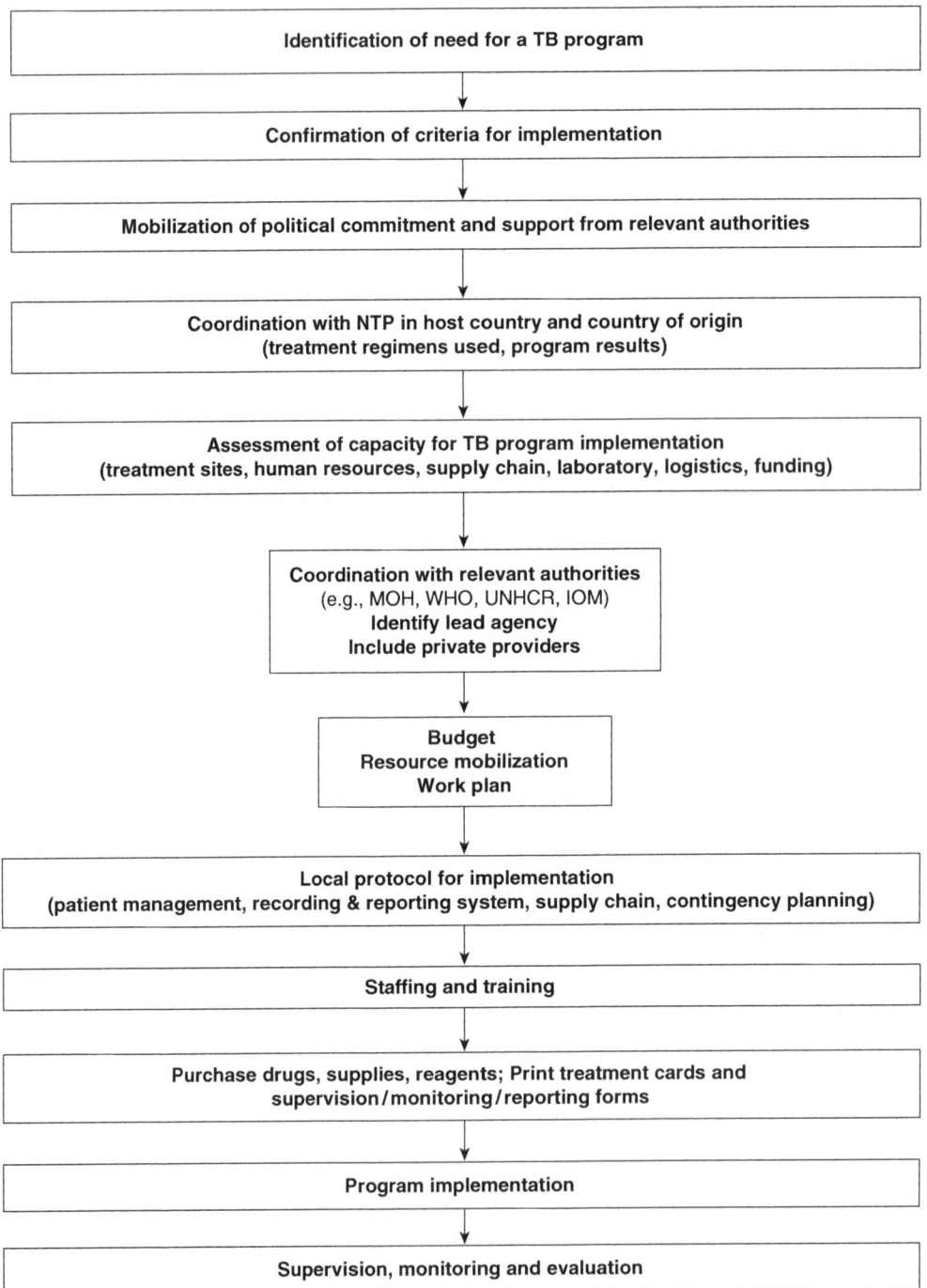

Figure 29.1 Key steps in implementation of a TB program in emergency settings (adapted from WHO 2007)

disruption or interruption, and their duration. The aim of minimizing treatment disruption is to prevent the development of anti-TB drug resistance, enhance patient cure and prevent transmission (WHO 2007).

Key events that may cause interruptions to treatment include:

- Natural disaster or conflict causing sudden population displacement/destruction of facilities, records, supplies

- Transfers in and out of TB programs
- Repatriation
- Cross-border movements
- Migrating and nomadic populations

Some actions to ensure continuity of treatment include:

- In case of recurrent conflict or natural disaster, prepositioning or mechanisms should be arranged for fast track procurement.
- A buffer stock of drugs and supplies could be ordered, imminent disruptions anticipated, and patients given a supply of drugs to keep with them.
- In the case of transfers in and out between countries, and cross-border movements, each country's National TB program should coordinate to make sure treatment protocols are aligned; ideally, the protocol the patient started should be completed, and patients should only transfer out after they have completed their intensive phase.
- For migrating populations and transfers, patients should have personal records of treatment and treatment plan, and at least one month's supply of drugs.
- Communicate between clinic staff in the different programs to alert them to migrations and transfers is ideal, although may be difficult in practice.
- Ensure that regular cross-border movements do not constrain treatment – e.g., patients have personal treatment cards and plans, which allow providers on either side to administer correct treatment and keep records.
- Make sure there are appropriate and reliable administrative systems for transfers of records.
- Arrange pick-up at borders and close follow-up in countries of return.
- In the event that patient records are not available for the receiving program, protocols should be followed after determining the duration of the treatment and performing two sputum smears on all patients.
- Stop new recruitments into programs if repatriation or transfers out are planned.

Monitoring and Evaluation

The purpose of any program evaluation should be to identify areas needing improvement and determine if the program is achieving its goals or objectives. The goal of TB control programs should be to lower the morbidity and mortality from TB and ultimately obtain eradication of the disease, for a defined population. Multiple tools and guidelines have been developed by United Nations agencies, and governmental and nongovernmental organizations for monitoring and evaluating TB control programs. As previously mentioned, the specific objectives of any TB control program are to detect at least 90 percent of all new smear-positive TB cases existing in a defined population and to cure at least 90 percent of them. This may not always be possible in the emergency setting but the objectives must still stand.

To aid in monitoring success toward these objectives, a cohort review (a systematic review of patients with TB disease and their contacts) should be conducted on a regular basis, usually every three months. Cohort reviews can motivate staff, reveal program strengths and weaknesses, indicate staff training and professional education needs, increase staff accountability for treatment completion of both patients with TB disease and LTBI, and improve TB case management (WHO 2010a). In addition to conducting a cohort review, the Centers for Disease Control and Prevention has developed an instruction guide (CDC 2006b) as well as WHO (WHO 2014b). To monitor the quality of the data within a cohort, the WHO manual on the use of Routine Data Quality Audit (RDQA) for TB monitoring at the peripheral TB control program level (WHO 2010b) may be used. WHO has also developed guidance on how best to use the TB data to determine the effectiveness of programmatic efforts (WHO 2014c).

Finally, to aid in evaluating the whole TB control program in resource-limited, refugee- and postconflict settings, CDC have revised their evaluation tool. This tool is inclusive, easy to use, and user-friendly (CDC 2013). In addition, it is adaptable, thorough, and field-tested.

The tool is for evaluators at national or regional headquarters of implementing partners that provide healthcare services or for the United Nations High Commissioner for Refugees (UNHCR). In addition, it is for medical and laboratory refugee camp staff or others in postconflict, resource-limited settings, who plan, organize, conduct, and supervise TB activities. The 2013 revision, version 2, incorporated items pertaining to drug-resistant TB in both the laboratory and clinical evaluation components. With the Syrian crisis, this tool is now available and has been used in Arabic.

The tool includes worksheets, references and resources, posters, and a patient charter for four components:

1. Laboratory
2. Health education
3. Clinical case management and treatment
4. Data management and logistics

Conclusion

Criteria now exist for establishing TB control programs in humanitarian emergencies (WHO 2007, WHO, Eastern Mediterranean Region 2015). These emergencies often last for long periods of time and delays in TB control implementation can result in increased morbidity and mortality (Coninx 2010). Multiple projects have shown that TB can be treated in refugee settings and even in unstable conditions. These projects are now known and the experiences have led to the criteria. However, one must weigh the pros and cons of delay in program implementation and the disruption in care that can lead to multiple drug-resistant TB with the ever-rising prevalence of TB. Until anti-TB regimens of shorter duration can be developed and confirmed as efficacious, these cons need remembering. However, programs to address the care of people with TB, especially continuation of medication, must be part of the emergency response.

Notes from the Field

Jordan (2013)

The WHO criteria for implementing a TB program in an emergency setting were evaluated by the Hashemite Kingdom of Jordan National TB Program, the United Nations High Commissioner for Refugees (UNHCR)-Jordan, and the International Organization for Migration (IOM)-Jordan with the technical assistance of WHO and the Centers for Disease Control and Prevention for determining additional intervention needs among Syrian refugees in Jordan. From the available data, among the Syrian refugees (the comparison that follows refers to the countries overall, not to the Syrian refugees), TB was an important health problem: in 2011 per WHO estimates, the TB prevalence of Syria was threefold greater than that of Jordan. Although Syrian refugees continue to arrive in Jordan and other neighboring countries, the mortality estimates among the refugees has remained below emergency levels with the health response increasingly focused on chronic disease management. The Syrian crisis is a protracted conflict; therefore, the refugees in Jordan and elsewhere can be expected to remain in place for the full length of an anti-TB regimen. Finally, both basic and essential clinic services for the refugees have been made available by UNHCR, local and international nongovernmental organizations (NGOs), and the Jordanian government.

Therefore, these organizations in close partnership developed a cohesive strategy for refugees in camps and in Jordan communities to:

1. Increase TB awareness and knowledge of treatment services among Syrian refugees and healthcare workers
2. Increase TB screening among Syrian refugees
3. Increase TB diagnosis among Syrian refugees
4. Maximize treatment success/completion of Syrian refugees, and
5. Support developing and implementing national guidelines for effective management and treatment of LTBI among Syrian refugees

Jordanian Public Health Strategy for Syrian Refugees, 2013 (Hashemite Kingdom of Jordan Ministry of Health et al. 2013).

Kenya (2007–2008)

In December 2007, civil unrest and violence in Kenya following national elections displaced 350,000 people. Health services including supply chains were temporarily disrupted. A study was conducted in March 2008 of 336 IDPs in nine camps and 1,294 patients in 35 health facilities. Findings showed that more than 85 percent of patients on long-term therapies for HIV, TB, diabetes, or hypertension avoided treatment interruptions compared with 2007. The proportion of TB patients who received a more than 45-day supply of drugs increased to 69 percent in December 2007 from 5 percent in November 2007. It was concluded that treatment interruptions were limited due to clinicians anticipating the potential disruption and providing patients with medications for an extended period.

Subsequently the Kenyan Ministry of Health considered this idea of "runaway" or "go" bags, similar to what was proposed by the Louisiana and Texas TB programs in advance natural disasters such as hurricanes, for their patients (CDC 2006a).

Postelection violence Kenya, 2007–08 (Bamrah et al. 2013).

Philippines (2013)

Typhoon Haiyan that struck the Philippines in November 2013 destroyed many medical records. The Department of Health (DOH), WHO, and health partners established a system to locate TB patients and to direct these individuals to the nearest treatment center. Local health staff compiled a list of their TB patients from memory. TB treatment centers, including those for MDR–TB, and diagnostic laboratories were mapped and assessed for functionality to enable the appropriate referral of patients for reinstitution of therapy as soon as possible. Facility maps were distributed to the numerous Foreign Medical Teams (FMTs) that arrived in the days to months post typhoon, to ensure they referred patients quickly to appropriate facilities. WHO and the DOH also rapidly prepared and distributed a basic field manual to assist NGOs, FMTs, and health centers in diagnosing and treating TB. The TB culture laboratory in Tacloban, which was completely destroyed, was quickly repaired.

Over this initial one-month period, almost one hundred percent of TB patients who were still present in typhoon-affected areas were receiving treatment again. However, those who had migrated to other areas in the country had not yet been traced after six months, and work continued to locate these people. After the initial priority to locate and reinstitute those already on treatment, the program was expanded to restart diagnosis of new TB suspects. Given the large geographical scale of the damage, functionality assessments of treatment centers and laboratories were continued six months posttyphoon, along with provision of further equipment and GeneXpert® training for health care professionals.

Philippines Typhoon Haiyan, 2013 (WHO, Western Pacific Region 2014).

Syria (2014)

In order to mitigate the higher risk of TB (and MDR TB) transmission and to reduce the increased burden on health care systems due to displacement of populations in seven countries affected by the Syria crisis, a regional TB project was developed in 2014 by IOM, United Nations Development Program, UNHCR, WHO and refugee-hosting governments, and several NGOs, which included: improving communication and coordination between TB control programs in affected countries, establishing effective systems for notification and management of TB (and MDR TB) patients who crossed borders; education and advocacy for TB patients (e.g., treatment compliance, follow-up); ensuring continuity of treatment; multilateral TB surveillance; a cross-country follow-up/referral system on detection and treatment to increase continuity of care, compliance and response to treatment and tracing of cases, particularly of MDR TB cases; a subregional standard for TB case management (e.g., screening, diagnostic, case definition, treatment of TB and MDR-TB); and a subregional communication strategy to increase awareness on transmission risks and TB prevention and control efforts. However, despite the importance of this strategy to combat TB regionally, because it was a multilateral organization proposal for regional implementation, it did not meet the eligibility criteria and was rejected.

Syria Crisis Regional TB project, 2014 (Aidspan, July 2014)

Note

1. In 2014, GeneXpert® (Cepheid Corp. Sunnyvale, CA, USA) was the only rapid molecular test approved by WHO for initial diagnostic use of TB. Use of trade names and commercial sources is for identification only and does not imply endorsement by the Centers for Disease Control and Prevention or the U.S. Department of Health and Human Services.

References

Aidspan. (2014). Regional pitch to fight TB in Syrian refugees rejected by Global Fund. Available at: www.aidspan.org/gfo_article/regional-pitch-fight-tb-syrian-refugees-rejected-global-fund-1 (Accessed July 14, 2017).

Bamrah, S., Mbithi, A., Mermin, J. H., et al. (2013). The impact of post-election violence on HIV and other clinical services and on mental health-Kenya, 2008. *Prehosp Disaster Med*, **28**(1), 43–51.

Barr, R. G. and Menzies, R. (1994). The effect of war on tuberculosis. *Tubercle Lung Dis*, **75**, 251–259.

Bhatia, S., Dranyi, T., and Rowley, D. (2002). Tuberculosis among Tibetan refugees in India. *Soc Sci Med*, **54**, 423–432.

Brudey, K., Gordon, M., Moström, P., et al. (2004). Molecular epidemiology of Mycobacterium tuberculosis in western Sweden. *J Clin Micro*, **42**(7), 3046–3051.

Cain, K. P., Marano, N., Kamene, M., et al. (2015). The movement of multidrug-resistant tuberculosis across borders in East Africa needs a regional and global solution. *PLOS Med*, 12(2), e1001791. doi:10.1371/journal.pmed.1001791 (Accessed July 13, 2017).

Callister, M. E., Barringer, J., Thanabalasingam, S. T., et al. (2002). Pulmonary tuberculosis among political asylum seekers screened at Heathrow Airport, London, 1995–9. *Thorax*, 57, 152–156.

Cegielski, J. P. and McMurray, D. N. (2013). Nutrition and susceptibility to tuberculosis, in B. Caballero, ed. *Encyclopedia of Human Nutrition*, 3rd edition, Volume **3**. Waltham, MA: Academic Press, pp. 309–314.

Centers for Disease Control and Prevention. (2006a). Tuberculosis control activities after Hurricane Katrina—New Orleans, Louisiana, 2005. *MMWR*, **296**(3), 275–276.

Centers for Disease Control and Prevention. (2006b). Understanding the TB cohort review process: Instruction guide. Available at: www.cdc.gov/tb/publications/guide stoolkits/cohort/Cohort.pdf (Accessed June 6, 2014)

Centers for Disease Control and Prevention and International Rescue Committee. (2013). Evaluation tool for tuberculosis programs in resource-limited, refugee and post-conflict settings. Version 2. Available at: www.cdc.gov/globalhealth/gdder/ierh/researchandsurvey/tbtool.htm (Accessed June 6, 2014).

Colditz, G. A., Brewer, T. F., Berkey, C. S., et al. (1994). Efficacy of BCG vaccine in the prevention of tuberculosis. Meta-analysis of the published literature. *JAMA*, **271**(9), 698–702.

Coninx, R. (2010). Tuberculosis in complex emergencies. *Bull WHO*, **85**(8), 637–640.

Cookson, S. T., Abaza, H., Clarke, K. R., et al. Impact of and response to increased tuberculosis prevalence among Syrian refugees compared with Jordanian tuberculosis prevalence: case study of a tuberculosis public health strategy. *Confl Health*, **9**, 18. doi:10.1186/s13031-015-0044-7

Cookson, S. T. and Jarvis, W. R. (1997). Prevention of nosocomial transmission of Mycobacterium tuberculosis. *Infect Dis Clin N Amer*, **11**, 385–409.

Cookson, S. T. and Maloney, S. A. (2017). Keeping up with a world in motion : Screening Strategies for migrating populations. *Clin Infect Dis*, 65(8), 1410–1411.

Curry International Tuberculosis Center. (2016). *Drug-resistant tuberculosis – A survival guide for clinicians*, 3rd edition. Available at: www.currytbcenter.ucsf.edu/products/view/drug-resistant-tuberculosis-survival-guide-clinicians-3rd-edition (Accessed July 7, 2017).

Dhavan, P., Dias, H. M., Creswell, J., et al. (2017). An overview of tuberculosis and migration. *Intern J Tuberc Lung Dis*, **21**(6), 610–23.

Gagnidze, l (2012). *IOM experience with Xpert MTB/RIF roll-out*. Fourth Green Light Initiative (GLI) Meeting, 17–19 April 2012, Annecy, France. Available at: www.stoptb.org/wg/gli/assets/html/day%202/Gagnidze%20-%20IOM%20projects.pdf (Accessed June 5, 2014).

Gele, A. A. and Bjune, G. A. (2010). Armed conflicts have an impact on the spread of tuberculosis: the case of the Somali Regional State of Ethiopia. *Conflic Health*, **4**, 1. Available at: www.conflictandhealth.com/content/4/1/1 (Accessed June 4, 2014).

Githui, W. A., Hawken, M. P., Juma, E. S., et al. (2000). Surveillance of drug-resistant tuberculosis and molecular evaluation of transmission of resistant strains in refugee and non-refugee populations in North-Eastern Kenya. *Int J Tuberc Lung Dis*, **4**(10), 947–955.

Gustafson, P., Gomes, V. F., Vierira, C. S., et al. (2001). Tuberculosis mortality during a civil war in Guinea-Bissau. *JAMA*, **286**(5), 599–603.

Hadzibegovic, D. S., Maloney, S. A., Cookson, S. T., et al. (2005). Determining TB rates and TB case burden for refugees. *Int J Tuberc Lung Dis*, **9**(4), 409–414.

Hashemite Kingdom of Jordan National Tuberculosis Program, United Nations High Commissioner for Refugees, International Organization for Migration. Public Health Strategy for Tuberculosis among Syrian Refugees in Jordan. Available at: https://data.unhcr.org/syrianrefugees/download.php?id=3791 (Accessed July 14, 2017).

Hehenkamp, A. and Hargreaves, S. (2003). Tuberculosis treatment in complex emergencies: South Sudan. *Lancet*, 362 **Supp**, s30–1.

Heldal, E., de Araujo, R. M., Martins, N., et al. (2007). The case of the Democratic Republic of Timor-Leste. *Bull WHO*, **85**(8), 641–642.

Keus, K., Houston, S., Melaku, Y., et al. (2003). Treatment of a cohort of tuberculosis patients using the Manyatta regimen in a conflict zone in South Sudan. *Trans R Soc Trop Med Hyg*, **97**, 614–618.

Kimbrough, W., Saliba, V., Dahab, M., et al. (2012). The burden of tuberculosis in crisis-affected populations: A systematic review. *Lancet Infect Dis*, **12**, 950–965.

Kipp, A. M., Pungrassami, P., Nilmanat, K., et al. (2011a). Socio-demographic and AIDS-related factors associated with tuberculosis stigma in southern Thailand: A quantitative, cross-sectional study of stigma among patients with TB and healthy community members. *BMJ Public Health*, **11**, 675. doi:10.1186/1471-2458-11-675.

Kipp, A. M., Pungrassami, P., Stewart, P. W., et al. (2011b). Study of tuberculosis and AIDS stigma as barriers to tuberculosis treatment adherence using validated stigma scales. *Int J Tuberc Lung Dis*, **15**(11), 1540–1545.

Liddle, K. F., Elema, R., Thi, S. S., et al. (2013). TB treatment in a chronic complex emergency: treatment outcomes and experiences in Somalia. *Trans R Soc Trop Med Hyg*, **107**, 690–698.

Ljubic, B. and Hrabac, B. (1998). Priority setting and scarce resources: case of the Federation of Bosnia and Herzegovina. *Croatian Med J*, **39**(3), 276–280.

Lönnroth, K., Jamamillo, E., Williams, B. G., et al. (2009). Drivers of tuberculosis epidemics: the role of risk factors and social determinants. *Soc Sci Med*, **68**, 2240–2246.

Martins, N., Kelly, P. M., Grace, J. A., et al. (2006). Reconstructing tuberculosis services after major conflict: experiences and lessons learned in East Timor. *PLOS Medicine*, **3**(10), e383. Available at: https://doi.org/10.1371/journal.pmed.0030383 (Accessed July 7, 2017).

M'Boussa, J., Yokolo, D., Pereira, B., et al. (2002). A flare-up of tuberculosis due to war in Congo Brazzaville. *Int J Tuberc Lung Dis*, **6**(6), 475–478.

Médecins Sans Frontières and Partners in Health. (2014). Tuberculosis: Practical guide for clinicians, nurses, laboratory technicians and medical auxiliaries. Available at: http://refbooks.msf.org/msf_docs/en/tuberculosis/tuberculosis_en.pdf (Accessed July 7, 2017).

Murray, E. J., Bond, V. A., Marais, B. J., et al. (2013). High levels of vulnerability and anticipated stigma reduce the impetus for tuberculosis diagnosis in Cape Town, South Africa. *Health Policy Plan*, **28**(4), 410–8.

Ndongosieme, A., Bahati, E., Lubamba, P., et al. (2007). Collaboration between a TB control programme and NGOs during humanitarian crisis: Democratic Republic of the Congo. *Bull WHO*, **85**(8), 642–643.

Oeltmann, J. E., Varma, J. K., Ortega, L., et al. (2008). Multidrug-resistant tuberculosis outbreak among US-bound Hmong refugees, Thailand, 2005. *Emerging Infect Dis*, **14**(11), 1715–1721.

Rodrigues, L. C. and Smith, P. G. (1990). Tuberculosis in developing countries and methods for its control. *Trans R Soc Trop Med Hyg*, **84**, 739–744.

Rysstad, O. G. and Gallefoss, F. (2003). TB status among Kosovar refugees. *Int J Tuberc Lung Dis*, **7**(5), 458–463.

Sarivalasis, A., Zellweger, J. P., and Faouzi, M. (2012). Factors associated with latent tuberculosis among asylum seekers in Switzerland: A cross-sectional study in Vaud County. *BMC Infect Dis*, **12**, 285. Available at: www.biomedcentral.com/1471-2334/12/285 (Accessed July 13, 2017).

Sphere Project. (2011). *The Sphere Handbook: Humanitarian Charter and Minimum Standards in Humanitarian Response*. Available at: www.sphereproject.org/handbook/ (accessed September 20, 2014).

Stop TB Partnership, UNOPS. (2015). The Paradigm Shift, 2016-2020: Global Plan to End TB. Geneva, Switzerland. Available at: http://www.stoptb.org/assets/documents/global/plan/GlobalPlanToEndTB_TheParadigmShift_2016-2020_StopTBPartnership.pdf (Accessed January 29, 2018).

TB CARE I. (2014). *International standards for tuberculosis care*, 3rd edition. The Hague, Netherlands: TB CARE I. Available at: www.istcweb.org/ISTC_Documents.html (Accessed May 30, 2014).

Turpie, I. D. (2008). Tuberculosis in Somalia. *Scot Med J*, **53**(2), 7–8.

United Nations High Commissioner for Refugees. (2016). Global trends, Forced displacement in 2015. Available at: www.unhcr.org/en-us/statistics/unhcrstats/576408cd7/unhcr-global-trends-2015.html (Accessed July 12, 2017).

Walker, T. M, Merker, M., Knoblauch, A. M., et al. (2018). A cluster of multidrug-resistant *Mycobacterium tuberculosis* among patients arriving in Europe from the Horn of Africa: a molecular epidemiological study. *Lancet Inf Dis*, 2018; DOI: http://dx.doi.org/10.1016/S1473-3099(18)30004-5.

Weinstock, D. M., Hahn, O., Wittkamp, M., et al. (2001). Risk for tuberculosis infection among internally displaced persons in the Republic of Georgia. *Int J Tuberc Lung Dis*, **5**(2), 164–169.

World Health Organization. (2006). The Stop TB Strategy, Vision, goal, objectives and targets. Available at: www.who.int/tb/strategy/stop_tb_strategy/en/ (Accessed June 5, 2014).

World Health Organization. (2007). *TB care and control in refugee and displaced populations. An interagency field manual.* 2nd edition. Connolly M., et al. ed. Available at: http://whqlibdoc.who.int/publications/ 2007/9789241595421_eng.pdf?ua=1 (Accessed May 30, 2014).

World Health Organization. (2008). WHO Three I's Meeting – Report of a Joint World Health Organization HIV/AIDS and TB Department Meeting. 2–4 April, 2008, Geneva, Switzerland. Available at: www.who.int/hiv/pub/meetingreports/WHO_3Is_meeting_report.pdf (Accessed June 5, 2014).

World Health Organization. (2010a). Treatment of tuberculosis guidelines, 4th edition. Available at: http://apps.who.int/iris/bitstream/10665/44165/1/9789241547833_eng.pdf (Accessed May 30, 2014).

World Health Organization. (2010b). WHO Stop TB Department, March 2010. Manual on use of Routine Data Quality Audit (RDQA) tool for TB monitoring. Available at: www.who.int/tb/dots/planning frameworks/RDQA_Tool_guideline_final.pdf (Accessed June 6, 2014).

World Health Organization. (2011). Guidelines for the programmatic management of drug-resistant tuberculosis – 2011 update. Available at: http://apps.who.int/iris/bitstream/10665/44597/1/9789241501583_eng.pdf (Accessed July 7, 2017).

World Health Organization. (2014a). Companion handbook to the WHO guidelines for the programmatic management of drug-resistant tuberculosis. Available at: http://apps.who.int/iris/bitstream/10665/130918/1/9789241548809_eng.pdf (Accessed July 7, 2017).

World Health Organization. (2014b). Standards and benchmarks for tuberculosis surveillance and vital registration systems, Checklist and user guide. Available at: www.who.int/tb/publications/standardsandbenchmarks/en/ (Accessed July 14, 2017).

World Health Organization. (2014c). Understanding and using tuberculosis data. Available at: www.who.int/tb/publications/understanding_and_using_tb_data/en/ (Accessed July 14, 2017).

World Health Organization. (2016a). Global tuberculosis report, 2016. Available at: www.who.int/tb/publications/global_report/en/ (Accessed July 10, 2017).

World Health Organization. (2016b). The end TB Strategy, Global strategy and targets for tuberculosis prevention, care and control after 2015. Available at: www.who.int/tb/post2015_TBstrategy.pdf?ua=1 (Accessed July 7, 2017).

World Health Organization. (2016c). The stop TB strategy, building on and enhancing DOTS to meet the TB-related millennium development goals. Available at: http://apps.who.int/iris/bitstream/10665/69241/1/WHO_HTM_STB_2006.368_eng.pdf (Accessed July 7, 2017).

World Health Organization. (2017a). The top 10 causes of death. Available at: www.who.int/mediacentre/factsheets/fs310/en/ (Accessed July 12, 2017).

World Health Organization. (2017b). TB detection and diagnosis, Available at: www.who.int/tb/areas-of-work/laboratory/en/ (Accessed July 14, 2017).

World Health Organization, Eastern Mediterranean Region. (2015). Tuberculosis control in complex emergencies. Available at: http://applications.emro.who.int/dsaf/EMROPUB_2015_EN_1913.pdf?ua=1 (Accessed July 7, 2017).

World Health Organization, Western Pacific Region. (2014). WHO Philippines response to typhoon Haiyan (Yolanda): The first six months. Available at: www.who.int/hac/crises/phl/sitreps/philippines_six_months_from_haiyan_may2014.pdf?ua=1 (Accessed May 30, 2014).

Zachariah, R., Harries, A.D., Srinath, S., et al. (2012). Language in tuberculosis services: can we change to patient-centred terminology and stop the paradigm of blaming the patients? *Intern J TB Lung Dis*, **16**(6), 714–717.

Chapter 30

Injuries and Trauma

Benjamin Levy, David Sugerman, Mark Anderson, and Charles Mock

Introduction

Injury prevention is a relatively new public health discipline and many developing countries have little injury prevention infrastructure. Complex humanitarian emergencies (CHEs) stress and often overwhelm what injury prevention systems do exist and expose the affected population to bodily harm before, during, and after the crisis. Injuries associated with natural disasters are exacerbated by poorly constructed buildings, inadequate shelter, crowded conditions, and a lack of public preparedness or evacuation measures (Alderman et al. 2012). Conflict and war can produce injuries through direct military action, as well as through indirect exposure of civilians to social violence and military ordinances (Hossain 2014, Roberts et al. 2001). In an immediate postdisaster setting, traumatic injuries that would be otherwise survivable can be fatal without medical attention and inadequate triage systems can impede access to potentially scarce medical resources. Among those that survive, long-term physical disability can negatively impact a family, community, or national workforce for a generation (Sudaryo et al. 2012). Furthermore, psychological wounds can persist for lifetimes with both mental illness and poor social outcomes being associated with injuries (Bryant et al. 2010).

In a disaster environment, many responding organizations focus on the provision of shelter, food, clean water, and waste disposal (Hanquet, 1997). While these measures are appropriate from the perspective of infection control, the provision of services for wounds and injuries are often overlooked or left to an uncoordinated collection of healthcare organizations (Brennan and Nandy 2001). The lack of injury surveillance and trauma system recovery can compound the morbidity of the injuries suffered during and after a disaster, which can hinder recovery efforts. It is thus important to understand injury epidemiology and use a public health approach to injury prevention in natural disasters and conflict.

Epidemiology

Natural disasters

Natural disasters include a range of climatologic and geophysical events that cause anything from minor local damage to catastrophic transnational humanitarian emergencies. As the global population grows, with increasing urbanization and coastal population density, the human and material effects of these disasters continues to rise. According to the EM-DAT International Disaster Database, there have been nearly 7,000 major recorded natural disasters in the past twenty years (1994–2014) causing over 1.3 million deaths, and over $2 trillion in damage (OFDA/CRED 2015). The largest impact disasters in terms of lives lost and damage done are generally considered to be windstorms, earthquakes, and inundations (floods or tsunamis). In this section we will discuss the epidemiology of injuries caused directly and indirectly by these natural phenomena.

Wind Disasters

The major types of wind disasters are tornadoes and cyclones, including hurricanes in the western hemisphere and typhoons in the eastern hemisphere. Both tornadoes and cyclones are immensely powerful storms with the ability to generate wind speeds in excess of 300 kph. Direct wind trauma includes blunt force injuries caused by victims being lifted or thrown, crush injuries from collapsing structures and falling debris, and lacerations or penetrating injuries from projectile debris. Head and upper body injuries are most commonly seen during wind storms (Rotheray et al. 2012). Eye injuries are common from dust and small debris. The indirect effects of the wind must also be considered and include injuries caused by falling trees, road traffic accidents, and drowning. In many settings, injury rates will begin to rise before the arrival of high wind speeds, as the population scrambles to evacuate or shelter, resulting in falls, traffic accidents, and occupational injuries.

Risk factors for direct injury from wind include sheltering in poorly constructed homes, such as those found in shanty towns on the periphery of most global cities. Children and smaller adults are at increased risk for severe injury and death due to their low body mass and increased likelihood of being thrown by the wind. Elderly victims are also at increased risk of death after a wind storm. These risk factors often coincide, and high death rates have been documented when tornadoes strike lower socioeconomic communities, whether they are mobile homes in the American heartland or rural farming villages in Bangladesh (Sugimoto et al. 2011, Chiu et al. 2013). However, paradoxically, men of working age may be the ones to suffer higher rates of bodily injury if they are outside during the event and more directly exposed to force of the wind. One example of this occurred when typhoon Saomei struck the southern Chinese coastline in August 2006. This windstorm injured 4.5 percent of the local population, and 87 percent of injuries were caused directly by flying or falling debris. In this typhoon, males, fishermen, and those living close to the ocean were at highest risk of injury and death. Thus, injury patterns seen after a windstorm can be highly variable depending on the context of the local population, and the size, intensity, and duration of the storm.

In addition to high wind speeds, cyclonic storms typically move from water onto land and push a large volume of water in front of them. This wall of water, a storm surge, may be a major source of damage and injury in the affected coastal area. Prior to the implementation of shelter and evacuation systems, 90 percent of cyclone-related mortality was directly related to storm surge (Shultz et al. 2005). An example of the damage wrought by storm surge took place during typhoon Haiyan in the Eastern Philippines in November of 2013. The typhoon pushed a storm surge in excess of 5 meters in height onto land in a major coastal city. Despite evacuation procedures having been implemented, over six thousand people died after many of the municipal shelters were inundated by the unexpected flooding (NDRRMC 2014).

Ongoing effects in the aftermath of a windstorm will likely include injuries sustained in the debris field, including electrocutions from downed wires, building collapse, and falls on uneven surfaces. In such a post–wind disaster setting, up to 80 percent of injuries may occur to the feet and lower extremities. In the absence of electricity, the use of candles and campfires can increase the risk of burn injuries. Chemical exposures and carbon monoxide poisonings are also more common due to ruptured pipe lines and an increased use of gasoline generators (Goldman et al. 2014). Respondents to these disaster settings should be prepared for the changing nature of injuries that may begin to rise immediately before the storm and continue during the clean-up and recovery phase.

Earthquakes

From 2001 to 2010, over 750,000 people died globally as a direct result of earthquakes, accounting for approximately 60 percent of all natural disaster-related deaths (Bartels and VanRooyen 2012). Earthquakes differ from windstorms in that they strike without warning and last no more than a few minutes. There are typically no injuries prior to the event, and most injuries will be suffered as a direct result of the earthquake. Falls may occur during the earthquake itself and cause lacerations, fractures, and soft-tissue injuries. However, the collapse of standing structures is a far greater source of injuries. Collapsing buildings can cause bony fractures, tearing of skin and tissues, limb entrapment, and other crush injuries. An estimated 80 percent of surgeries needed in an earthquake region will be orthopedic in nature (Bartels and VanRooyen 2012). Fractures that have open skin wounds have a very high rate of bone infection (osteomyelitis) unless surgical care and antibiotics are provided rapidly. Spinal fractures are common with either immediate paralysis or secondary nerve damage occurring upon movement. The danger posed by collapsing structures indicates that the population density and quality of building construction in an affected region are important predictors of injury, alongside earthquake intensity. In the Haitian post-earthquake response, higher rates of both nonfatal and fatal injuries were found in the crowded, poorly constructed living camps situated outside the city than in the more affluent, less densely crowded neighborhoods within Port-au-Prince (Doocy et al. 2013).

Relief workers responding to an earthquake need to be aware that the active urban search and rescue phase may continue for several weeks. In the aftermath of an earthquake, survivors who remain buried or entrapped in rubble face a second type of injury. Crush injuries affect a reported 3–20% of earthquake trauma victims, and represent the second most frequent cause of death after direct trauma (Bartels and VanRooyen 2012, Lu-Ping et al. 2012). Limbs that have been pinched or crushed by heavy debris lose their blood flow and begin to die within 4–6 hours. If a dead limb is released from entrapment, the resumption of blood flow can cause a release of toxins that have accumulated in the dying tissue, flowing into the central circulation and causing immediate shock, kidney damage, and even death (Genthon and Wilcox 2014). Entrapped limbs will often require surgical care or amputations; the need for advanced medical and surgical capacity can be enormous in the aftermath of a large earthquake. The 2010 Haitian earthquake caused as many as three hundred thousand injuries, of which at least 1,500 required surgical amputations (Bhattacharjee and Lossio 2011, Knowlton et al. 2011). Initial needs assessments should take into consideration the percent of buildings destroyed and the estimated population density of a given area, as this may directly influence the crush injuries that are discovered in the days to weeks after the event.

In the response to earthquakes, special attention should be given to vulnerable populations. Children are particularly at risk after earthquakes, as their small mass is particularly prone to injury from falling debris or collapsing structures. Children are also much more likely than working adults to be inside during an earthquake. In the Haitian earthquake, 53 percent of deaths were younger than 20 years old and 25 percent were under five (Bartels and VanRooyen 2012). The elderly population is also at particular risk in any disaster setting. They may be slower to evacuate buildings, increasing their likelihood of injury by falling debris or entrapment. Furthermore, elderly persons are at increased risk for fractures due to age-related bone fragility and are more prone to medical complications following injuries. An analysis of injuries and deaths after the earthquake in Wenchuan, China (2008) showed that the mean age for nearly two thousand injured patients was 46 years, but the median age for deaths was 64 years, with most elderly deaths occurring by fracture followed by delayed infection and organ failure (Xie et al. 2008).

Inundations

Inundations, including floods and tsunamis, are among the most common and destructive natural disasters in the world (Alderman et al. 2012). Tsunamis such as that following the 2011 Japanese Tohoku earthquake or the 2004 Indian Ocean tsunami captured international attention due to their dramatic nature and massive damage. However, flooding is far more common and often underappreciated as a cause of economic damages and loss of human life. Between 1994–2014 there were over three thousand recorded floods, leaving 53 million people homeless, and costing over US$500B in property damages (OFDA/CRED 2015). In comparison, there were 25 recorded tsunamis during the same period, leaving approximately one million people homeless and costing US$200B, more damaging than floods on an event-by-event basis, but far less common.

Floods often have a strong socioeconomic disparity in their injury patterns and death rates. In a review of 53,000 flood-based deaths, there was a 23:1 ratio of deaths in low- and middle-income countries as compared to wealthier nations (Alderman et al. 2012). Increased mortality and trauma are seen in poor communities that are often located in low-lying areas peripheral to city centers, near agricultural sources of water, in known flood zones, or in substandard dwellings. The age extremes are at increased risk for death following flooding as they are more likely to be inside unstable dwellings and have less ability to evacuate and/or swim to safety. In contrast, nonfatal injury rates are often higher in the middle age ranges, likely due to activities in postdisaster debris fields (Doocy et al. 2009). Societal gender roles also play a role in postflooding injury risk. In the 2004 Indian Ocean tsunami, some communities reported 80 percent female deaths, as most men were at sea fishing during the event (Oxfam International 2005). In contrast, men were at increased risk of injury and death after Hurricane Katrina struck the gulf coast of the United States in 2006 largely due to their activities in the debris fields in the immediate postdisaster phase (Brunkard et al. 2008).

While the general assumption is that inundation disasters will cause fewer injuries than earthquakes or wind storms, wound complications can cause excessive mortality in the days or weeks following the disaster (Sphere Project 2011). Strong currents carrying debris and brackish water hiding hazards create an environment where lacerations, contusions, and

443

fractures are the most common immediate injury patterns (Sullivent et al. 2006). In the days and weeks after the disaster, wound complications begin to rise in prominence. A condition known as Tsunami Lung, characterized by severe pulmonary infections, is thought to be a late complication of inhaling contaminated flood waters (Inoue et al. 2012). Wound infections are especially prevalent as open wounds are poorly cleaned and repeatedly exposed to contaminated water (Lim et al. 2005). These infections are characterized by the growth of multiple and often rare organisms that may not be susceptible to standard antibiotic therapy (Guha-Sapir and van Panhuis 2009, Tam and Nayak 2012, Miskin et al. 2010). The need for surgical and advanced wound care may be more important than first suspected from immediate aftermath injury reports.

There are several important factors to consider in those exposed to flood waters. Immunization status should be assessed due to the high risk of contaminated injuries. Even those previously vaccinated may need a tetanus vaccine booster (Faul et al. 2011). This applies to disaster response volunteers and workers as well as affected locals. Flood-impacted communities may also be at increased risk of exposure to toxic chemicals as industrial or agricultural areas are often affected by flooding (Foulds et al. 2014). Early needs assessments should consider commercial, agricultural, and industrial zones to assess potential toxic exposures and risks.

War and Conflict

A 2001 International Rescue Committee study of 22 months of conflict in eastern Congo found that an estimated 1.7 million excess deaths were directly attributable to the fighting, most suffered by civilians rather than soldiers (Roberts et al. 2001). The impact of armed conflict can be staggering and undermining to every component of an affected society. Public health practitioners deployed to a postconflict zone will likely find themselves dealing with a public health system that is fundamentally disrupted, a populace that has been traumatized, and a burden of injuries and wounds that require a coordinated response.

Blast Injuries

Blast injuries have been declared the "signature injury" of the modern era of warfare (Institute of Medicine Report 2014). However, blast injuries are not limited to active war zones. Land mines were used as weapons of civilian control, land denial, and border security through much of the twentieth century (Bilukha et al. 2008). In postconflict zones, unexploded ordnance, either by accident or by design, have exposed generations to the threat of indiscriminate detonation. The public health practitioner must understand these wounds in both the immediate and long-term setting.

Blast injuries occur in four major patterns (Institute of Medicine Report 2014, Mitka 2014). The first is caused by the blast wave itself. High-powered explosives cause a high-pressure wave called the blast wave, which expands from the epicenter in concentric circles. The blast wave causes trauma to gas or fluid filled organs, and can result in ruptured eardrums, eye injuries, lung injuries, and internal organ injury (Champion et al. 2009). Furthermore, the initial blast wave can ricochet and intensify if it occurs in a confined space (Wightman and Gladish 2001). A study in Israel found that closed space "bus bombings" had an average 50 percent mortality, while open-air bombings had average mortality rates under 10 percent (Leibovici et al. 1996). The second pattern is due to shrapnel that flies outward from the explosion. Many explosive devices are constructed to disperse shrapnel widely. These injuries are characterized by penetrating and tearing wounds that can rupture viscera or amputate limbs (Wightman and Gladish 2001). The range for these injuries typically extends farther than the danger from the blast wave itself. For this reason, secondary blast injuries, or penetrating shrapnel injuries, are the most common type of injury pattern seen in survivors after explosive blasts (Champion et al. 2009). The third pattern of injury from a blast is caused by the blast wind, which will throw objects and people outward (Champion et al. 2009). Injuries occur as the thrown body hits the ground or other immobile object, producing external injuries, fractured bones, or rupturing solid organs such as the kidneys, spleen, or liver. This pattern also includes the effects of falling debris and the collapse of surrounding buildings (Wightman and Gladish 2001). The fourth pattern of injury seen in explosions is through exposure to the by-products of the blast. Burns are a very common fourth pattern of blast injury. Hazardous toxins may be released by the blast, either as a byproduct, or by design.

Recognizing the four patterns of injury caused by blasts can help the public health worker determine the types of explosives being used, the resources needed in the event of further detonations, and develop a healthcare delivery system to manage future injuries.

In the last decade, traumatic brain injury has been recognized as a critical fifth injury pattern seen in blasts. Brain injuries can be caused by any one of the earlier categories of injury; by blast wave, by shrapnel, or by blast wind forces. The majority of traumatic brain injuries are concussions or brief losses of consciousness (Hoge et al. 2008). A minority of traumatic brain injuries will be more severe and display open head wounds, skull fractures, and symptoms such as persistent unconsciousness, seizures, or dense confusion. Mild brain injuries and concussions may be difficult to detect in the immediate setting, as many survivors may act disoriented or confused. However, recent studies have linked mild traumatic brain injuries to the development of posttraumatic stress disorder and other long-term health problems (Hoge et al. 2008). In an environment where blast injuries are common, the public health worker should consider monitoring and recording the rates of minor and major traumatic brain injuries for the purposes of long-term disability assessments and mental health interventions.

Years after the end of major military activities, the people of Afghanistan continue to suffer high rates of blast injuries (Bilukha et al. 2008). The nation contains an estimated five to seven million unmapped Soviet landmines. In addition, aerial bombardment by coalition forces in late 2001 to 2002 left a new threat of unexploded ordnance across the landscape. An epidemiologic review of explosive injuries from 2002 to 2006 found that 92 percent of deaths were in civilians and the most common age group was 10–14 years. Thirty-eight percent of victims suffered traumatic amputations of limbs. The most common activity associated with unexploded ordnance injuries was when children played with the devices. The effects upon a civilian population by these types of injuries can be devastating to a community and a local economy not only through deaths and disabilities, but also through the land denial associated with minefields.

Ballistics Injuries

Ballistics injuries can be caused by any fast moving projectile. Explosive shrapnel or wind driven debris can result in ballistic wounds but the term is typically applied to gunshot wounds. Ballistic injuries are characterized as either low-velocity / low-energy injuries or high-velocity / high-energy injuries. High-powered rifles, with a muzzle velocity above 750 m/s, result in the archetypal high-velocity ballistic injuries, while other projectiles, including handguns or shrapnel with velocities less than 250 m/s fall into the category of low velocity (Fackler 1996). Recognizing these injury patterns will help public health workers assess healthcare needs and implement healthcare delivery systems.

Low velocity

The damage caused by low-velocity ballistics relate directly to the path and tumble of the projectile. Thus, a wound through a muscle will only cause localized bleeding and bruising, while a wound that enters the thoracic or abdominal cavity has a high likelihood of causing wounds to internal organs (Fackler 1996). For this reason, surgical exploration is generally the rule for penetrating ballistics injuries to the thorax or abdomen, and any penetrating wound to the trunk should be rapidly referred to a center with surgical capacity. On the other hand, bullet retrieval is a misconception, and stable gunshot wounds to the extremities typically do not require advanced care. These wounds are not typically at risk for infection; however, tetanus immunization should be provided in all cases.

High velocity

High-velocity injuries most commonly occur due to long barrel military rifles, such as the American M-16 or Russian AK-47. The major difference in high-velocity ballistic injuries is a pressure wave cavitation that occurs. Cavitation is caused when a bullet enters with such velocity as to cause a focalized shock wave, which can massively disrupt and tear surrounding tissues. These bullets not only cause a primary track of injury, but also disrupt tissues widely around their path. Furthermore, the negative pressure caused by the shock wave has a much higher tendency to draw debris into the entry wound, causing high rates of infection. For these reasons, high-velocity ballistic injuries tend to require extensive surgery and nearly always require referral to advanced medical care where available.

It is important to understand that the epidemiology of war wounds will vary greatly by context and will evolve rapidly within a context. Ballistics injuries are not limited to combatants, and civilian populations are highly vulnerable. A study of a field hospital in an active conflict zone on the Persian Gulf in 2003 found that 34 percent of war wounds occurred in noncombatants, of which a significant portion were children under the age of 16 (Hinsley et al. 2005). A study of Red Cross Hospitals during a conflict found that gunshot wounds, blast injuries, and all-cause mortality rose during the conflict but remained elevated after the cessation of active military operations (Meddings 1997).

Interpersonal Violence

Populations in proximity to active conflict are at greatly increased risk for violence and intentional injuries. A cross-sectional study performed in two civilian hospitals in the West Bank of Palestine in 2000 found only 23 intentional injuries. In late 2000, the Second Intifada occurred, marked by a period of increased civil strife, protests, and riots. The study was repeated in 2001 and found that the same two hospitals saw a volume of 740 violent injuries in the same time period (Helweg-Larsen et al. 2004). This rise in civilian on civilian violence in times of conflict was also demonstrated in Iraq during 2003–08, when investigators found that most killings of women and children were occurring by unknown or nonmilitary perpetrators as opposed to deaths by direct military action (Hicks et al. 2011).

While it is perhaps not surprising that violent injuries rise during armed conflict, the available research indicates that violence also increases in the immediate wake of natural disasters as well. Research on this topic is limited, and a review of the available literature concluded that there is insufficient evidence to link increases in societal violence after natural disasters (Rezaeian 2013). However, disasters disrupt social support systems and lead to critical resource shortages, unemployment, and family displacement. There is evidence that these economic stressors do drive increases in property crime in the aftermath of disasters (Bailey 2009 and Roy 2010). Violent crime may also increase in the immediate aftermath of a disaster, such as was seen in the two years after Hurricane Katrina struck New Orleans (Bailey 2009). It is unclear whether these immediate events lead to long-term changes in baseline social violence.

However, specific vulnerable populations, such as children and women, are at increased risk of violence during CHEs (Roberts et al. 2009). Gender-based violence, intimate partner violence, and child abuse have all been shown to increase during times of crisis. Rape has been closely associated with military conflict, but rates of domestic sexual violence also rise in conflict regions (Hossain et al. 2014). Refugee and displaced populations in conflict areas also have higher rates of violence against women (Marsh et al. 2006). A review of reports from refugees of 19 different conflicts over 17 years found that approximately 20 percent of women reported sexual violence during their displacement; however, rates varied widely, with over 80 percent of women sexually assaulted in some contexts (Vu et al. 2014). Transactional and exploitative sex can also rise in prevalence as families face immediate survival needs (UNHCR 2011).

Child abuse may surge, as families under duress may lash out at the vulnerable members of the family. A study examining the effects of the 2007 floods in Bangladesh found an increased rate of domestic abuse in families suffering food and resource shortages during the flooding. Lower socioeconomic status and a worse financial situation were found to be contributing risk factors (Biswas et al. 2010). Evaluating and halting the victimization of populations at risk should be of the upmost priority for humanitarian workers in conflict and disaster zones. Protection is discussed in detail in Chapter 15.

Environmental Injuries

Disrupted or displaced populations are vulnerable to numerous environmental hazards, and injury rates seen in postdisaster and displaced populations remain elevated far after the event itself (Sugerman et al. 2005, Uscher-Pines et al. 2009). Unnaturally crowded conditions may occur after the large-scale destruction of homes by a natural or manmade disaster. Furthermore, refugees are often concentrated in camps for the efficiency of aid delivery. A disruption of the normal community structure, including childcare and schools, may lead to a large number of unattended children left to play amongst rubble, open fires, or the military remnants left by departing combatants. The population may be exposed to the elements, living in temporary shelters or abruptly migrating. The loss of normal protective barriers, such as sidewalks, roads, and pedestrian walkways may lead to an increase in pedestrian vehicular injuries. Water management systems may fail, leading to delayed or recurrent flooding raising the risk of drownings. Washed out or destroyed roads may increase vehicular crashes and injuries. Rubble may create pedestrian hazards as well as reroute traffic in unexpected ways. The loss of the electrical grid will create community hazards from dark areas, as well as promote the use of unconventional and unsafe cooking, heating, and lighting sources. Police presence will likely be diverted and limited in affected communities, and a rise in criminal activity may result. Chemicals used in homes or industry may spill out into the environment, polluting civic water sources in residential areas. A careful evaluation of environmental conditions is critical to the context of an immediate needs assessment as well as the development of longer-term planning for recovery from these events.

Public Health Activities

Disaster preparedness is a vital function of a public health system and, when possible, the public health worker can be involved in ongoing capacity building and response planning. Even when disasters strike without warning, such as earthquakes, well-trained disaster response teams can bring rapid order and efficiency to the chaos and confusion of the early postdisaster environment. A rapid needs assessment should be performed to identify major injury patterns, mortality estimates, and healthcare capacity. A health information system should be utilized to facilitate resource allocation and form the core of an ongoing injury surveillance system. The overarching goal should be the rapid direction of healthcare resources and the identification and mitigation of risk factors for further trauma and injury.

Disaster Preparedness

The World Health Organization (WHO) has established guidelines for disaster preparedness (WHO 2007). Preparedness plans should be evidence-based, have clear lines of responsibility and command, be scalable, take into account all healthcare sectors, involve multiple civic agencies, and enable local decision-making. National policy should encourage strong local capacity for disseminating public advisories in an emergency, providing adequate shelter, and ensuring access to emergency medical care. Different localities and environments will have a variety of material resources; however, all localities can, at baseline, develop an emergency organization plan. Such a plan should have clear lines of authority, points of communication, and a logistic hub. The lessons learned in wealthy nations, in response to recent terrorist attacks, have highlighted the need for this type of coordinated disaster preparedness. After the September 2001 attacks, the United States adopted a National Incident Management System (NIMS) that serves as a platform for the coordination and response to domestic disasters (NIMS 2015). Similarly, the United Nations has designated the Office of the Coordination of Humanitarian Affairs (OCHA) as a focal point for the multiagency response to humanitarian emergencies (OCHA 1999). The lessons learned and the systems developed by the large agencies can be replicated on any level, and the development of a sound emergency response plan is a key public health activity.

Rapid Needs Assessment

A rapid needs assessment should be performed as soon as logistically possible, preferably within 48 hours of a major event (WHO 1999). In terms of injuries, the purpose of a rapid injury needs assessment should be to both qualitatively describe the context of the injuries, as well as to quantitatively determine the morbidity, mortality, and the need for external resources. As part of the assessment, questionnaires should be developed that track demographics of the affected population, deaths, current health conditions, and access to resources. A thorough assessment should focus on more than the affected populations but also examine the environment with special attention to physical hazards that may contribute to further violent or unintentional injuries. For instance, it would be important to note unstable buildings, brackish water hiding sharp metal edges, minefields, or the current frontlines of conflict. Finally, the assessment should also document the movement of survivors, whether an influx of refugees or an efflux of disaster survivors, as these population shifts can massively alter postdisaster demographics (WHO 1999). All rapid assessments should conclude with a list of specific priority actions that should be undertaken as soon as possible in response to the emergency. An example of a rapid assessment following a sudden impact disaster such as a hurricane or earthquake is shown in Figure 30.1. Rapid assessments are discussed in detail in Chapter 7.

Health Information System

After a rapid needs assessment, the next major goal for the public health response is the development and implementation of a standardized data collection and reporting system. Injury surveillance requires such standardization, and its importance cannot be overstated in promoting an adequate, measured, and appropriate emergency response. A public health worker may need to collaborate directly with the domestic authorities to ensure the early adoption of a data reporting system across multiple agencies. In developing these systems, local reporting mechanisms should be utilized and adapted wherever possible.

To maximize data quality, the system should be simple, practical, and easy for partners to work with. The system must be affordable, unless the implementing agency can guarantee adequate funding. Finally, the system should be designed for stability and sustainability with an eye on long-term regional recovery as well as the immediate response needs. A core minimum data set (MDS) should be agreed upon as the bare minimum information that should be collected on each injury. An optional data set (ODS) may be added as the capacity or need for data collection increases. Figure 30.2 provides suggested data elements to incorporate into both an MDS and an ODS health information system.

The injuries selected for monitoring should be consistent with results of the first rapid assessments. Supplemental datasets may be considered as specific situations arise and context specific or highly sensitive information is needed. Examples might include gathering information on violence, rape, toxic exposures, or other unexpected injuries. Initial health information will often need to be gathered by hand, but automated data collection should be implemented early to maintain high quality continuous injury surveillance. A simple alphanumeric system should be used to uniquely identify each record to avoid duplicate record entry. Results should be prepared and reported in a clear format with easily interpreted findings. Identify stakeholders and plan information distribution. Ensure that results are being used for the formation of results oriented activities and interventions. Finally, the system should be constantly reevaluated and improved as the context evolves and the postdisaster needs change.

Phase 1: Immediate response
- Simultaneously assess and respond to the crisis (field and emergency care)
- Obtain injury estimates from health centers for the first day
- Estimate crude mortality by body counts, family reports, and health center reports
- Plan the logistics of a full assessment

Phase 2: Extension of immediate response to affected areas
- Gain access to and establish emergency response to less accessible areas
- Survey the availability of primary healthcare resources
- Assess secondary needs such as shelter, food, water
- Assess external resource needs (healthcare capacity, medical supplies, equipment)

Phase 3: Establish healthcare services and provide shelter
- Assess environmental health issues, security, safety
- Identify and assess the needs of vulnerable groups
- Work to reestablish primary healthcare network and referral system
- Design distribution plan for incoming supplies and resources

Phase 4: Implement healthcare needs, assess recovery needs
- Identify established surveillance systems and adapt to new environment
- Evaluate injury patterns and identify long-term needs
- Identify long-term resource needs (disability, rehabilitation, psychosocial counseling)

Figure 30.1 Rapid assessment of injuries in sudden onset disasters
Adapted from WHO, 2009 and MSF, 2006

Minimum Data Set (MDS)

- Unique record identifier
- Demographics (gender, age)
- Incident details
  - Activity involved
  - Intent (unintentional, intentional-self harm, intentional-assault)
- Injury details
  - Mechanism of injury (motor vehicle crash, fall, building collapse)
  - Nature of injury (broken leg, burn, lacerations, chest trauma)
- Outcome (death, admission, discharge)

Optional Data Sets (ODS)

- Extended demographics
  - Race, occupation, location of home
  - Postdisaster status (refugee, displaced, at home, with family)
  - Degree of damage to home (total, major, minor, undamaged)
  - Military involved or civilian war victim
- Extended incident details
  - Setting (house, work, school, public area)
  - Location, date, and time
  - Injury mechanism details (driver, passenger, type of gun, fall height)
  - If assault, by whom (friend, intimate partner, family, stranger)
  - Involvement of drugs or alcohol
- Clinical data
  - Time to healthcare (delays, access, transport?)
  - Method of arrival to health facility
  - Arrival vital signs (blood pressure, pulse, respirations, alertness)
  - Clinical diagnoses (indicate major or minor)
- Facility information
  - Typical volume and capacity (outpatient, inpatient, surgeries)
  - Functional status (personnel, structure, electrical supply, medical supplies)
  - Immediate resources needed (stang, equipment, pharmacy)
  - Health system function (communication, referral network, transportation)
  - Evacuation procedures (plan in place, site identified, barriers)
- Medical interventions (early quality indicators and capacity assessment)
  - Medical procedures performed (wound care, splint, drain abscess)
  - Surgeries (number of procedures, types of surgery, outcomes, anesthesia)
  - Admissions, discharges, and inpatient deaths from injuries

Adapted from Holder et al., 2001

Figure 30.2 Suggested data elements to incorporate into both an MDS and ODS health information system for postdisaster injury monitoring

Injury Surveillance System

The long-term public health goal for injury prevention in a complex humanitarian emergency should be the establishment of a robust injury surveillance system. Currently, it is common for an EWARN (Early Warning and Response Network) system to be established to identify and control communicable diseases (WHO 2012). However, injury surveillance should also be incorporated into the early development of a sustainable surveillance system to appropriately direct prevention efforts as well as medical and surgical resources. In the wake of Hurricane Katrina on the Gulf Coast of the United States in 2005, a large infectious disease surveillance system was established to detect outbreaks of diarrheal and respiratory disease; however, communicable disease outbreaks were infrequent and sporadic (MMWR 2005). Physical injuries, meanwhile, suffered during flooding as well as during the relief operations, were far more prevalent, and approximately half of all evacuees required tetanus immunization (Brunkard et al. 2005, Faul et al. 2011).

The best injury surveillance systems will include data collected from multiple sources, including field assessments, clinical data from healthcare facilities, behavioral data from surveys and interviews, and demographic data from external sources such as OCHA or other humanitarian agencies (Horan and Mallonee 2003). Such injury data can inform the delivery of aid, prioritize the rebuilding of healthcare delivery systems, and avoid compounding tragedy through misallocation of resources and the complications of poor wound care. Figure 30.3 provides an injury surveillance questionnaire that can be modeled and adapted for use in most contexts. Surveillance is discussed in detail in Chapter 9.

Emergency Health System Management

The Humanitarian Charter and Minimum Standards in Humanitarian Response advises that wound care and injury prevention be considered part of the essential health services to be rapidly prioritized within the emergency setting (Sphere Project 2011). Mass triage, field first aid, and medical resource mobilization should begin immediately and require direction and coordination. Tetanus vaccine must be made available, for both disaster victims and aid workers who receive wounds in the course of recovery efforts. Patient evacuation and referral procedures must be clarified and universally adopted by all health agencies. The existing trauma care infrastructure should be identified and operational surgical care facilities should be established as referral centers. Posttrauma and rehabilitative care should be considered early to mitigate the effects of long-term disability. The public health worker entering the emergency environment must be ready to evaluate these essential health services and assert these immediate priorities in a chaotic environment where competing interests are the rule instead of the exception.

Referral System

The wound care capabilities of healthcare facilities will be an important consideration in the development of a postemergency medical system (Brennan and Nandy 2001). Assess the native healthcare infrastructure, taking into consideration the level of disruption to facilities, infrastructure, and staffing. The top level of healthcare provision is the referral hospital, that should meet the needs of approximately one hundred thousand affected persons (Hanquet 1997). Services at these facilities should, at a minimum, include diagnostic capacity and a surgical team capable of performing damage control surgeries including amputations and large wound management. The next tier of service is provided at central health facilities that should be equipped and provisioned for populations of 10–30 thousand affected persons. These facilities should have physician oversight, sizeable outpatient departments, and some inpatient bed capacity. Aseptic facilities should be maintained for minor surgical procedures such as wound care, abscess drainage, and fracture reductions. Intravenous fluids and antibiotics should be available and 24-hour staffing is optimal at this level. Peripheral health clinics, typically managed by nurses or health officers, are used for the decentralization of primary healthcare services for populations of three to five thousand affected persons. Services provided at these decentralized clinics can involve basic wound care, provision of oral antibiotics, and early referral to advanced health centers in the event of wound complications. Ambulatory care and home visitations should be offered when resources permit as simple follow up wound care and rehabilitation can be done from home. The public health practitioner can be vitally important in identifying contact points at these facilities, coordinating resource allocation and care delivery, and identifying gaps and needs within this framework.

Triage

Triage is the process of rapidly determining how to utilize limited medical resources. Modern western emergency departments run triage as a standard operating procedure, with more ill patients being preferentially seen while less ill patients wait. In a humanitarian emergency, the assumption is that the health system is overwhelmed, necessitating a triage system. There are a variety of triage systems

DISASTER XYZ INJURY SURVEILLANCE TOOL

INJURY SURVEILLANCE COORDINATING OFFICE: _____
INJURY SURVEILLANCE COORDINATOR: _____
COORDINATOR CONTACT INFORMATION: _____

OFFICE USE ONLY
RECORD NUMBER

SECTION 1: DEMOGRAPHICS

GENDER: ☐ MALE ☐ FEMALE ☐ OTHER
RACE: ☐ UNKNOWN ☐ _____ ☐ _____ ☐ _____
AGE: _____ YEARS _____ MONTHS (IF <1Y)
OCCUPATION:
☐ NONE (CHILD) ☐ FULL TIME PARENT
☐ VENDOR ☐ BIZ OWNER ☐ DRIVER ☐ CIVIL SERVANT ☐ LABORER
☐ STUDENT ☐ EDUCATOR ☐ ADMINISTRATOR ☐ GEN. ASSISSTANT ☐ HOUSEKEEPER
☐ CHILD CARE ☐ FARMER ☐ POLICE ☐ MILITARY ☐ UNEMPLOYED
☐ _____

LOCATION OF HOME: _____ _____ _____
NEAREST ADDRESS CITY/TOWN REGION

SECTION 2: INCIDENT DETAILS

LOCATION OF THE INCIDENT: _____ _____ _____
NEAREST ADDRESS CITY/TOWN REGION

SETTING:
☐ HOME ☐ WORK ☐ SCHOOL ☐ STREET ☐ SHOP/STORE
☐ BAR ☐ RESTAURANT ☐ GOV. BLDG. ☐ POLICE STA. ☐ MILITARY BASE

INJURY DATE: _____

INJURY MECHANISM:
☐ CAR CRASH: DRIVER ☐ CAR CRASH: OCCUPANT ☐ CAR CRASH
☐ PEDESTRIAN HIT BY MOTOR VEHICLE ☐ MOTORCYCLE CRASH ☐ BICYCLE CRASH
☐ FALL ☐ BUILDING COLLAPSE ☐ FALLING DEBRIS
☐ LACERATION: DEBRIS ☐ LACERATION: BITE WOUND ☐ LACERATION: BLADE
☐ BURN: THERMAL ☐ BURN: CHEMICAL ☐ BURN: ELECTRICAL
☐ SUN EXPOSURE ☐ COLD EXPOSURE ☐ DROWNING
☐ GUNSHOT WOUND ☐ BEATEN WITH BLUNT OBJECT ☐ STABBING
☐ _____ ☐ _____ ☐ _____
☐ _____

TIMING OF THE INJURY TO THE DISASTER:
☐ INJURED BEFORE DISASTER ☐ INJURED DURING DISASTER ☐ UNKNOWN
☐ INJURED AFTER DISASTER

INCIDENT INVOLVED POST-DISASTER RECOVERY OPERATIONS:
☐ NO ☐ PAID LABOR ☐ VOLUNTEER ☐ PERSONAL RECOVERY ACTIVITIES

INTENT:
☐ UNINTENTIONAL ☐ UNKNOWN ☐ INTENTIONAL: SELF-HARM
☐ INTENTIONAL: ASSAULT
BY: ☐ STRANGER ☐ FRIEND ☐ FAMILY ☐ UNKNOWN ☐ INTIMATE PARTNER

WERE ALCOHOL OR DRUGS INVOLVED IN THE INCIDENT:
☐ YES ☐ NO ☐ UNKNOWN

Figure 30.3 Injury surveillance questionnaire

---

that may be employed, but all systems divide the patients into three key groups, including those who need immediate help, those for which help may be delayed, and those who cannot be helped due to the severity of their injuries or illness. The triage process should start at the scene of the injury, especially in the case of the multiple casualty incidents. The triage system should be designed to prioritize care for those who need it most, and will benefit most. Inherent to the triage process is also the difficult decision to deprioritize care to those who have suffered catastrophic or inevitably fatal injuries. Comfort measures can always be provided, but when lives are at risk, responders must be educated and empowered

Section 3: Illness and Injury

SECTION 3: CLINICAL DATA

DID THE VICTIM SEEK IMMEDIATE HEALTH CARE:
- [ ] YES
- [ ] NO
- [ ] UNKNOWN

IF NO, WHY NOT:
- [ ] MINOR INJURIES
- [ ] DEATH
- [ ] CARED FOR OTHERS
- [ ] LACK OF FACILITIES
- [ ] LACK OF TRANSPORTATION
- [ ] LACK OF KNOWLEDGE
- [ ] TRAPPED/PINNED
- [ ] OTHER: _____

ARRIVAL TO HEALTH CARE DATE: _____

ARRIVAL METHOD:
- [ ] HIRED VEHICLE
- [ ] OWN VEHICLE
- [ ] WALK
- [ ] AMBULANCE
- [ ] NON-MOTORIZED CART

MEDICAL EVALUATION PERFORMED BY:
- [ ] MD AT HOSP.
- [ ] OTHER AT HOSP.
- [ ] MD AT CLINIC
- [ ] OTHER AT CLINIC
- [ ] NON-MEDICAL SETTING

PAST MEDICAL HISTORY / PRE-EXISTING CONDITIONS:
- [ ] NO
- [ ] YES: (specify) _____

ARRIVAL VITAL SIGNS: (if available)
BLOOD PRESSURE: _____ PULSE: _____ RESPIRATORY RATE: _____
GLASGOW COMA SCALE: Eyes: ___ Verbal: ___ Motor: ___ Total: ___

MAJOR DIAGNOSES: (check all that apply)
- [ ] LACERATION: MINOR
- [ ] LACERATION: MAJOR
- [ ] TRAUMATIC AMPUTATION
- [ ] CONTUSION / BRUISE
- [ ] CRUSH INJURY
- [ ] RENAL FAILURE
- [ ] CHEST TRAUMA: MINOR
- [ ] CHEST TRAUMA: MAJOR
- [ ] WOUND INFECTION
- [ ] ABDOMINAL TRAUMA: MINOR
- [ ] ABDOMINAL TRAUMA: MAJOR
- [ ] BURN
- [ ] HEAD TRAUMA: MINOR
- [ ] HEAD TRAUMA: MAJOR
- [ ] SPINAL INJURY
- [ ] FRACTURE: UPPER EXTREMITY
- [ ] FRACTURE: LOWER EXTREMITY
- [ ] PELVIC FRACTURE
- [ ] OTHER: (specify) _____

PROCEDURES PERFORMED:
- [ ] WOUND CARE
- [ ] SUTURE
- [ ] SPLINT/CAST
- [ ] CHEST DRAIN
- [ ] REMOVE FOREIGN BODY
- [ ] LIMB SURGERY
- [ ] CHEST SURGERY
- [ ] ABD. SURGERY
- [ ] AMPUTATION
- [ ] ABCESS DRAINED
- [ ] OTHER: (specify) _____

OPERATION:
- [ ] YES
- [ ] NO
- [ ] UNKNOWN

REFERRAL TO OTHER FACILITY:
- [ ] YES
- [ ] NO
- [ ] UNKNOWN

PATIENT OUTCOME:
- [ ] TREATED AND RELEASED
- [ ] ADMITTED
- [ ] DEAD ON ARRIVAL
- [ ] TRANSFERRED
- [ ] LEFT AGAINST ADVICE
- [ ] DIED IN DEPARTMENT

DISABILITY ANTICIPATED:
- [ ] NO DISABILITY
- [ ] UNKNOWN
- [ ] DEATH: NOT APPLICABLE
- [ ] UNABLE TO WORK <1 MONTH
- [ ] UNABLE TO WORK <1 YEAR
- [ ] UNABLE TO WORK PERMANENTLY
- [ ] NEEDS CARE <1 MONTH
- [ ] NEEDS CARE <1 YEAR
- [ ] NEEDS CARE PERMENENTLY

OTHER DETAILS NOT COVERED ABOVE:

DATA FORM COMPLETED BY: _____

DATE COMPLETED: _____

Figure 30.3 (cont.)

to make difficult triage decisions. A firm, preplanned triage system can dramatically improve operational efficiency and healthcare utilization in these events.

Most medical systems in the United States have now adopted a uniform triage system, called the Model Uniform Code Criteria for Mass Casualty Incident Triage (Disaster medicine and public health preparedness 2011). This multilateral agreement is designed to maintain consistent triage protocols across jurisdictions, agencies, and organizations.

International organizations or national health ministries may have their own triage protocols, but knowing a standardized set of triage guidelines will help the public health practitioner design, implement, and assess any operational emergency health system. The Model Uniform Code Criteria is based on the SALT algorithm, which stands for Sorting, Assessing, performing Lifesaving therapies, and Transporting (Disaster medicine and public health preparedness 2008 and Lerner 2008. The SALT algorithm is shown in Figure 30.4. Global sorting involves a rapid categorization of victims by those who are laying still, those who can make purposeful movements, and those who are upright or walking. The assessment involves rapid individualized assessments for life-threatening injuries. Immediate lifesaving interventions are performed on those who may be saved, including control of major bleeding, breathing assistance, or decompressing chest wounds. Finally, transport to medical facilities is prioritized to those who will benefit most and delayed or withheld from those with either minor wounds or nonsurvivable injuries. It should be clear that not all lifesaving intervention will be possible in every setting. Furthermore, the criteria for transport will change from setting to setting. However, the fundamentals of the Model Uniform Code Criteria can be applied to any triage and health delivery system in the CHE setting.

Evacuation

The triage mechanisms established should inform the development of safe evacuation plans for those with serious but survivable injuries. Safe evacuation involves providing appropriate patient care as well as addressing logistical and security concerns of transit. An evacuation plan must be laid out at the

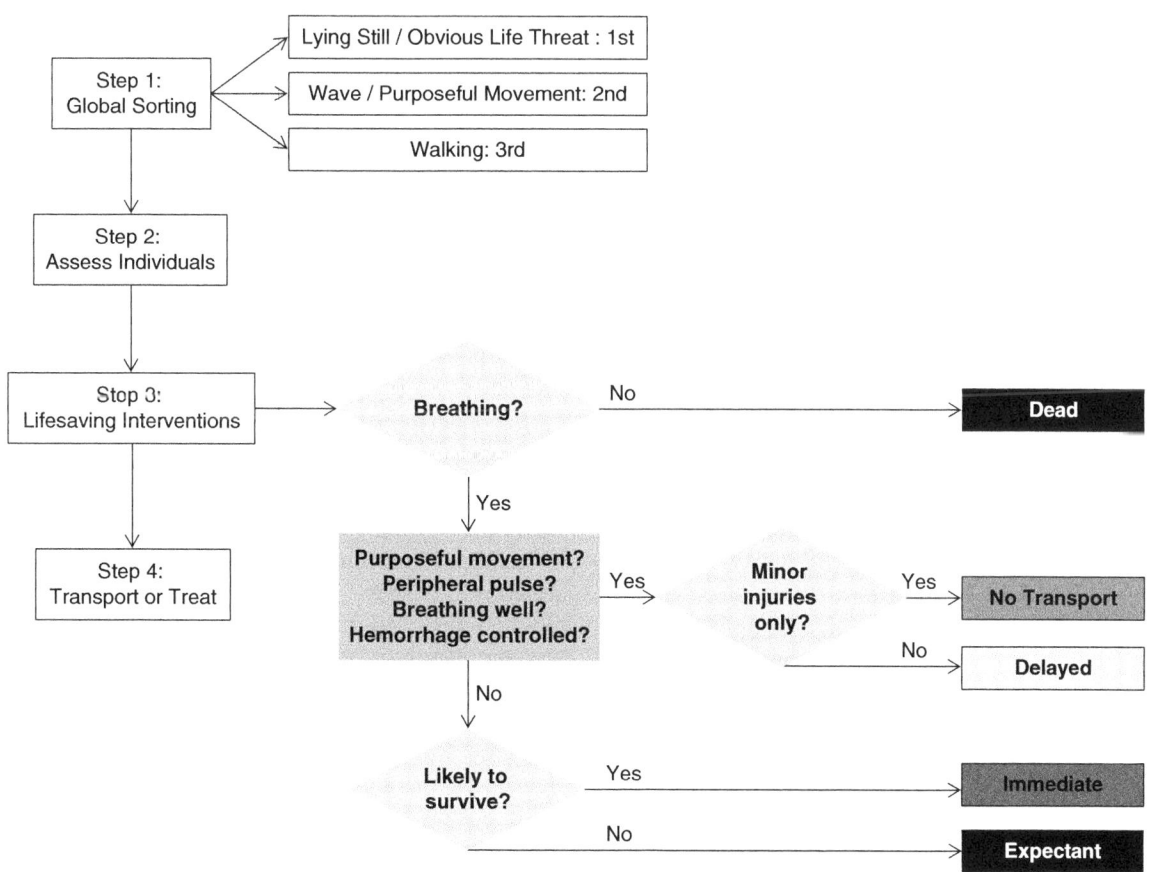

Figure 30.4 SALT Mass Casualty Triage Algorithm (Sort, Assess, Lifesaving actions, Transport) Disaster medicine and public health preparedness, 2008

earliest opportunity. Means of transportation and infrastructural capacity for patient transport must be assessed and identified. Whenever possible, advanced medical care facilities with surgical capabilities should be identified. The logistics of patient transport directly affect evacuation protocols, as roads may be rough, time of transport may be unpredictable, and security may shift rapidly. The evacuation plans must be made in coordination with involved medical facilities and be equipped with alternative plans, in the event of logistical challenges.

Wound Care and Tetanus Immunization

Emergency environments often lead to poor wound care. Complications of poor wound care can involve poor fracture healing, wound infections, tetanus, and contracted scarring. These avoidable wound complications can produce further mortality and long-term disability in an affected population. The role of the public health worker should be to attempt to minimize these complications by assuring a coordinated and effective medical mobilization, implementing a supplemental tetanus immunization program, and promoting healthy wound care practices through education and messaging. The first tenet of wound care is wound stabilization. Fractures should be appropriately splinted and immobilized. Open lacerations should be thoroughly cleaned (foreign debris and dead tissue removed) and wrapped in clean bandages, which should be changed daily. A tetanus immunization campaign should be initiated early in the emergency intervention, especially in environments where lacerations are expected in any significant number (Kouadio et al. 2012). Tetanus immunization should be provided to all wounded patients, regardless of the severity of their wounds. Measures should be in place to provide tetanus immunization to relief workers who will be active in debris fields and very likely to suffer lacerations in the course of recovery efforts. When making initial assessments of supplies needed, the public health worker should consider the immunization rates of the local population, the amount of foreign assistance personnel that will be arriving, and the expected number of wounds to ensure that the appropriate amount of tetanus vaccine is procured. Finally, wound care messages should be disseminated to both disaster victims, as well as emergency responders. Individuals in the emergency environment may ignore seemingly small injuries and fail to receive appropriate medical care. Encouraging and educating appropriate wound care and injury stabilization even outside the health delivery system can reduce the impact of these wounds upon recovery effort.

Coordination

Agencies providing trauma care and surgical capabilities must be in constant communication with each other. Capacity will change as teams move in and out, as specialty surgeons arrive on brief deployments, and as shipments arrive and infrastructure is rebuilt. The "4-W's" of who, where, when, and what are an important component of a functioning trauma system. A clear line of communication should be established between all agencies, and clearly delineated service provision should be available to all health cluster organizations. A referral system is a critical component of evolving triage, as the movement and evacuation of priority patients depends on service availability and transport capacity. Coordination of medical teams is further discussed under Emergency Medical Teams in Chapter 4.

Also, as the early recovery begins, expect services to expand in waves, with urban centers often receiving a restoration of services rapidly while outlying communities face significant delays. This is similarly true in refugee settings, where camps become the centers where services are provided, and the host community and those who arrive later often experience ongoing delays in services. Thus the need for reassessments will continue as the emergency response shifts and affected populations receive humanitarian assistance.

Long-Term Consequences

The long-term consequences of humanitarian emergencies bring additional considerations in the field of injury prevention. The building or rebuilding of public health systems must take new demographic, infrastructural, and geographic realities into consideration. As the postemergency phase gives way, the energy and money flowing through the international aid agencies and domestic departments of health will begin to focus elsewhere. Money for new programs will dissipate and personnel will be reassigned elsewhere. The public health aid worker in these postdisaster environments must understand that this phase should look past the systems most immediately affected by the emergency. There is opportunity to improve the public health system in the long-term, and energy should be applied to addressing long-standing causes of injury such as road traffic collisions, burns, and violence. Long-term determinants of health and social well-being such as physical disability, mental health, and social violence are intimately linked to traumatic injuries, and will be explored here.

Physical Disability and Rehabilitation

In the rush to provide services in the immediate aftermath of an emergency, the problems of chronic disability are frequently relegated to low priority. There has been much discussion regarding the gap in services between the immediate surgical care of Haiti's earthquake victims and the long-term disability that followed after thousands of lifesaving amputations were performed (Arie 2012). In the postdisaster setting, the issues of disability rise in prominence as one considers economic recovery, work force capacity, and the long-term health of disaster survivors (Hermansson et al. 1996). In a study conducted after a 2009 earthquake off the coast of Sumatra, Indonesia, researchers found consistently higher disability scores, chronic pain, and a lower quality of life among victims who had survived traumatic injuries, even when controlled for actual symptoms and chronic illness (Sudaryo et al. 2012). Even injuries that might be considered relatively minor in developed health systems can become debilitating in the resource poor context (Wu and Poenaru 2013). Proper burn care, provision of orthotic devices, and physical rehabilitative services can ameliorate much of the morbidity associated with post-traumatic disability. It is within the purview of the public health practitioner to advocate for the provision of these services and to examine the epidemiology and public impact of these issues in the postdisaster setting.

Mental Health

The long-term consequences of trauma on the mental health of an affected population cannot be overstated. Mental health is discussed in detail in Chapter 28, including an overview of the numerous psychosocial stressors that contribute to the strong link between complex humanitarian emergencies and poor mental health outcomes of a population. In addition, physical injuries also predispose victims to worse mental health outcomes and quality of life outcomes (Michaels et al. 2000). Whether unintentional or violent, the victims of traumatic injuries deal with long-term and sometimes severe mental health difficulties including post-traumatic stress disorder (PTSD), depression, and substance abuse. Traumatic brain injury, as discussed earlier, is also a risk factor for the development of mental health problems (Bryant et al. 2010). Refugee populations have been documented with elevated rates of depression, and those with a history of torture or physical abuse are at even further increased risk for mental health disorders and poor life outcomes (Hermansson et al. 2000, Buhmann 2014).

Studies examining Bhutanese refugees found elevated rates of mental illness whether the refugee populations had been permanently relocated to the United States or chronically interned in Nepal (Mills et al. 2008, Vonnahme et al. 2014). Child soldiers in particular have been identified to have particularly high rates of mental illness in the aftermath of their activities during the conflict (Kohrt et al. 2008). Suicide is also a concern in the wake of disaster and civil upheaval. Though not a universal phenomenon, increased suicide rates have been documented after natural disasters in certain cultures such as Japan and Taiwan (Kolves et al. 2013). Furthermore, PTSD and depression have been strongly linked to suicides in conflict survivors from Bhutan and Kosovo (MMWR 2013, Wang et al. 2012).

Societal Violence

There is firm evidence to show that populations in conflict regions are at increased risk of violent injuries. There is also some evidence that violent injuries increase in the immediate aftermath of natural disasters. There is less clarity on whether these types of crises directly contribute to chronic rates of violent crime. However, there is no doubt that exposure to violence can affect long-term outcomes. The victims of child abuse are at increased risk of becoming perpetrators of physical child abuse (Thornberry and Henry 2013). The victims of violent injuries are at risk of violent reinjury even in the absence of war, conflict, or natural disasters (Cunningham et al. 2014). In South Kivu, Democratic Republic of the Congo, after a decade of severe disruption to civil society, rates of sexual violence in the civilian population nearly doubled from documented pre–civil war rates (Bartels et al. 2013). Monitoring rates of violence and victimization are crucial to understanding longitudinal impacts of CHE's long after the immediate risk of infectious outbreaks and active military conflict have ended.

Conclusion

In the aftermath of a conflict or disaster, the public health response is critical. In the immediate postdisaster context, injuries and wounds are often viewed as a medical problem, and are therefore overlooked by the public health response. However, injuries have identifiable epidemiologic patterns that can be anticipated and responded to effectively. Failing to respond to injury patterns can result in the misallocation of vital health resources and can compound the disaster by exposing both victims and aid workers to further sources of injury. Therefore, injury prevention and control should be prioritized by the humanitarian public health response in the same manner as other health concerns such as measles, cholera, and malnutrition.

Rapid assessments of injury patterns can inform the primary and secondary healthcare needs in the immediate aftermath. Appropriate training of local personnel in wound care, field triage, and safe evacuation procedures can help decrease morbidity from injuries and minimize delays in treatment to those who most need care. Attention to environmental hazards can minimize postdisaster complications such as wound infections, road traffic injuries, poisonings, falls, and burns. Tetanus immunization is an important measure to protect those with minor wounds from more serious, life-threatening infections. Injury prevention and control for recovery workers is also critical.

The anticipated increase in traumatic injuries in the postdisaster or conflict setting can be ameliorated by early recognition and adoption of an aggressive public health platform that seeks to engage stakeholders and survivors in primary prevention efforts. Land mine awareness training, road traffic safety education, drowning prevention, safe handling of fire equipment, electrocution prevention, poison prevention, and community psychological assistance, should all be considered in the same context as the provision of clean water, waste disposal, vector control, and immunization campaigns in humanitarian emergencies.

References

Alderman, K., Turner, L. R., Tong, S. (2012). Floods and human health: a systematic review. *Environment International*, **47**, 37–47.

Arie, S. (2012). Work of 125 aid agencies failed to create lasting rehabilitation services in Haiti, study shows. *BMJ (Clinical research ed.)*, **344**, e2952.

Bailey, K. (2009). An evaluation of the impact of Hurricane Katrina on crime in New Orleans, Louisiana: Applied Research Projects, Texas State University-San Marcos. Doctoral Thesis.

Bartels, S. A., Scott, J. A., Leaning, J., et al. (2011). Sexual violence trends between 2004 and 2008 in South Kivu, Democratic Republic of Congo. *Prehospital and disaster medicine*, **26**(6), 408–413.

Bartels, S. A. and VanRooyen, M. J. (2012). Medical complications associated with earthquakes. *Lancet*, **379** (9817), 748–757.

Bhattacharjee, A. and Lossio, R. (2011). Evaluation of OCHA response to the Haiti earthquake: final report: United Nations Office for the Coordination of Humanitarian Affairs. Available at: www.unocha.org/what-we-do/policy/thematic-areas/evaluations-of-humanitarian-response/reports.

Bilukha, O. O., Brennan, M., and Anderson, M. (2008). The lasting legacy of war: Epidemiology of injuries from landmines and unexploded ordnance in Afghanistan, 2002–2006. *Prehospital and Disaster Medicine*, **23**(06), 493–499.

Biswas, A., Rahman, A., Mashreky, S., Rahman, F., and Dalal, K. (2010). Unintentional injuries and parental violence against children during flood: A study in rural Bangladesh. *Rural and Remote Health*, **10**(1), 1199.

Brennan, R. J. and Nandy, R. (2001). Complex Humanitarian Emergencies: A Major Global Health Challenge. *Emergency Medicine*. **13**(2), 147–156.

Brunkard, J., Namulanda, G., and Ratard, R. (2008). Hurricane Katrina deaths, Louisiana, 2005. *Disaster Medicine and Public Health Preparedness*, **2**(4), 215–223.

Bryant, R. A., O'Donnell, M. L., Creamer, M., McFarlane, A. C., Clark, C. R., and Silove, D. (2010). The psychiatric sequelae of traumatic injury. *The American Journal of Psychiatry*, **167**(3), 312–320.

Buhmann, C. B. (2014). Traumatized refugees: Morbidity, treatment and predictors of outcome. *Danish Medical Journal*, **61**(8), B4871.

Champion, H. R., Holcomb, J. B., and Young, L. A. (2009). Injuries from explosions: physics, biophysics, pathology, and required research focus. *The Journal of Trauma*, **66**(5), 1468–1477.

Chiu, C. H., Schnall, A. H., Mertzlufft, C. E., et al. (2013). Mortality from a tornado outbreak, Alabama, April 27, 2011. *American Journal of Public Health*, **103**(8), e52–58.

Cunningham, R. M., Carter, P. M., Ranney, M., et al. (2014). Violent reinjury and mortality among youth seeking emergency department care for assault-related injury:

A 2-year prospective cohort study. *JAMA Pediatrics*, **169**(1), 63–70.

Doocy, S., Jacquet, G., Cherewick, M., and Kirsch, T. D. (2013). The injury burden of the 2010 Haiti earthquake: a stratified cluster survey. *Injury*, **44**(6), 842–847.

Doocy, S., Robinson, C., Moodie, C., and Burnham, G. (2009). Tsunami-related injury in Aceh Province, Indonesia. *Global public health*, 4(2), 205–214.

EM-DAT: The OFDA/CRED International Disaster Database. Available at: www.emdat.be (Accessed January 2015).

Evelyn-Depoortere, V. B. (2006). Rapid health assessment of refugee or displaced populations, 3rd edition. Paris: Medécins Sans Frontières. Available at: refbooks.msf.org/msf_docs/en/rapid_health/rapid_health_en.pdf.

Fackler, M. L. (1996). Gunshot wound review. *Annals of Emergency Medicine*, **28**(2), 194–203.

Faul, M., Weller, N. F., and Jones, J. A. (2011). Injuries after Hurricane Katrina among Gulf Coast Evacuees sheltered in Houston, Texas. *Journal of Emergency Nursing: The Official Publication of the Emergency Department Nurses Association*, 37(5), 460–468.

Foulds, S. A., Brewer, P. A., Macklinm M. G., Haresignm W., Betson, R. E., and Rassner, S. M. (2014). Flood-related contamination in catchments affected by historical metal mining: an unexpected and emerging hazard of climate change. *The Science of the Total Environment*, **476**–477, 165–180.

Genthon, A. and Wilcox, S. R. (2014). Crush syndrome: A case report and review of the literature. *The Journal of Emergency Medicine*, **46**(2), 313–319.

Goldman, A., Eggen, B., Golding, B., and Murray, V. (2014). The health impacts of windstorms: a systematic literature review. *Public Health*, **128**(1), 3–28.

Guha-Sapir, D. and van Panhuis, W. G. (2009). Health impact of the 2004 Andaman Nicobar earthquake and tsunami in Indonesia. *Prehospital and Disaster Medicine*, 24 (6), 493–499.

Hanquet, G., ed. (1997). Refugee Health: An Approach to Emergency Situations. Paris: Medécins Sans Frontières.

Helweg-Larsen, K., Abdel-Jabbar, Al-Qadi, A. H., Al-Jabriri, J., and Bronnum-Hansen, H. (2004). Systematic medical data collection of intentional injuries during armed conflicts: a pilot study conducted in West Bank, Palestine. *Scandinavian Journal of Public Health*, **32**(1), 17–23.

Hermansson, A. C., Thyberg, M., and Timpka, T. (1996). War-wounded refugees: The types of injury and influence of disability on well-being and social integration. *Medicine, conflict, and survival*, **12**(4), 284–302.

Hermansson, A. C., Timpka, T., and Thyberg, M. T. (2002). The mental health of war-wounded refugees: An 8-year follow-up. *The Journal of Nervous and Mental Disease*, **190** (6), 374–380.

Hicks, M. H., Dardagan, H., Guerrero-Serdan, G., Bagnall, P. M., Sloboda, J. A., and Spagat, M. (2011). Violent deaths of Iraqi civilians, 2003–2008: Analysis by perpetrator, weapon, time, and location. *PLoS medicine*, 8 (2), e1000415.

Hinsley, D. E., Rosell, P. A., Rowlands T. K., and Clasper J. C. (2005). Penetrating missile injuries during asymmetric warfare in the 2003 Gulf conflict. *The British Journal of Surgery*, **92**(5), 637–642.

Hoge, C. W., McGurk, D., Thomas, J. L., Cox, A. L., Engel, C. C., and Castro, C. A. (2008). Mild traumatic brain injury in U.S. Soldiers returning from Iraq. *The New England Journal of Medicine*, **358**(5), 453–463.

Holder, Y. M., Peden, E., Krug, J., Lund, G., and Gurura-Kobusingye, O., eds. (2001). *Injury Surveillance Guidelines*. Geneva: World Health Organization.

Horan, J. M. and Mallonee, S. (2003). Injury surveillance. *Epidemiologic Reviews*, **25**, 24–42.

Hossain, M., Zimmerman, C., Kis, S. L., et al. (2014). Men's and women's experiences of violence and traumatic events in rural Cote d'Ivoire before, during and after a period of armed conflict. *BMJ*, **4**(2), e003644.

Inoue, Y., Fujino, Y., Onodera, M., et al. (2012). Tsunami lung. *Journal of Anesthesia*, **26**(2), 246–249.

Institute of Medicine. (2014). Gulf War and Health, Volume 9: Long-Term Effects of Blast Exposures: The National Academies Press; Institute of Medicine Report. Available at: www.iom.edu/Reports.aspx.

Kohrt, B. A., Jordans, M. J., and Tol, W. A., et al. (2008). Comparison of mental health between former child soldiers and children never conscripted by armed groups in Nepal. *JAMA*, **300**(6), 691–702.

Kolves, K., Kolves, K. E., De Leo, D. (2013). Natural disasters and suicidal behaviors: a systematic literature review. *Journal of Affective Disorders*, **146**(1), 1–14.

Knowlton, L. M., Gosney, J. E., and Chackungal, S., et al. (2011). Consensus statements regarding the multidisciplinary care of limb amputation patients in disasters or humanitarian emergencies: report of the 2011 Humanitarian Action Summit Surgical Working Group on amputations following disasters or conflict. *Prehospital and Disaster Medicine*, **26**(6), 438–448.

Kouadio, I. K., Aljunid, S., Kamigaki, T., Hammad, K., and Oshitani, H. (2012). Infectious diseases following natural disasters: prevention and control measures. *Expert review of anti-infective therapy*, **10**(1), 95–104.

Leibovici, D., Gofrit, O. N., Stein, M., et al. (1996). Blast injuries: Bus versus open-air bombings—a comparative study of injuries in survivors of open-air versus confined-space explosions. *The Journal of Trauma*, **41**(6), 1030–1035.

Lerner, E. B., Schwartz, R. B., Coule, P. L., et al. (2008). Mass casualty triage: an evaluation of the data and development of a proposed national guideline. *Disaster Med Public Health Prep.* **2** Suppl 1:S25–S34.

Lim, J. H., Yoon, D., Jung, G., Joo Kim, W., Lee. H. C. (2005). Medical needs of tsunami disaster refugee camps. *Family Medicine,* **37**(6), 422–428.

Lu-Ping, Z., Rodriguez-Llanes, J., Qi, W., et al. (2012). Multiple injuries after earthquakes: a retrospective analysis on 1,871 injured patients from the 2008 Wenchuan earthquake. *Critical Care,* **16**(3), R87.

Marsh, M., Purdin, S., and Navani, S. (2006). Addressing sexual violence in humanitarian emergencies. *Global Public Health,* **1**(2), 133–146.

Meddings, D. R. (1997). Weapons injuries during and after periods of conflict: Retrospective analysis. *BMJ,* **315**(7120), 1417–1420.

Michaels, A. J., Michaels, C. E., Smith, J. S., Moon, C. H., Peterson, C., and Long, W. B. (2000). Outcome from injury: General health, work status, and satisfaction 12 months after trauma. *Journal of Trauma and Acute Care Surgery,* **48**(5), 841–850.

Mills, E., Singh, S., Roach, B., and Chong, S. (2008). Prevalence of mental disorders and torture among Bhutanese refugees in Nepal: a systemic review and its policy implications. *Medicine, Conflict, and Survival,* **24**(1), 5–15.

Miskin, I. N., Nir-Paz, R., Block, C., et al. (2010). Antimicrobial therapy for wound infections after catastrophic earthquakes. *The New England Journal of Medicine,* **363**(26), 2571–2573.

Mitka, M. (2014). IOM addresses ongoing effects of blast injury on soldiers. *JAMA,* **311**(11), 1098–1099.

MMWR. (2005). Infectious disease and dermatologic conditions in evacuees and rescue workers after Hurricane Katrina–multiple states, August-September, 2005. *Morbidity and Mortality Weekly Report,* **54**(38), 961–964.

MMWR. (2013). Suicide and suicidal ideation among Bhutanese refugees–United States, 2009–2012. *Morbidity and mortality weekly report,* **62**(26), 533–536.

Model uniform core criteria for mass casualty triage. (2011). *Disaster medicine and public health preparedness,* **5**(2), 125–128.

National Incident Management System (NIMS). (2015). Federal Emergency Management Agency website. Available at: https://www.fema.gov/national-incident-management-system (Accessed: January 2015).

NDRRMC UPDATE: Updates re the Effects of Typhoon "YOLANDA" (HAIYAN). Camp Aguinaldo, Quezon city, Philippines: National Disaster Risk Reduction and Management Council; April 17, 2014. Available at: www.ndrrmc.gov.ph.

OCHA. (1999). Orientation handbook on complex emergencies. Geneva, Switzerland. Relief Web website.

Available at: reliefweb.int/report/world/ocha-orientation-handbook-complex-emergencies.

Oxfam Briefing Note. (2005). The tsunami's impact on women. Oxfam International; March 2005. Available at: www.oxfam.org/sites/www.oxfam.org/files/women.pdf.

Rezaeian, M. (2013). The association between natural disasters and violence: A systematic review of the literature and a call for more epidemiological studies. *Journal of Research in Medical Sciences: The Official Journal of Isfahan University of Medical Sciences,* **18**(12), 1103–1107.

Roberts, B., Felix-Ocaka, K., Browne, J., Oyok, T., and Sondorp, E. (2009). Factors associated with the health status of internally displaced persons in northern Uganda. *Journal of Epidemiology and Community Health,* **63**(3), 227–232.

Roberts, L., Belyakdoumi, F., et al. (2001). Mortality in eastern Democratic Republic of Congo: Results from eleven mortality surveys, 2001. *International Committee for the Red Cross.*

Rotheray, K. R., Aitken, P., Goggins, W. B., Rainer, T. H., Graham, C. A. (2012). Epidemiology of injuries due to tropical cyclones in Hong Kong: A retrospective observational study. *Injury,* **43**(12), 2055–2059.

Roy, S. (2010). The impact of natural disasters on crime. College of Business and Economics: Department of Economics and Finance, University of Canterbury. Doctoral Thesis; 2010.

SALT mass casualty triage: concept endorsed by the American College of Emergency Physicians, American College of Surgeons Committee on Trauma, American Trauma Society, National Association of EMS Physicians, National Disaster Life Support Education Consortium, and State and Territorial Injury Prevention Directors Association. (2008). *Disaster medicine and public health preparedness,* **2**(4), 245–246.

Shultz, J. M., Russell, J., and Espinel, Z. (2005). Epidemiology of tropical cyclones: the dynamics of disaster, disease, and development. *Epidemiologic Reviews,* **27**, 21–35.

The Sphere Project. (2011). Humanitarian Charter and Minimum Standards in Humanitarian Response. 3rd edition. Available at: www.sphereproject.org/handbook.

Sudaryo, M. K., Besral-Endarti, A. T., et al. (2012). Injury, disability and quality of life after the 2009 earthquake in Padang, Indonesia: a prospective cohort study of adult survivors. *Global Health Action,* 5, 1–11.

Sugerman, D. E., Hyder, A. A., and Nasir, K. (2005). Child and young adult injuries among long-term Afghan refugees. *International Journal of Injury Control and Safety Promotion,* **12**(3), 177–182.

Sugimoto, J. D., Labrique, A. B., Ahmad, S., et al. (2011). Epidemiology of tornado destruction in rural northern Bangladesh: Risk factors for death and injury. *Disasters,* **35**(2), 329–345.

Sullivent, E. E., West, C. A., Noe, R. S., Thomas, K. E., Wallace, L. J., and Leeb, R. T. (2006). Nonfatal injuries following Hurricane Katrina–New Orleans, Louisiana, 2005. *Journal of Safety Research*, **37**(2), 213–217.

Tam, V. and Nayak, S. (2012). Isolation of Leclercia adecarboxylata from a wound infection after exposure to hurricane-related floodwater. *BMJ Case Reports*, 2012.

Thornberry, T. P. and Henry, K. L. (2013). Intergenerational continuity in maltreatment. *Journal of Abnormal Child Psychology*, **41**(4), 555–569.

UNHCR. (2011). Driven by desperation: Transactional sex as a survival strategy in Port-au-Prince IDP Camps: United Nations High Commissioner for Refugees.

Uscher-Pines, L., Vernick, J. S., Curriero, F., Lieberman, R., and Burke, T. A. (2009). Disaster-related injuries in the period of recovery: the effect of prolonged displacement on risk of injury in older adults. *The Journal of Trauma*, **67**(4), 834–840.

Vonnahme, L. A., Lankau, E. W., Ao, T., Shetty, S., and Cardozo, B. L. (2014). Factors Associated with Symptoms of Depression Among Bhutanese Refugees in the United States. *Journal of Immigrant and Minority Health / Center for Minority Public Health*.

Vu, A., Adam, A., Wirtz, A., et al. (2014). The Prevalence of Sexual Violence among Female Refugees in Complex Humanitarian Emergencies: A Systematic Review and Meta-analysis. *PLoS Currents*, **6**.

Wang, S. J., Rushiti, F., Sejdiu, X., et al. (2012). Survivors of war in northern Kosovo (III): The role of anger and hatred in pain and PTSD and their interactive effects on career outcome, quality of sleep and suicide ideation. *Conflict and Health*, 6(1), 4.

Wightman, J. M. and Gladish, S. L. (2001). Explosions and blast injuries. *Annals of Emergency Medicine*, **37**(6), 664–678.

World Health Organization. (1999). Rapid health assessment protocols for emergencies. Geneva: World Health Organization. Available at: www.wpro.who.int/vietnam/publications/rapid_health_assessment_protocols.pdf.

World Health Organization. (2007). Mass casualty management systems: strategies and guidelines for building health sector capacity. Geneva: World Health Organization; 2007. Available at: www.who.int/hac/techguidance/tools/mcm_guidelines_en.pdf.

World Health Organization. (2012). Outbreak surveillance and response in humanitarian emergencies. Geneva: World Health Organization. Available at: www.who.int/diseasecontrol_emergencies/publications/who_hse_epr_dce_2012.1/en/.

Wu, V. K. and Poenaru, D. (2013). Burden of surgically correctable disabilities among children in the Dadaab Refugee Camp. *World journal of surgery*, **37**(7), 1536–1543.

Xie, J., Du, L., Xia, T., Wang, M., Diao, X., and Li, Y. (2008). Analysis of 1856 inpatients and 33 deaths in the West China Hospital of Sichuan University from the Wenchuan earthquake. *Journal of Evidence Based Medicine*, **1**, 20–26.

Chapter 31

Noncommunicable Diseases

Bayard Roberts, Holly Williams, and Sonia Angell

Introduction

Today, noncommunicable diseases (NCDs) are responsible for more deaths than any other diseases. About two-thirds of all deaths are due to NCDs, largely cardiovascular disease, cancer, diabetes, and chronic lung disease (responsible for 30%, 15%, 7%, and 2% of all deaths respectively) (Lozano et al. 2012). The majority of these deaths occur in low- and middle-income countries. The epidemiologic transition to NCDs from maternal, nutritional, and infectious disease as the leading cause of death is complete in all regions of the world except in sub-Saharan Africa, where NCDs are expected by 2030 to surpass all other causes (Lozano et al. 2012).

Converging global conditions are responsible for changing the global burden of disease. As the benefits of investments in health and related technologies accrue worldwide, the number of infectious, maternal, and child deaths is decreasing and life expectancy is increasing (Jamison et al. 2013). This trend is concurrent with globalization that has resulted in rapid urbanization and associated lifestyles that increase exposure to NCD risk factors. As the population ages in these evolving environments, so does its likelihood for risk accumulation. For example, travel is increasingly by motorized vehicle and work life is more sedentary, contributing to decreased physical activity. The so-called "nutrition transition" to processed foods throughout the world is resulting in diets often high in saturated and trans fat, sodium, and sugar, and low in fresh fruits, vegetables, and whole grains. Low- and middle-income countries, in particular, are increasingly targeted by industry for the marketing of alcohol, tobacco, and processed foods, resulting in greater numbers of daily smokers, increased exposure to secondhand smoke, harmful use of alcohol, and consumption of unhealthy foods.

Hypertension

The global impact of these trends is striking. For example, elevated blood pressure, or hypertension, a leading cause of stroke and heart attack, is now the leading risk for death worldwide. Over nine million people died due to this condition in 2012 (Lim et al. 2012). A recent study of 1.25 million people demonstrated that having this condition at 30 years of age confers a lifetime risk for a cardiovascular event of 63.3 percent compared with 46.1 percent in those without the condition (Rapsomaniki et al. 2014). This predicts substantial impact globally, as over one-third of adults worldwide have this condition. Effective treatment varies considerably by country. In the United States, only a little over half of all people with the condition have it under control, while in lower income countries like Albania and Armenia, control has been reported as low as 4.4 percent and 8.6 percent respectively (Ikeda et al. 2014). While some countries are doing better, the need for improvement is shared.

Tobacco Use

Tobacco use is the second leading cause of death globally, responsible for over 6 million deaths per year (Lim et al. 2012). An estimated 31 percent of adults (defined as over the age of 15) smoke daily (Ng et al. 2014). Use varies, including by country and by sex. Extremes in prevalence of daily smoking are as low as 5 percent in adult women in some African countries, and as high as 55 percent of adult men in Timor-Leste and Indonesia and 60 percent of men in Russia (Ng et al. 2014, Giovino et al. 2012). While a study assessing trends since 1980 demonstrated decreasing use, the rate of decline from 2006 to 2012 slowed when compared to the prior decade (Ng et al. 2014). Furthermore, as the world's population has expanded the total number of daily smokers has increased, from 721 million in 1980 to 967 million in 2012, highlighting the continued expansion of marketing and sales of tobacco products. Data on smokeless tobacco use is limited, but in countries like India and Bangladesh at least one quarter of adults use these products (Giovino et al. 2012).

Diabetes

Diabetes is also an important contributor to global NCD related deaths with 3.4 million deaths attributed to diabetes in 2010 (Lim et al. 2012). Globally, this is expected to increase significantly as the number of people with the diabetes is expected to grow from 382 million now to 592 million in 2035 (IDF 2013). As an underlying condition, diabetes increases the risk of micro- and macrovascular disease, including but not limited to cardiovascular, renal, and retinal disease. Diabetes is associated with an increased risk for infections. The risk for tuberculosis is two to three times higher in those with diabetes. Conversely, some infections, such as hepatitis C, also appear to increase the risk for diabetes. Diabetes also complicates pregnancy. In 2013, over 21 million live births were affected by diabetes during pregnancy and, as the epidemic grows, so will the rates of maternal diabetes (IDF 2013). An increased risk of certain cancers is associated with diabetes, although the specific biologic mechanisms remain the subject of investigation (Shi and Hu 2014).

Global Response

In 2011, the United Nations responded to this growing crisis, hosting a High-Level Meeting on NCDs. This resulted in the 2013 World Health Assembly endorsing a set of global voluntary targets to be achieved by 2025 that focus national efforts on reducing NCD risk, morbidity, and mortality; improving related health systems elements; and an NCD Action Plan aimed at realizing these targets (WHO 2013). These documents assumed that the NCD response will occur largely under relatively stable national conditions, including referring to the broad scale and sustainable implementation of programming and policies that support healthy lifestyles and facilitate access to effective treatment and control measures. Amongst the recommendations were policy and environmental change actions, such as those that change the physical and food environment, making regular activity an increased part of daily living and access to healthful foods more common. There are recommendations to decrease tobacco smoking by banning its use in public places and reducing the harmful use of alcohol by decreasing points of access.

Such measures will have less relevance, however, when a population is forced to migrate out of the place of implementation because of conflict or when enforcement wanes due to government instability from political and social unrest. Similarly, recommended health system improvements in the diagnosis, treatment, and control of NCD risk factors, such as hypertension and diabetes, will have almost no impact when the population no longer has access to the infrastructure that regularly delivers care and provides access to vital medications. The NCDs and risk factors that are common in a population in a stable setting will also be common in an unstable setting such as a humanitarian emergency. The existing framework to respond that is anchored in stable environments may no longer provide support when stability is lost.

Continuity of Care

Planning for continuity of care for NCDs is a major challenge in Humanitarian emergencies (Arrieta et al. 2008). Ideally, predisaster planning would include the following:

- Understanding the epidemiological profile of the projected affected area
- Assessing the local health infrastructure and the ability to provide healthcare including the provision of medications
- Preidentification of vulnerable populations and special medical needs that require continuous care
- Stockpiling adequate medications and supplies

While the burden from NCDs is now better acknowledged globally, there remains a paucity of research examining the impact of NCDs in the context of humanitarian emergencies. Prior to hurricane Katrina in 2005, priority was given to preventing the spread of infectious diseases, treating injuries, and managing environmental concerns during humanitarian emergencies (Demaio et al. 2013, Evans 2010, Rottman 2008, Arrieta et al. 2008, Chan and Sondorp 2007). In addition to a lack of published literature, few operational emergency guidelines and policies exist for NCDs in humanitarian emergencies and disasters, including in published global minimum standards for humanitarian responses such as the Sphere Guidelines (Demaio et al., 2013).

Lessons learned from previous disasters have identified gaps in preparedness and response in high-income countries. Examples include lack of patient education and preparation in relation to healthcare needs during disasters (for example, patients in postdisaster settings could not accurately recount the medications they were taking), failure to recognize a need for shelters in which medical needs could be addressed, and a lack of backup medical records (Arrieta et al. 2008). Postdisaster, it was found that having multiple means by which one could contact patients was critical to ensure continuity of care (Arrieta et al. 2008). In disaster planning for NCDs, thought should be given to how the type of disaster may affect NCDs differentially (Rottman 2008). For example, large fires, earthquake-induced structural collapses, or volcanic eruptions may trigger or exacerbate pulmonary disorders due to the particulate matter in the air, while conflicts pose a greater threat for access to NCD services and continuity of care.

Types and examples of NCDs commonly seen in humanitarian emergencies include diabetes, cardiovascular disorders (hypertension), respiratory illnesses (chronic obstructive pulmonary disease and asthma), and mental health conditions. An examination of the impact of disasters between 1995 and 2005 on long-term health issues and NCDs noted that exacerbations of NCDs following disasters were not random. Rather, they followed a predictable pattern with worsening of underlying respiratory and cardiovascular disease and instability in preexisting diabetes patients (Evans 2010). Issues such as disruptions in access medications, altered activity/rest cycles, biological stress responses, and changes to dietary intake can negatively affect NCDs and cause additional morbidity and negative health outcomes. Some NCDs necessitate regular follow-up with healthcare providers and this is often disrupted during humanitarian emergencies. The stress of such situations may also cause individuals who could normally cope with the daily demands of their illnesses to deteriorate with more acute morbidity and, thus, increased dependency on external sources of healthcare (Demaio et al. 2013).

In order to plan adequately for management of NCDs during humanitarian emergencies, it is important to understand that the demographics of populations affected by humanitarian emergencies have changed over time, with increasingly older populations more likely to have NCDs (Leaning et al. 2011, Spiegel et al. 2010). In addition, humanitarian emergencies have become more protracted and thus, health needs are extending beyond basic primary care traditionally provided by humanitarian response agencies. A growing proportion of refugees and internally displaced persons (IDPs) now arise from middle-income countries, such as Iraq and Syria, with longer life expectancies, compared with lower-income countries. Furthermore, approximately half of displaced persons now live in urban areas, rather than traditional refugee camps or settlements (Spiegel et al. 2010). Urban refugees and IDPs pose challenges for humanitarian response agencies. In many settings, these agencies struggle to access urban refugees and IDPs and monitor their health needs. Health information system for urban refugees and IDPs are often inadequate or not functioning at all (Leaning et al. 2011).

The Balkans conflict in the 1990s was perhaps the first recognition by the humanitarian response community that health issues in conflict settings were shifting and attention needed to be given to a new epidemiological profile manifested by chronic disease and psychosocial trauma (Waldman and Martone 1999). The current crisis in Syrian mirrors the profile of refugees presenting with NCDs, notably, diabetes, hypertension, cardiovascular disease, and chronic obstructive pulmonary disease. This is also reflected in findings from other humanitarian emergencies (Amara and Aljunid 2014).

Preparedness and Response

In terms of preparedness and response, issues in higher-income countries may not adequately capture the reality on the ground for less-developed, low- and middle-income countries. Many of these low- and middle-income countries are in the nascent phases of emergency preparedness, mitigation, prevention, planning, response, and recovery. Many are struggling just to provide adequate health services to national populations, without the added burden of a humanitarian emergency within their borders or in a neighboring country.

Many of the common challenges in responding to humanitarian emergencies carry over to NCDs. This includes the chaotic and fluid environment, often with little information initially about the size of the affected population or their epidemiological profile. Identifying and counting the population in need and planning adequate healthcare services is easier if the displaced population is located in a camp or settlement area. If, however, the displaced population relocates to urban areas, reaching them with healthcare services is a much larger challenge. In these situations, fear related to possible deportation, user-fees, indirect health costs (such as transportation), lack of legal status, and cultural and ethnic differences may inhibit the displaced population from seeking medical care (Spiegel et al. 2010).

Displacement during a humanitarian emergency may occur very quickly and, often, healthcare personnel flee early in the emergency. This may mean leaving without documentation of their credentials. Once resettled, this may limit their ability to work as a healthcare professional, even in situations where healthcare capacity is stretched from a lack of adequate personnel. For those that remain, they may become exhausted, emotionally stressed, and grieving from experiencing the crisis firsthand. This is especially true in a conflict setting.

Affected populations are often mobile, affected by changing security situations and lack of resources in certain and shifting environmental threats. Establishing healthcare facilities where maintenance therapy can be offered is difficult if the population is mobile or difficult to access. Unlike high-income countries in which medical records are systematized, many low- and middle-income countries have inadequate medical records. Patients may have no medical information with them or perhaps a small handwritten card from a health dispensary containing medical information. This information is often inadequate or incomplete. This lack of adequate medical and pharmaceutical information is especially problematic for the continued care of NCDs.

Nutrition

It is a challenge to meet the nutritional needs of patients with NCDs during humanitarian emergencies. Displaced populations are often given food assistance or rations that are standardized to meet basic protein, energy, and fat requirements and micronutrient and mineral composition for survival aimed at providing 2,100 kcal/person/day (Sphere Project 2011). Trying to address special dietary needs resulting from NCDs (such as a low-salt or diabetic diet) is not realistic, particularly in the early stages of a humanitarian emergency. Nutrition is discussed in detail in Chapter 12.

Medications, Supplies, and Equipment

The types of healthcare, including medications, available during a humanitarian emergency will reflect the capacity of the responding agencies, with variations between what international nongovernmental organizations (NGO) provide compared with in-country NGOs. Traditionally, medications available to address NCDs are minimal, at best. For example, during the 1990s Balkans conflict there were prepackaged medical kits utilized, but they did not include antihypertensive drugs or insulin despite a high incidence of NCDs in the population.

The Inter-Agency Emergency Health Kit (IEHK) is designed as a reliable, standardized, quickly available, and affordable mechanism to obtain essential medications, supplies, and equipment that are urgently needed to address medical needs in disaster settings (WHO 2011). However, to date, drugs and supplies needed to treat NCDs in humanitarian emergencies remain minimal in the IEHK. For example, while the IEHK includes nine antibiotics, three cardiovascular drugs, two diuretics, and two medications that work on the respiratory tract, insulin, oral agents and glucose testing supplies are not routinely provided.

The changing demographic of affected populations in humanitarian emergencies requires a response that includes accurate estimates of the displaced population, providing healthcare services that may include the public sector, disaggregating surveillance data by nationality in order to improve humanitarian planning, strengthening referral systems, reducing financial costs of care for urban-based refugees, and developing and financing systems of care to address the care issues associated with NCDs (Doocy et al. 2013, Spiegel et al. 2010). It is essential in planning management of NCDs in any humanitarian emergency for continuation of care and transition from emergency to longer-term sustainable care for the affected populations.

Understanding the shifting demographic of their populations of concern, the United Nations High Commissioner for Refugees (UNHCR) adapted policies during the past decade to better meet healthcare needs resulting from NCDs. In 2008, UNHCR finalized referral guidelines to address referrals to specialty care (UNHCR 2008). In 2009, they developed an Urban Refugee Policy in which they outlined strategies to address healthcare for urban refugees, including specialized care (UNHCR 2009). In their updated

Global Strategy for Public Health 2014–2018, one of six strategic objectives, to "facilitate access to integrated prevention and control of non-communicable diseases, including mental health services," explicitly addresses NCDs (UNHCR 2014a).

Surveillance and Monitoring

Reliable surveillance and monitoring data is essential in tackling NCDs but remains scarce in many countries globally and are even scarcer during humanitarian emergencies due to factors including insecurity, damaged health systems, limited resources, and large population movement (WHO 2010a). In addition, guidance on NCD surveillance and monitoring during humanitarian emergencies is limited (Demaio et al. 2013). For example, the specific guidance on NCD surveillance and monitoring in the Sphere standards is essentially limited to identifying individuals with NCDs who were receiving treatment before the emergency and ensuring that they continue to do so to avoid sudden discontinuation of treatment, ensuring that people with acute complications and exacerbations of NCDs that pose a threat to their life and individuals in pain receive treatment, and sharing data on NCD prevalence (Sphere Project 2011). The WHO Health Cluster Guide is also limited in providing guidance on NCD surveillance and monitoring (WHO 2009). In addition, individual agencies do not yet appear to have published guidelines on NCD surveillance and monitoring, although agencies such as Médecins Sans Frontières (MSF) are currently developing new guidelines for managing NCDs, including monitoring and surveillance components.

In the absence of detailed surveillance and monitoring guidelines for NCDs in humanitarian crises, core elements of recommended programs for national NCDs surveillance in more stable, but resource poor settings, such as the WHO STEPwise Approach to Surveillance (STEPS) of NCD Risk Factors could be adapted and applied to humanitarian emergencies (WHO 2016). These core elements include (WHO 2016):

- Monitoring exposures such as: behavioral risk-factors of alcohol use, tobacco use, food intake/salt intake; physiological and metabolic risk factors such as elevated blood glucose, elevated cholesterol; social risk-factors such as household income, access to health services and; mental health risk-factors such as exposure to stress and existence of mental disorders.
- Monitoring outcomes such as: cause-specific mortality; NCD incidence and prevalence; NCD related complications; NCD treatment outcomes; continuity of NCD care.
- Monitoring health system capacity and response such as: availability of services and medicines on the essential medicine list; availability and capacity of staff; existence of policies and plans.

Early response planning, before data can be collected in the field, could use WHO STEPS data for that country, if available. The ability to then collect data for some or all of the above elements would clearly be influenced by local contextual factors such as security, capacity, and resources, prior existence of surveillance system before the crisis, and setting. For example, surveillance systems may be much easier to establish and maintain in well-established camps than in urban areas.

The incremental stepwise approach noted above could be applied to scaling up the monitoring and surveillance system from initially collecting minimum monitoring of key outcomes and service availability in more acute and insecure environments to collecting more comprehensive data on outcomes, exposures and health system capacity as security and resources improve. For example, cause of death data may initially be derived from the use of verbal autopsy methods but, as the situation stabilizes, cause of death can be identified from more reliable clinically confirmed data. Similarly, hospital-based cancer registries may be initially used but these should be scaled-up towards the establishment of population-based cancer registries, which provide a less biased description of the cancer patterns and trends in a population.

Where possible, data collection methods should include prospective surveillance of mortality and NCD incidence. Cohort monitoring, in which all the patients diagnosed with a certain condition within a particular catchment area over a period of time are registered and standard clinical outcomes regularly reported, could provide an important means of systematically evaluating NCD programs. This has been shown to be effective in large-scale interventions for chronic infectious diseases of tuberculosis and HIV/AIDS, and similar approaches could be applied to NCDs (WHO 2008, Maher 2012, Harries et al. 2008, Maher et al. 2009).

For example, cohort monitoring has been used for managing diabetes and hypertension in Palestinian refugees in Jordan, and this provided valuable real-time data on the burden of diabetes and hypertension, and their management at the primary clinic level (Khader et al. 2014, Khader et al. 2012a, Khader et al. 2012b). Similarly, comprehensive cancer reporting, ideally through the establishment of population-based electronic cancer registries, provides vital information sources for tracking cancer incidence and outcomes over time and understanding and addressing the cancer burden in a population. The data from cohort monitoring and cancer registries also provide important operational research data on the introduction of new medications, new diagnostic technologies, and new models of healthcare delivery (Kapur and Harries 2013). However, examples of comprehensive surveillance systems remain rare in low- and middle-income countries, and many conflict and postconflict countries do not have any kind of NCD surveillance systems in place (WHO 2010a). The existence of operational policy, strategy, or action plan for key NCDs, risk factors, and surveillance for selected countries affected by armed conflict over the past decade is shown in Table 31.1.

Other potential sources of information on NCDs include cross-sectional population-based household surveys which, although quite resource-intensive, provide valuable population-level data such as NCD prevalence, exposure to risk-factors, and access to services (Doocy et al. 2013). Greater use can also be made of routine data collected by agencies, as done by UNHCR with their "exceptional care committees" data on expensive medical treatment for refugees in host countries (Spiegel et al. 2014). Health system and policy research, including health economics research, is also important for understanding the impact of crises on patients with NCDs, and broader health system capacity, financing and policy issues (Fonseca et al. 2009).

These monitoring and surveillance activities should be coordinated between different agencies and also integrated into broader health surveillance activities where possible. National health authorities in humanitarian emergencies may not have the capacity to monitor NCD control activities given the insecurity, poor resources, and damaged health system in such settings. However, individual UN agencies and humanitarian NGOs can perform vital NCD monitoring and surveillance activities. Ideally, they should also be made openly available online, as is the case with UNHCR's integrated online public health information platform, TWINE (UNHCR 2013).

The knowledge base on NCDs needs and responses in humanitarian emergencies is further hampered by the limited research that has taken place on NCDs in humanitarian emergencies. A search of peer-reviewed articles published between 1993 and 2013 of cancer diagnoses in refugees identified only six articles (Spiegel et al. 2014). A review of the literature on the prevalence and distribution of NCDs among urban refugees living in developing countries identified only eight studies, with six from the Middle East (Amara and Aljunid 2014). Information on the effectiveness of NCD interventions in humanitarian emergencies is also extremely limited, with a systematic review conducted identifying only three studies on diabetes interventions and two on cardiovascular disease interventions in humanitarian emergencies (Ruby et al. 2015). The review also highlighted the need for more evidence on the feasibility of NCD interventions in humanitarian emergencies. Therefore, experimental, quasi-experimental and descriptive study designs should also incorporate outcomes of cost, adherence, availability, and acceptability.

Prevention

Efforts to prevent the increase of NCDs globally target the main modifiable risk-factors of tobacco use, harmful alcohol use, lack of exercise, and unhealthy diet (WHO 2010a). However, evidence on these risk-factors in humanitarian emergencies remains very limited (Grijalva-Eternod et al. 2012, Ezard 2012, Weaver and Roberts 2010), with very few studies addressing the effectiveness of efforts to address these key risk-factors in humanitarian emergencies (Lo et al. 2014, Roberts and Ezard 2015).

Prevention activities in humanitarian emergencies should recognize WHO's "best buys" for NCD prevention in LMICs which most successfully meet criteria of health impact, cost-effectiveness, cost of implementation, and feasibility of scale-up, particularly in resource-poor settings (WHO/WEF 2011). The best-buys identified to address NCDs in these countries are listed in Table 31.2.

The ability to implement and enforce these best buys in humanitarian emergencies will clearly be influenced by contextual constraints in the

Table 31.1 Existence of operational policy/strategy/action plan for key NCDs, risk-factors, and surveillance, for selected countries affected by armed conflict over the past decade (WHO 2010)

Country	Major NCDs			Risk-factors and prevention					Monitoring and surveillance	
	Cancer	CVD	Resp. diseases	Diabetes	Alcohol	Tobacco	Insufficient physical activity	Unhealthy diet/ overweight/ obesity	Fiscal interventions[1]	Cancer registry	Risk surveillance[4]
Afghanistan	no	no	yes	no	no	no	no	no	no	no	no
CAR	no	no	no	no	no	no	no	no	no	no	no
DRC	no	no	yes	no	no	yes	no	yes	no	no	no
Georgia	no	no	no	no	no	no	no	no	no	yes[2]	no
Iraq	yes	no	yes	yes	DK	yes	yes	yes	no	yes[2]	no
Liberia	no	no	no	no	no	no	no	no	DK	no	no
Libya	DK	no	DK	no	yes	no	no	no	no	yes[3]	yes
Myanmar	yes	yes	yes	DK	DK	yes	DK	yes	yes	yes[3]	yes
Nepal	yes	yes	yes	no	yes	yes	no	no	yes	yes[2]	yes
Somalia	no	no	no	no	no	no	no	no	yes	no	no
Sri Lanka	yes	yes	yes	yes	yes	yes	yes	yes	yes	yes[2]	yes
Syria	no	no	no	no	no	no	no	no	no	yes[2]	no
Uganda	no	no	no	no	no	no	no	no	yes	yes[3]	no

Abbreviation: CAR, Central African Republic; DRC, Democratic Republic of the Congo; CVD, cardiovascular disease; DK, Don't Know (data not provided to WHO), Resp., respiratory.
[1] Implementation of fiscal interventions to influence behavior change for NCDs.
[2] National cancer registries
[3] Subnational cancer registries
[4] Surveillance of key risk factors of harmful alcohol use, diet, physical inactivity, and tobacco use.

Data from 2010.
Source: World Health Organization. Global Health Observatory. Available at: http://apps.who.int/gho/data/view.main.2473 (accessed May 26, 2014)

Table 31.2 WHO recommended 'best buys' for the prevention of NCDS in low- and middle-income countries

Tobacco use	• Protect people from tobacco smoke and banning smoking in public places • Warn about the dangers of tobacco use • Enforce bans on tobacco advertising, promotion and sponsorship • Raise taxes on tobacco
Harmful alcohol use	• Restrict access to retailed alcohol • Enforce bans on alcohol advertising • Raise taxes on alcohol
Unhealthy diet and insufficient physical inactivity	• Reduce salt intake and salt content of food • Replace trans-fat in food with polyunsaturated fat • Promote public awareness about diet and physical activity, including via mass media

Source: WHO/WEF (2011), From Burden to "Best Buys": Reducing the Economic Impact of Non-Communicable Diseases in Low- and Middle-Income Countries (WHO/WEF, 2011).

humanitarian emergency and the target populations, particularly with regards to government capacity and willingness. The limited data available suggest that NCD prevention policies are weak in a number of humanitarian emergencies, as reflected in the sample of conflict-affected countries shown in Table 31.1. While the fiscal prevention interventions are largely beyond the scope of humanitarian agencies, they can support activities to control tobacco and harmful alcohol use, particularly given some evidence of their higher use among conflict-affected populations and those with greater levels of trauma exposure and mental disorders (Lo et al. 2014, Weaver and Roberts 2010). However, as noted above, humanitarian agencies have extremely weak guidelines on NCDs. The guidelines they do have are focused on the treatment of NCDs and virtually ignore activities to prevent NCDs (Sphere Project 2011, WHO 2009, Demaio et al. 2013).

The gaps in NCD policies significantly impede progress in effectively preventing and treating NCDs in humanitarian emergencies. They also provide opportunities for multinational tobacco, alcohol, and food companies to expand activities and potentially influence policies in ways that undermine efforts to control tobacco and harmful alcohol use or improve unhealthy diets in transitional countries such as those emerging from conflict (Roberts et al. 2012). This may be further exacerbated by weak policy enforcement given the weak governance and policing observed in many humanitarian emergencies and postconflict settings, for example, with regard to the manufacture of illicit alcohol or smuggling of cigarettes (Nakkash and Lee 2008, Titeca et al. 2011).

Treatment

Similar to the state of guidance for NCD surveillance, monitoring, and prevention, clear guidance for treatment of NCDs in humanitarian emergencies is lacking. For example, the Sphere Standards have less than one page specific to NCDs (Sphere Project 2011). Medications recommended during the emergency response in key guidance, such as the Interagency Emergency Health Kit, are not sufficient for the most common NCDs (WHO 2011).

Treating NCDs in humanitarian emergencies creates ethical issues that need consideration. In displaced populations coming from countries with well-established healthcare systems and disease profiles characterized by a high number of NCDs, expensive tertiary care, such as renal dialysis, cancer treatments, or complex cardiac surgeries, may be the norm. A guiding principle used by UNHCR and other humanitarian agencies when establishing and providing healthcare to displaced populations is to follow the policies and treatment guidelines from the host government whenever possible, trying to make sure that equity of access to and quality of care is similar across refugees and host populations (Leaning et al. 2011). However, this means that in areas such as the Middle East, the relative resource allocation for refugees is higher than for refugees in other areas of the world where infectious diseases may predominate (Leaning et al. 2011).

The decision of whether or not to include or initiate new treatment of NCDs in the acute or prolonged emergency response may draw from related discussions for HIV/AIDS. Similar to a number of chronic diseases, HIV/AIDs requires lifetime treatment once initiated and, if not continued in the humanitarian emergency setting, may have serious immediate and long-term consequences for the individual and his/her family as well as the community. The Inter-Agency Standing Committee (IASC) guidance for treatment of HIV/AIDs provides an action framework that delineates a minimum initial response for the early stages of response regardless of the epidemiology of disease in the emergency-affected population, and an expanded response that would take into account local conditions. The initial response includes continuing or reinitiating antiretroviral therapy for those who were previously on treatment, while counseling, testing and scale-up is initiated later (IASC 2010). HIV/AIDs is discussed in detail in Chapter 23. While beyond the scope of this chapter, defining the scope of recommended treatment of NCDs, including differentiation in the acute and prolonged emergency response setting, is greatly needed. Until formal comprehensive guidance is available, however, there are some existing tools and actions that may be undertaken to assure that the urgent treatment needs of this vulnerable population are not compromised.

Public Health Data

One immediate action is to assess existing public health data and address gaps in information needed to design rational, effective, and sensitive health services delivery systems for NCDs in humanitarian emergencies (Sphere Project 2011). As described earlier, surveillance and monitoring of NCDs in humanitarian emergencies is generally lacking, and the area of health services delivery is no exception. The Sphere Project provides sample data collection forms designed to identify and inform health services delivery. In these forms, however, NCDs are not listed as a specific cause of death for mortality surveillance, and the morbidity surveillance form lists NCDs as a single aggregate disease (Sphere Project 2011). Amendment of these forms to include NCDs known to be both prevalent in the population and sensitive to deterioration during humanitarian emergencies is critical. The Sphere Project is discussed in greater detail in Chapter 4.

Ideally, diseases added in these data collection tools would be guided by prior knowledge of prevalence of NCDs in the affected population. Where this is lacking, general assumptions based upon similar populations with data available may serve as a starting point. To further prioritize which diseases to include, the concept of ambulatory care sensitive conditions may provide insight. Originally defined and currently used to assess the quality of highly functioning healthcare delivery systems during nonhumanitarian emergencies, ambulatory care sensitive conditions are those for which escalation to hospitalization could be avoided if appropriate ambulatory care is given. They include angina, asthma, chronic obstructive pulmonary disease, diabetes, grand mal and other epileptic convulsions, heart failure and pulmonary edema, and hypertension. In humanitarian emergencies, these treatment-sensitive conditions are similarly likely to deteriorate without continued treatment, resulting in preventable morbidity or mortality. The capacity to detect and diagnose these conditions in the humanitarian emergency setting will vary, but this list may inform which NCD conditions are vital to track, monitor, and to prioritize for treatment in the initial stages of emergency response.

Guidance

For detailed treatment guidance for NCDs beyond that currently included in the Sphere Project, one may refer to a general Sphere Project guidance, which notes that when any care is provided, it should reflect the standards of the country where the disaster response is being conducted (Sphere Project 2011). In 2010, the World Health Organization put forward the Package of Essential Noncommunicable (PEN) Disease Intervention for Primary Health Care in Low-Resource Settings (WHO 2010b). It is a prioritized set of cost-effective interventions, a minimum standard that countries should implement to address cardiovascular disease, diabetes, cancer, asthma, and chronic obstructive pulmonary diseases (COPD) in primary care settings. Countries are encouraged to add other interventions to this set of interventions depending upon the specific NCD profile of the country and the availability of cost effective interventions.

As this is the expected minimum standard, responses to humanitarian emergencies should include at least the PEN list of essential interventions covering elements of primary, secondary, and acute treatment for select cardiovascular diseases, diabetes, kidney disease, asthma, COPD, and cancer. Essential technologies and tools for implementing these interventions, such as blood pressure measuring devices and glucometers, are outlined in the PEN and may serve as a foundation for planning (WHO 2010b).

Medications

The Interagency Emergency Health Kit (IEHK) 2011 is a package of medicines and medical devises intended to meet the initial primary health-care needs of ten thousand people with disrupted or no medical facilitates for three months (WHO 2011). Although it was developed through a process facilitated by the World Health Organization, it does not include the basic medications listed in the PEN list (WHO 2010b). The PEN medication list was prepared in 2009, and is derived from the WHO Model List of Essential Medicines. Responders to humanitarian emergencies may consider supplementing the IEHK medications, drawing preferably from national formularies of the country in which the response is occurring. If a national formulary does not exist, response planners may refer to the most current WHO Model List of Essential Medicines, which is updated every two years. This will assure that treatment meets the basic minimum global guidance, and that once affected populations return to stable conditions, they are able to continue treatment with minimal disruption due to differences in the specific medications available.

Care Delivery

Because NCDs share with HIV/AIDs and tuberculosis the need for sustained lifetime management and continued access to medications, effective NCD care delivery models can learn from HIV/AIDs and tuberculosis treatment in LMICs, where scale-up was made possible through the introduction of cohort monitoring, simplifying, and standardizing treatment protocols, and ensuring a supply of medication at no cost (Kapur and Harrison, 2013). In Palestinian refugee camps, for example, this approach has been used to improve care for the treatment of hypertension and diabetes and may provide a model for the nonacute humanitarian emergency context (Khader et al. 2012b). One important takeaway is that parallel systems for treatment of chronic diseases and long term infectious diseases, such as HIV/AIDs and tuberculosis in humanitarian emergencies, may not be needed. Instead, building upon existing health delivery systems in humanitarian emergencies to facilitate the needs of NCD treatment will improve efficiency of the response.

While much remains to be defined in the area of treating NCDs in humanitarian emergencies, key NCD treatment guidance developed outside the humanitarian emergency context can be applied to humanitarian emergencies, understanding they will need to be adapted, tested, and evaluated to ensure they are effective and feasible in the context of humanitarian emergencies.

Conclusion

The humanitarian response community must address the healthcare needs resulting from NCDs of people affected by humanitarian emergencies. This includes advocating for displaced populations to receive healthcare at limited to no cost, developing and testing guidelines on NCDs, improving surveillance for NCDs, integrating refugees into host country healthcare systems whenever possible and avoiding the development of parallel healthcare systems, enhancing equity in healthcare, and providing support to host countries to bolster their healthcare systems. Other strategies include integrating training on NCDs as part of public health training for humanitarian workers; developing easy to use home-based care guidelines for diabetes and heart disease, and treatment kits for refugees and IDPs in areas in which there are limited healthcare services and/or insecurity; and planning ahead to ensure sufficient funding to cover disease of long duration, expensive tests and treatments, and specialist consultations (Spiegel et al. 2010). For example, as part of its strategic public health plan for 2014–18, UNHCR is proposing developing integrated approaches to target common risk factors for diabetes, cardiovascular disease, and chronic respiratory disease, using primary care and prevention as a way to reduce expensive secondary and tertiary care (UNHCR 2013).

In addition to addressing NCDs during the humanitarian emergency, efforts should address ways to ensure that therapy is maintained during the transition phase from the emergency to a more sustainable healthcare system that would provide long-term management and continuity of care. Given the higher cost of secondary and tertiary care, the issues of providing healthcare financing to fragile, post-conflict countries and the provision of equity of care within the context of budgetary constraints needs to be addressed (Leaning et al. 2011).

Additionally, research is needed to quantify the burden of NCDs in humanitarian emergencies, to better understand short- and long-term sequelae that arise from interruptions in NCD care and management, and to identify innovative and cost-effective methods of NCD care delivery during humanitarian emergencies.

The challenges in NCD management during humanitarian emergencies are many and complex, characterized by insecurity, restricted access, limited resources, fragmented healthcare systems, and lack of standardized health indicators and data collection. There is an urgent need to develop improved NCD guidelines, surveillance and research activities, and health systems capacity in order to support decision-making and increase the effectiveness and feasibility of NCD interventions during humanitarian emergencies.

Notes from the Field

Syria (2014)

The Syrian conflict is now entering its fourth year, with 9.3 million persons affected, 625,000 injured and 6.5 million displaced as of March 2014 (WHO 2014a). Of those displaced, approximately 2.8 million Syrians have fled to the neighboring countries of Jordan, Iraq, Lebanon, and Turkey (USAID 2014). The impact on the health system of Syria and surrounding countries is enormous, resulting in 73% of Syrian healthcare facilities, including 27% of primary healthcare facilities and 65–70% of pharmaceutical companies, being nonfunctional (WHO 2014a).

Prior to the conflict that started in January 2011, noncommunicable diseases (NCDs) were a major burden in Syria, with 44 percent of proportional mortality accounted for by cardiovascular disease (WHO 2014b). As NCDs play a larger role in population health, even in conflict-free countries, LMICs struggle to address the growing scale and impact of NCDs (Sen et al. 2013). The inability to address NCDs becomes an even greater challenge in conflict-affected countries, such as Syria.

Humanitarian law has been violated throughout the conflict, with bombing attacks on health facilities and blood banks, targeted attacks on health personnel that treat patients from the opposition areas, and blockage of humanitarian deliveries of medications and supplies (Lynch 2014). In spite of the February 2014 United Nations Security Council Resolution 2139 that directed all parties to allow delivery of humanitarian aid, access to such aid remains limited (UN 2014). Over time, WHO is beginning to make inroads in delivery of essential medications and supplies. For example, on April 4, 2014, WHO was able to deliver 40 metric tons of life-saving drugs, including for NCDs, as well as other medical and surgical supplies, to a besieged governorate, Ar-Raqqah, in north central Syria, which was used to support over 117,000 people in the affected area, but more is needed (WHO 2014c).

The impact is felt not only on Syrians but also on the estimated 540,000 Palestinian refugees residing in Syria (UNRWA 2014a). The NCD profile indicated 26,113 registered Palestinian refugees in Syria presented with a NCD-related health problem, including 3,762 with diabetes, 12,753 with hypertension, and 9,598 with a combination of diabetes and hypertension. The government of Syria has stopped referring these patients to Ministry of Health hospitals but violence, damage, and insecurity have forced closure of United Nations Relief and Works Agency (UNRWA) clinics, with only 14 of the original 23 open (UNRWA 2014b).

Meeting the health needs of Syrian refugees with NCDs is causing stress on the health systems of neighboring countries that are hosting these refugees. From January to March 2013, UNHCR reported that diabetes, cardiovascular disease, and lung disease were the most commonly reported NCDs for refugees in the neighboring countries of Iraq, Jordan, and Lebanon (UNHCR 2013a). NCDs accounted for 7.4%, 21.8%, and 8.3% of all primary healthcare visits in refugee camps in Iraq, Jordan and Lebanon, respectively (UNHCR 2014b). The large number of refugees that have settled outside refugee camps, in urban areas, has placed a further strain on country health systems, but data on urban refugees with NCDs in these host countries is minimal to nonexistent. To compound the challenge, humanitarian funding has been limited, while costs of more expensive referral treatment, such as cancer care or dialysis, have increased (UNHCR 2013b).

Lebanon is hosting more Syrian refugees than any other country, straining their ability to provide healthcare services. The number of refugees in Lebanon has increased 434 percent between January 28, 2013 and January 28, 2014, with all refugees living outside camps. Data from UNHCR's Health Information Systems (HIS) in Lebanon indicate that 52 percent of all healthcare consultations for persons aged 18–59 years were for NCDs (UNHCR, 2014c). The healthcare system in Lebanon is highly fragmented, privatized, and depends on user fees, with some refugees receiving healthcare through a UNHCR-run program, while, for others, UNHCR must pay for the costs of their care from the private sector. Given the shortfall of funding, UNHCR has had to decrease its funding of healthcare in this situation and now prioritizes care using a public health approach that emphasizes basic primary healthcare and emergency care, which means that the costliest care, such as medications and kidney dialysis, must be borne by the patient (Amnesty International 2014).

A Médecins Sans Frontières (MSF) colleague conducted a household survey focused during the winter of 2013/14, on access to medical care among Syrian refugees displaced in the Bekaa Valley on the Lebanon-Syria border. She shared an experience that highlights the difficulties faced by refugees in the Syrian humanitarian crisis:

"In a border village called 'Majda Anjar,' I remember a man walking up to me, slowly and arduously, as I was cross-checking a form. His name escapes me now but his face is clear. He was older, maybe late 50s, and flashed a grim smile devoid of several teeth as he approached my translator and me. That smile quickly evolved into rushed Arabic as he pleaded with us for medical services. He saw the MSF logo on the side of our car and knew that we were healthcare providers. He continued to speak rapidly as he needed care for his kidney condition immediately. He could not tell us the specific health condition but said he could not access desperately needed dialysis in Lebanon, which he previously had access to in Syria. He was scared that he was going to die as a result of not being able to access care. He needed a ride to a dialysis clinic, money to pay for the dialysis service, and medications. He begged and pleaded and had a look of fear throughout that I still remember. I handed the man a flyer that contained a map and contact information for MSF clinics in the Bekaa, although I knew he would throw this in the trash as he walked away. He had no transportation available to him in order to access these clinics and, even if he did manage to find a vehicle, none of the clinics in the Bekaa were providing dialysis. I wanted to help but it was beyond what my mission could provide. It felt like a lost battle from the start and – somehow, he also seemed to feel that as well. The last I remember of him is the flyer, somewhat crumpled, in his right hand as he hobbled down a dirt path in the freezing cold towards his informal tented settlement and a future that looked dim. His story is not unique among the millions of displaced Syrians throughout the Middle East. His story, and the countless others with a similar plight, represents the new reality for the consequences of war-torn middle-income countries" (personal communication contributed by Jesse Erin Berns, MPH).

References

Amara, A. H. and Aljunid, S. M. (2014). Noncommunicable diseases among urban refugees and asylum-seekers in developing countries: a neglected healthcare need. *Global Health*, **10**, 24.

Amnesty International. 2014. *Agonizing choices. Syrian refuges in need of healthcare in Lebanon*. Amnesty International: London, England.

Arrieta, M. I. et al. (2008). Insuring continuity of care for chronic disease patients after a disaster: Key preparedness elements. *Am J Med Sci*, **336**, 128–133.

Chan, E. Y. and Sondorp, E. (2007). Interventions following natural disasters: missing out on chronic medical needs. *Asia Pac J Public Health*, 19 spec no, 45–51.

Demaio, A. et al. (2013). Non-communicable diseases in emergencies: a call to action. *Plos Curr*, 5.

Doocy, D. et al. (2013). Chronic disease and disability among Iraqi populations displaced in Jordan and Syria. *Int J Health Plann Manage*, 28, e1–e12.

Evans, J. (2010). Mapping the vulnerability of older persons to disasters. *Int J Older People Nurs*, **5**, 63–70.

Ezard, N. (2012). Substance use among populations displaced by conflict: a literature review. *Disasters*, **36**, 533–557.

Fonseca, V. A. et al. (2009). Impact of a natural disaster on diabetes: exacerbation of disparities and long-term consequences. *Diabetes Care*, **32**, 1632–1638.

Giovino, G. A. et al. (2012). Tobacco use in 3 billion individuals from 16 countries: An analysis of nationally representative cross-sectional household surveys. *Lancet*, **380**, 668–679.

Grijalva-Eternod, C. S., et al. (2012). The double burden of obesity and malnutrition in a protracted emergency setting: A cross-sectional study of western Sahara refugees. *Plos Med*, **9**, e1001320.

Harries, A. D. et al. (2008). Adapting the dots framework for tuberculosis control to the management of non-communicable diseases in sub-Saharan Africa. *Plos Med*, **5**, e124.

IASC. (2010). Guidelines for addressing HIV in humanitarian settings. *IASC*, Geneva, Switzerland.

IDF. (2013). IDF diabetes atlas. 6th ed. *International Diabetes Federation*; Brussels, Belgium.

Ikeda, N. et al. (2014). Control of hypertension with medication: a comparative analysis of national surveys in 20 countries. *Bull World Health Organ*, **92**, 10-19c.

Jamison, D. T. et al. (2013). Global health 2035: A world converging within a generation. *Lancet*, **382**, 1898–1955.

Kapur, A. and Harries, A. D. (2013). Cohort monitoring – as a tool to improve diabetes care services. *Diabetes Res Clin Pract*, **102**, 260–264.

Kapur, A. and Harrison, J. E. (2013). Cohort monitoring – as a tool to improve diabetes care services. *Diabetes Res Clinl Pract*, **102**, 260–264.

Khader, A. et al. (2012a). Cohort monitoring of persons with diabetes mellitus in a primary healthcare clinic for Palestine refugees in Jordan. *Tropl Med Int Health*, **17**, 1569–1576.

Khader, A. et al. (2012b). Cohort monitoring of persons with hypertension: An illustrated example from a primary healthcare clinic for Palestine refugees in Jordan. *Trop Med Int Health*, **17**, 1163–1170.

Khader, A. et al. (2014). Treatment outcomes in a cohort of Palestine refugees with diabetes mellitus followed through use of e-health over 3 years in Jordan. *Trop Med Int Health*, **19**, 219–223.

Leaning, J., Spiegel, P., and Crisp, J. (2011). Public health equity in refugee situations. *Conf Health*, **5**, 6.

Lim, S. S. et al. (2012). A comparative risk assessment of burden of disease and injury attributable to 67 risk factors and risk factor clusters in 21 regions, 1990–2010: a systematic analysis for the global burden of disease study 2010. *Lancet*, **380**, 2224–2260.

Lo, J., Patel, P., and Roberts, B. 2014. A systematic review on tobacco use among civilian populations affected by armed conflict. *Tob Control*, 13 March 2015 [online first].

Lozano, R. et al. (2012). Global and regional mortality from 235 causes of death for 20 age groups in 1990 and 2010: a systematic analysis for the global burden of disease study 2010. *Lancet*, **380**, 2095–2128.

Lynch C. (2014). Syria's War on Medicine. Available at: http://thecable.foreignpolicy.com/posts/2014/04/24/syrias_war_on_medicine (accessed May 10, 2014).

Maher, D. (2012). The power of health information–the use of cohort monitoring in managing patients with chronic non-communicable diseases. *Trop Med Int Health*, 17, 1567–1568.

Maher, D., Harries, A.D., Zachariah, R., and Enarson, D. (2009). A global framework for action to improve the primary care response to chronic non-communicable diseases: a solution to a neglected problem. *BMC Public Health*, **9**, 355.

Nakkash, R. and Lee, K. (2008). Smuggling as the "key to a combined market": British American tobacco in Lebanon. *Tob control*, **17**, 324–331.

Ng, M., Freeman, M. K., Fleming, T. D., Robinson, M., Dwyer-Lindgren, l., Thomson, B., Wollum, A., Sanman, E., Wulf, S., Lopez, A. D., Murray, C. J., and Gakidou, E. (2014). Smoking prevalence and cigarette consumption in 187 countries, 1980–2012. *JAMA*, **311**, 183–192.

Rapsomaniki, E., Timmis, A., George J., Pujades-Rodriguez, M., Shah, A.D., Denaxas, S., White, I.R., Caulfield, M. J., Deanfield, J. E., Smeeth, l., Williams, B., Hingorani, A., and Hemingway, H. (2014). Blood pressure and incidence of twelve cardiovascular diseases: lifetime risks, healthy life-years lost, and age-specific associations in 1·25 million people. *Lancet*, **383**, 1899–1911.

Roberts, B. and Ezard, N. (2015). Why are we not doing more for alcohol use disorder among conflict-affected populations? *Addiction*, **110**, 889–90.

Roberts, B., Patel, P., and McKee, M. (2012). Noncommunicable diseases and post-conflict countries. *Bull World Health Organ*, **90**, 2, 2a.

Rottman, S. J. (2008). Pharmaceuticals and chronic diseases in disaster preparedness. *Prehospital and Disaster Medicine*, **23**, 459–60.

Ruby, A., Knight, A., Perel, P., Blanchet, K, and Roberts, B. (2015). The effectiveness of interventions for non-communicable diseases in humanitarian crises: a systematic review. *Plos One*, October 2015.

Sen, K., Al-Faisal, W., and Al Saleh, Y. (2013). Syria: effects of conflict and sanctions on public health. *J Public Health* (Oxford), **35**, 195–199.

Shi, Y. and Hu, F. B. (2014). The global implications of diabetes and cancer. *Lancet*, **383**, 1947–1948.

Sphere Project. (2011). *Sphere handbook: Humanitarian charter and minimum standards in humanitarian response.* The Sphere Project; Geneva, Switzerland.

Spiegel, P., Khalifa, A., and Mateen, F. J. (2014). Cancer in refugees in Jordan and Syria between 2009 and 2012: challenges and the way forward in humanitarian emergencies. *Lancet Oncol*, 15, e290–e297.

Spiegel, P. B., Checchi, F., Colombo, S., and Paik, E. (2010). Health-care needs of people affected by conflict: future trends and changing frameworks. *Lancet*, **375**, 341–345.

Titeca, K., Joossens, I., and Raw, M. (2011). Blood cigarettes: cigarette smuggling and war economies in central and eastern Africa, *Tob Control*, **20**, 226–232.

UN. (2014). Available at: www.un.org/News/Press/docs/2014/sc11292.doc.htm (accessed May 10, 2014).

United Nations High Commissioner for Refugees. (2008). *UNHCR's principles and guidance for referral healthcare for refugees and other persons of concern.* United Nations High Commissioner for Refugees: Geneva, Switzerland.

United Nations High Commissioner for Refugees. (2009). *UNHCR policy on refugee protection and solutions in urban areas*. United Nations High Commissioner for Refugees: Geneva, Switzerland.

United Nations High Commissioner for Refugees. (2013a). Inter-agency regional response for Syrian Refugees Health and Nutrition Bulletin, Iraq, Jordan and Lebanon, January–March 2013.

United Nations High Commissioner for Refugees. (2013b). UNHCR Briefing Notes (April 26,2013): UNHCR report shows healthcare services for Syrian refugees increasingly overstretched, Available at: www.unhcr.org/517a58af9.html (accessed May 10, 2014).

United Nations High Commissioner for Refugees. TWINE. (2013). Available at: http://twine.unhcr.org/app/.

United Nations High Commissioner for Refugees. (2014a). *Global strategy for public health*. United Nations High Commissioner for Refugees; Geneva, Switzerland.

United Nations High Commissioner for Refugees. (2014b). At a glance: Health data for Syrian refugees. *Iraq, Jordan and Lebanon*. United Nations High Commissioner for Refugees; Geneva, Switzerland.

United Nations High Commissioner for Refugees. (2014c). HIS Syrian Annual Report 2013. At a glance: Health data for Syrian refugees. *Iraq, Jordan and Lebanon*. United Nations High Commissioner for Refugees; Geneva, Switzerland.

United Nations Relief and Works Agency for Palestine Refugees in the Near East. (2014a). Syria crisis: United Nations Relief and Works Agency for Palestine Refugees. Available at: www.unrwa.org/syria-crisis (accessed November 3, 2014).

United Nations Relief and Works Agency for Palestine Refugees in the Near East. (2014b). Available at: www.unrwa.org/activity/health-syria (accessed May 10, 2014).

United States Aid for International Development. (2014). Available at: www.usaid.gov/sites/default/files/documents/1866/syria_ce_fs14_05-08-2014.pdf (accessed May 10, 2014).

Waldman, R. and Martone, G. (1999). Public health and complex emergencies: new issues, new conditions. *Am J Public Health*, **89**, 1483–1485.

Weaver, H. and Roberts, B. (2010). Drinking and displacement: A systematic review of the influence of forced displacement on harmful alcohol use. *Substance Use and Misuse*, **45**, 2340–2355.

World Health Organization. (2008). *Global tuberculosis control—surveillance, planning, financing: WHO report 2008*. World Health Organization; Geneva, Switzerland.

World Health Organization. (2009). *Health cluster guide*. World Health Organization; Geneva, Switzerland.

World Health Organization. (2010a). *Global status report on noncommunicable diseases 2010*. World Health Organization; Geneva, Switzerland.

World Health Organization (2010b). Package of essential noncommunicable (pen) disease intervention for primary healthcare [online]. Available at: www.who.int/cardiovascular_diseases/publications/pen2010/en/ (accessed June 13, 2014).

World Health Organization. (2011). Interagency emergency health kit. World Health Organization. Available at: www.who.int/medicines/publications/emergencyhealthkit2011/en/ (accessed April 18, 2014).

World Health Organization. (2013). *Global action plan for the prevention and control of ncds 2013–2020*. World Health Organization; Geneva, Switzerland.

World Health Organization. (2014a). Available at: www.who.int/hac/crises/syr/sitreps/syria_country_fact_sheet_13march2014_final.pdf (accessed May 10, 2014).

World Health Organization. (2014b). Available at: www.who.int/nmh/countries/syr_en.pdf?ua=1 (accessed 10 May 2014).

World Health Organization. (2014c). Press release, May 6, 2014, WHO EMRO office: WHO delivers life-saving medicines and surgical supplies to Ar-Raqqah governorate.

World Health Organization. Global Health Observatory. Available at: http://apps.who.int/gho/data/view.main.2473 (accessed May 26, 2014).

World Health Organization. STEPS. (2016). Available at: www.who.int/chp/steps/en/.

World Health Organization / World Economic Forum. (2011). *From burden to "best buys": reducing the economic impact of non-communicable diseases in low- and middle-income countries*. World Health Organization / World Economic Forum; Geneva, Switzerland.

Index

Abdallah, S., 1, 2, 298, 299
abortion care, 204
acute malnutrition, community-based management (CMAM), 365–366
acute respiratory infections (ARIs)
 blood cultures, 306
 case definitions, 298–299
 challenges, 300
 clinical presentation, course, 304–305
 complete blood counts (CBC), 306
 data collection, 299–300
 diagnosis, 305
 epidemiology, 296–297
 etiology, 295
 imaging, 306
 Kenya, 2006, 307
 nasopharyngeal, oropharyngeal swabs, 305–306
 outbreak detection, 300
 outbreak response, control, 301–304
 prevention, 297–298
 rates, types, affected populations, 295–296
 surveillance, 298
 transmission risk factors, 297
 treatment, 306
Afghanistan, 2002, 75–76
African famines, 17–18
Afshar, M., 234
Ager, A., 418, 419
Agte, V. V., 377
Ahlström, C., 7
Ahmed, J. A., 296, 305
Ahmed, T., 362
Aiello, A. M., 150
Albu, M., 190
Alderman, K., 63, 441, 443
Alexander, J. P., Jr., 239
Aljunid, S. M., 462, 465
Amara, A. H., 462, 465
American Red Cross, 11. *See also* International Committee of the Red Cross
Amin, N., 151
Anda, R. F., 417
Andemicael, A., 256
Annan. R. A., 370
Anon, 4

Ardalan, A., 284, 288, 289
Argenal, E., 268
Arie, S., 455
armed conflict, direct/indirect consequences, 63
Arrieta, M. J., 461
Art of War (Sun Tzu), 10
Ashworth, A., 362
Assessment Capacities Project (ACAPS), 84–86
assessments, 275
attack rate (AR), 322
Australian Aid, 49
Azman, A. S., 316

Babcock, C., 42
Baggaley, R., 338
Bailey, K., 446
Baker, K. K., 145
Baker, M., 401, 402
Bakewell, O., 255
Bamberger, M., 132
Bamrah, J., 132
Bamrah, S., 337, 345
Barnett, M. N., 9, 16
Barr, G., 427, 428
Barré-Sinoussi, F., 336
Bartels, S. A., 442, 443
Barth, J., 415
Barton, C., 11
Barzilay, E. J., 323
Bass, J. K., 416
Bausch, D. G., 285
Beauchamp, T., 73
bed requirement estimation, 321
Bellos, A., 295, 297
Benca, J., 400
Benjamin, E., 35, 42
Berendes, D., 147
Berkelman, R. L., 109
Berry, K, 69
Bhatia, S., 427
Bhatt, K. M., 230
Bhattacharjee, A., 443
Bhattacharya, S. K., 316
Bhutta, Z. A., 167–168, 176, 177, 376, 379
Bilukha, O. O., 171, 376, 444, 445
Bisson, J. I., 415

Biswas, A., 446
Bitar, D., 199
Bjun, 428
Black, M. M., 16, 169
Black, R., 68
Black, R. E., 162, 167–168
Blanton, L. V., 363
Bloland, P., 351
Boccia, D., 311
Bolton, P., 415
Bonwick, A., 214, 215
Borton, J., 9, 12, 122
Bosnan, A., 389
Boss, L. P., 233
Brauman, R., 11, 16, 20
Brazilay, E. J., 61
Brennan, R. J., 36, 59, 63, 295, 441, 450
Briseño, S., 284, 286
Brown, V., 246
Bruce, M. G., 401
Brudey, K., 428
Brunkard, J., 443, 450
Bryant, R. A., 441, 455
Bryce, J., 167–168
Buhmann, C. B., 455
Burki, T., 323
Burkle, F. M., 36, 43, 48, 50, 64
Burnham, G., 1, 2
Burtsher, D., 366

Cain, K. P., 428
Cairns, K. L., 57
Calhoun, C., 20
Callister, M. E., 428
Camaschella, C., 378
Cambodia, 17
camp management
 camp layout, 250
 self-rule systems, 255
 shelter, 250
 site planning, 249–250
 support systems, 244, 256
camp management, community and public facilities
 centers of worship, 255
 markets, 255
 recreational facilities, 255
 schools, 255

474

Index

camp management, displacement scenarios, 244–245
  camps, 245–246
  initial site assessment, 246
  Sphere Handbook, 246
camp management, management systems, 251–253
  administration, 253
  food distribution, 253
  health systems, facilities, 254–255
  non-food item (NFI) distribution, 253–254
  registration, 253
  water, sanitation, 254
camp management, site selection, 246–247
  accessibility, 248
  land ownership, usage, 247–248
  resources, 248–249
  security, protection, 248
  soil conditions, 248
  topography, 248
camp management, social groups
  professional associations, 256
  sports associations, 256
  women's groups, 255–256
Campagne, D. A., 400
Carballo, M., 418
CARE International, 31
Cartwright, E. J., 323
case definitions, inconsistent application, 116
case fatality rate (CFR), 322
Castillo-Salgado, C., 306
Caugant, D. A., 401
Caverzasio, S. G., 217
Cegielski, J. P., 429
Centers for Disease Control and Prevention (CDC), 30, 50
Cerda, M., 62
Chaignat, C. L., 233
chain of custody, medical commodities, 280
Champion, H. R., 444
Chan, E. Y., 461
Chan, M., 285
Chapman, L. E., 233
Checchi, F., 57, 58, 59, 295
Chew, L., 417
Chiu, C. H., 442
cholera, 323–325
  treatment, 328–329
cholera treatment center (CTC), 320
cholera treatment unit (CTU), 320
Chow, A. W., 305
Chris, B., 351
Churchill, Winston, 13
civil war, 18–19
Clasen, T., 136, 141, 142, 313, 314
Clemens, J., 232

clolera treatment centers, other health facilities, 315
Cochran, 408
Code of Ethics for Emergency Nurses, 72
Coghlan, B., 64
Cohn, A. C., 400, 402
Cohn, J., 227
cold chain, medical commodities, 278
Colditz, R., 431
Colindres, R. E., 313, 314
Collins, S., 170, 370, 373
Colllins, S., 370
commodities movement
  essential medicines, 276
  kits, 275–276
community information, education, communication, 321–322
"Complex Emergencies and the Crisis of Developmentalism" (Duffield), 6
complex humanitarian emergencies (CEs), 4–6, 19–20
  armed conflict and, 6–8
complex humanitarian emergencies (CHE), 35–36
Complicated Severe Acute Malnutrition (SAM), 363
Compton, J., 172
Concern Worldwide, 16–17, 31
Coninx, R., 429
Connolly, M. A., 136, 229, 298, 323, 389, 391
containments, 268
context analysis, 188–189
Contzen, N., 157
Cookson, S. T., 427, 428, 431
Corsellis, T., 245, 249, 250, 251, 252
Cosgrave, J., 122, 126, 127
crop protection, 193–194
crop recovery, 194–195
Culbert, H., 345
Cunningham, R. M., 455
Curtis, V. A., 149

Dabelstein, N., 131
Dafur, 65
Dahab, M., 200
Dahinden, M., 287
Danel, D., 343
D'Aoust, O., 55, 57
Darcy, J., 87
Das, P., 323
data, data collection. *See* surveillance
data analysis, interpretation, 116
Davey, E., 9, 12
Davidson, F. R., 376
Davidson, J., 124
Davis, J., 138, 259
de Boer, H., 306
de Jong, K., 409, 414

De Jong J. T., 410
de Onis, M., 364
De Roo, A., 408
de Villiers, G., 271, 278
De Waal, A., 17
De Wals, P., 401
Degomme, O., 63
Demaio, A., 51, 62, 461, 462
Deng, F., 215
Department for International Development (DFID), 30
Department for International Development (DFID), UK, 49
Desal, S. N., 238
Dhavan, P., 432
diabetes, 461
diarrheal diseases
  clinical presentation, treatment, 323
  clolera treatment centers, other health facilities, 315
  epidemiology, 310–311
  episodes, treatment, prevention, 310
  food handing, 314
  household disinfection, 315
  hygiene promotion, 315
  prevention, 313–314
  prevention programs targeting, 316
  risk factors, transmission, 311–313
  sanitation, waste management, 314–315
  surveillance, outbreak detection, 316–318
  vaccination, 316
  Zimbabwe, 2008, 330–332
diarrheal diseases, case management, 319–320
  bed requirement estimation, 321
  case fatality rate (CFR), 322
  cases expected determination, 320–321
  cholera treatment center (CTC), 320
  cholera treatment unit (CTU), 320
  community information, education, communication, 321–322
  fluid requirements estimation, 321
  oral rehydration point (ORP), 320
diarrheal diseases, epidemic prone enteric diseases
  cholera, 323–325
  cholera treatment, 328–329
  diagnosis, 326–327
  shigella dysenteria type 1, 325
  treatment, 327–328
  typhoid fever, 325–326
  typhoid fever treatment, 329
diarrheal diseases, special considerations, 315
  funerals, 313
  prisons, orphanages, military barracks, enclosed quarters, 313

Index

diarrheal diseases outbreak response.
  control, 318
  initial investigation, 318–319
  response organization, objectives, 319
diarrheal diseases outbreak surveillance, monitoring/evaluation
  data analysis, attack rate (AR), 322
  data analysis, case fatality rate (CFR), 322
  data analysis, weekly incidence rate (WIR), 322
  data collection, 322
Diaz, J. H., 63
Dick, M. H., 326
disaster risk management cycle, 38–39
disaster risk reduction (DRR)
  development, 285
  Global Platform, 286–287
  health care systems, 287–288
  health facilities, 288–289
  Hyogo Framework for Action (HFA), 286
  International Strategy for Disaster Reduction (ISDR), 285–286
  origins, 284
  post-2015 framework, 287
  public health, 289
  risk management, health, 289
disaster risk reduction (DRR), challenges
  coordination, implementation, 291
  limited resources, 290–291
disaster risk reduction (DRR), implementation
  local communities, 290
  national governments, 289–290
  private sector, 290
disasters
  classification of, 1–2
  complex emergencies, 2
  disease, epidemics and, 2
  fragile states and, 1
  impact, vulnerability and, 1
  incidence of, 1
  industrial, 2
  onset of, 2
  sudden onset, 2
  UNISDR definition, 1
diseases, vaccine preventable
  decision framework, goal, 227–228
Docey, 443
Dolan, C., 168
donors, 274
Doocy, D., 463
Doocy, S., 61, 62, 442
Doolan, D. L., 351
Dossa, N. I., 416
Dreibelbis, R., 151

Dubus, B., 55
Ducusin, M. J., 390
Duffield, M., 6, 7, 20
Durant, H., 10–11
Durheim, D. N., 387, 390
Dye, T. D., 376

edematous malnutrition, Kwashiorkor, 362–363
Edwards, M. S., 402
Eftekhari, A., 416
Ejemot-Nwadiaro, R. I., 150
Ellsberg, M., 200
emergency medical teams (EMT) initiative, 42
emergency settlements, 262–263
emergency shelter, 261–262
emergency shelter kits, 261
emergency tents, 262
engineering, relief worker guide, 259
Ennis, J. G., 349
epidemiology
  affected populations, 55
  armed conflict, direct/indirect consequences, 63
  background, 53
  Dafur, 65
  Haiti, 62, 66
  indicators, 54
  infectious diseases, 61
  injury, non-communicable diseases, mental health, 61–64
  morbidity indicators, 59–60
  mortality, morbidity causes, 59–61
  mortality rates, 57–59
  public health impact, selected disasters, 59–61
  Rwanda, 65–66
  trends, use of, 53
epidemiology, persons affected numbers
  conflicts, 56–57
  natural disasters, 55–56
Eriksson, C. B., 418, 419
Ernst, E., 306
Estrada Garcia, T., 312
ethics of humanitarianism, 70. *See also* research ethics
Ethiopia, 17–18
European Community Humanitarian Office (ECHO), 30, 49
Evans, J., 461, 462
Evelyn-Depoortere, V. B., 65, 246
Ezard, N., 465

Fackler, M. L., 445
family planning, 205–206
Farré, S., 9, 16
Faul, M., 444, 450
Fazel, M., 409

fertility, family planning, 200–201
Fields, B. S., 306
Fijen, C. A., 401
File, T. M., 296
Fillol, F., 351
Fischer, M., 401
Fischer Walker, C. L., 310
Foley, M., 9, 12
Fonseca, V. A., 465
food aid, 192
Food and Agricultural Organization (FAO), 15
food cash, vouchers, 192–193
Food for Peace, 15
food handing, 314
food security
  globally, 181
  household livelihoods and, 182
  International Food Policy Research Institute (IFPRI) Global Hunger Index, 181–182
  Millennium Development Goal 1, 182
  Pakistan, 2010, 195–196
  UN Food and Agriculture Organization (FAO) definition, 181
food security, challenges
  context analysis, 188–189
food security, livelihood resilience, 187
  health, 187
  livelihood resilience, 187–188
food security, emergency interventions
  crop protection, 193–194
  crop recovery, 194–195
  food aid, 192
  food cash, vouchers, 192–193
  immediate needs, food assistance, 191–192
  livelihood protection, 193
  livelihood recovery, 194
  livelihood value chain protection, 194
  livelihoods needs assessments, 189–190
  livestock protection, 193
  livestock recovery, 194
  needs identified, response, 191
  value chain recovery, 195
food security, four pillars
  accessibility, 183–184
  availability, 183
  supply stability, 184
  utilization, 184
food security, livelihood resilience, 187
food security, risks
  accessibility, 186
  availability, 184–186

Index

supply stability, 186–187
utilization, 186
Foote, A., 147
Ford, N., 73, 74
Foulds, S. A., 444
Frechtling, J., 128
Fuller, I. A., 145
funerals, 313

Gage, A. J., 417
Gagnidze, I., 429
Gallagher, M., 380
Gallefoss, 427
Gallo, R. C., 336
Garcia-Pando, C. P., 401
Garfield, R. M., 64, 88
Gayer, M., 109, 297
Gele, A. A., 428
gender based violence (GBV), 205
Geneva Convention, 11
Genthon, A., 443
Giovino, G. A., 461
Githui, W. A., 428
Gladish, S. L., 444
global food security. *See* food security
Global Platform, 286–287
global response, 461
Golden, M. H., 168, 176, 362, 363, 364, 377
Goldman, A., 442
Goodson, J. L., 388
Goodwin, R., 408
Goossens, S., 170
Gorstein, J., 171
governmental organizations, funding agencies, 29–30
Graham, S. M., 306
Grais, R. F., 239, 392, 393
Granoff, D. M., 405
Greenwood, B., 400
Grellety, E., 364
Griffith, D. C., 312
Griffiths, K., 336, 337, 343
Grijalva-Eternod, C. S., 169, 465
Groce, N., 146
Guerin, P. J., 320, 322, 325
Guerrero, S., 367, 375
Guerrier, G., 389
Guevart, E., 313
Guha-Sapir, D., 55, 57, 62, 63, 64
Gunnlaugsson, G., 313, 315
Gutchinson, P. L., 417

Hadzibegovic, D. S., 427
Haelterman, E., 400
Hailey, P., 380
Haiti, 62, 66
Haiti, 2010, 89, 118, 359
Hallam, A. H., 122, 133

Halperin, S. A., 400
Hanquet, G., 441, 450
Hanson, B. W., 345
Hargreaves, S., 430
Harries, A. D., 464
Harris, J. B., 390
Harvey, P., 144, 147, 254
Haskew, C., 395
Hatem, M., 416
Health and Nutrition Tracking Service (HNTS), 83
health events prioritization, 110–111
Hehenkamp, A., 430
Heijnen, M., 144
Heldal, E., 430
HelpAge International, 31
Helwig-Larsen, K., 446
Henry, K. L., 455
Hermansson, A. C., 455
Heymann, D. L., 297, 388, 389, 390, 391
Heymann, S. N., 228, 229, 230, 231, 232, 233
Hicks, M. H., 446
High Commissioner for Refugees (HCR), 12
Hilhorst, D., 21
Hill, K., 200–201, 206
Hinsley, D. E., 446
Hinton, D. E., 416
HIV patients, acute malnutrition, 373
HIV/Aids, 204–205
Hodge, J. G., 73
Hoge, C. W., 445
Holder, Y. M., 449
Holguín-Veras, P. E., 270
Holmes, J., 286
Holmgren, J., 232
Holtz, T. H., 418
Horan, J. M., 450
Hornik, R. C., 153
Hossain, M., 441, 446
host nation, 272–273
hosting support, 264
House, S., 146
house repairs, 264–265
household disinfection, 315
Howe, P., 174
Hrabac, B., 427
Hu, F. B., 461
Hulland, K., 149
human immunodeficiency virus (HIV)
 clinical presentation, 340–341
 Democratic Republic of the Congo (DRC), 345
 diagnosis, 341
 effective treatment, 336
 epidemiology, risk factors, transmission, 336–337
 informed consent, 341–342

prevention, 337–340
quality assurance, diagnosis, 342
surveillance, 340
treatment, 342–344
treatment program preparedness, humanitarian emergencies, 344–345
virology, antibody tests, 341
humanitarian emergencies
 definition, scope of, 2–3
 Inter-Agency Standing Committee (IASC), 3
 OCHA Handbook, 6–7
 population displacement, 4–6
humanitarian emergencies, models, 64
 developed countries, 65
 developing countries, 64
 smoldering, chronic countries, 64–65
humanitarian emergencies, phases
 acute emergency phase, 4
 crude mortality rate (CMR) and, 4
 post-emergency phase, 4
 pre-emergency phase, 3–4
 recovery phase, 4
humanitarian movement
 history, 9
 19th century, 10–11
 prior to 19th century, 9–10
 religious tradition and, 9–10
 20th century, 11–21
 21st century, 21–22
humanitarian organizations
 categories, 25
 resources, 25
 types, 25
humanitarian organizations, UN
 Food and Agricultural Organization, 27
 Inter-Agency Standing Committee (IASC), 26
 Office for the Coordination of Humanitarian Affairs (OCHA), 26
 Office of the United Nations High Commissioner for Human Rights (OHCHR), 28
 United Nations Children's Fund (UNICEF), 26–27
 United Nations Development Programme (UNDP), 27–28
 United Nations High Commissioner for Refugees (UNHCR), 26
 United Nations Population Fund (UNFPA), 27
 World Food Programme (WFP), 27
 World Health Organization (WHO), 27

477

Index

humanitarian principles
  humanity, 36
  impartiality, 36
  independence, 36
  neutrality, 36
humanitarian professionalism
  independence, 36
Humanitarian Response Review (HRR) recommendations, 44
humanitarian supply chain, 273–274
Humphries, V., 44, 47
Hunt, M., 68
Hunter, P. R., 230, 400
Husain, F., 150, 410
Hutson, R. A., 417
hygiene. *See* water, sanitation, hygiene
hygiene promotion, 315
Hyman, S., 204
Hynes, M., 199, 200
Hyogo Framework for Action, 50
Hyogo Framework for Action (HFA), 286
hypertension, 460

Imanishi, M., 325
implementation delays, 115
Imran, 140, 141, 142
inconsistent reporting, 116
in-country processing, 277–278
indicator minimization, 110
indoor residual spraying (IRS), 355–356
infants, 365
  with acute malnutrition, 373
Initial Rapid Assessment (IRA), 83
injuries and trauma, 441
  coordination, 454
  disaster preparedness, 447
  emergency health system management, 450
  evacuation, 453–454
  health information system, 448
  injury surveillance system, 449–450
  long term consequences, 454–455
  mental health, 455
  physical disability, rehabilitation, 455
  public health activities, 447
  rapid needs assessment, 447
  referral system, 450
  societal violence, 455–456
  triage, 450–453
  wound care, tetanus immunization, 454
injuries and trauma, epidemiology, 441
  ballistics injuries, 445–446
  blast injuries, 444–445
  earthquakes, 442–443
  environmental injuries, 446–447
  interpersonal violence, 446
  inundations, floods, tsunamis, 443–444
  war, conflict, 444
  wind disasters, 441–442
Inoue, Y., 444
inpatient stabalization center, 370–371
InterAction, 29
Interagency Emergency Health Kit (IEHK), 469
Inter-Agency Standing Committee (IASC), UN, 20
  Transformative Agenda, 22
international assistance, 38
International Center for Migration and Health and Development (ICMHD), 31
International Committee of the Red Cross (ICRC), 10–11, 28
International Federation of Red Cross and Red Crescent Societies (IFRC), 12, 28
International Federation of the Red Cross and Red Crescent Movement (IFRC), 49
International Food Policy Research Institute (IFPRI) Global Hunger Index, 181–182
International Medical Corps Worldwide (IMC), 31–32
International Monetary Fund (IMF), 13
International Movement for Migration (IOM), 29
international non-governmental organizations (NGOs), 31–33
International Red Cross and Red Crescent Movement, 21, 28
International Refugee Organization (ICO), 14
International Rescue Committee, 32
International Search and Rescue Advisory Group (INSARAG), 43–44
International Strategy for Disaster Reduction (ISDR), 285–286
inventory management, 279–280
iodine, 378–379
iron deficiency anemia, 378
Isanaka, S., 372
Islam, M. A., 142
Islamic Relief Worldwide (IRW), 32
Israel, A. D., 380
Ivers, L. C., 233
Iwane, M. K., 296

Jackson, B. R., 328–329
Jamieson, D. J., 199
Jamison, D. T., 460
Jarvis, 431
Jeffreys, M., 416

Jennings, B., 69
Jeremijenko, A., 234
Johnson, L. F., 336
Jones, K., 415
Jong, E. C., 295
Jordon, 2013, 435–436
Juan-Giner, A., 239

Kadir, K., 140, 141
Kagwanja, P. M., 244
Kahn, 379
Kahn, J. S., 296
Kaiser, R., 229, 391, 396
Kalter, H., 199
Kamadjeu, R., 230
Kamat, D., 238
Kamugisha, C., 229, 389, 391, 394
Kandji, S., 201
Kanj, S. S., 240
Karakochuk, C., 370
Keddy, K. L., 327
Kenya, 2006, 307
Kerac, M., 169, 365, 372
Kerneis, S., 322, 325
Kessler, R. C., 409
Keus, K., 430
Khader, A., 465
Khan, A. A., 234
Khara, T., 168
Kim, C., 306
Kimbrough, W., 427
Kinzie, J. D., 417
Kipp, A. M., 428
Klein, B. P., 370
Knowlton, L. M., 443
Kohrt, B. A., 411, 455
Kolbe, A. R., 417
Kolves, K., 455
Kotloff, K. L., 310
Kouadio, K., 387, 388, 389, 392, 393, 454
Kouchner, B., 16
Kovacs, P., 285
Kremastinou, J., 401
Kriss, J. L., 390
Kriz, P. M., 401
Kulin, H. E., 364
Kutty, P., 394
Kwasnicka, D., 149

Lam, E., 386, 390
Lambert, R., 259
Lancet, 418
Lantagne, D. S., 141, 142, 313, 314
Lautze, S., 43
Lawn, J. E., 199, 204, 206, 208
Layover, J. P., 280
League of Nations, 12
League of Red Cross Societies, 12
Leaning, J., 64, 462

Leborgne, P., 378
Lee, K., 467
Lee, L., 72
Leibovici, D., 444
Levey, T., 313
Levin, M. J., 304, 305
Levine, M. M., 312, 327
Levy, J. A., 336
Lewis, C., 415
Liberia, 2007, 209–210
Liddle, B., 430
Lim, J. H., 444
Lim, S. S., 460, 461
Liu, L., 199, 310, 386
Liu, W., 349
livelihood
 needs assessments, 189–190
 protection, 193
 recovery, 194
 resilience, 187–188
 value chain protection, 194
livestock
 protection, 193
 recovery, 194
Ljubic, 427
Lo, J., 465, 467
local and national humanitarian partners, 33
local response, 37–38
logistics
 definition, 270
 goal, 270
logistics, challenges
 damaged infrastructure, 281
 Indonesia, 2009, 281–282
 language, cultural differences, 281
 limited resources, 281
 neutrality, 281
 unsolicited donations, 280
logistics, commercial vs. humanitarian, 270–271
 assessments, 275
 chain of custody, medical commodities, 280
 cold chain, medical commodities, 278
 commodities movement, essential medicines, 276
 commodities movement, kits, 275–276
 coordination, 272
 dispatch, 280
 donors, 274
 host nation, 272–273
 humanitarian supply chain, 273–274
 in-country processing, 277–278
 inventory management, 279–280
 Logistics Cluster Approach, 272
 personnel deployment, 276–277
 pre-deployment processing, equipment, 277
 prepositioning, 275
 procurement, 274–275
 professionalism, 271–272
 safety, security, 278
 warehousing, 278–279
Logistics Cluster Approach, 272
Loharikar, A., 323
long lasting insecticide treated nets (LLIN), 354–355
long-term needs, budgets, 268–269
Lönnroth, K., 428
Lopes Cardozo, B., 409, 410–412, 418, 419
Lopez, A. D., 408
Lossio, R., 443
Lovon, M., 89
Lozano, R., 296, 460
Lubbers, R., 200
Lu-Peng, Z., 443
Luque Fernandez, M. A., 331
Luquero, F. J., 233, 316
Lutterloh, E., 325
Lynch, C., 470

MacDonald, G., 125, 128
Machel, G., 225
Mackintosh, K., 15
MacQueen, K. M., 73
Mahamud, A., 61, 389, 391, 393
Maher, D., 464
Maine, D., 203
Makoka, D., 166
Malaney, P., 348
malaria
 case definitions, indicators, 353
 clinical malaria overview, 356–357
 complicated (severe) malaria, 357
 control, prevention, 351–352, 354–356
 disease burden, 349–351
 Haiti, 2010, 359
 health services, 352
 indoor residual spraying (IRS), 355–356
 life cycle, transmission, 348–349
 long lasting insecticide treated nets (LLIN), 354–355
 outbreak response, 354
 prevalence, 348
 surveillance, 352–353
 surveillance limitations, 353–354
 treatment, 349–351
malaria, diagnosis
 clinical diagnosis, 358
 microscopy, 357
 rapid diagnostic tests (RDT), 357–358

Malfait, P., 377
Mallonee, S., 450
malnutrition. *See also* nutrition
malnutrition, acute
 Complicated Severe Acute Malnutrition (SAM), 363
 edematous malnutrition, Kwashiorkor, 362–363
 wasting, Maramus, 362
malnutrition, diagnosis and classification
 adults, 364–365
 children 6–59 months, MUAC, 364
 children 6–59 months, weight-for-height, 363–364
 infants, 365
 older children, adolescents, 364
 pregnant, lactating women, 365
malnutrition, micronutrient malnutrition, 375–376
 vitamin A deficiency, 376
 vitamin B (thiamin) deficiency, 376–377
 vitamin B2 (riboflavin) deficiency, 377
 vitamin B3/PP (niacin) deficiency, 377
 vitamin C deficiency, scurvy, 377–378
malnutrition, mineral deficiencies
 iodine, 378–379
 iron deficiency anemia, 378
 zinc, 379
malnutrition, monitoring and evaluation
 coverage, 375
 defaulter rate, 374
 mortality rate, 374
 non-recovery rate, 374–375
 performance statistics, 373–375
 recovery rate, 373–375
malnutrition, treatment and management, 365
 acute malnutrition, community-based management (CMAM), 365–366
 adolescents, adults, older people, 373
 community mobilization, outreach, 366–368
 emotional, physical stimulation, 372
 HIV patients, acute malnutrition, 373
 infants with acute malnutrition, 373
 inpatient stabilization center, 370–371
 medical treatment, therapeutic care, 372
 medical treatment, tSFPs, 368–370

malnutrition, treatment (cont.)
  national health systems and, 380–381
  nutritional treatment, outpatient therapeutic programs, 371–372
  outpatient therapeutic care, 370
  patient discharge, 372
  prevention, treatment, 379–380
  targeted supplementary feeding programs (tSFPs), 368–370
  treatment programs, strategic shift, 380
Maloney, S. A., 428
Manary, M. J., 372
Marc Laforce, F., 402
Marsh, M., 446
Martins, N., 425
Martone, G., 462
maternal, newborn health, 202–204
maternal morbidity, mortality, 198–199
Mathison, S., 128
Mati, E., 306
Maxwell, D. G., 9–10, 11, 12, 13, 14, 15, 16, 17, 18, 19, 22, 189, 190–191
Mayo-Wilson, E., 379
M'Boussa, J., 427, 428
McCall, M., 419
McCall, V., 50
McDonald, S. M., 53
McGinn, T., 198, 201
McMurray, D. N., 429
McNallly, L. M., 297
measles
  case fatality rate (CFR), 389
  clinical presentation, 387–388
  epidemiology, 388
  eradication, 386
  outbreaks, 386–387
  risk, vaccine introduction, 386
  risk assessment, 389–390
  risk factors, 388–389
measles, outbreak preparedness and response
  treatment, 393
  vaccination campaigns, 391–393
  vaccination strategies, 391
  vaccine, 389–391
measles, surveillance, 393–394
  case-based, 394
  community-based, 395
  Early Warning and Response Network (EWARN), 394–395
  Global Measles and Rubella Laboratory Network (GMRLN), 394
  Health Information System (HIS), 395
  Horn of Africa, 2010, 395–396

Medair International, 32
Meddings, D. R., 7, 446
Médecins Sans Frontières (MSF), 16–17, 32–33
"A Memory of Solferino" (Durant), 11
Mendelsohn, J., 200
meningitis
  Central Africa Republic (CAR), 2013, 405
  classification, 400
  clinical presentation, course, 402
  diagnosis, 402–403
  epidemiology, meningitis belt, 400
  outbreak response, 405
  prevention, 402
  risk factors, 401–402
  surveillance, outbreak detection, 403–405
  treatment, 403
Mensaes, R., 427, 428
mental health
  burden of disease, 408–409
  chronic disease, 417
  gender-based violence, women's health, 417–418
  Global Burden of Disease Study, 408
  international humanitarian aid workers, 418–419
  Kosovo, 1999, 420
  mental health and psychosocial (MHPS) needs, 409–412
  national humanitarian aid workers, 419
  suicide, 408
mental health, best practices
  emergency risk communication, 412
  guidelines, 412–413
mental health, DST mental health disorders treatment, 415
  depression, anxiety, 415
  post traumatic stress disorder (PATS), acute stress disorder (ADS), 416–417
mental health, humanitarian aid workers, 418
mental health, risk and mitigating factors
  community, 409
  individual, 409
mental health, treatment approaches
  community, 414
  counseling, 414–415
  mental health care integration, 413–414
Michaels, A. J., 455
military and paramilitary humanitarian support, 33–34
military forces, 50
Millennium Development Goal 1, 182
Mills, E., 455

Minimum Initial Service Package (MISP), 201–202
Miskin, I. N., 444
Mitchell, T., 288, 291
Mitka, M., 444
Mollica, R. F., 408, 409, 410–411, 417
monitoring, evaluation
  challenges, limitations, 131–133
  data collection, sources, 126–127
  evaluation methods, 122–123
  evaluation vs. monitoring, 123–124
  evaluations vs. assessment, 124–125
  Kenya, 2012, 133
  key initiatives, 122
  methods, 126–127
  OECD-DAC definitions, 123–124
  public health program evaluation, framework, 125
  purposes, examples, 125–127
  results, dissemination, recommendations, 130–131
  standards, indicators, criteria selection, 128–130
Montclos, M. A. P. D., 244
Moodley, K., 239
Moore, J., 207
Moore, P. S., 311, 400, 401, 402
Morgan, O., 37
Morgenstern, S., 11
Morinière, L., 127
Morof, D. F., 200, 208, 323, 395
Morris, E. K., 167–168
mortality system, data sources, 111
Mosler, H. J., 157
Munford, R. S., 401
Mupere, E., 391
Murray, C. J., 408
Murray, E. J., 428
Myanmar, 2008, 88–89
Myatt, M., 375
myths and realities, 37

Nackers, F., 370
Naheed, A., 325
Nair, H., 296
Nakkash, R., 467
Nandy, R., 36, 59, 63, 441
Nathoo, K. J., 297
Naugle, D. A., 153
Navarro-Colorado, C., 229, 364, 389, 391, 393, 396
Nawaz, J., 157
Nayak, S., 444
Ndekha, M., 370
Ndongosieme, A., 430
Neal, D., 151
needs assessment, 79
needs assessment, challenges, 86–87
  agreement on indicators, 88
  information overload, 87–88

Index

needs assessment, common (CNA), 80–81
  public health survey methodologies, 81
  quality, challenges, 81
needs assessment, information
  accuracy *vs.* precision, 82
  original, secondary data, 82–83
  valuable, 81–82
needs assessment, objectives
  response decisions influence, 79
  response decisions justification, appeal for funds, 79–80
needs assessment, tools
  Assessment Capacities Project (ACAPS), 84–86
  Health and Nutrition Tracking Service (HNTS), 83
  Initial Rapid Assessment (IRA), 83
  multi-cluster/sector initial rapid assessment (MIRA), 84–85
  phases specific assessment tools, 83–84
neighborhood approach, 266
Neil, K. P., 325
Nelson, E. J., 232, 329
neonatal morbidity, mortality, 199
Newell, M., 340
Ng, M., 460
Nichols, E. K., 169
Nieburg, P., 23
Nigeria, 2012, 118–119
1951 Refugee Convention, 14
Nizame, F. A., 151
Noji, E. K., 23, 37, 288
non-communicable diseases (NCDs)
  care delivery, 469
  continuity of care, 461–462
  diabetes, 461
  global response, 461
  guidance, Sphere Project, 468–469
  hypertension, 460
  incidence, global burden, 460
  medications, Interagency Emergency Health Kit (IEHK), 469
  medications, supplies, equipment, 463–464
  nutrition, 463
  preparedness, response, 462–463
  prevention, 465–467
  public health data, 468
  surveillance, monitoring, 464–465
  Syria, 2014, 470–471
  tobacco use, 460–461
  treatment, 467–468
non-governmental organizations (NGOs), 48–49
Nordquist, K.-Å., 7
nutrition
  Africa, 2016, 177–178
  emergency nutrition agencies, 162–164
  non-governmental organizations, 164
  nutritional, food security emergencies classification, 174
  nutritional crisis, 172–173
  UN agencies, 162–164
nutrition, epidemiology
  malnutrition, 168–169
  overnutrition, 169
nutrition, malnutrition types
  acute, 166–167
  chronic, 167–168
  malnutrition definitions, 167
  micronutrient malnutrition, 168
  stunting-wasting linkages, 168
  underweight, 168
nutrition, nutrients and food groups
  food groups, 162
  macronutrients, 161
  malnutrition causes, 163
  micronutrients, 161–162
nutrition, nutritional status measurement
  anthropometry, body parameters, MUAC, 169–170
  community mobilization, screening, 170
  population nutritional status assessment, 170–172
  rapid assessment (RA), 171
  surveillance, 171–172
  surveys, 171
nutrition, risk factors
  malnutrition-infection cycle, 165
  seasonalitiy, 166
  social, care environment, 166
  vulnerable populations, 164–165
  water, sanitation, hygiene, health services, 165–166
nutrition response, control
  Blanket Supplementary Feeding Program (BSFP), 173–175
  complementary feeding, 176–177
  infant and young child feeding (IYCF), 175–176
  micronutrient supplementation, 177

O'Brien, K. L., 297
Oeltmann, J. E., 428
Office for the Coordination of Humanitarian Affairs (OCHA), UN, 43
Office of US Foreign Disaster Assistance (OFDA), 49
O'Heir, J., 198, 199
O'Laughlin, K. N., 341
Oliver, M. L., 133
Olofin, I., 167, 168
oral rehydration point (ORP), 320
overcrowding, 266
Owais, A., 239

Page, A. L., 326
Pakistan, 2008, 89
Pakistan, 2010, 89, 118, 195–196
Palmieri, D., 11
Panjabi, 298, 299
Paquet, C., 66, 229, 388
Parekh, B. S., 342
Park, S. E., 380
Parry, C. M., 325
partner coordination, 117
Patel, D., 147, 223
Patel, M. P., 370
Patel, P., 337
Pelling, M., 285, 287
Perez-Exposito, A. B., 370
performance, non-standard reporting forms, 115
Perry, R. T., 386, 394
personnel deployment, 276–277
pest infestations, 267
Petevi, M., 412
Pettersson, T., 1, 7
Philippines, 2013, 118–119
Phillips, R. M., 152
Pickering, A. J., 151
Pickering, L. K., 228, 230, 233, 388
Plotkin, S. A., 231, 232, 394
Pluess, B., 355
Poenaru, D., 455
Pollitzer, R., 314
Polonsky, J. A., 60, 61, 228, 300
Porta, M. I., 233
Potts, M., 201
Powers, H. J., 377
pre-deployment processing, equipment, 277
pregnant, lactating women, 365
prepositioning, 275
prisons, orphanages, military barracks, enclosed quarters, 313
procurement, 274–275
professionalism, 271–272
protection
  background, 214–215
  do's, don'ts, 221
  frameworks, 217–218
  in humanitarian setting, 214
  interventions, 217
protection, child-focused needs, 224
  key actions, 225
  UN Security Council Resolution 1612, 225–226
  UN Security Council Resolution 1882, 226

protection, child-focused (cont.)
  violations monitoring, reporting, 225
protection, gender-based violence (GBV), 218–219
  key actions, compassionate/ confidential treatment, 219
  key actions, forensic evidence collection, 219–220
  key actions, physical examination, 219
  key actions, prepare survivor, 219
  psychosocial distress and, 220
protection, key groups
  internally displaced persons, 215
  refugees, 215
  stateless, 216
protection, mental health and psychosocial support (MHPSS), 220–221
  alcohol, substance abuse, 224
  community mobilization, support, 221
  essential knowledge, 223
  health information systems (HIS), 224
  institutionalized persons, 224
  other healing systems linkage, 224
  psychological considerations, 221–223
  psychotropic medications, 223
  severe mental illness, health care, 223
protection, principles
  available resources, capacities, 216–217
  do no harm, 216
  human rights, equity, 216
  participation, 217
Prudhon, C., 59
public health action, 116
public health response, 21st century, 22–23
Puett, C., 367

Qadri, F., 312

Ragunathan, L., 402
Ramdas, K. N., 417
Rapsomaniki, E., 460
Reichhold, U., 215
Reis, 325
relative humidity (RH), 267
Rencoret, N., 89
reproductive health (RH)
  abortion care, 204
  adolescents, 206
  concepts, refugee populations, 201
  family planning, 205–206

fertility, family planning, 200–201
gender based violence (GBV), 205
glossary of terms, 210
HIV/Aids, 204–205
Liberia, 2007, 209–210
maternal, newborn health, 202–204
Minimum Initial Service Package (MISP), 201–202
reproductive health (RH), challenges and controversies
  programs, 207
  research, data collection, 206–207
reproductive health (RH), epidemiology
  maternal morbidity, mortality, 198–199
  neonatal morbidity, mortality, 199
reproductive health (RH), next steps
  programs, 208
  research, 207–208
Republic of Biafra, 15–16
Requejo, J. H., 199, 204
research ethics, 69–70
  beneficence, 70
  justice, 70
  respect for persons, 70
research ethics, challenges and controversies
  decision making considerations, 72–73
  research gaps, 73
  research in emergencies, 70–72
  research vs. non-research, 73–74
response
  Australian Aid, 49
  Centers for Disease Control and Prevention (CDC), 50
  complex humanitarian emergencies (CHE), 35–36
  coordination, 43–44
  Department for International Development (DFID), UK, 49
  displaced populations, 36
  emergency medical teams (EMT) initiative, 42
  European Community Humanitarian Office (ECHO), 49
  government agencies, 49–50
  healthcare/clinical response organizations, 42
  humanitarian relief organizations, 47–50
  Hyogo Framework for Action, 50
  international organizations, 49
  International Search and Rescue Advisory Group (INSARAG), 43–44
  military forces, 50
  non-governmental organizations (NGOs), 48–49

Office for the Coordination of Humanitarian Affairs (OCHA), UN, 43
Office of US Foreign Disaster Assistance (OFDA), 49
public organizations, 40–42
rapid onset natural disasters, 35
slow onset natural disasters, 35
Transformative Agenda, 50
United Nations Disaster Assessment and Coordination (UNDAC), 43–44
United Nations organizations, 48
WHO Emergency Response Network, 48
response, cluster approach
  country level, 45–47
  criticism, challenges, 47
  global level, 45
  Humanitarian Response Review (HRR) recommendations, 44
  lead agencies and, 44
response priorities, 39
Reynolds, B., 412
Rezaeian, M., 446
Riaz, H., 239
Roberts, B., 59, 417, 441, 444, 446, 465, 467
Robertson, R. C., 314
Rodrigues, L. C., 431
Rogers, E., 367, 375
Roosevelt, Franklin, 13, 15
Rosborough, S., 323
Rose, B., 414
Rothbaum, B. O., 416
Rotheray, K. R., 441
Rottman, S. J., 461, 462
Rouzier, V., 233
Roy, S., 446
Ruby, A., 465
Rudan, I., 297
Rwanda, 19, 65–66
Rysaback-Smith, H., 11, 15
Rysstad, O. G., 427

Sabin, C. A., 340
Sabin, M., 409
Sachs, J., 348
Sadler, K., 370
safety, security, 278
Salama, P., 165, 229, 391, 419
Sanahuja, H., 290
sanitation. See water, sanitation, hygiene
sanitation, waste management, 314–315
Santaniella-Newton, A., 230, 400
Sarivalasis, A., 428
Save the Children Fund (SCF), 12–13, 33

Sazawal, S., 378, 379
Schaible Ue, K. S., 165
Schipper, L., 285, 287
Schopper, D., 74
Schuller, M., 313
Schwartz, L., 72, 285
Seal, A. J., 379
Sejvar, L., 325
Selen, A., 379
Semrau, M., 89
Sen, A., 17
Sen, K., 470
Setchell, C. A., 268
settlement camps. *See* camp management
settlements approach, 258
Shah, D., 379
Sharara, S. L., 240
Sharp, T. W., 311
Shear, M. K., 417
Shears, P., 389
Sheik, M., 418
shelter and settlements (SS)
    assistance activities, Disaster Risk Reduction (DRR), 259–261
    engineering, relief worker guide, 259
    health linkage, 258–259
    long-term needs, budgets, 268–269
    settlements approach, 258
    Sphere Project, 259
shelter and settlements, emergency assistance
    emergency settlements, 262–263
    emergency shelter, 261–262
    emergency shelter kits, 261
    emergency tents, 262
shelter and settlements, healthy shelter/settlements, 266
    containments, 268
    neighborhood approach, 266
    overcrowding, 266
    pest infestations, 267
    relative humidity (RH), 267
    temperature, 267–268
    ventilation issues, 266–267
shelter and settlements, traditional assistance
    hosting support, 264
    house repairs, 264–265
    technical assistance, 265
    traditional shelter, 263–264
    transfers assistance, 265
    Transit Centers (TC), 265–266
    transitional settlements, 265
Shi, Y., 461
shigella dysenteria type 1, 325
Shikanga, O. T., 323
Short, Clare, 21
Shulman, S. T., 306
Shultz, A., 312

Shultz, J. M., 416, 442
Sida, L., 127
Siddique, A. K., 109
Simoes, E. A. F., 295, 306
Sledjeski, E. M., 417
Slim, H., 214, 215
slow onset natural disasters, 35
Small, M. J., 417
Smillie, I., 16
Smith, 431
Smith, M. B., 122, 126, 127
Somalia, 2011, 118
Sommer, A., 376
Sondorp, E., 461
Sozzi, E., 155
Spangaro, J., 208
Sphere Handbook, 40
Sphere Project, 21, 39–40, 259
Spiegel, P., 59, 200, 337, 351, 417, 462, 463, 465, 469
Spitzer, C., 417
Staveteig, S., 201
Steele, S., 128
Steketee, R. W., 23
Stelmach, R. D., 136
Stevens, D., 295, 376
Stoianova, V., 89
Strebel, P. M., 386, 387, 390
Sugerman, D. E., 446
Sugimoto, J. D., 442
Sullivent, E. E., 63, 444
Sumner, S. A., 312
Sun Tzu, 10
surveillance
    activities, system components, 112
    case definition, 112
    coordination, 111
    data analysis, 113–114
    global health security and, 117
    Somalia, 2011, 118
surveillance challenges, potential pitfalls, 114
    case definitions, inconsistent application, 116
    data analysis, interpretation, 116
    data collection, 93
    data collection, active surveillance, 113
    data collection, passive surveillance, 113
    data collection coverage, exhaustive/universal, 113
    data collection coverage, sentinel, 113
    data interpretation, dissemination, 114
    data reporting, transmission, 113
    data sources, 112–113
    early implementation, 110
    exit strategy, 111

Haiti, 2010, 118
health events prioritization, 110–111
implementation delays, 115
inconsistent reporting, 116
indicator minimization, 110
laboratory support, 117
mortality system, data sources, 111
Nigeria, 2012, 118–119
overview, methods, goal, 109–110
Pakistan, 2010, 118
partner coordination, 117
performance, non-standard reporting forms, 115
Philippines, 2013, 118–119
public health action, 116
simplicity, flexibility, acceptance, 111
Somalia, 2011, 118
supplies, logistical support, 117
syndromic, 111
Syria, 2012, 119–120
untimely reporting, 115–116
Sutiono, A. B., 326
Swerdlow, D. L., 323, 328–329
Swiss, S., 200
Syria, 2012, 119–120
Syria, 2013, 89
Syria, 2014, 470–471

Tam, C. W. C., 408
Tam, V., 444
Tappero, J., 288
targeted supplementary feeding programs (tSFPs), 368–370
Tauxe, R., 288
Taylor, D. L., 153
Taylor-Powell, E., 128
temperature, 267–268
Terre des Hommes International Federation, 33
Teutsch, S., 110
Tewolderberha, D., 380
Thacker, S. B., 109
Thaddeus, S., 203
Thiele, B., 258
Thieren, M., 69
Thomas, C. F., 297
Thompson, M. J., 402
Thornberry, T. P., 455
Titeca, K., 467
tobacco use, 460–461
Tol, W. A., 414
Tomczyk, B., 200, 209
Toole, M. J., 18, 23, 37, 39, 59, 60, 109, 228, 229, 386, 391
traditional shelter, 263–264
transfers assistance, 265
Transformative Agenda, 50
Transformative Agenda (IASC), 22

483

Index

Transit Centers (TC), 265–266
transitional settlements, 265
trauma. *See* injuries and trauma
treatment programs, strategic shift, 380
tuberculosis (TB)
 Jordon, 2013, 436
 Kenya, 2007–2008, 437
 monitoring, evaluation, 435–436
 Philippines, 2013, 437
 Syria, 2014, 437
tuberculosis (TB), clinical course
 diagnosis, treatment, 429–430
 infection *vs.* disease, 428–429
 signs, symptoms, 429
 stigma, 428
tuberculosis (TB), control
 contingency planning, 433–435
 disruptions to ongoing programs, 433
 implementation criteria, 432
 implementation steps, 432–433
 Jordon, 2013, 435–436
 need identification criteria, 432
 strategy, guidelines, tools, 431–432
tuberculosis (TB), epidemiology
 contributing factors, 428
 emergency affected populations, 426–428
 global, 425–426
tuberculosis (TB), prevention
 healthcare setting, 431
 individual, 430
 infant, 430–431
Turner, P., 297, 299
Turpie, I. D., 428
typhoid fever, 325–326
 treatment, 329

UN Food and Agriculture Organization (FAO) definition, 181
UN Security Council Resolution 1612, 225–226
UN Security Council Resolution 1882, 226
United Nations (UN) humanitarian principles, 20–21
United Nations Disaster Assessment and Coordination (UNDAC), 43–44
United Nations Disaster Relief Organization (UNDRO), 1
United Nations High Commissioner for Refugees (UNHCR), 1, 14
United Nations International Children's Emergency Fund (UNICEF), 14–15
United Nations organizations, 48

United States Agency for International Development (USAID)/Office of US Foreign Disaster Assistance (OFDA), 30–31
untimely reporting, 115–116
Ursano, R. J., 418
Uscher-Pines, L., 446

vaccination, 316
vaccine preventable diseases (VPDs)
 cholera, 232–233
 diphtheria, 233–234
 Jordon, 2013, 240
 measles, 228–229
 meningococcal disease, 230–231
 poliomyelitis, 229–230
 risk assessment, 235
 risk factors mitigation, 227
 tetanus, 233–234
 yellow fever, 231–232
vaccine preventable diseases (VPDs), control measures
 organizations, 239
 outbreak response, 236
 surveillance, 235–236
 vaccination campaigns, 236–238
Van Emmerick, A. R. P., 414
van Soest, M., 66
VanRooyen, 442, 443
Varaine, F., 405
ventilation issues, 266–267
Ververs, M. T., 170
Victora, C. G., 167–168, 176
Vincent, M., 215
Vishwanatham, K., 75
Vitale, A., 245, 249, 250, 251, 252
vitamin A deficiency, 376
vitamin B (thiamin) deficiency, 376–377
vitamin B2 (riboflavin) deficiency, 377
vitamin B3/PP (niacin) deficiency, 377
vitamin C deficiency, scurvy, 377–378
Vonnahem, L. A., 455
Vu, A., 446

Waila, I., 166
Waldman, R. J., 23, 39, 59, 60, 109, 228, 229, 386, 391, 462
Walker, P., 9–10, 11, 12, 13, 14, 15, 16, 17, 18, 19, 22
Wallensteen, P., 1, 7
Wang, S. J., 455
warehousing, 278–279
wasting, Maramus, 362
water, sanitation, hygiene (WASH)
 alcohol-based hand rub, 151
 ash as handwashing alternative, 151
 boiling, 141
 buckets, with lid/tap, 150
 challenging environments, 146

 chemical toilets, 146–147
 children's excreta, 146
 chlorination, 139–140, 141
 communal latrines, 144
 community mobilization, 152–153
 composting toilets, 147
 defecation fields, 144
 disabilities, 146
 disposable biodegradable bags, 147
 Ethiopia, 2012, 157
 filtration, 141–142
 flocculation, disinfectant sachets, 141
 Haiti, 2010, 157
 hand hygiene, chlorine solution, 151
 handwashing bags, 150
 handwashing hardware, 150
 handwashing products, 151
 healthcare facilities, 153
 healthcare facilities, excreta/waste disposal, 154–155
 healthcare facilities, handwashing, 154
 healthcare facilities, waste management, 155
 healthcare facilities, water quality/access, 153–154
 hygiene, acute phase, 151–152
 hygiene, key items, 149–150
 hygiene, protracted emergencies, 153
 hygiene messaging in emergencies, 149
 hygiene promotion, 148–149, 152
 latrines, pit, 145
 latrines, pour-flush, 145–146
 latrines, shared *vs.* household, 144–145
 mass media, social media, 153
 Pakistan, 2005, 157
 point-of-collection disinfection, 140
 Point-of-Use (PoU), household water treatment, 140–141
 populations affected, 136
 sanitation, 142–144
 sanitation, during acute phase, 144
 sanitation, middle/long-term phases, 145
 sanitation disposal, 147
 septic tanks, 146
 shock chlorination, 140
 soapy water, 151
 Solar Disinfection (SODIS), 142
 solid waste control, 148
 Tanzania, 2015, 156–157
 tippy taps, 150
 urine diversion dry (dehydration) toilets (UDDTs), 147
 visual aids, print materials, 153

WASH data sources/methods, 155–156
WASH distribution, resources monitoring, 156
WASH indicators, 155
WASH monitoring, 155
water access, 137
water quality, 142
water sources, 138
water storage, 137–138
water supply, 136–137
water treatment, 138–142
water trucking, 138
women, 146
Watt, J. P., 297
Weaver, H., 465, 467
Weber, 296
Weinberg, A., 296, 304, 305
Weinstock, D. M., 427
Weiss, C. H., 126
Weiss, T. G., 18
Welton-Mitchell, C. E., 418
WHO Emergency Response Network, 48
Wightman, J. M., 444
Wilcox, S. R., 443
Williams, B. G., 68, 296
Williams, H. A., 351
Wolfe, M. K., 151
Wong, V. K., 402
Woodward, A., 200, 338
World Association for Disaster and Emergency Management (WADEM), 33
World Bank, 13
World Food Programme (WFP), 15
World Health Organization (WHO), 27
World Humanitarian Summit, 22
World Vision International, 33

Wright, J., 140
Wu, V. K., 455

Xavier, S., 388
Xie, J., 443

Yarbrough, D. B., 129
Yates, R., 370
Yates, T. M., 140
Yazdankhah, S. P., 401
Yee, E. L., 311
Yip, R., 311
Young, H., 375, 377, 378
Yugoslavia, 18

Zachariah, R., 428
Zenner, D., 228, 387
Zimbabwe, 2008, 330–332
Zimmerman, L., 199
zinc, 379